Absolute Dermatology Review

Hugh Morris Gloster, Jr. • Lauren E. Gebauer
Rachel L. Mistur

Absolute Dermatology Review

Mastering Clinical Conditions on the Dermatology Recertification Exam

Springer

Hugh Morris Gloster, Jr.
Professor of Dermatology
University of Cincinnati School of Medicine
Cincinnati, Ohio
USA

Rachel L. Mistur
College of Medicine
University of Cincinnati
Cincinnati, Ohio
USA

Lauren E. Gebauer
Department of Dermatology
University of Cincinnati Dermatology Surgical
Fellow
Cincinnati, Ohio
USA

ISBN 978-3-319-03217-7 ISBN 978-3-319-03218-4 (eBook)
DOI 10.1007/978-3-319-03218-4

Library of Congress Control Number: 2015941104

Springer Cham Heidelberg New York Dordrecht London

Printed on acid-free paper

Springer International Publishing AG Switzerland is part of Springer Science+Business Media (www.springer.com)

Contents

Chapter IV Adnexal Diseases

Chapter V Autoimmune Disorders

Chapter VI Metabolic and Deposition Diseases

Chapter I

Papulosquamous and Eczematous Dermatoses

1 Psoriasis Vulgaris

a. Chronic Plaque Psoriasis

Chronic plaque psoriasis

A. Most common variant
B. Chronic course, but remissions can occur
C. Symmetric distribution of sharply demarcated red plaques with thick silvery scale
D. Auspitz sign: pinpoint bleeding after scale removal
E. Most common on the scalp, extensor surfaces (elbows, knees), sacrum, umbilicus, hands, feet, genitalia (usually involves the glans penis in men)
F. Nail changes (also see Chap. 11, section 641)
   1. Thickening and yellow discoloration of nail plate
   2. Distal onycholysis
   3. Pitting
   4. Red, spotted lunula
   5. Subungual hyperkeratosis
   6. Oil spots (pink-yellow)
G. Arthritis (sausage digits)

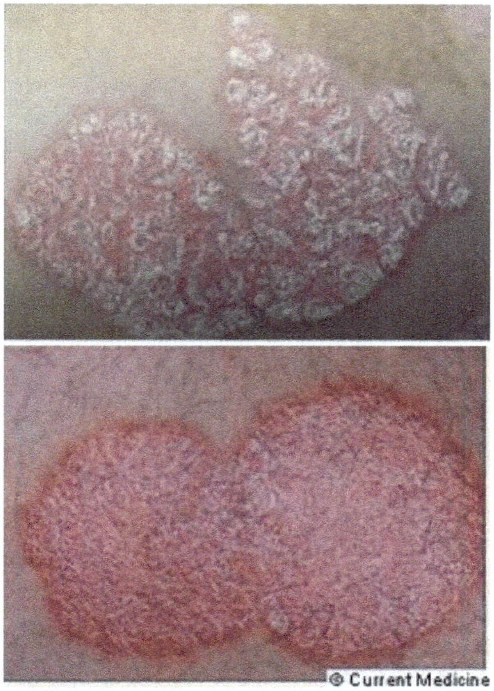

Chronic plaque psoriasis
Photograph courtesy of SpringerImages Database, Springer Publishing Company

Chronic plaque psoriasis

A. Sharply demarcated red plaque with thick silvery scale

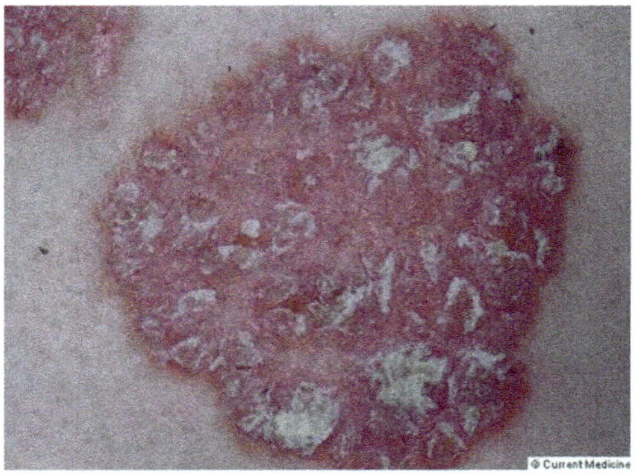

Chronic plaque psoriasis
Photograph courtesy of SpringerImages Database, Springer Publishing Company

H.M. Gloster, Jr. et al., *Absolute Dermatology Review: Mastering Clinical Conditions on the Dermatology Recertification Exam*, DOI 10.1007/978-3-319-03218-4_1, © Springer International Publishing Switzerland 2016

Chronic plaque psoriasis
A. Sharply demarcated, erythematous plaques with silvery-white, micaceous scales on lower chest, abdomen, and pubic area

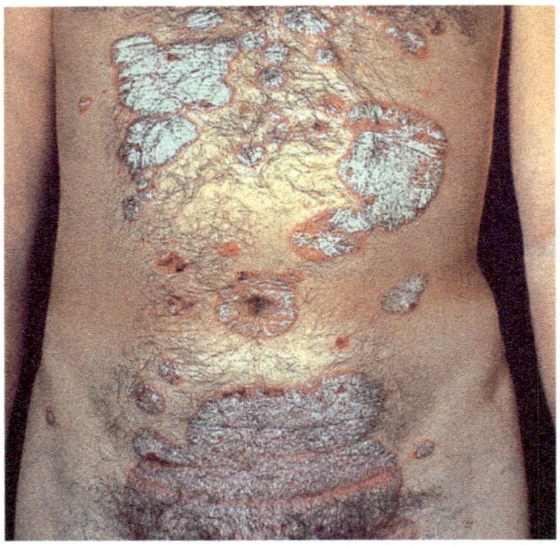

Chronic plaque psoriasis
Photograph courtesy of SpringerImages Database, Springer Publishing Company

b. Erythrodermic Psoriasis

Erythrodermic psoriasis
A. Severe form of psoriasis characterized by generalized erythema and scaling
B. Often associated with systemic illness including fever, hypotension, insensible fluid losses, and hypoalbuminemia
C. Can be spontaneous but usually is associated with a trigger factor such as abrupt discontinuation of corticosteroids or medications known to flare psoriasis such as lithium or beta-blockers, and infection

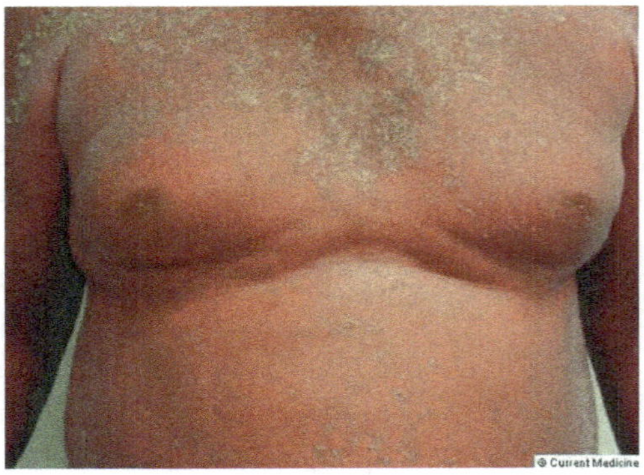

Erythrodermic psoriasis
Photograph courtesy of SpringerImages Database, Springer Publishing Company

Erythrodermic psoriasis
A. Generalized erythema, scaling, and occasionally pustules

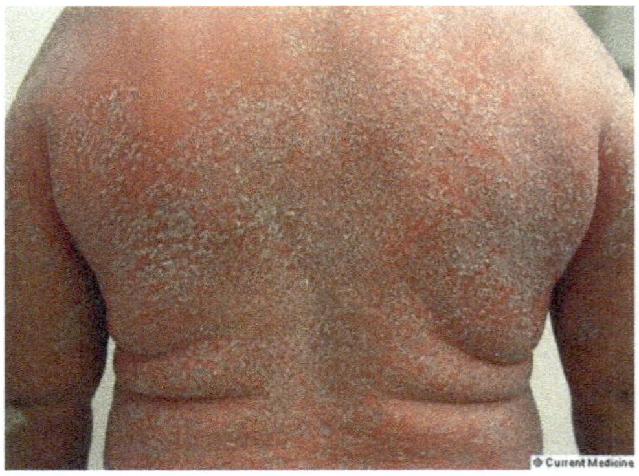

Erythrodermic psoriasis
Photograph courtesy of SpringerImages Database, Springer Publishing Company

c. Generalized Pustular Psoriasis

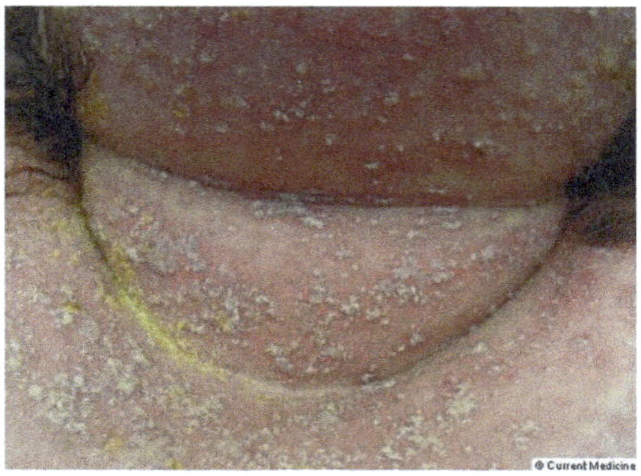

Generalized pustular psoriasis
Photograph courtesy of SpringerImages Database, Springer Publishing Company

Generalized pustular psoriasis

A. Large areas of erythema with numerous sterile pustules forming lakes of pus
B. Triggering factors include pregnancy, rapid tapering of steroids, hypocalcemia, infections
C. Four patterns of pustular psoriasis
   1. Von Zumbusch
      a. Generalized onset of erythema and pustules which resolves in several days with extensive scale
      b. Skin is painful
      c. Patients are ill with fever and chills
   2. Annular
      a. Annular inflammatory plaques with erythema and scale and pustules at the advancing edge
      b. Lesions expand centrifugally and heal with central clearing with scale
   3. Exanthematic
      a. Acute eruption of small pustules which disappear over a few days (looks like acute generalized exanthematous pustulosis)
   4. Localized
      a. Pustules appear within or at the edge of existing psoriatic plaque
      b. Can be seen after the application of irritants like tars

d. Palmoplantar Psoriasis

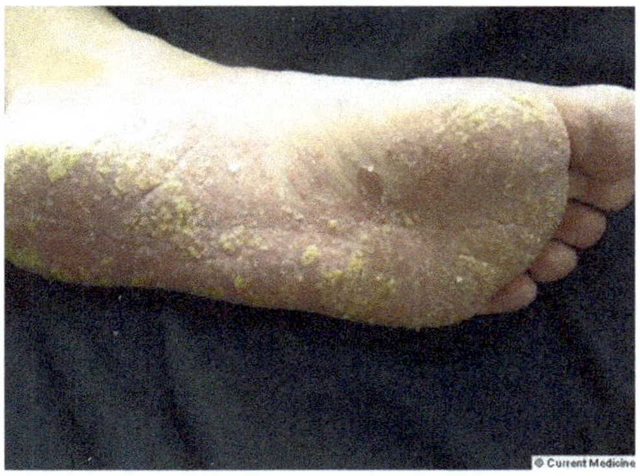

Palmoplantar psoriasis
Photograph courtesy of SpringerImages Database, Springer Publishing Company

Palmoplantar psoriasis

A. Non-pustular variant
   1. Well-demarcated hyperkeratotic plaques with scaling and fissuring
   2. Can be difficult to differentiate from other diseases such as hand eczema and contact dermatitis

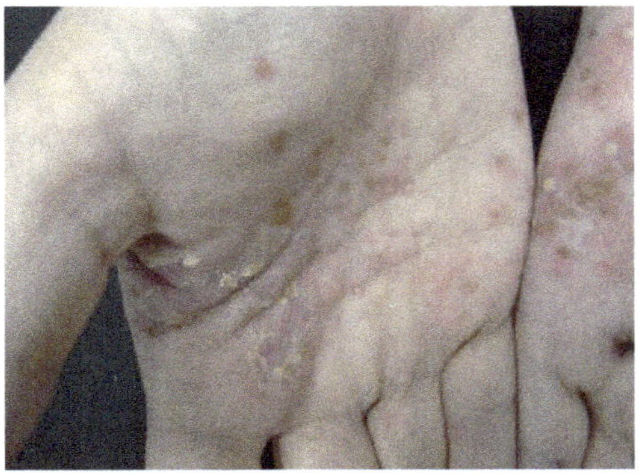

Palmoplantar psoriasis
Photograph courtesy of SpringerImages Database, Springer Publishing Company

Palmoplantar psoriasis

A. Pustular variant
   1. Sterile pustules of the palmoplantar surfaces mixed with yellow-brown macules and scaly plaques
   2. Chronic course
   3. Associated with sterile inflammatory bone lesions

e. Guttate Psoriasis

Guttate psoriasis

A. Most common in children and adolescents
B. Frequently preceded by triggers including streptococcal pharyngitis, viral infections, medications, major stressors, or abrupt withdrawal of treatments (particularly corticosteroids or cyclosporine)
C. Numerous widely disseminated, bright red, discrete "drop shaped" small scaly papules and plaques
D. Most common on the trunk

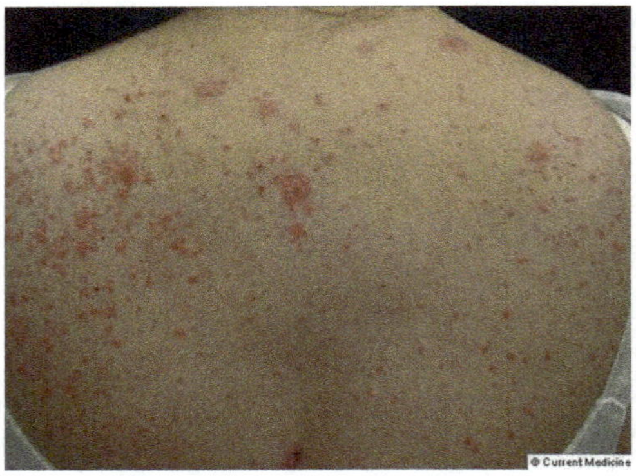

Guttate psoriasis
Photograph courtesy of SpringerImages Database, Springer Publishing Company

Lichen Planus 2

a. Lichen Planus

Lichen planus

A. Flat-topped, polygonal, violaceous, pruritic papules and plaques
B. Surface of papules are shiny and transparent with a network of fine lacy white lines called Wickham's striae
C. Favors flexor wrists and forearms, genitals, distal anterior lower extremities (ankles), presacral area
D. May koebnerize and form linear lesions

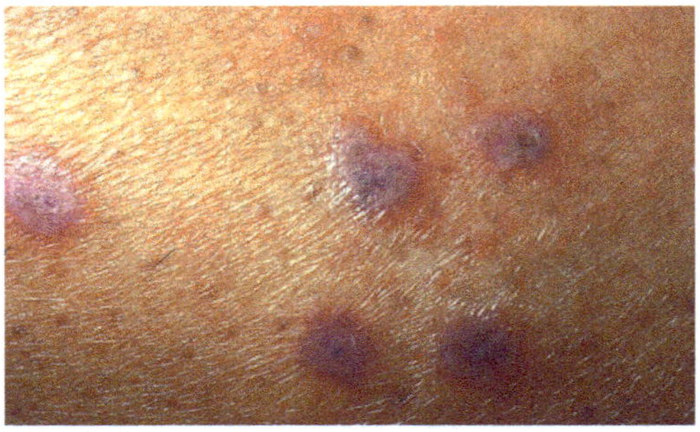

Lichen Planus
Photograph courtesy of SpringerImages Database, Springer Publishing Company

b. Hypertrophic Lichen Planus

Hypertrophic lichen planus

A. Extremely pruritic, thick plaques covered with fine adherent scale on the shins and dorsal feet, usually symmetrical

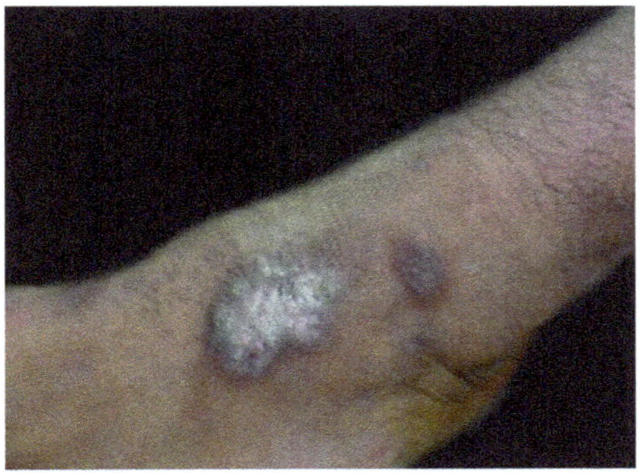

Hypertrophic lichen planus
Photograph courtesy of SpringerImages Database, Springer Publishing Company

H.M. Gloster, Jr. et al., *Absolute Dermatology Review: Mastering Clinical Conditions on the Dermatology Recertification Exam*, DOI 10.1007/978-3-319-03218-4_2, © Springer International Publishing Switzerland 2016

c. Mucosal Lichen Planus

Mucosal lichen planus

A. The oral mucosa affected in over 50 %, 15–20 % only have mucosal involvement
B. May be related to chronic liver disease, hepatitis C virus
C. Violaceous plaques with white, reticular, linear lines in a lacy pattern or in rings with radiating spines usually on buccal mucosa

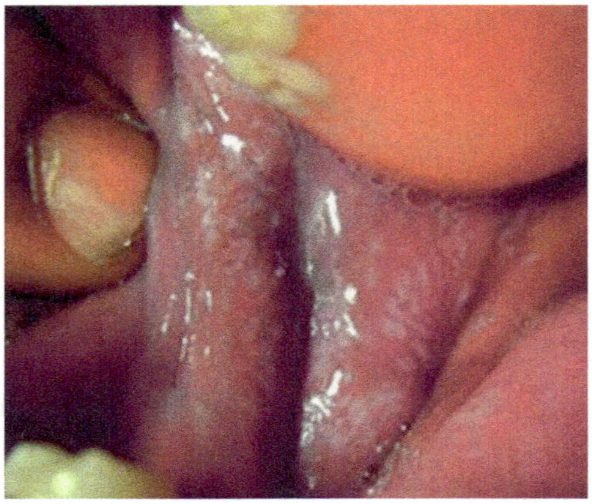

Mucosal lichen planus
Photograph courtesy of SpringerImages Database, Springer Publishing Company

d. Lichen Planus of the Nails

Lichen planus of the nails

A. Nail changes are secondary to damage to the nail matrix
B. Lateral thinning of the nail plate with lateral loss
C. Longitudinal ridging (onychorrhexis) and fissuring of the nail plate with distal splitting
D. Dorsal pterygium—proximal nail fold fuses with nail bed
E. Trachyonychia (20 nail dystrophy)—nail plate roughness resembling sandpaper due to excessive longitudinal ridging, often associated with thinning (the nails look like they have been sandpapered in a longitudinal direction)

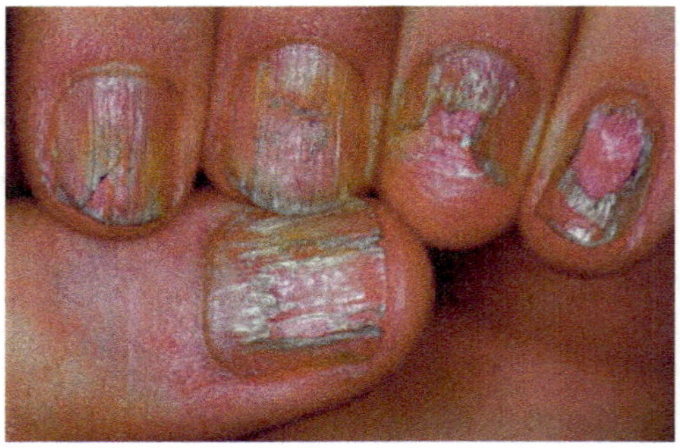

Lichen planus of the nails
Photograph courtesy of SpringerImages Database, Springer Publishing Company

e. Erosive Lichen Planus (Vulvovaginal)

Erosive lichen planus Vulvovaginal

A. Oral mucosal disease often coexists: vulvovaginal—gingival syndrome
B. Most common in peri- and postmenopausal women
C. Erosive or desquamative painful plaques that may involve some combination of the vulval, vaginal, or gingival surfaces
D. Fine, very subtle white lacy reticulated Wickam's striae may be present

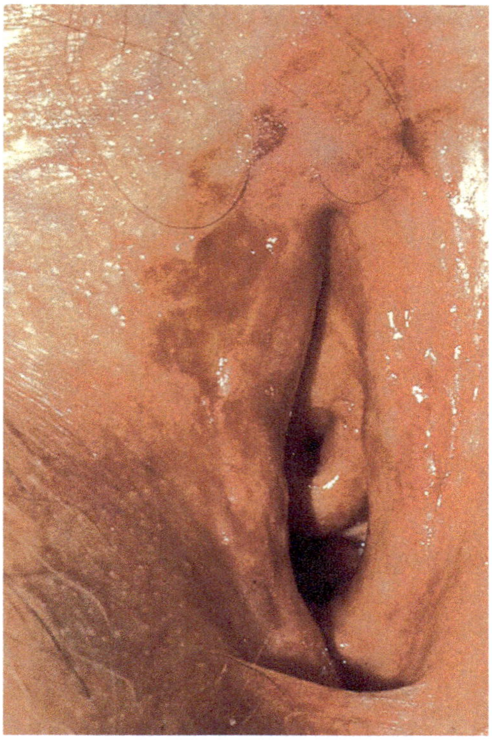

Erosive lichen planus (vulvovaginal)
Photograph courtesy of SpringerImages Database, Springer Publishing Company

Erosive lichen planus (vulvovaginal)

A. Erosive or desquamative painful plaques that may involve some combination of the vulval, vaginal, or gingival surfaces

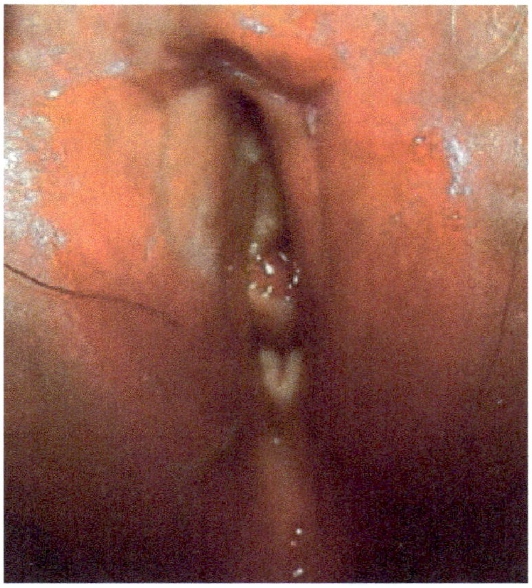

Erosive lichen planus (vulvovaginal)
Photograph courtesy of SpringerImages Database, Springer Publishing Company

f. Annular Variant of Lichen Planus

Annular variant of lichen planus

A. Papules spread peripherally resulting in a central hyperpigmented area with an annular edge that is purple white and raised

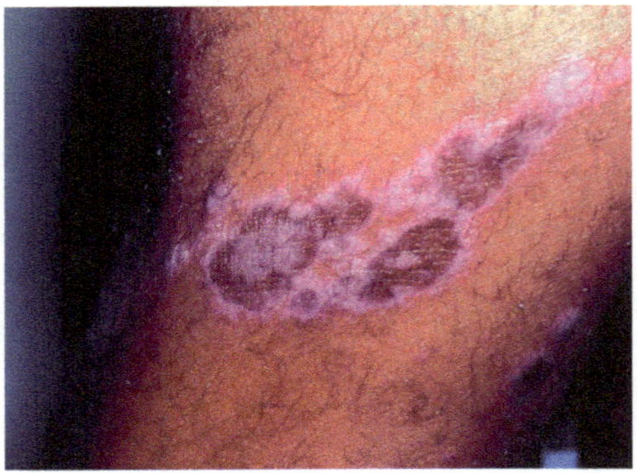

Annular variant of lichen planus
Photograph courtesy of SpringerImages Database, Springer Publishing Company

g. Drug Induced Lichen Planus

Drug-induced lichen planus

A. Usually generalized, spares classic sites
B. Eczematous, psoriasiform, or pityriasis rosea-like lesions may be present in addition to violaceous flat-topped papules
C. Wickham striae may be absent
D. Postinflammatory hyperpigmentation is very common and persistent
E. Photodistribution is common
F. Mucous membranes are usually spared
G. There may be a latent period of several months before the eruption occurs
H. Most commonly associated with angiotensin-converting enzyme inhibitiors, thiazide diuretics, antimalarials, quinidine, gold

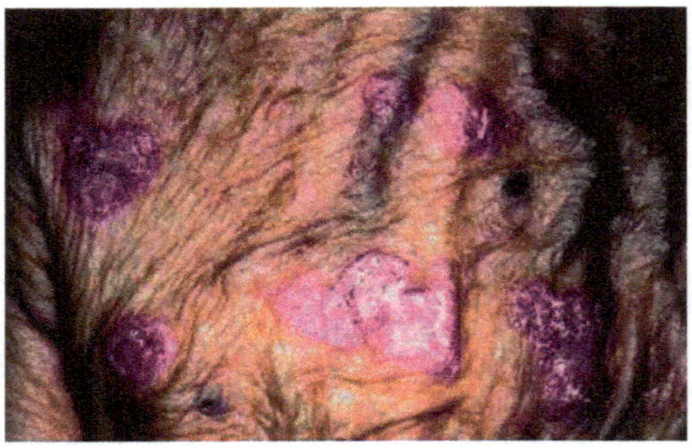

Drug-induced lichen planus
Photograph courtesy of SpringerImages Database, Springer Publishing Company

3 Dermatitis

a. Contact Dermatitis

i. Allergic Contact Dermatitis

Allergic contact dermatitis

A. Delayed-type hypersensitivity reaction when the skin contacts a chemical to which it is previously sensitized
B. Well-demarcated (confined to area of contact), sharp, streaky, erythematous, pruritic, vesicular patch or plaque with scale
C. May be acute (blistering, weeping, edema) or chronic (lichenified or scaly plaques)
D. Localized to site of contact forming geometric or well-circumscribed patterns (e.g., foot dermatitis to shoes, hand dermatitis to gloves, perioral dermatitis to dentures or lip balm, linear to a leaf or branch)

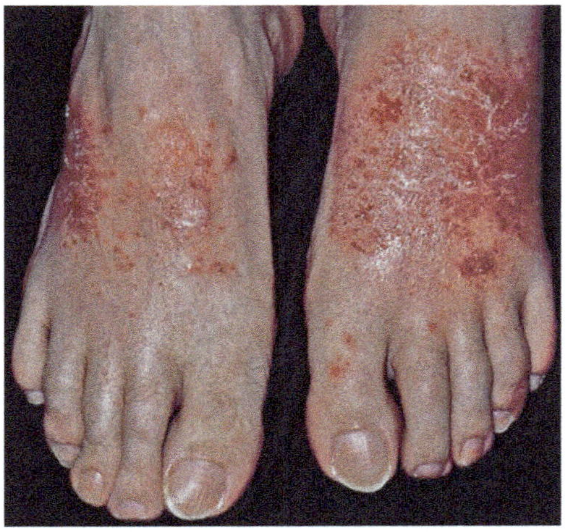

Allergic contact dermatitis
Photograph courtesy of SpringerImages Database, Springer Publishing Company

Allergic contact dermatitis

A. Well-demarcated sharp, erythematous, pruritic, vesicular plaque with scale localized to site of contact on the lower abdomen as a result of allergy to nickel in pants or belts

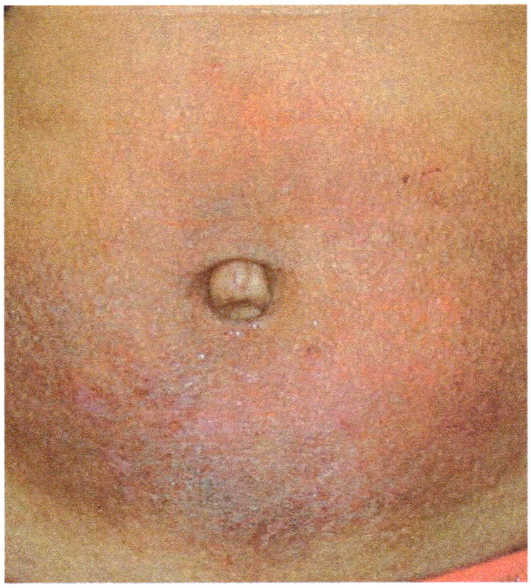

Allergic contact dermatitis
Photograph courtesy of SpringerImages Database, Springer Publishing Company

H.M. Gloster, Jr. et al., *Absolute Dermatology Review: Mastering Clinical Conditions on the Dermatology Recertification Exam*, DOI 10.1007/978-3-319-03218-4_3, © Springer International Publishing Switzerland 2016

Allergic contact dermatitis

A. Well-demarcated erythematous, edematous, vesicular plaque with linear streaks due to Rhus toxicodendron

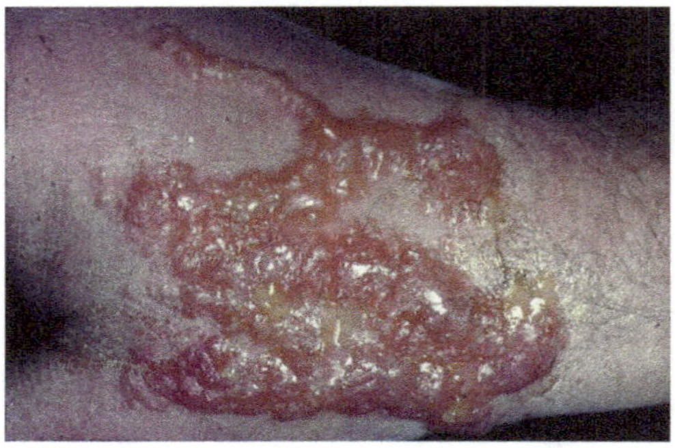

Allergic contact dermatitis
Photograph courtesy of SpringerImages Database, Springer Publishing Company

ii. Irritant Contact Dermatitis

Irritant contact dermatitis

A. Local toxic effect of an irritant on the skin
B. Erythematous scaly papules and plaques confined to area of contact after application of tretinoin and urea cream

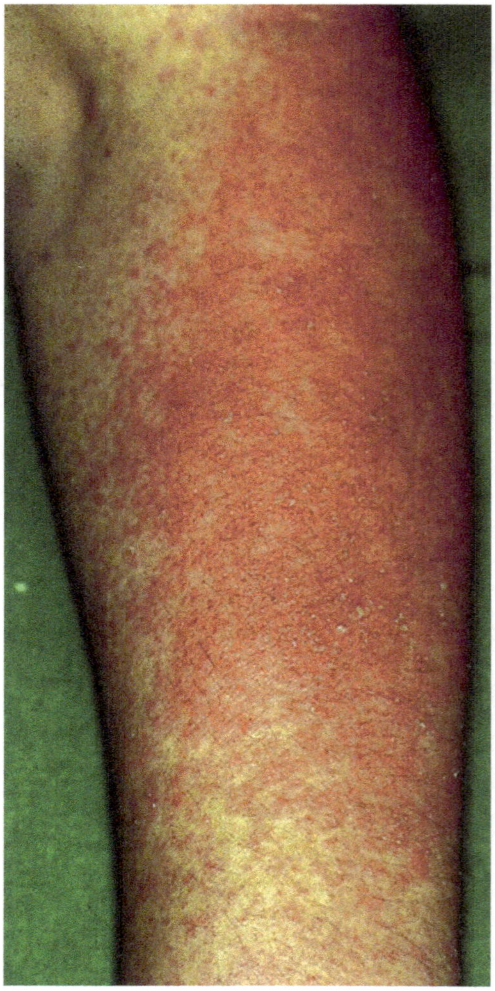

Irritant contact dermatitis
Photograph courtesy of SpringerImages Database, Springer Publishing Company

Irritant contact dermatitis

A. Pruritic, discretely painful, sharply demarcated plaque of the dorsum of the hand due to repeated contact with household detergents

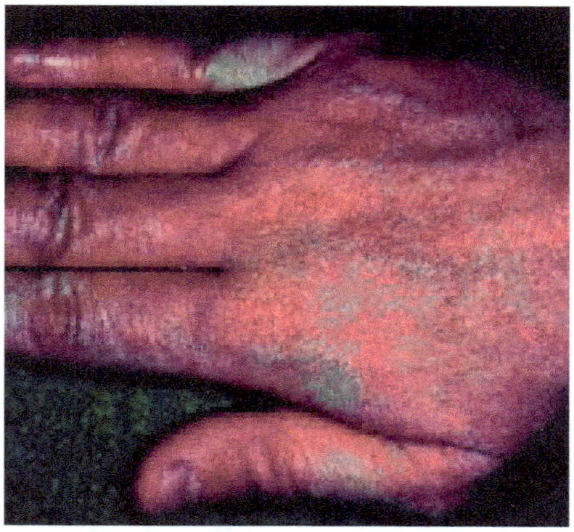

Irritant contact dermatitis
Photograph courtesy of SpringerImages Database, Springer Publishing Company

b. Seborrheic Dermatitis

Seborrheic dermatitis

A. Sharply demarcated, yellow, red, or red–brown patches or thin plaques with bran-like flaky greasy adherent scales
B. Develops in areas rich in sebaceous glands such as the scalp, midface and nasolabial folds (figure a), eyebrows, behind the ears (figure b), and central chest
C. May be hypopigmented in patients with darker skin (especially on the face)

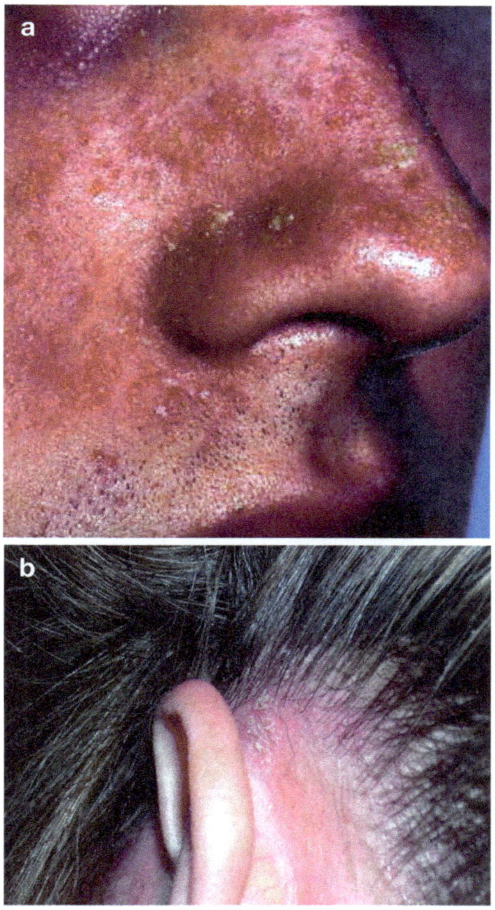

Seborrheic dermatitis
Photograph courtesy of SpringerImages Database, Springer Publishing Company

Seborrheic dermatitis

A. Pink thin plaque with bran-like flaky greasy adherent scales along the hairline

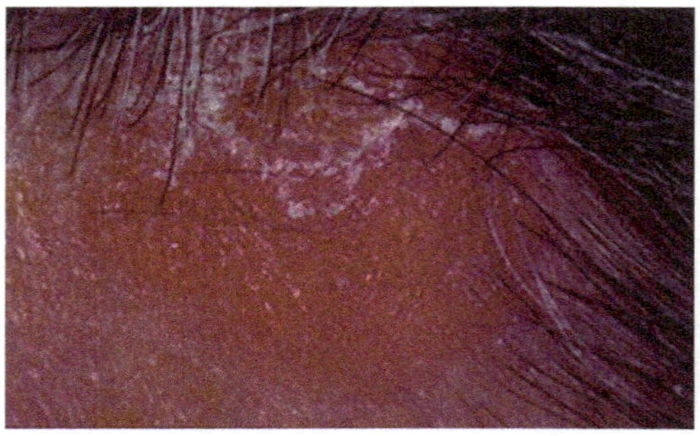

Seborrheic dermatitis
Photograph courtesy of SpringerImages Database, Springer Publishing Company

i. Infantile Seborrheic Dermatitis

Infantile seborrheic dermatitis

A. Begins 1 week after birth, persists several months
B. Greasy scales on the scalp, may develop inflammation and oozing and result in coherent crusty scale over entire scalp (cradle cap)
C. Disseminated lesions may occur on the face, retroauricular folds, neck, trunk, proximal extremities (axillary and inguinal folds may be acutely inflamed)

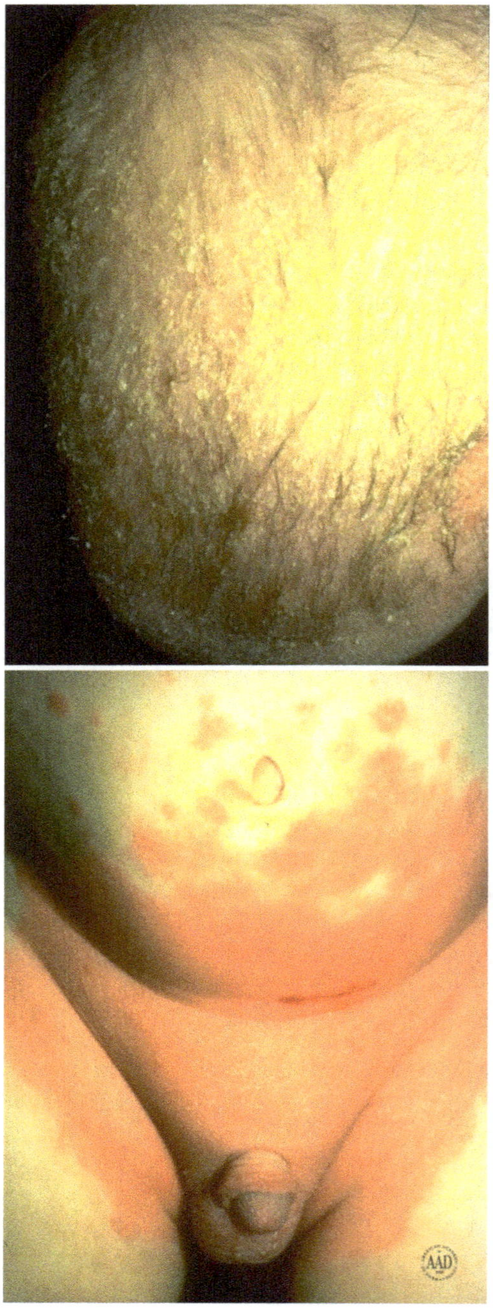

Infantile seborrheic dermatitis
Photograph courtesy of the American Academy of Dermatology

c. Atopic Dermatitis

i. Infantile Atopic Dermatitis

Infantile atopic dermatitis

A. Develops after second month of life and before 2 years of age
B. Acute lesions present with edematous, erythematous papules and plaques with vesiculation, oozing, and crusting
C. Initially appears on the cheeks sparing central face, then spreads to the scalp, neck, and extensor extremities
D. The face (especially around the mouth) and neck are affected in over 90 % of infants

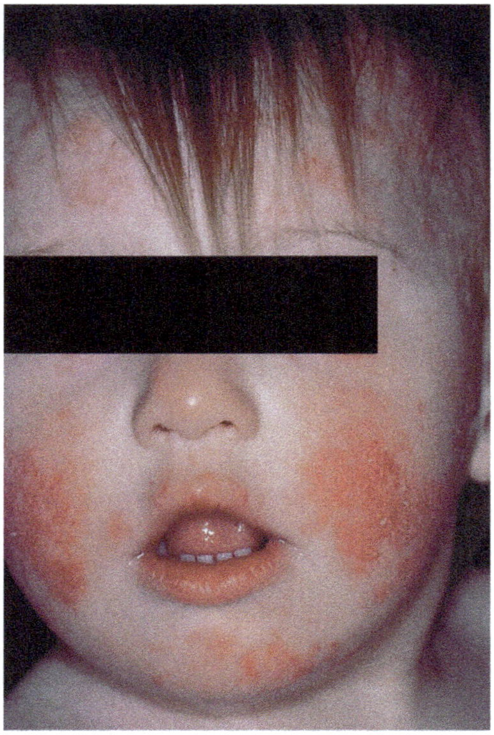

Infantile atopic dermatitis
Photograph courtesy of SpringerImages Database, Springer Publishing Company

ii. Childhood Atopic Dermatitis

Childhood atopic dermatitis

A. Onset 2–12 years of age
B. Less exudative than infantile atopic dermatitis, more lichenified with widespread xerosis
C. The antecubital and popliteal fossa are classic sites (flexural eczema)
D. May also involve the head (especially periorificial areas), neck, wrists, hands, ankles, and feet

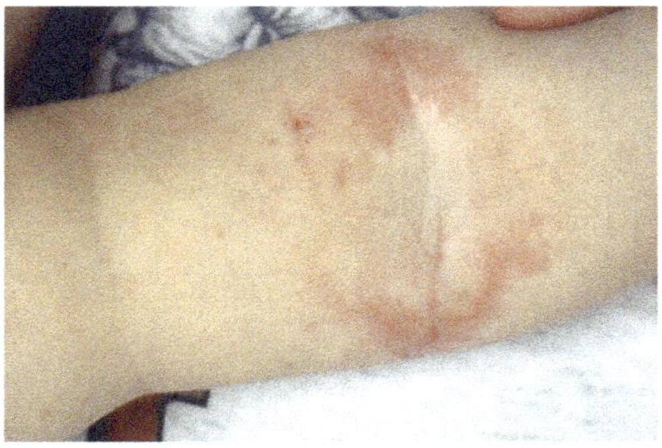

Childhood atopic dermatitis
Photograph courtesy of SpringerImages Database, Springer Publishing Company

Childhood atopic dermatitis

A. Lichenified plaques in the popliteal fossa

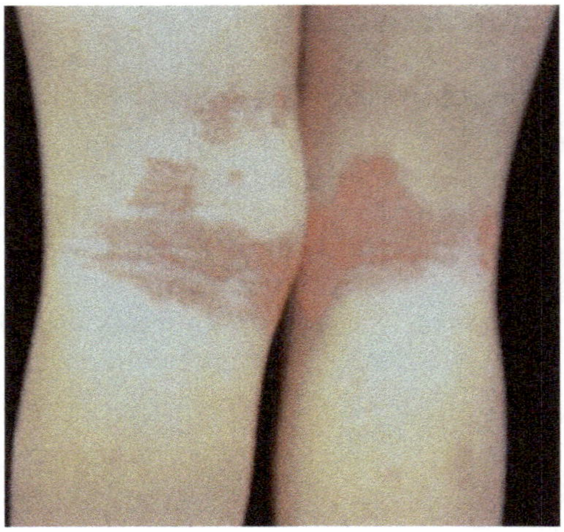

Childhood atopic dermatitis
Photograph courtesy of SpringerImages Database, Springer Publishing Company

iii. Adult Atopic Dermatitis

Adult atopic dermatitis

A. Seen in individuals greater than 12 years of age
B. Subacute to chronic, lichenified plaques with involvement of flexural areas as well as the head, neck, and chest
C. Facial dermatitis with severe eyelid involvement may also be seen

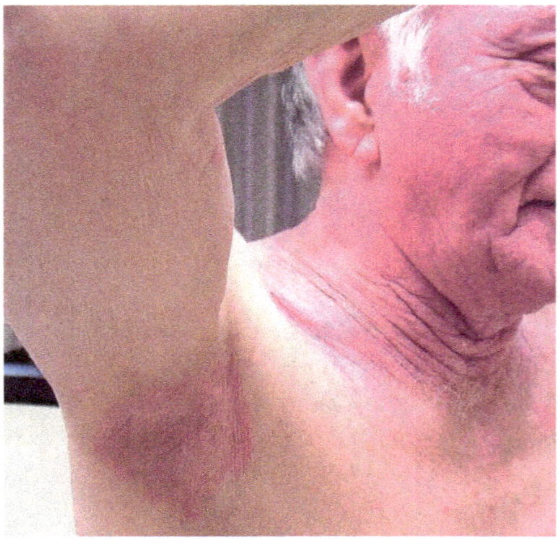

Adult atopic dermatitis
Photograph courtesy of SpringerImages Database, Springer Publishing Company

Adult atopic dermatitis

A. May also involve the wrists, arms, knees, ankles

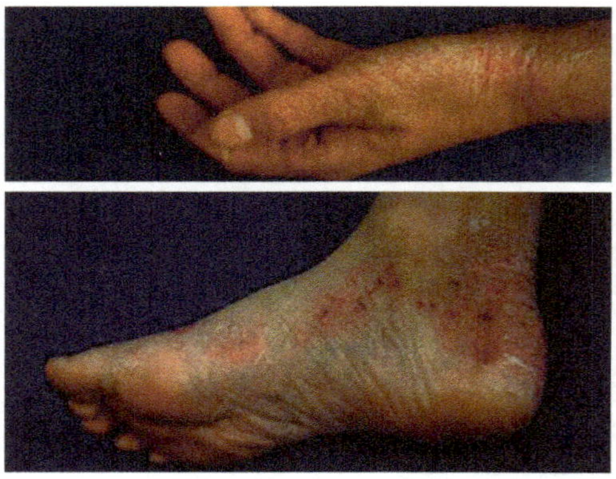

Adult atopic dermatitis
Photograph courtesy of SpringerImages Database, Springer Publishing Company

Adult atopic dermatitis
A. Chronic hand dermatitis may occur

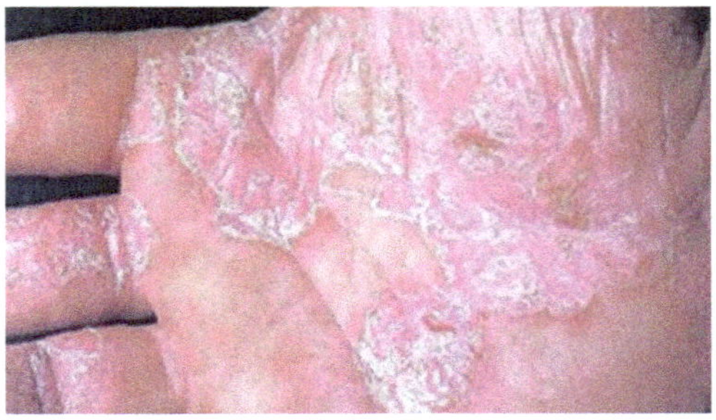

Adult atopic dermatitis
Photograph courtesy of SpringerImages Database, Springer Publishing Company

d. Periorificial Dermatitis

Perioral dermatitis
A. Discrete papules and/or pustules on an erythematous and sometimes scaly base around the mouth

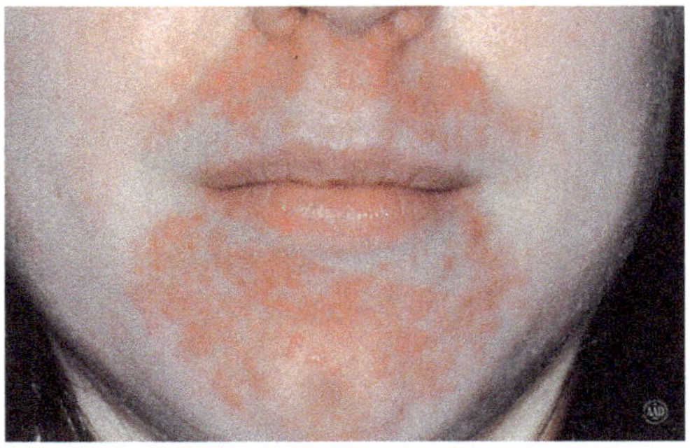

Periorificial dermatitis
Photograph courtesy of the American Academy of Dermatology

Perioral dermatitis
A. Discrete papules and/or pustules on an erythematous and sometimes scaly base around the mouth

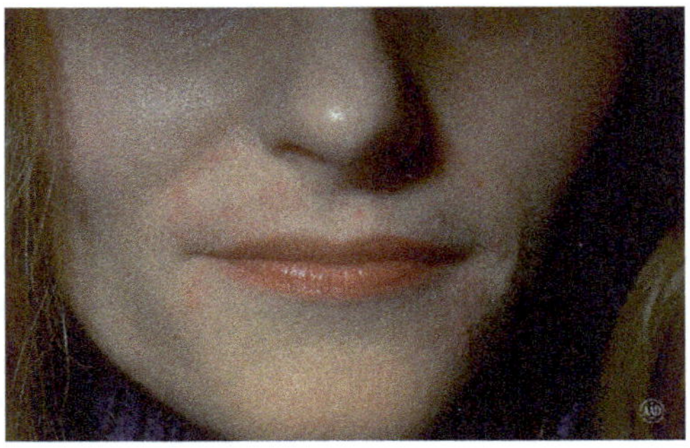

Periorificial dermatitis
Photograph courtesy of the American Academy of Dermatology

e. Stasis Dermatitis

Stais dermatitis

A. Eczematous dermatitis on the lower legs caused by venous insufficiency
B. Ulcerations (secondary to venous insufficiency) may occur on medial lower leg associated with changes of chronic venous insufficiency (edema, red–brown discoloration, fibrosis)

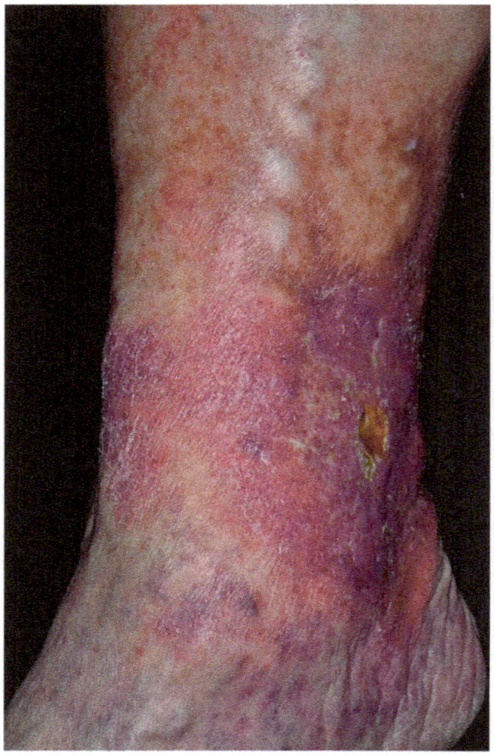

Stasis dermatitis
Photograph courtesy of SpringerImages Database, Springer Publishing Company

f. Asteatotic Dermatitis

Asteatotic dermatitis

A. Pruritic, dry, cracked, and polygonally fissured skin with irregular scaling resembling a "dry cracked river bed"
B. Usually occurs on the shins of elderly patients during winter months, especially in cold climates (also extensor arms, lower flanks, posterior axillary line)
C. Most common cause of pruritus in the elderly

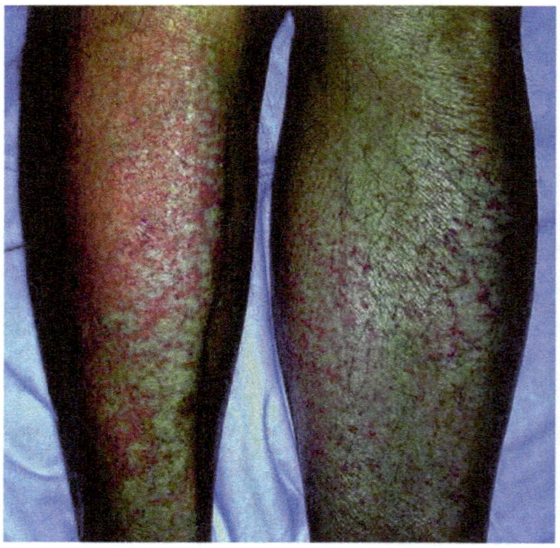

Asteatotic dermatitis
Photograph courtesy of SpringerImages Database, Springer Publishing Company

g. Dyshidrotic Dermatitis

Dishydrotic eczema (pompholyx)

A. Occurs on the palms and soles, especially the lateral fingers and toes
B. Scaly patches and deep-seated small 1–2 mm vesicles resembling tapioca pudding

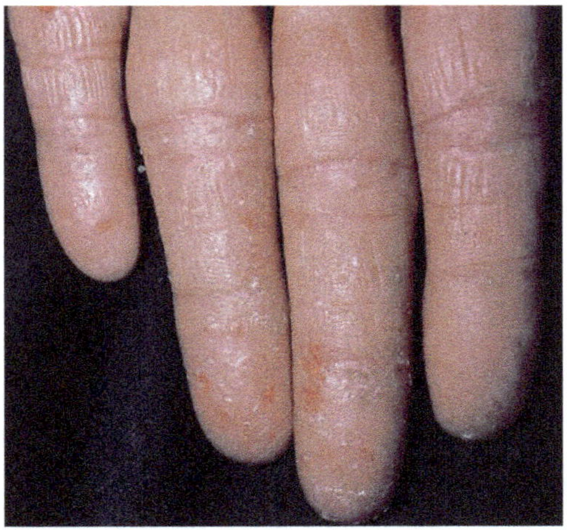

Dyshidrotic dermatitis
Photograph courtesy of SpringerImages Database, Springer Publishing Company

Dishydrotic eczema (pompholyx)

A. Scaly patches and deep-seated small 1–2 mm vesicles resembling tapioca pudding

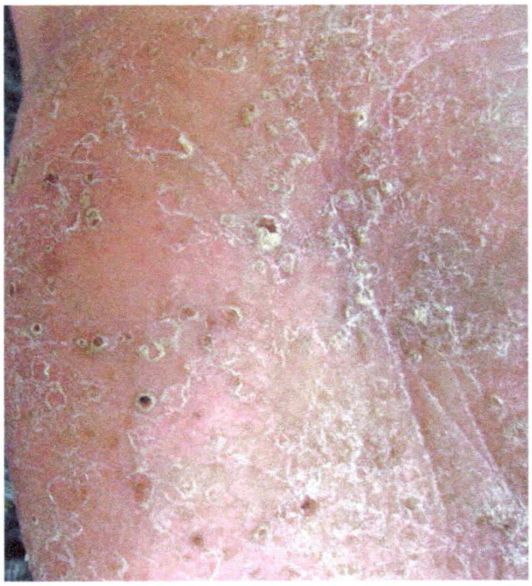

Dyshidrotic dermatitis
Photograph courtesy of SpringerImages Database, Springer Publishing Company

4 Keratosis Pilaris

Keratosis Pilaris

A. Common condition, autosomal dominant, affects over 40 % of patients with atopic dermatitis and over 75 % with ichthyosis vulgaris
B. Onset childhood, may improve with puberty (especially facial involvement)
C. Discrete rough follicular keratotic papules with a rim of erythema
D. Most commonly occurs on the lateral surface of upper arms, thighs, buttocks, and cheeks
E. In children occurs on the lateral cheeks more commonly than the trunk and extensor surfaces of distal extremities

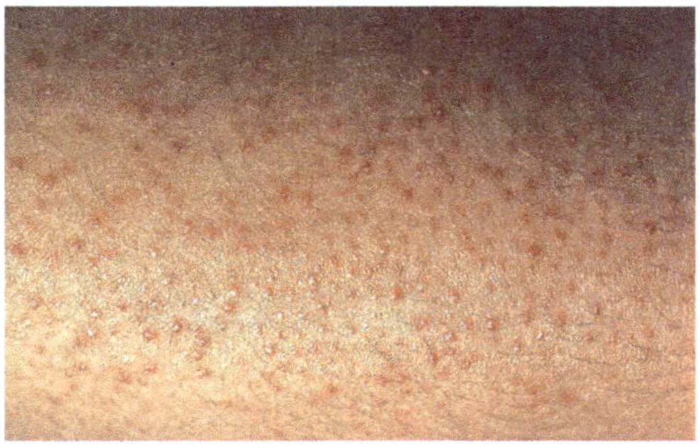

Keratosis pilaris
Photograph courtesy of SpringerImages Database, Springer Publishing Company

H.M. Gloster, Jr. et al., *Absolute Dermatology Review: Mastering Clinical Conditions on the Dermatology Recertification Exam*, DOI 10.1007/978-3-319-03218-4_4, © Springer International Publishing Switzerland 2016

5 Lichen Simplex Chronicus

Lichen Simplex Chronicus

A. Secondary to chronic, habitual rubbing and scratching
B. Well-defined, hyperpigmented to erythematous, leathery plaques with exaggerated skin lines (lichenification)
C. Posterior neck, extensor arms and legs, genitalia

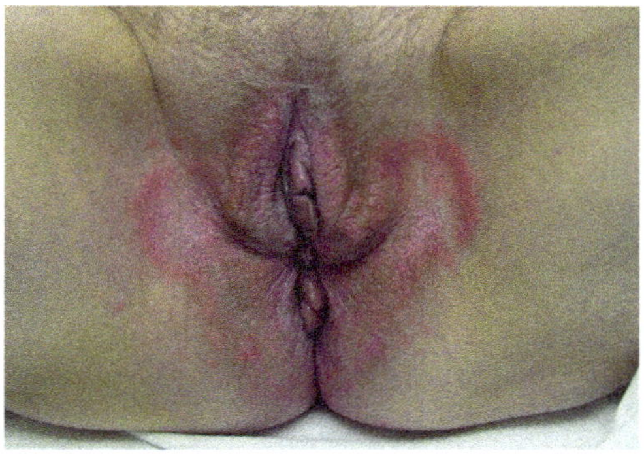

Lichen simplex chronicus
Photograph courtesy of SpringerImages Database, Springer Publishing Company

Lichen simplex chronicus

A. Erythematous, leathery lichenified plaque of the posterior neck

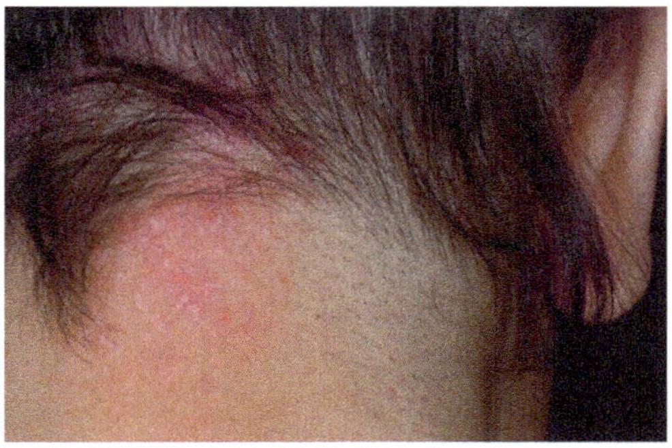

Lichen simplex chronicus
Photograph courtesy of SpringerImages Database, Springer Publishing Company

H.M. Gloster, Jr. et al., *Absolute Dermatology Review: Mastering Clinical Conditions on the Dermatology Recertification Exam*, DOI 10.1007/978-3-319-03218-4_5, © Springer International Publishing Switzerland 2016

Lichen Striatus

6

Lichen striatus

A. Asymptomatic linear dermatosis mainly affecting children under the age of six
B. Continuous or interrupted linear band of small (2–4 mm) flat-topped slightly scaly red to hypopigmented papules
C. Usually there is a single unilateral streak on an extremity along Blashko's lines
D. Most common on the extremities, then trunk, then head and neck
E. Develops rapidly, spontaneously resolves in months–years with hypopigmentation
F. Digital involvement may be associated with nail dystrophy

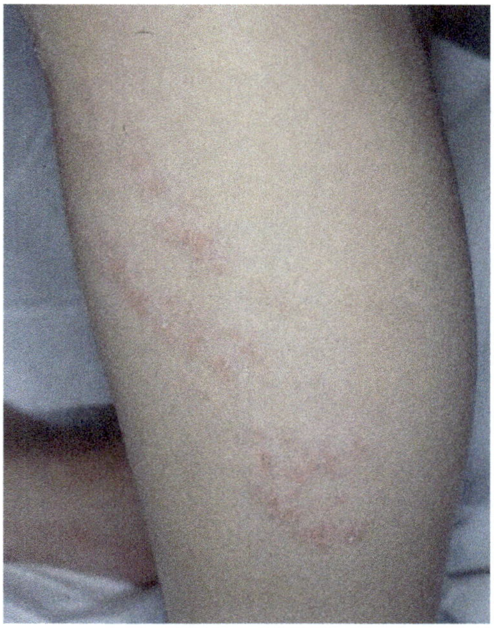

Lichen striatus
Photographs courtesy of SpringerImages Database, Springer Publishing Company

H.M. Gloster, Jr. et al., *Absolute Dermatology Review: Mastering Clinical Conditions on the Dermatology Recertification Exam*, DOI 10.1007/978-3-319-03218-4_6, © Springer International Publishing Switzerland 2016

Lichen striatus

A. Linear band of small (2–4 mm) flat-topped slightly scaly red to hypopigmented papules on an extremity along Blashko's lines

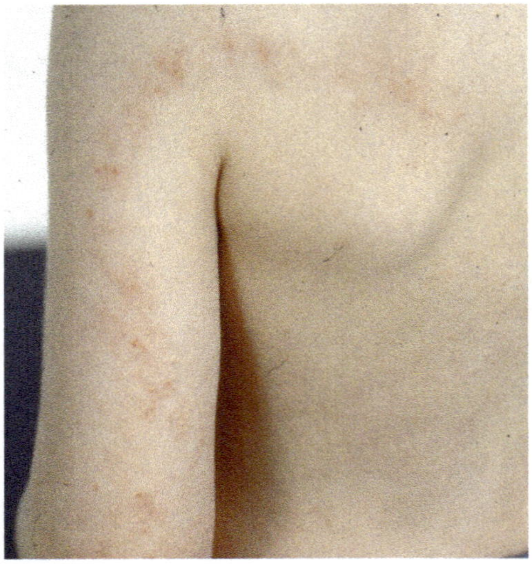

Lichen striatus
Photographs courtesy of SpringerImages Database, Springer Publishing Company

7 Pityriasis Lichenoides

a. Pityriasis Lichenoides Et Varioliformis Acuta

Pityriasis Lichenoides Et Varioliformis Acuta

A. Abrupt onset of crops of asymptomatic red–brown papules that evolve into vesicles and pustules with erythematous halos which may ulcerate and form hemorrhagic necrotic crusts
B. Older lesions may form varioliform depigmented scars
C. Lesions are present in different stages of development
D. Most commonly develops on the trunk, buttocks, and proximal extremities
E. Resolves in weeks to months

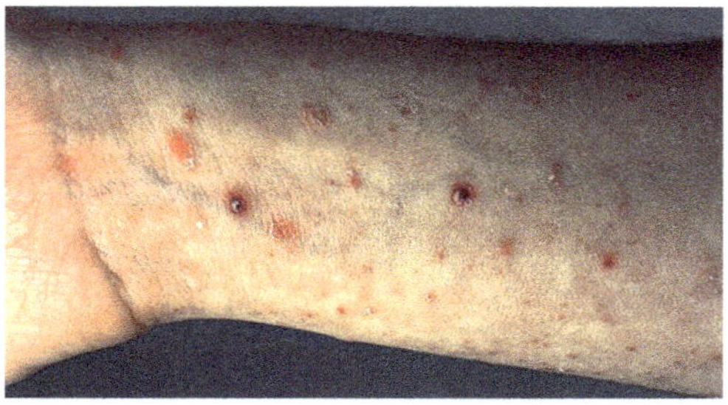

Pityriasis lichenoides et varioliformis acuta
Photograph courtesy of SpringerImages Database, Springer Publishing Company

H.M. Gloster, Jr. et al., *Absolute Dermatology Review: Mastering Clinical Conditions on the Dermatology Recertification Exam*, DOI 10.1007/978-3-319-03218-4_7, © Springer International Publishing Switzerland 2016

Pityriasis Lichenoides Et Varioliformis Acuta

A. Red–brown papules that evolve into vesicles and pustules with erythematous halos which may ulcerate and form hemorrhagic necrotic crusts

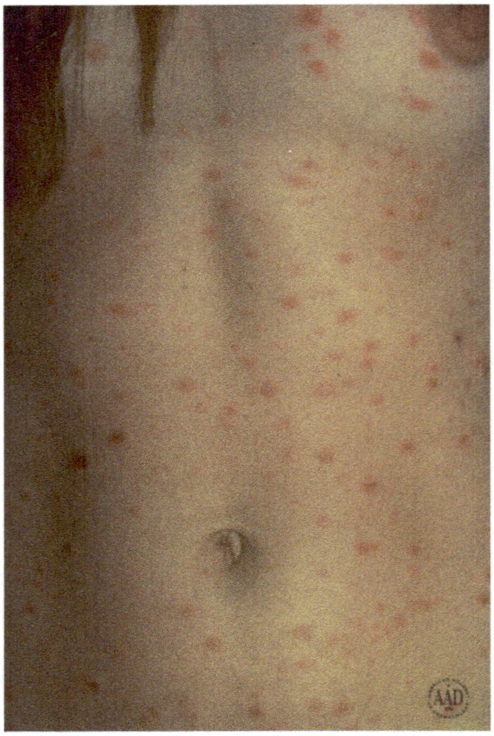

Pityriasis lichenoides et varioliformis acuta
Photograph courtesy of American Academy of Dermatology

b. Pityriasis Lichenoides Chronica

Pityriasis lichenoides chronica

A. Monomorphous, red–brown, pink to violaceous scaly papules which resolve to form hypopigmented macules
B. Slower onset than pityriasis lichenoides et varioliformis acuta
C. Distributed along Langer's lines (may resemble pityriasis rosea)
D. May regress over weeks to months (more indolent course than pityriasis lichenoides et varioliformis acuta) or may relapse
E. CD 4 clonality

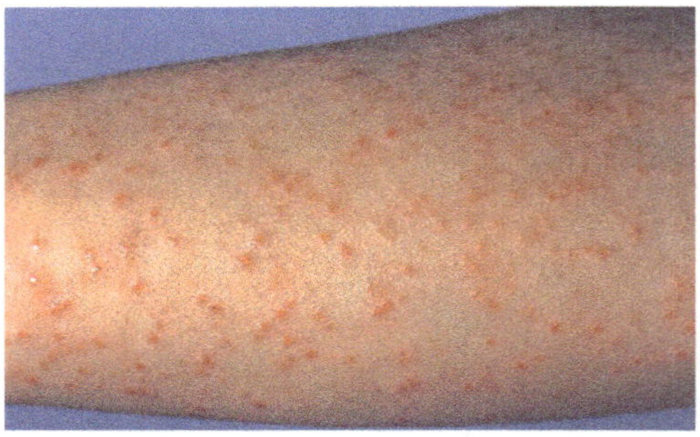

Pityriasis lichenoides chronica
Photograph courtesy of SpringerImages Database, Springer Publishing Company

Pityriasis lichenoides chronica

A. Monomorphous, red–brown, pink to violaceous scaly papules which resolve to form hypopigmented macules

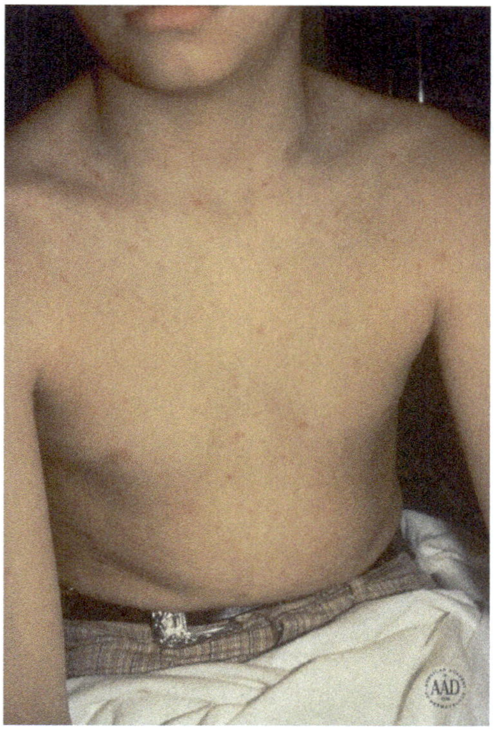

Pityriasis lichenoides chronica
Photograph courtesy of American Academy of Dermatology

Pityriasis lichenoides chronica

A. Lesions may be distributed along Langer's lines similar to pityriasis rosea

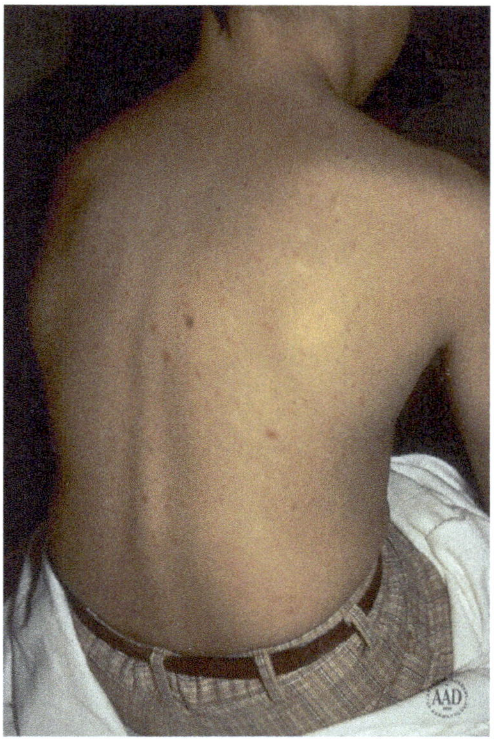

Pityriasis lichenoides chronica
Photograph courtesy of American Academy of Dermatology

Pityriasis Rosea

8

Pityriasis Rosea

A. Self-limited, acute papulosquamous eruption most common in adolescents and young adults
B. Herald Patch
   1. Predates more extensive lesions by hours to days
   2. Solitary, skin-colored to pink to salmon-colored patch or plaque with a slightly raised advancing margin with trailing scale and central fine scale
   3. Appears on the trunk and enlarges over several days
   4. Usually 2–4 cm in diameter but may be smaller or larger
C. Less common variants
   1. Inverse
      a. Involves axilla and inguinal areas
      b. More common in children, dark skin
   2. Vesicular
   3. Purpuric
   4. Pustular

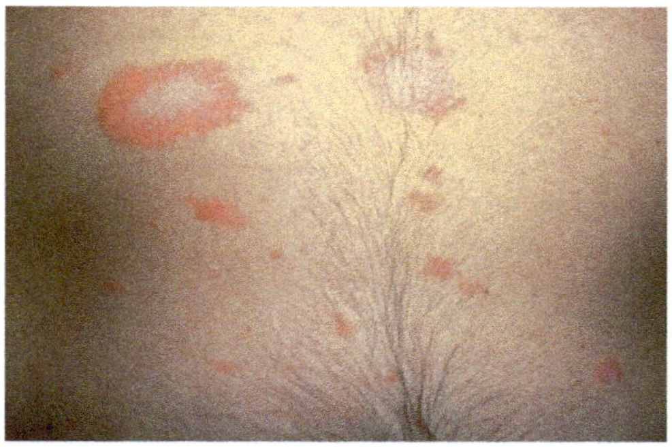

Pityriasis rosea
Photographs courtesy of SpringerImages Database, Springer Publishing Company

H.M. Gloster, Jr. et al., *Absolute Dermatology Review: Mastering Clinical Conditions on the Dermatology Recertification Exam*, DOI 10.1007/978-3-319-03218-4_8, © Springer International Publishing Switzerland 2016

Pityriasis rosea

A. Blossoming of salmon-colored oval scaly plaques with a collarette of scale (trailing scale) or central fine scale
B. Distributed with the long axis, which is oriented along Langer's lines of cleavage parallel to skin lines; on the back this creates a Christmas tree or fir tree pattern
C. Most commonly occurs on the trunk and extremities (face, palms, soles usually spared)
D. Spontaneous resolution 6–8 weeks

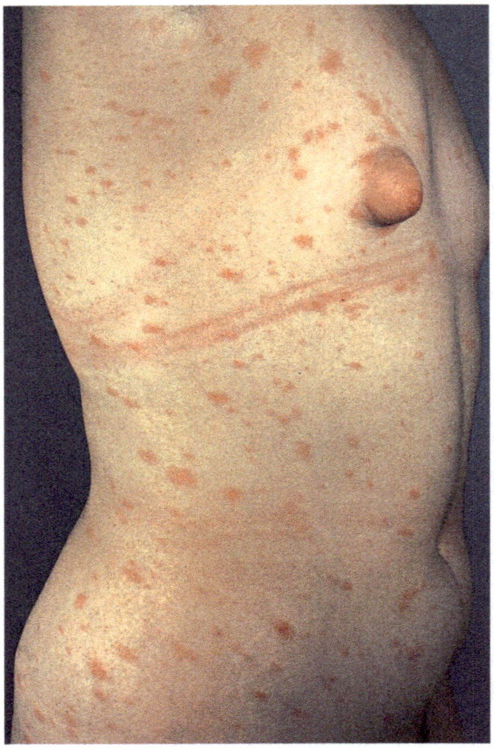

Pityriasis rosea
Photographs courtesy of SpringerImages Database, Springer Publishing Company

Pityriasis rosea

A. In dark skin, the lesions tend to be more papular peripherally and centrally hyperpigmented

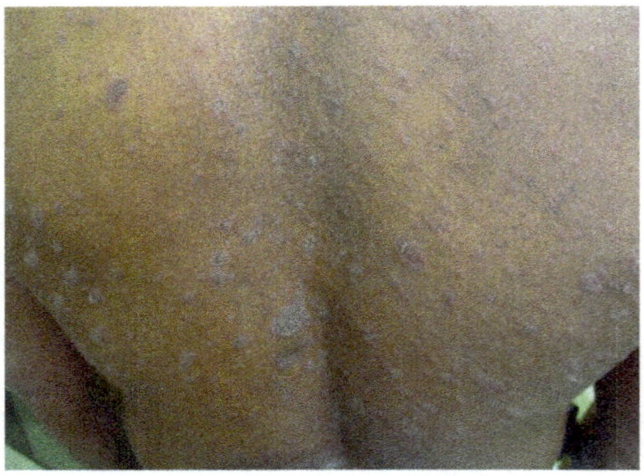

Pityriasis rosea
Photographs courtesy of SpringerImages Database, Springer Publishing Company

9 Pityriasis Alba

Pityriasis alba

A. Subclinical atopic dermatitis that presents in children as hypopigmented, poorly defined patches on the cheeks, upper arms, and trunk

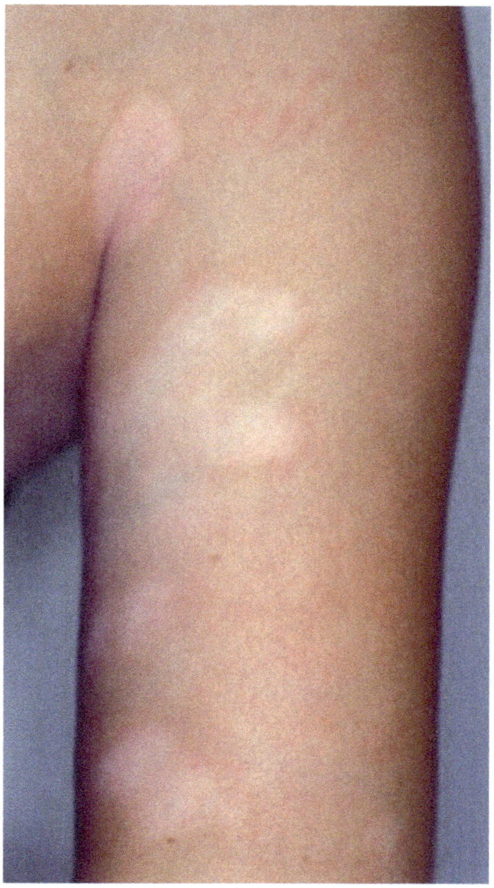

Pityriasis alba
Photographs courtesy of SpringerImages Database, Springer Publishing Company

H.M. Gloster, Jr. et al., *Absolute Dermatology Review: Mastering Clinical Conditions on the Dermatology Recertification Exam*,
DOI 10.1007/978-3-319-03218-4_9, © Springer International Publishing Switzerland 2016

Pityriasis alba

A. Hypopigmented, poorly defined patches on the cheeks

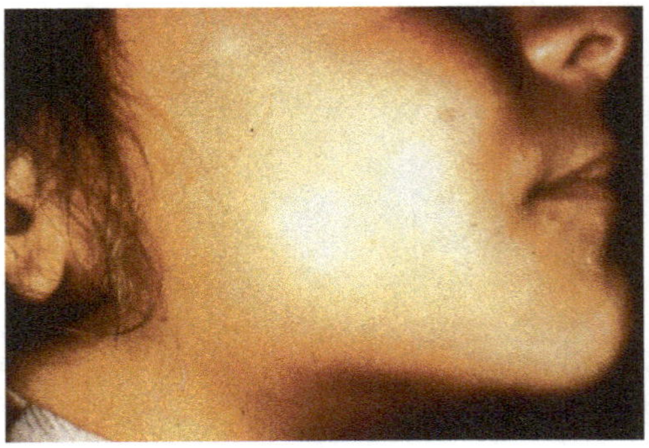

Pityriasis alba
Photographs courtesy of SpringerImages Database, Springer Publishing Company

10 Pityriasis Rubra Pilaris

Pityriasis rubra pilaris

A. Follicular hyperkeratotic papules on an erythematous base
   1. Dorsal fingers, trunk, and extremities
B. Coalescing red–orange (salmon-colored) plaques with intervening uninvolved skin ("islands of sparing")
   1. Plaques can progress to an erythroderma with varying degrees of exfoliation
C. Orange–red waxy palmoplantar keratoderma
D. Diffuse scaly scalp resembling seborrheic dermatitis
   1. May be initial presentation: PRP usually begins on head and progresses to trunk
E. Nail involvement
   1. Thick yellow–brown nails and subungual debris (subungual hyperkeratosis)
F. Eyes: ectropion, dryness

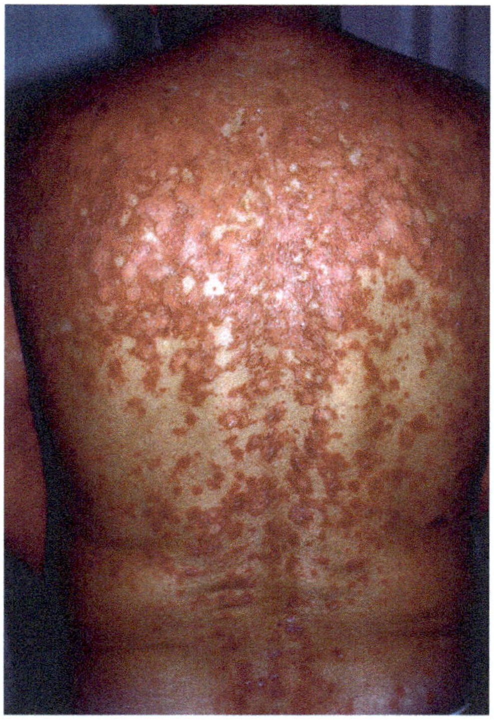

Pityriasis rubra pilaris
Photograph courtesy of SpringerImages Database, Springer Publishing Company

H.M. Gloster, Jr. et al., *Absolute Dermatology Review: Mastering Clinical Conditions on the Dermatology Recertification Exam*,
DOI 10.1007/978-3-319-03218-4_10, © Springer International Publishing Switzerland 2016

Pityriasis rubra pilaris

A. Coalescing red–orange (salmon-colored) plaques with intervening uninvolved skin ("islands of sparing")

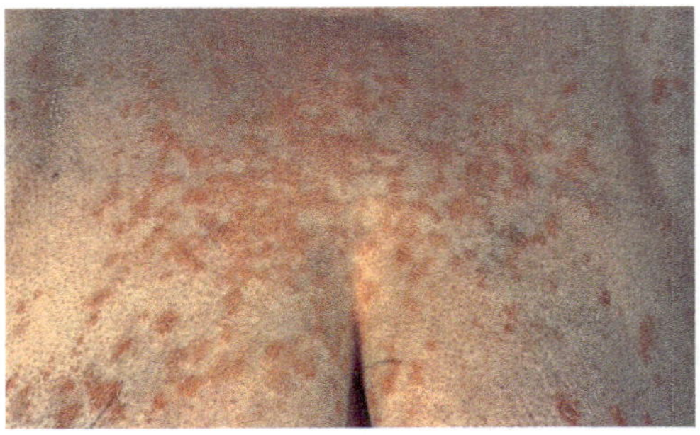

Pityriasis rubra pilaris
Photograph courtesy of SpringerImages Database, Springer Publishing Company

Pityriasis rubra pilaris

A. Orange–red waxy palmoplantar keratoderma

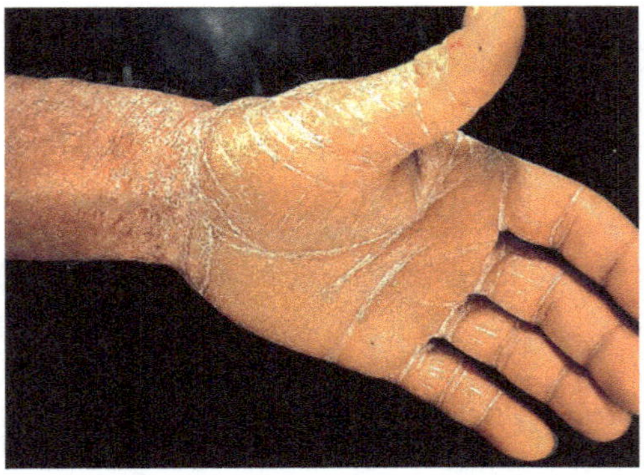

Pityriasis rubra pilaris
Photograph courtesy of SpringerImages Database, Springer Publishing Company

11 Granular Parakeratosis

Granular parakeratosis

A. Brownish red, pruritic keratotic papules that may coalesce into plaques, sometimes macerates, may flare with heat and sweat
B. Adult form (mainly in middle-age or elderly women): occurs mostly on the axilla but may involve other intertriginous areas such as the gluteal, inguinal, inframmamary, and abdominal fold
C. Infantile form: associated with diaper wearing and presents with bilateral plaques in inguinal folds or geometric plaques underlying diaper pressure points

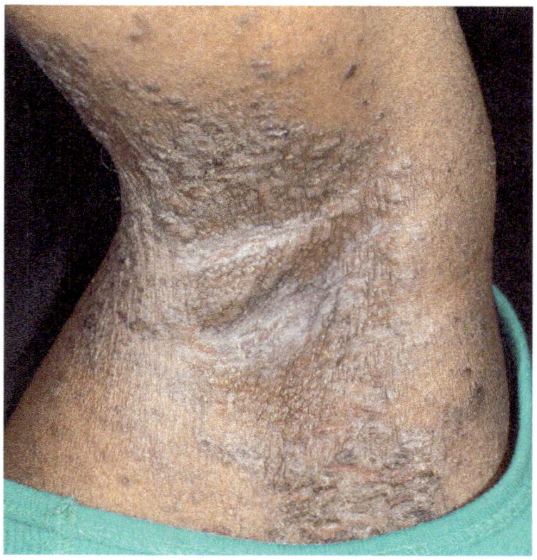

Granular parakeratosis
Photograph courtesy of Dr. Kara Shah, M.D, PhD, CCHMC (Cincinnati, OH), Department of Dermatology

H.M. Gloster, Jr. et al., *Absolute Dermatology Review: Mastering Clinical Conditions on the Dermatology Recertification Exam*, DOI 10.1007/978-3-319-03218-4_11, © Springer International Publishing Switzerland 2016

Chapter II

Cutaneous Vasculitis, Vasculopathy, and Microvascular Occlusion Sydromes

12 Small Vessel Vasculitis: Leukocytoclastic Vasculitis

a. Leukocytoclastic Vasculitis

A. Postcapillary venules of the dermis are involved with neutrophilic inflammation as a result of circulating immune complexes
B. Most cases resolve spontaneously within weeks to months
C. Causes: idiopathic, infection, autoimmune, or inflammatory disorder, drugs, neoplasm
D. Clinical signs usually appear 7–10 days after exposure
E. Stasis and hydrostatic pressure contribute to distribution: lesions tend to develop on dependent sites (lower extremities, especially ankles), areas under pressure points (tight clothes), and trauma sites (koebner phenomenon)
F. Most common lesions: palpable or macular purpura, which may undergo central necrosis with hemorrhagic infarcts

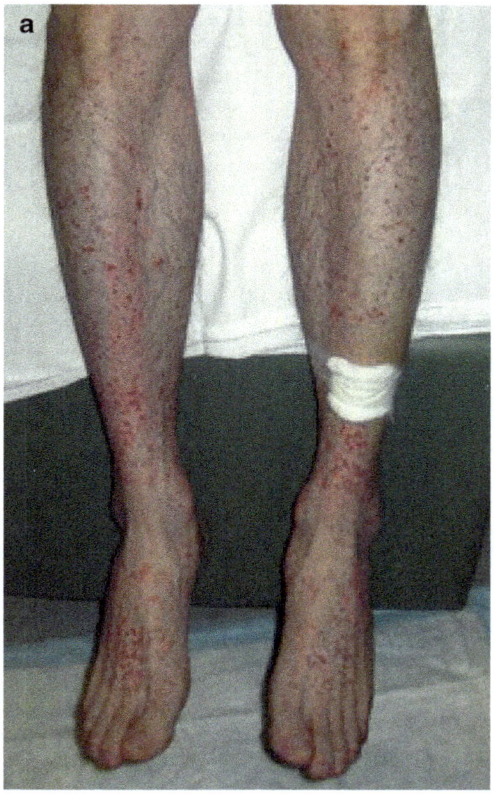

Leukocytoclastic vasculitis
Photograph courtesy of SpringerImages Database, Springer Publishing Company

H.M. Gloster, Jr. et al., *Absolute Dermatology Review: Mastering Clinical Conditions on the Dermatology Recertification Exam*, DOI 10.1007/978-3-319-03218-4_12, © Springer International Publishing Switzerland 2016

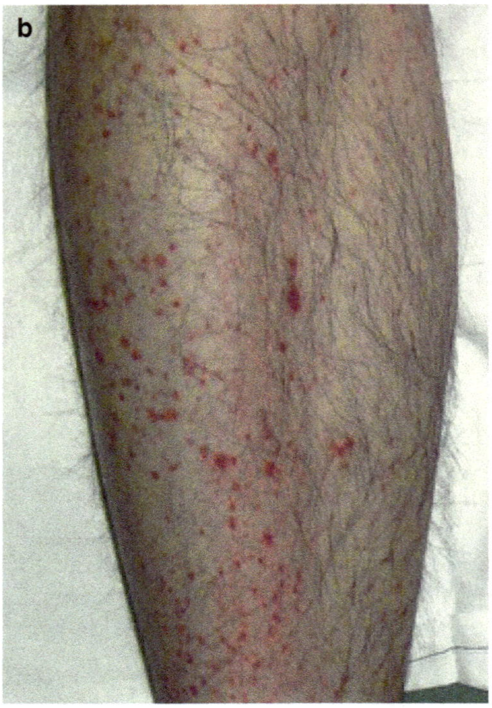

Leukocytoclastic vasculitis (*continued*)

Leukocytoclastic Vasculitis

A. Urticarial papules, pustules, vesicles, petechiae, and target lesions may occur
B. Extracutaneous involvement occurs but is uncommon
    1. Constitutional fever, weight loss, myalgias
    2. Systemic symptoms (if present should increase the suspicion of systemic vasculitis): arthralgias and arthritis (most common symptom), renal (second most common symptom), gastrointestinal, neurological

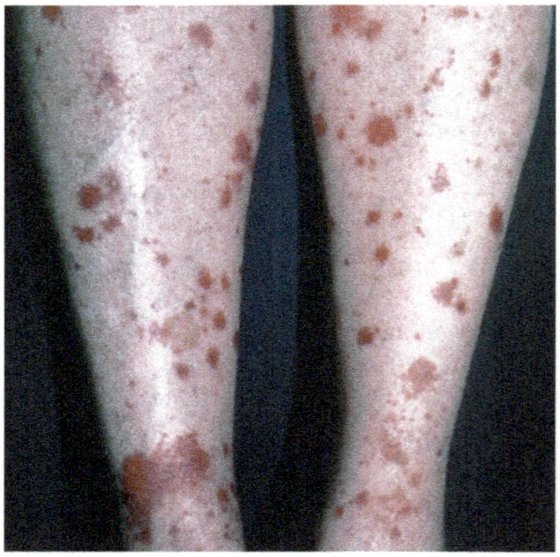

Leukocytoclastic vasculitis
Photograph courtesy of the American Academy of Dermatology

Leukocytoclastic vasculitis

A. Palpable or macular purpura, which may undergo central necrosis with hemorrhagic infarcts

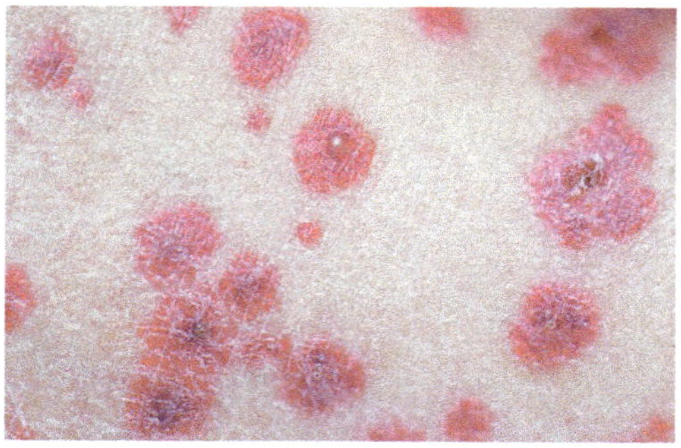

Leukocytoclastic vasculitis
Photograph courtesy of SpringerImages Database, Springer Publishing Company

b. Henoch-Schonlein Pupura

Henoch-Schonlein Purpura

A. IgA immune complexes in the walls of vessels (type of small vessel vasculitis)
B. Most commonly in children less than 10 years of age in association with preceding upper respiratory infection but may be seen in adults
C. Usually resolves weeks to months
D. Clinical signs
   1. Intermittent palpable purpura on extensor extremities and buttocks
   2. Urticarial, vesicles, bullae, necrosis can also be seen
   3. Abdominal pain and/or gastrointestinal bleeding and vomiting—50–75 %
   4. Arthralgias and arthritis (usually knees and ankles)—75 %
   5. Renal vasculitis with nephritis, hematuria, proteinuria—40–50 %

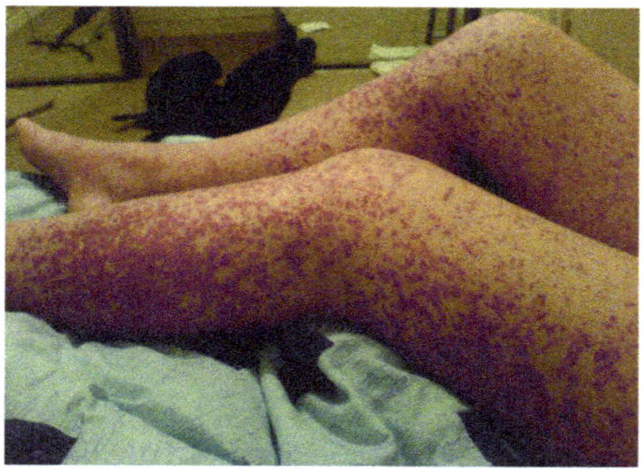

Henoch-Schonlein pupura
Photograph courtesy of SpringerImages Database, Springer Publishing Company

Henoch-Schonlein Purpura
  A. Intermittent palpable purpura on extensor extremities and buttocks

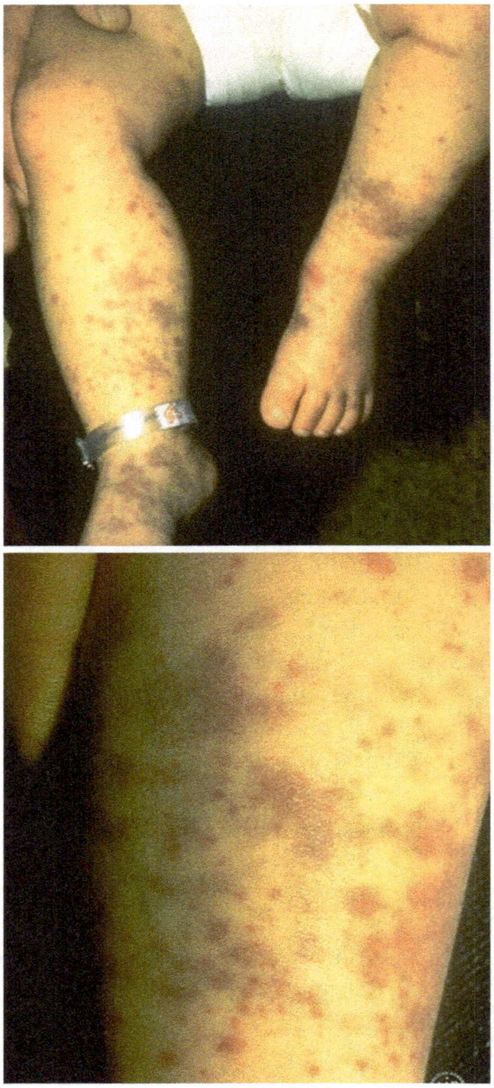

Henoch-Schonlein purpura
Photograph courtesy of the American Academy of Dermatology

c. Acute Hemorrhagic Edema of Infancy

Acute hemorrhagic edema of infancy
  A. Type of small vessel vascultis
  B. Well-appearing child less than 2 years of age, recent history of upper respiratory infection, antibiotic use, or both
  C. Abrupt onset of large, annular or targetoid purpuric plaques on face, ears, and extremities
  D. Tender nonpitting edema of acral sites (face, ears, hands, feet)
  E. Resolves 1–3 weeks

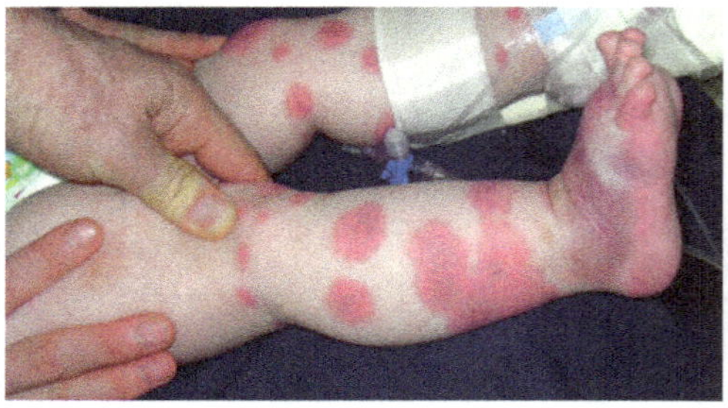

Acute hemorrhagic edema of infancy
Photograph courtesy of SpringerImages Database, Springer Publishing Company

Acute hemorrhagic edema of infancy

A. Large, annular or targetoid purpuric plaques on the face

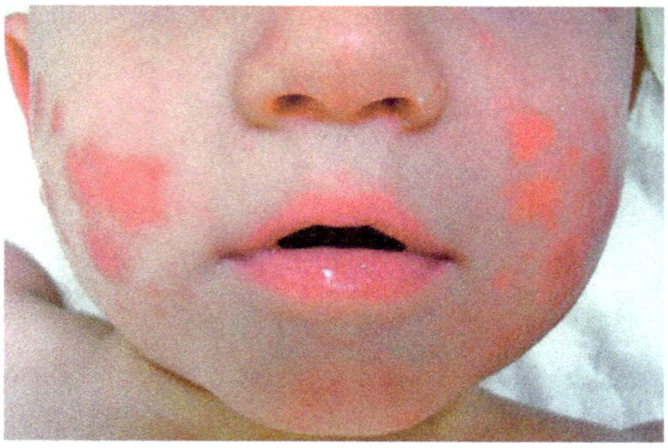

Acute hemorrhagic edema of infancy
Photograph courtesy of SpringerImages Database, Springer Publishing Company

d. Urticarial Vasculitis

Urticarial Vasculitis

A. Recurrent episodes of painful (not pruritic like urticaria), persistent urticarial plaques that last more than 24 hours and resolve with postinflammatory hyperpigmentation
B. May occur with or without angioedema
C. Most common on the trunk and proximal extremities
D. Constitutional symptoms and arthritis may be present
E. Systemic disease
   1. Arthralgia and arthritis—most common
   2. Uveitis or episcleritis
   3. Renal—hematuria, proteinuria
   4. Gastrointestinal—abdominal pain, nausea, vomiting, diarrhea
   5. Pulmonary
F. Associated disorders—viral infections, autoimmune connective tissue disease

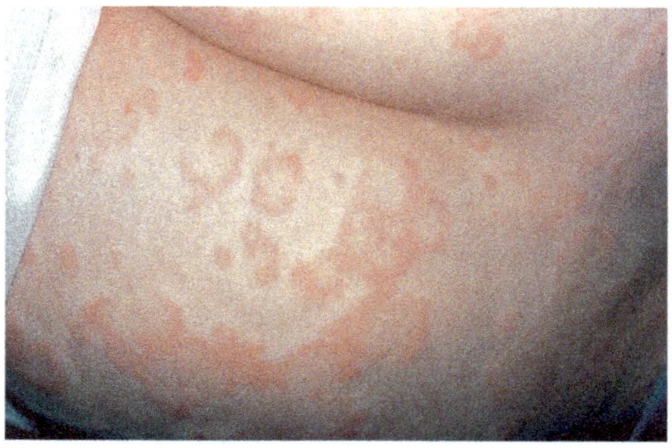

Urticarial vasculitis
Photograph courtesy of American Academy of Dermatology

Urticarial Vasculitis

A. Painful, persistent urticarial plaques on the lower extremities

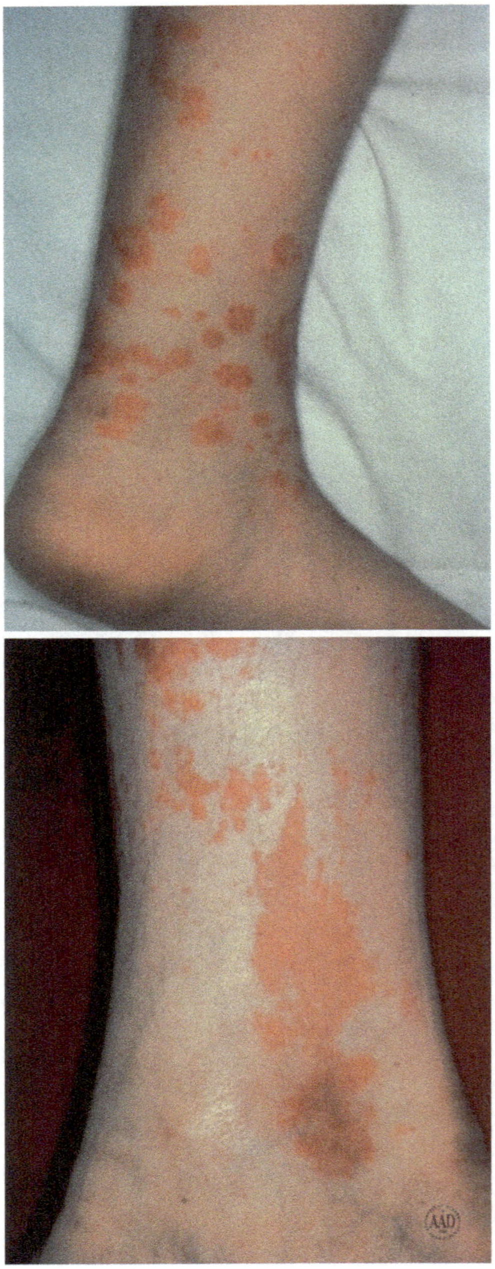

Urticarial vasculitis
Photograph courtesy of the American Academy of Dermatology

Urticarial Vasculitis

A. Painful, persistent urticarial plaques on the lower extremities

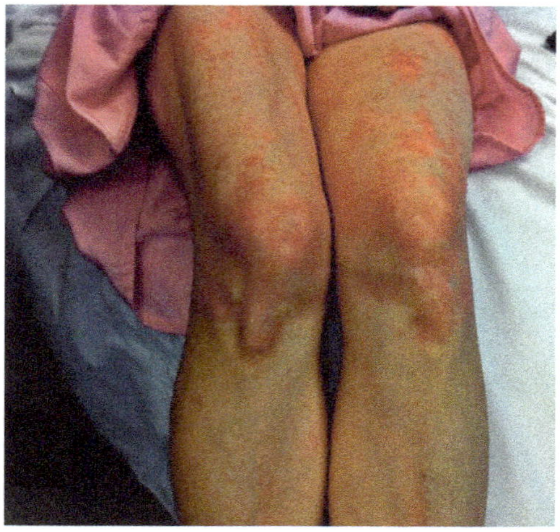

Urticarial vasculitis
Photograph courtesy of the American Academy of Dermatology

e. Erythema Elevatum Diutinum

Erythema elevatum diutinum

A. Symmetric, firm red–violet or red–brown papules and plaques on extensor extremities (knees, elbows, ankles, hands, fingers)
B. Ocular disease (keratitis, uveitis, blindness) is the most common extracutaneous manifestation
C. Usually occurs ages 30–60, earlier in patients with HIV
D. Leukocytoclastic vasculitis in early lesions
E. Associated conditions
   1. Infections—HIV, hepatitis B virus, tuberculosis, syphilis, beta hemolytic streptococcus
   2. Autoimmune disorders
   3. Monoclonal gammopathy (especially IgA paraproteinemia)

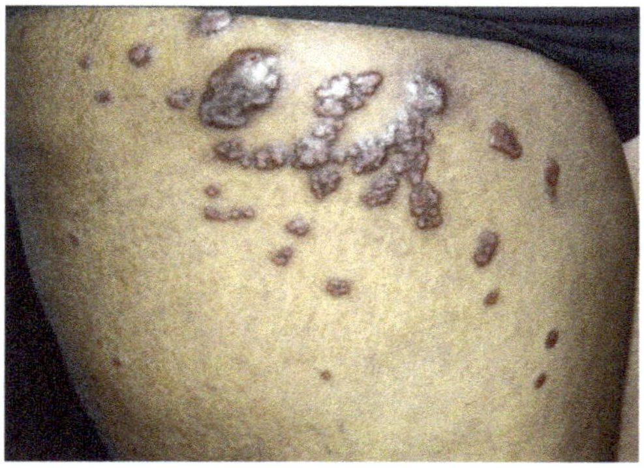

Erythema elevatum diutinum
Photograph courtesy of SpringerImages Database, Springer Publishing Company

Erythema elevatum diutinum

A. Symmetric, firm red–violet or red–brown papules and plaques on extensor extremities

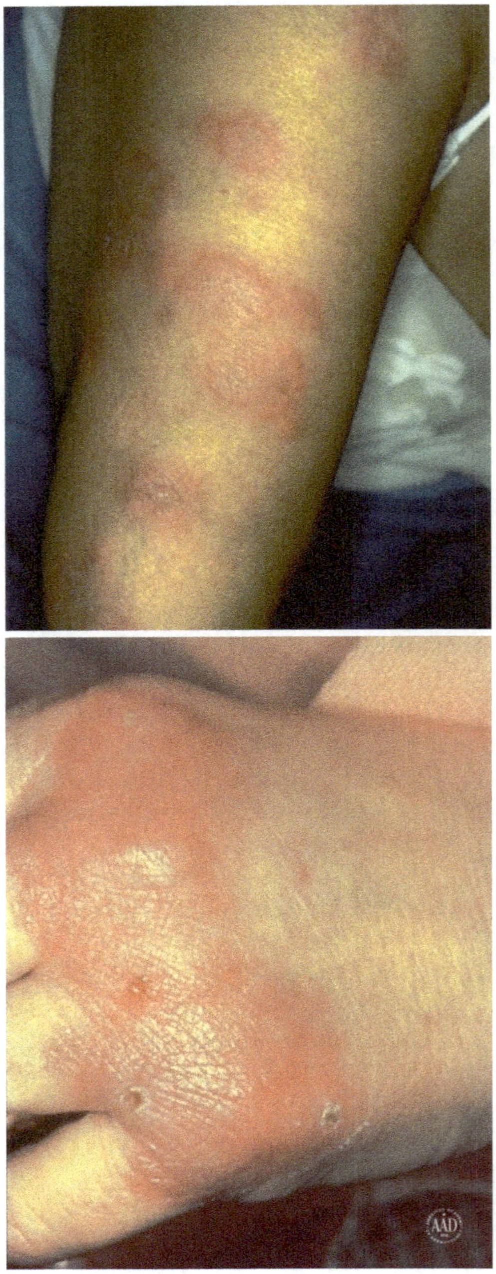

Erythema elevatum diutinum
Photograph courtesy of American Academy of Dermatology

13 Mixed Small and Medium Vessel Vasculitis

a. Cryoglobulinemic Vasculitis

Cryoglobulinemic vasculitis

A. Mixed small and medium vessel vasculitis
B. Detectable serum cryoglobulins—uncentrifuged serum after 48 hours at 4 °C with the arrow indicating cryoprecipitiate
C. Mixed serum cryoglobulins (IgG and IgM) most commonly in the setting of HCV infection
D. Affects skin, kidneys, peripheral nerves
E. Palpable purpura on lower extremities (90 %)
F. Myalgias, arthralgias (70 %), peripheral sensory neuropathy (40 %), hepatitis (30 %), and glomerulonephritis (25 %)
G. Associated with infections (hepatitis C infection), autoimmune connective tissue disease (rheumatoid arthritis), hematologic malignancy (non-Hodgkin B cell lymphoma)

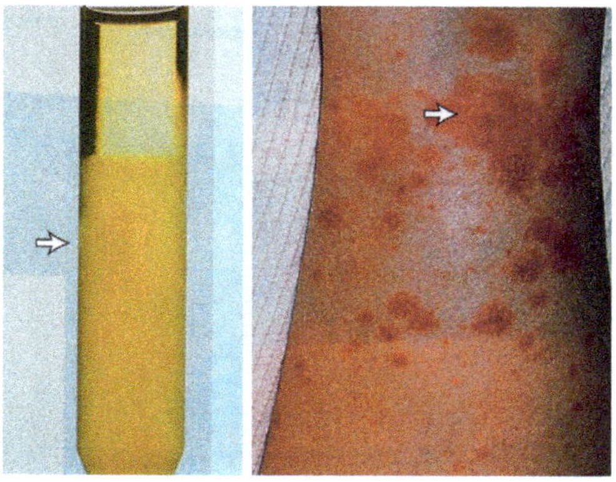

Cryoglobulinemic vasculitis
Photographs courtesy of SpringerImages Database, Springer Publishing Company

H.M. Gloster, Jr. et al., *Absolute Dermatology Review: Mastering Clinical Conditions on the Dermatology Recertification Exam*, DOI 10.1007/978-3-319-03218-4_13, © Springer International Publishing Switzerland 2016

b. ANCA-Associated Vasculitis

i. Wegener's Granulomatosis

Wegener's granulomatosis

A. Pulmonary—necrotizing granulomas of upper and lower respiratory tract, most common manifestation
B. Renal—glomerulonephritis
C. Systemic small vessel necrotizing vasculitis of skin and oral mucosa
D. Palpable purpura, painful subcutaneous nodules, and pyoderma gangrenosum–like ulcers

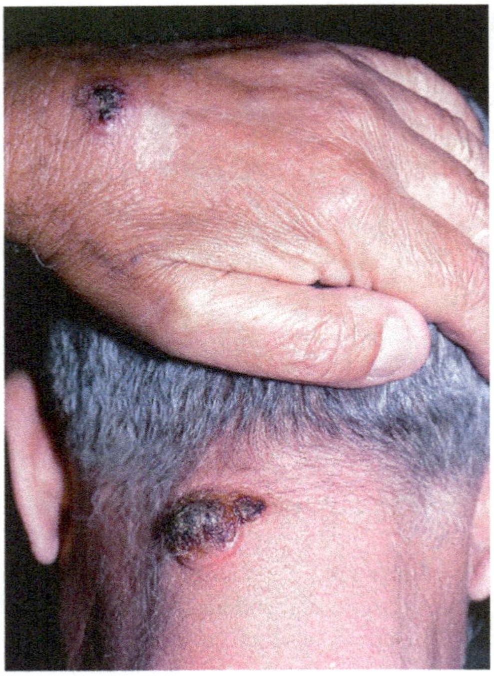

Wegener's granulomatosis
Photograph courtesy of SpringerImages Database, Springer Publishing Company

Wegener's granulomatosis

A. Saddlle nose deformity: cartilage necrosis and collapse occurs in systemic or localized Wegener's granulomatosis

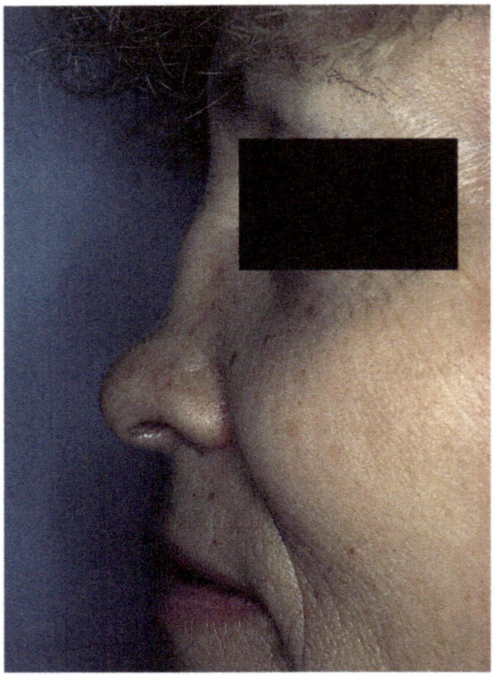

Wegener's granulomatosis
Photograph courtesy of SpringerImages Database, Springer Publishing Company

Wegener's granulomatosis
A. Strawberry gums—red inflamed gingiva due to gingival hyperplasia

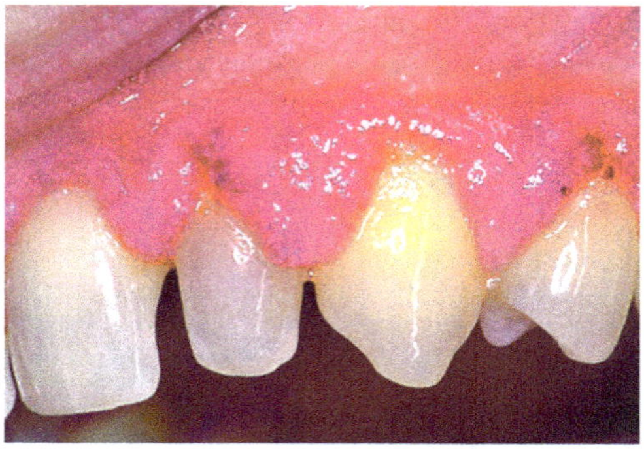

Wegener's granulomatosis
Photograph courtesy of SpringerImages Database, Springer Publishing Company

ii. Churg–Strauss Syndrome

Churg-Strauss syndrome
A. 1st phase—asthma, allergic rhinitis, nasal polyps; may persist for years; precedes vasculitis
B. 2nd phase—peripheral eosinophilia, respiratory tract infections, gastrointestinal symptoms
C. 3rd phase—several years to decades after phase 1
   1. Cutaneous vasculitis with granuloma formation in the skin
      a. Palpable purpura
      b. Subcutaneous nodules
   2. Cardiac
      a. Cardiomyopathy, pericarditis
      b. Leading cause of death
   3. Neurological
      a. Mononeuritis multiplex—sudden weakness, asymmetric foot or wrist drop, and sensory deficits

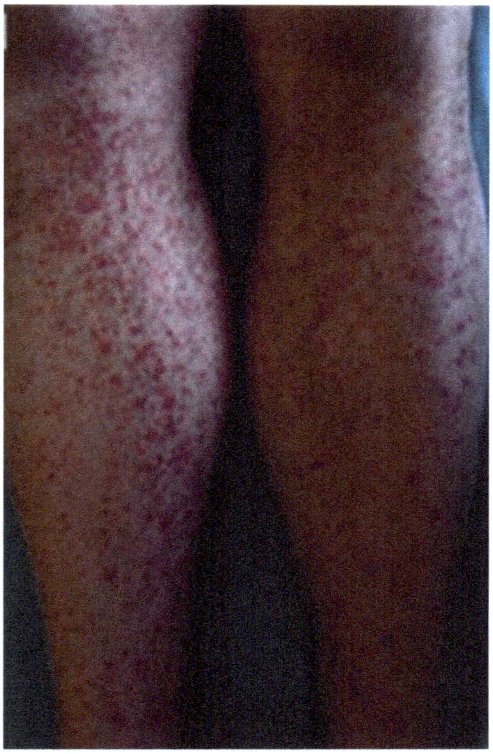

Churg-Strauss syndrome
Photograph Courtesy of SpringerImages Database, Springer Publishing Company

Churg-Strauss syndrome

A. Mononeuritis multiplex with asymmetric foot drop

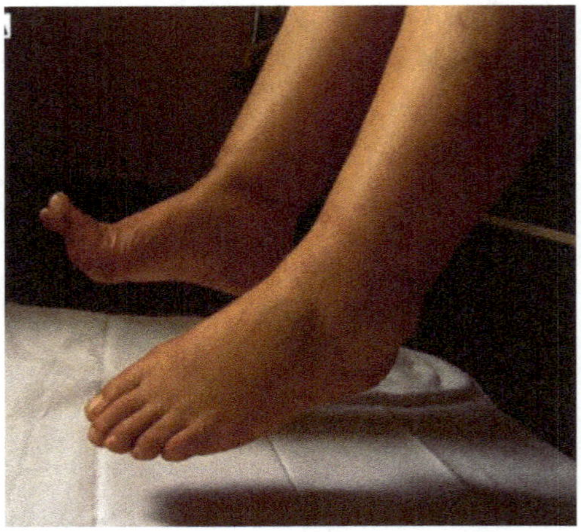

Churg-Strauss syndrome
Photograph courtesy of SpringerImages Database, Springer Publishing Company

14 Medium-Sized Vessel Vasculitis

a. Polyarteritis Nodosa

Polyarteritis nodosa (PAN)

A. Medium-sized vessel vasculitis
B. Association: infection (hepatitis B and C, HIV, streptoccal infections (especially in children), parvovirus B19); inflammatory diseases (inflammatory bowel disease, systemic lupus), medications (minocycline), malignancy (hairy cell leukemia)
C. Two variants
   1. Cutaneous—10 % of PAN cases, chronic, more benign course, most common form of PAN in children (most often associated with streptoccal infections)
      a. Palpable purpura—most common manifestation, may be pustular or ulcerative (see figure)
      b. Livedo reticularis
      c. Retiform purpura
      d. Punched-out ulcers
      e. Painful subcutaneous nodules on the lower extremities which may ulcerate
      f. Peripheral gangrene and ulceration of distal digits
      g. Mild systemic features—fever, myalgias, arthralgias, peripheral neuropathy with paresthesias
   2. Systemic (classic PAN)
      a. Skin features are the same as cutaneous PAN
      b. Systemic features
         i. Fever, myalgias, arthralgias, weight loss
         ii. Peripheral neuropathy (paresthesias), mononeuritis multiplex
         iii. Abdominal pain—mesenteric ischemia carries a poor prognosis
         iv. Orchitis—especially with hepatitis B
         v. Renovascular hypertension

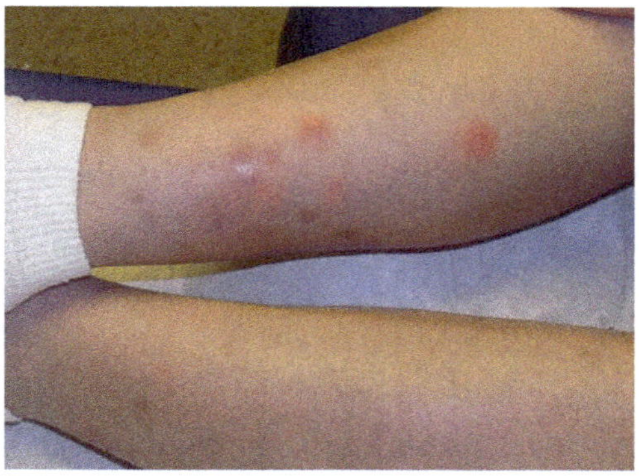

Polyarteritis nodosa
Photograph courtesy of SpringerImages Database, Springer Publishing Company

H.M. Gloster, Jr. et al., *Absolute Dermatology Review: Mastering Clinical Conditions on the Dermatology Recertification Exam*, DOI 10.1007/978-3-319-03218-4_14, © Springer International Publishing Switzerland 2016

Polyarteritis nodosa

A. Livedo reticularis

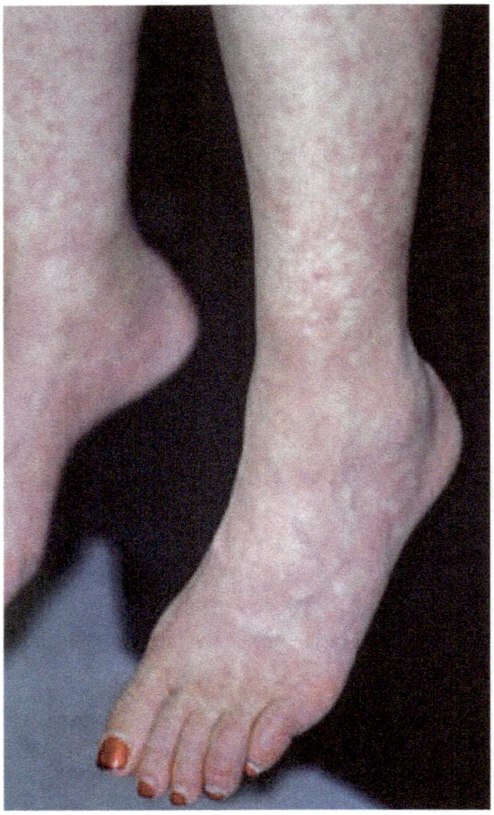

Polyarteritis nodosa
Photograph courtesy of SpringerImages Database, Springer Publishing Company

Polyarteritis nodosa

A. Painful subcutaneous nodules on the lower extremities which may ulcerate

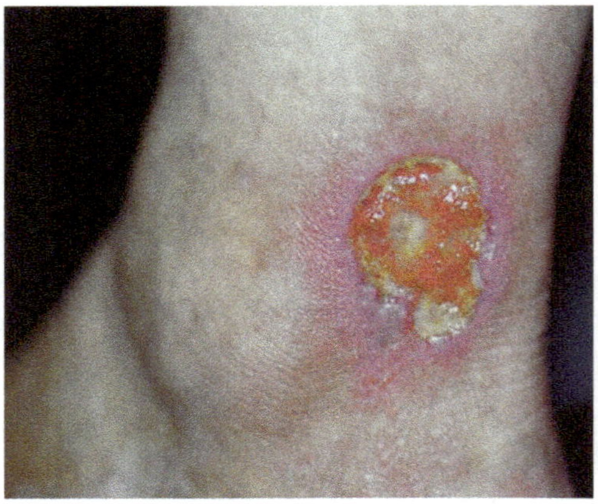

Polyarteritis nodosa
Photograph courtesy of SpringerImages Database, Springer Publishing Company

15 Livedoid Vasculopathy (Atrophie Blanche)

Livedoid vasculopathy (atrophie blanche)

A. More common in women
B. Painful punched-out ulcers most commonly on the distal lower extremities (especially the ankles)
C. Reticulated violaceous erythema may extend from the ulcers (livedo reticularis)
D. Lesions heal with white, round, or stellate scars (atrophie blanche) with peripheral telangiectasias
E. Chronic with episodes of recurrence and healing
F. Caused by alteration of coagulation resulting in fibrin thrombi within superficial dermal vessels (vasoocclusive hypercoagulation state)
G. Primary (idiopathic) or secondary (venous hypertension and varicocities or hypercoagulable states)

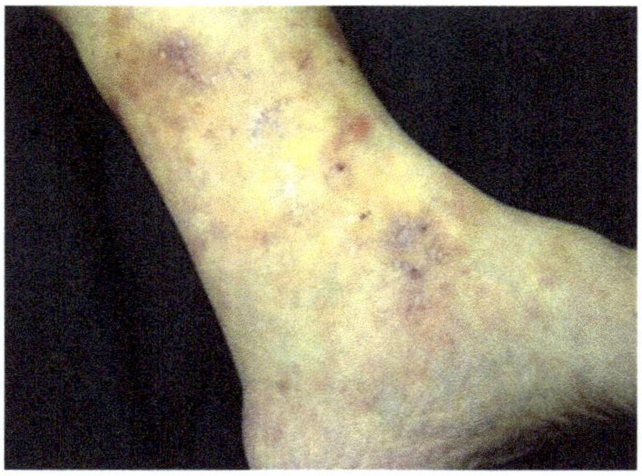

Livedoid vasculopathy (atrophie blanche)
Photograph courtesy of SpringerImages Database, Springer Publishing Company

H.M. Gloster, Jr. et al., *Absolute Dermatology Review: Mastering Clinical Conditions on the Dermatology Recertification Exam*, DOI 10.1007/978-3-319-03218-4_15, © Springer International Publishing Switzerland 2016

16 Coumadin Necrosis

Coumadin Necrosis

Coumadin necrosis

A. Develops 2–5 days after starting warfarin without heparin (especially loading doses) and is caused by occlusion of vessels of the dermis and subcutaneous tissue
B. Risk factors: female sex, obesity, advanced age (sixth to seventh decade)
C. Occurs on areas abundant in fat (breast, abdomen, buttocks, thigh)
D. Initially presents with pain and the development of well-demarcated erythema and edema
E. Progresses to petechiae and ecchymoses, hemorrhagic bullae, and full-thickness necrosis with deep ulceration with retiform branching purpura seen at periphery of cutaneous lesions
F. "Retiform purpura in plaques" describes palpable purpura in a livedoid or reticular pattern secondary to thrombotic occlusion of dermal and subcutaneous vessels, which leads to ischemic necrosis, red blood cell extravasation, and hemorrhage
G. "Retiform purpura in plaques" can also be seen in heparin necrosis, calciphylaxis, antiphospholipid antibody syndrome, septic emboli (meningococcemia, angioinvasive fungal infections), disseminated intravascular coagulation or purpura fulminans, and vasculopathies (cryoglobulinemia, cholesterol emboli, vasculitis)

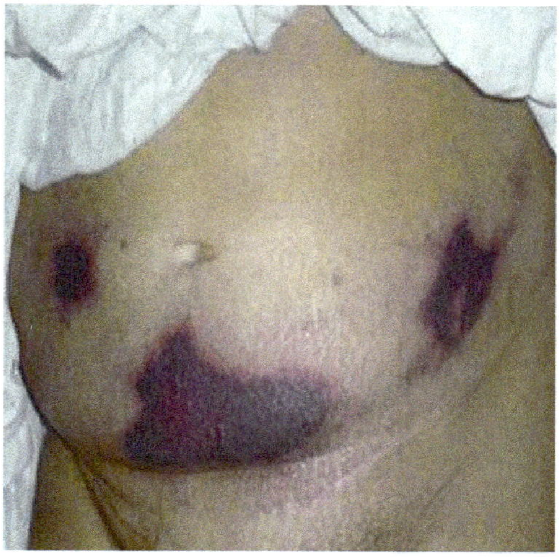

Coumadin necrosis
Photograph courtesy of SpringerImages Database, Springer Publishing Company

H.M. Gloster, Jr. et al., *Absolute Dermatology Review: Mastering Clinical Conditions on the Dermatology Recertification Exam*, DOI 10.1007/978-3-319-03218-4_16,

Chapter III

Vesiculobullous Diseases

17 Bullous Pemphigoid

Bullous pemphigoid

A. Most common autoimmune subepidermal blistering disease
B. Most commonly occurs in the elderly with chronic exacerbations and remissions
C. Early stages may be nonspecific and feature excoriated, eczematous, pruritic urticarial papules and plaques that may persist for months and remain as the only signs of the disease

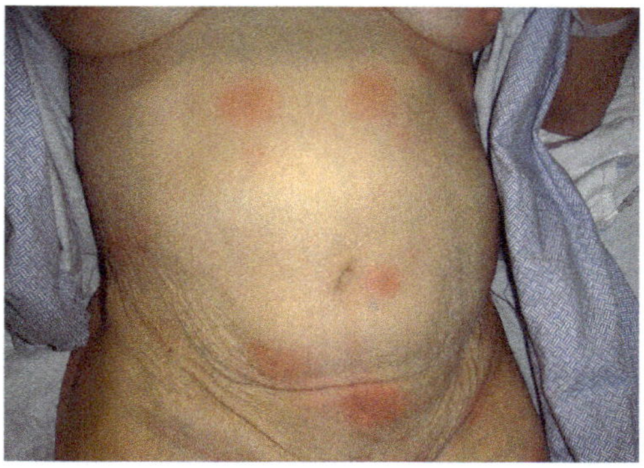

Bullous pemphigoid
Photograph courtesy of Dr. Adam Ingraffea, M.D., University of Cincinnati, Cincinnati, OH

Bullous pemphigoid

A. May evolve into pruritic, widespread tense vesicles and bullae arising on normal or erythematous skin; bullae rupture leaving erosions and crusts

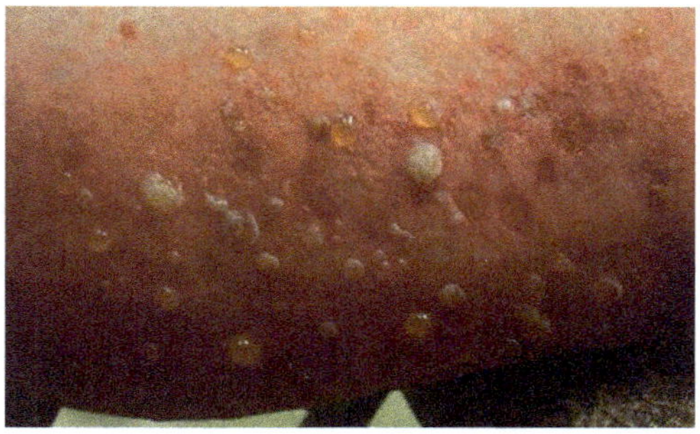

Bullous pemphigoid
Photograph courtesy of SpringerImages Database, Springer Publishing Company

H.M. Gloster, Jr. et al., *Absolute Dermatology Review: Mastering Clinical Conditions on the Dermatology Recertification Exam*,
DOI 10.1007/978-3-319-03218-4_17, © Springer International Publishing Switzerland 2016

Bullous pemphigoid

A. Vesicles and bullae may coexist with urticarial papules and plaques that may be annular or figurate

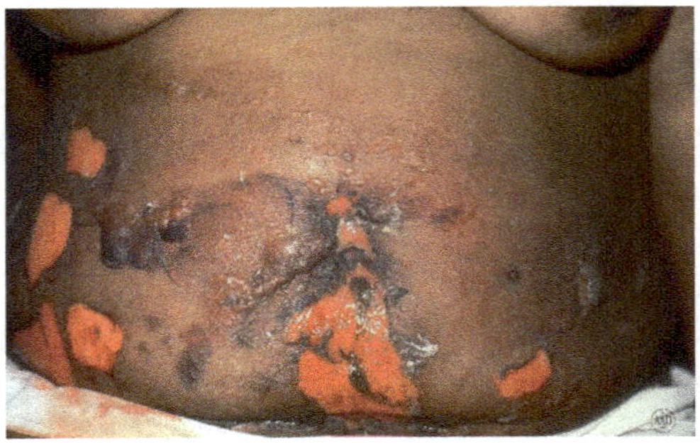

Bullous pemphigoid
Photograph courtesy of American Academy of Dermatology

Bullous pemphigoid

A. Tense blisters and erosions in the groin

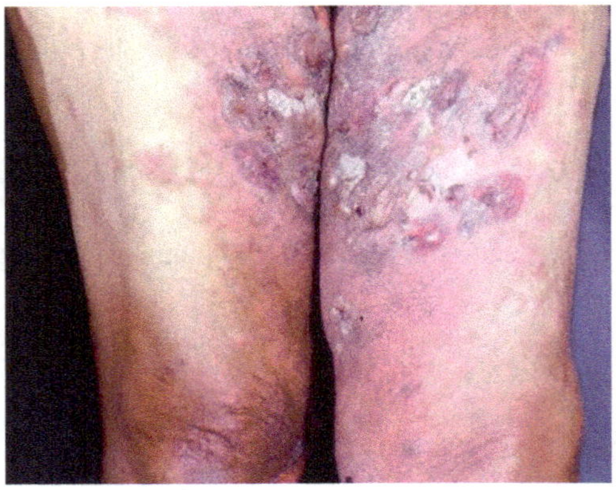

Bullous pemphigoid
Photograph courtesy of SpringerImages Database, Springer Publishing Company

Bullous pemphigoid

A. Tense blisters and erosions on the flexural aspects of limbs

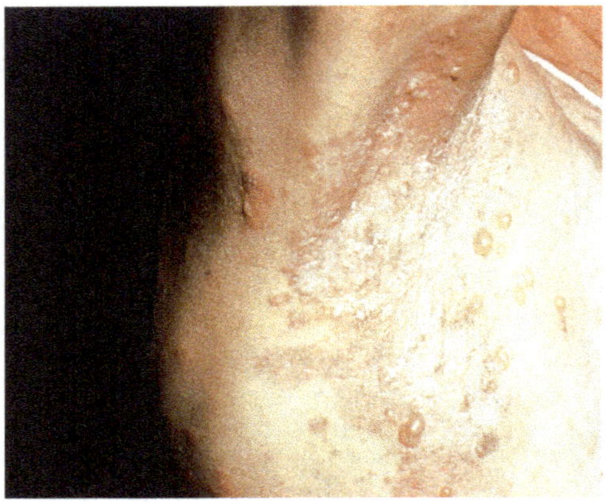

Bullous pemphigoid
Photograph courtesy of SpringerImages Database, Springer Publishing Company

18 Mucous Membrane (Cicatricial) Pemphigoid

Mucous Membrane (Cicatricial) Pemphigoid

A. Rare, chronic autoimmune disease associated with involvement of the external mucosal surfaces (oral and conjunctival) and subsequent scarring
B. Occurs most often in the elderly
C. Ocular disease: conjunctival inflammation and erosions resulting in scarring, fibrosis, ectropion, and blindness

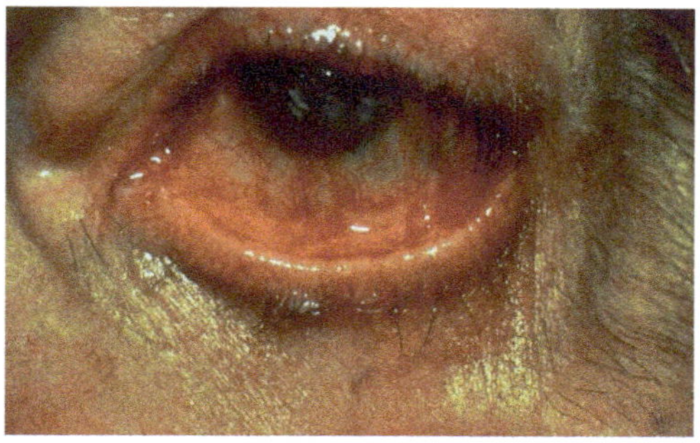

Mucous membrane (cicatricial) pemphigoid
Photograph courtesy of American Academy of Dermatology

Mucous Membrane (Cicatricial) Pemphigoid

A. Conjunctival inflammation and erosions resulting in scarring and fibrosis, ectropion

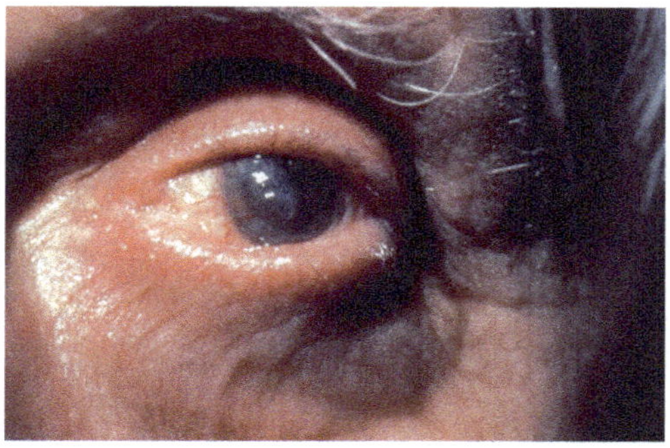

Mucous membrane (cicatrical) pemphigoid
Photograph courtesy of American Academy of Dermatology

H.M. Gloster, Jr. et al., *Absolute Dermatology Review: Mastering Clinical Conditions on the Dermatology Recertification Exam*,
DOI 10.1007/978-3-319-03218-4_18, © Springer International Publishing Switzerland 2016

Mucous Membrane (Cicatricial) Pemphigoid

A. Oral cavity disease: desquamative gingivitis and erosions of the buccal mucosa and palate
B. Occurs in 85 % of patients

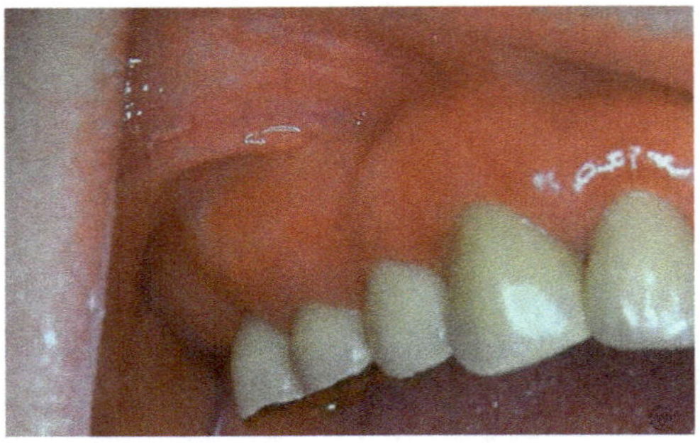

Mucous membrane (cicatrical) pemphigoid
Photograph courtesy of American Academy of Dermatology

Mucous Membrane (Cicatricial) Pemphigoid

A. Cutaneous disease
    1. 25–30 % of patients
    2. Red plaques evolve into blisters and erosions which result in atrophic scarring
    3. Most common on the scalp, face, neck, upper trunk
    4. Brunsting-Perry cicatricial pemphigoid: head and neck lesions with minimal mucosal involvement

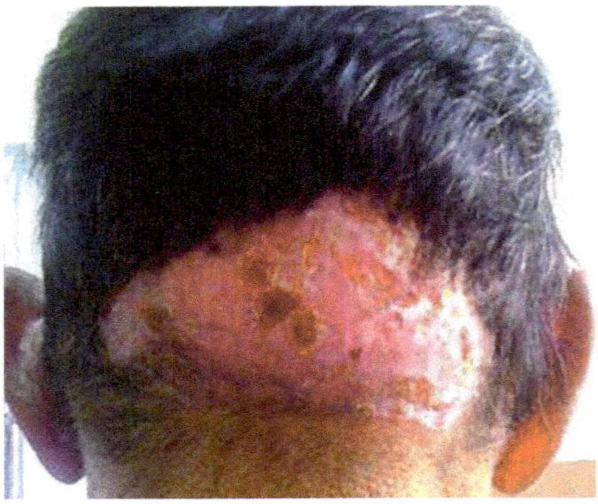

Mucous membrane (cicatrical) pemphigoid
Photograph courtesy of SpringerImages Database, Springer Publishing Company

19 Pemphigoid Gestationis

Pemphigoid gestationis

A. Variant of bullous pemphigoid
B. Develops during late pregnancy (third trimester) or immediate postpartum period
C. Lesions begin on the gravid abdomen, especially the periumbilical area, with rapid progression to generalized pemphigoid-like eruption (pruritic urticarial papules and plaques and clustered vesicles or tense bullae on a red base)
D. The eruption typically improves late in pregnancy but flares at the time of delivery
E. May flare with menstruation, oral contraceptives, or subsequent pregnancies
F. Increased risk of prematurity and small for gestational-age neonates (risk correlates with disease severity)

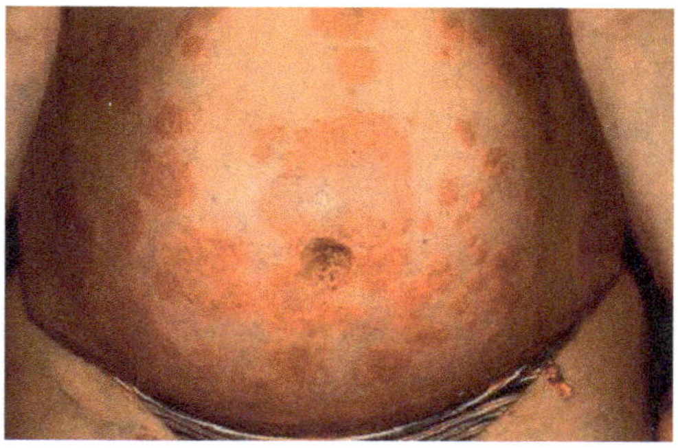

Pemphigoid gestationis
Photograph courtesy of SpringerImages Database, Springer Publishing Company

H.M. Gloster, Jr. et al., *Absolute Dermatology Review: Mastering Clinical Conditions on the Dermatology Recertification Exam*, DOI 10.1007/978-3-319-03218-4_19, © Springer International Publishing Switzerland 2016

Pemphigus Vulgaris

20

Pemphigus vulgaris

A. Two types
   1. Mucosal dominant with mucosal erosions but minimal skin involvement
   2. Mucocutaneous, with extensive skin blisters and erosions in addition to mucosal involvement

B. Painful erosions of the oral mucosa
   1. Precede skin disease in 60 %
   2. Buccal and palate mucosa most common
   3. May extend to vermilion lip with thick crusts
   4. Esophagus, conjunctiva, nasal mucosa, penis, vagina, anus and labia can be involved

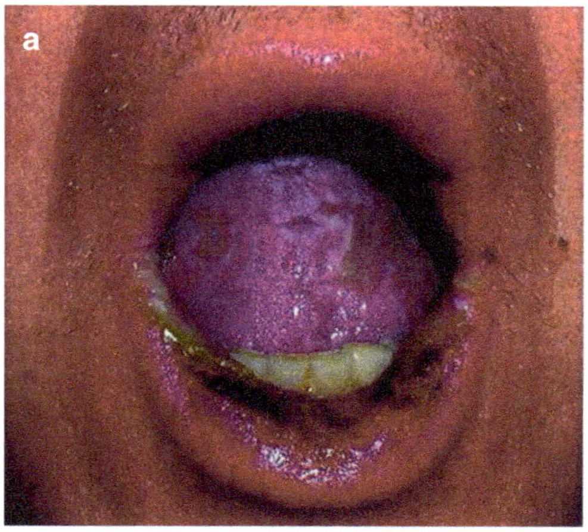

Pemphigus vulgaris
Photograph courtesy of SpringerImages Database, Springer Publishing Company

Pemphigus vulgaris

A. Painful erosions of the palate

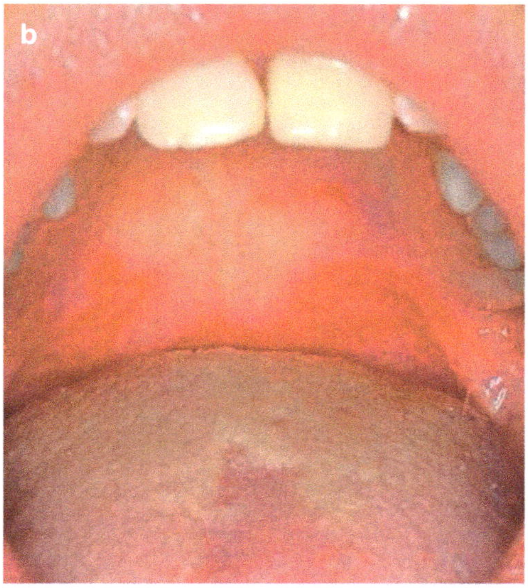

Pemphigus vulgaris
Photograph courtesy of SpringerImages Database, Springer Publishing Company

H.M. Gloster, Jr. et al., *Absolute Dermatology Review: Mastering Clinical Conditions on the Dermatology Recertification Exam*,
DOI 10.1007/978-3-319-03218-4_20,

Pemphigus vulgaris

A. Flaccid easily ruptured vesicles or blisters which soon rupture to form widespread painful erosions that may attain a large size and become generalized and crusted

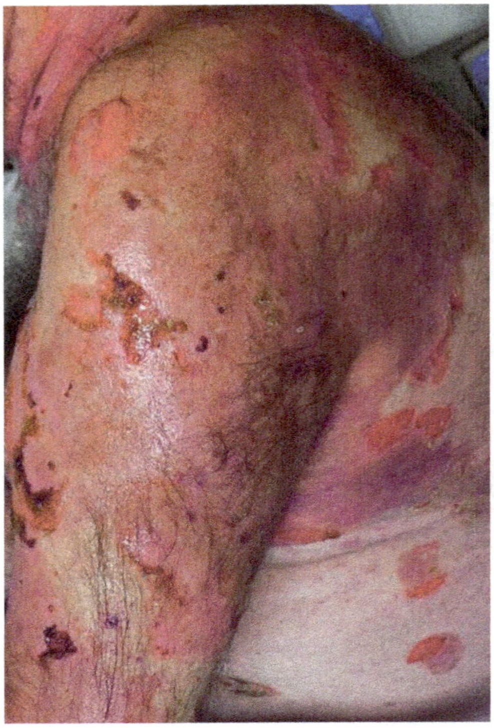

Pemphigus vulgaris
Photograph courtesy of SpringerImages Database, Springer Publishing Company

Pemphigus vulgaris

A. Flaccid easily ruptured vesicles or blisters which soon rupture to form widespread painful erosions (figures a and c)
B. Painful erosions of the palate (figure b)

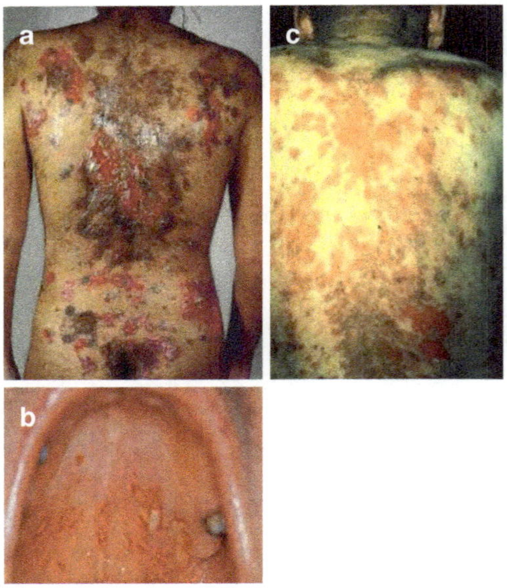

Pemphigus vulgaris
Photograph courtesy of SpringerImages Database, Springer Publishing Company

21 Pemphigus Foliaceous

Pemphigus foliaceous

A. Scaly, crusted, well-demarcated erosions on a red base
   1. Vesicle is superficial and fragile, and thus usually only erosions with crust and scale are present
   2. Seborrheic distribution is common (face, scalp, upper chest, and back)
   3. May stay localized or generalize to an exfoliative erythroderma
   4. Positive Nikolski sign

B. No mucosal involvement, and usually patients are not severely ill

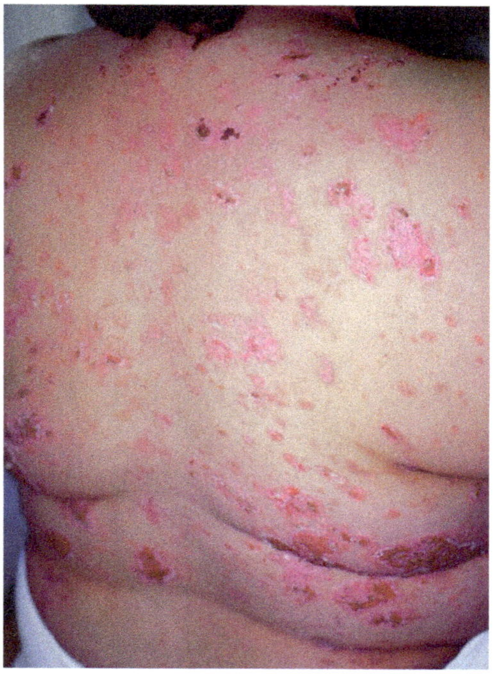

Pemphigus foliaceous
Photograph courtesy of SpringerImages Database, Springer Publishing Company

Pemphigus foliaceous

A. Scaly, crusted, well-demarcated erosions on a red base on the face

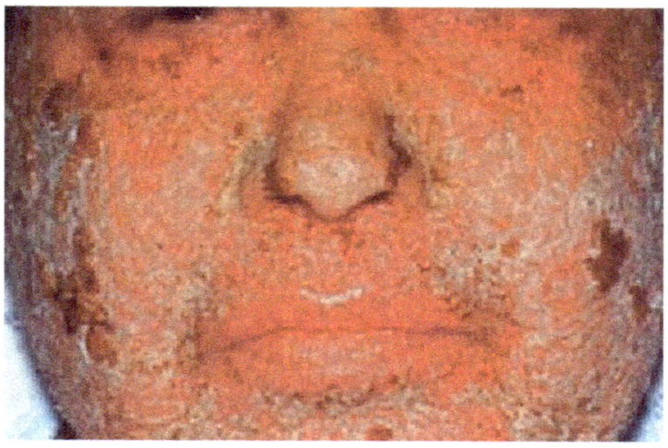

Pemphigus foliaceous
Photograph courtesy of SpringerImages Database, Springer Publishing Company

H.M. Gloster, Jr. et al., *Absolute Dermatology Review: Mastering Clinical Conditions on the Dermatology Recertification Exam*,
DOI 10.1007/978-3-319-03218-4_21, © Springer International Publishing Switzerland 2016

22 Pemphigus Vegetans

Pemphigus vegetans

A. Variant of pemphigus vulgaris
B. Erythematous bullae and erosions evolve into moist, fungating vegetations
C. Most commonly involves the intertriginous folds (groin, axilla), scalp, and face
D. Two subtypes
   1. Neumann
      a. Extensive disease similar to pemphigus vulgaris
      b. Flaccid blisters of pemphigus vulgaris become eroded and turn into vegetative plaques
   2. Hallopeau
      a. Localized disease
      b. Pustular lesions become vegetative plaques

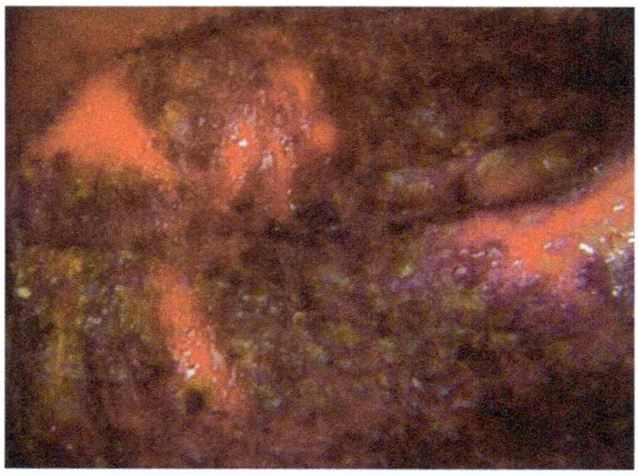

Pemphigus vegetans
Photograph courtesy of SpringerImages Database, Springer Publishing Company

H.M. Gloster, Jr. et al., *Absolute Dermatology Review: Mastering Clinical Conditions on the Dermatology Recertification Exam*, DOI 10.1007/978-3-319-03218-4_22, © Springer International Publishing Switzerland 2016

Hailey-Hailey Disease (Benign Familial Pemphigus) 23

Hailey-Hailey Disease (Benign Familial Pemphigus)

A. Autosomal dominant inheritance, usually develops in the second or third decade
B. Flaccid blisters and vesicles that easily rupture producing painful erosions at sites of friction on intertriginous areas (lateral neck, axilla, groin, and inframammary areas)
C. Moist, malodorous vegetative plaques and fissures may develop
D. Pain, pruritus, odor are the usual symptoms, and secondary bacterial infection may occur
E. Acantholysis occurs in the epidermis ("dilapidated brick wall" histologically)

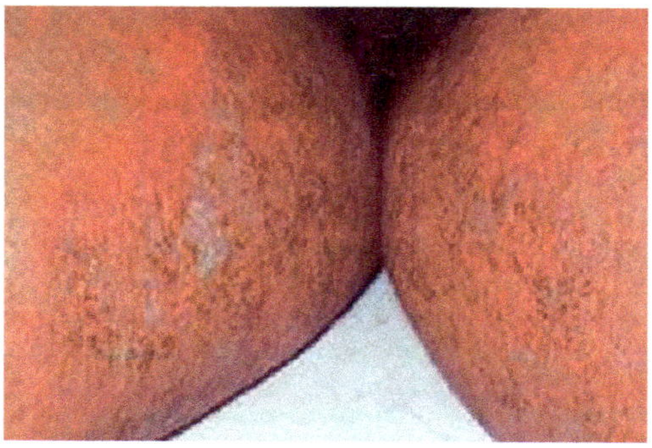

Hailey-Hailey disease (Benign familial pemphigus) Photograph courtesy of SpringerImages Database, Springer Publishing Company

Hailey-Hailey Disease (Benign Familial Pemphigus)

A. Flaccid blisters and vesicles that easily rupture producing painful erosions in the groin

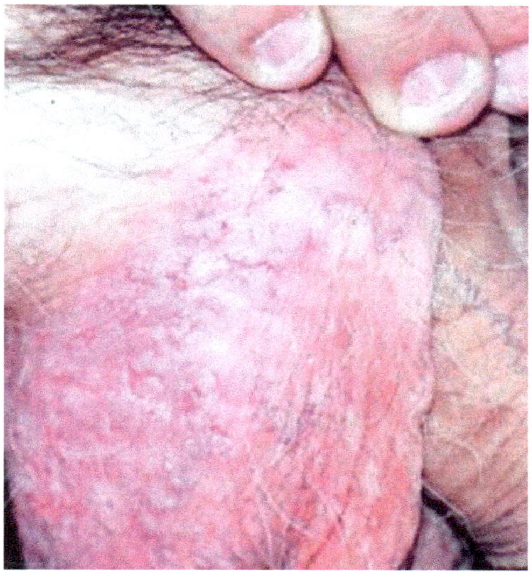

Hailey-Hailey (Benign familial pemphigus) Photograph courtesy of SpringerImages Database, Springer Publishing Company

H.M. Gloster, Jr. et al., *Absolute Dermatology Review: Mastering Clinical Conditions on the Dermatology Recertification Exam*, DOI 10.1007/978-3-319-03218-4_23, © Springer International Publishing Switzerland 2016

24 Paraneoplastic Pemphigus

Paraneoplastic pemphigus

A. Intractable stomatitis: most common clinical feature and usually the earliest sign; erosions and ulcerations affect all surfaces of the oropharynx and extend onto vermilion lip
B. Conjunctivitis
C. Esophageal, vaginal, labial, and penile lesions may also be seen
D. Cutaneous findings are polymorphic: red macules, flaccid blisters, erosions resembling pemphigus vulgaris; tense blisters resembling bullous pemphigoid; erythema multiforme like target lesions; lichenoid eruptions
E. Associated neoplasms: non-Hodgkins lymphoma (40 %), chronic lymphocytic leukemia (*30%*), Castelman's disease (10 %), malignant and benign thymomas (6 %), Waldenstrom's macroglobulinemia (6 %), sarcomas (6 %)

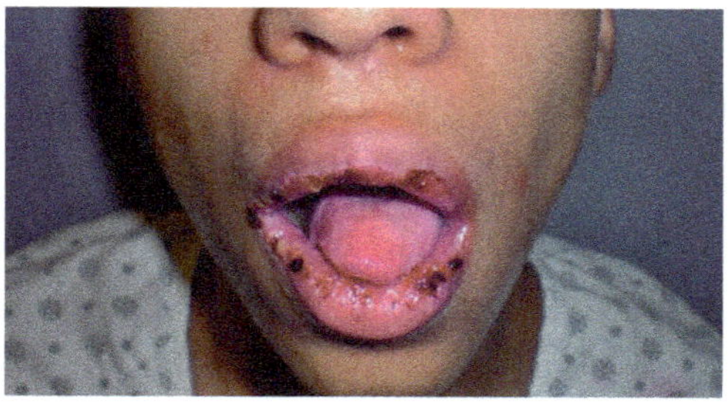

Paraneoplastic pemphigus
Photograph courtesy of SpringerImages Database, Springer Publishing Company

H.M. Gloster, Jr. et al., *Absolute Dermatology Review: Mastering Clinical Conditions on the Dermatology Recertification Exam*,
DOI 10.1007/978-3-319-03218-4_24,

25 Dermatitis Herpetiformis

Dermatitis herpetiformis (DH)

A. Symmetric, intensely pruritic grouped or herpetiform papules and vesicles with an erythematous base
B. Rarely are vesicles intact, usually only excoriated papules
C. Extensor surfaces of the arms, legs, buttocks, and back
D. Cutaneous manifestation of gluten sensitivity (90 % of DH patients have gluten-sensitive enteropathy)
E. Patients have levated antitransglutaminase antibodies
F. Granular IgA is deposited in the dermal papillae of clinically normal adjacent skin

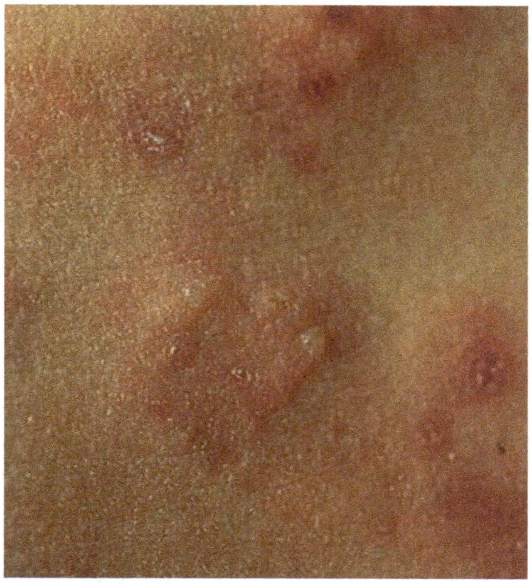

Dermatitis herpetiformis
Photograph courtesy of SpringerImages Database, Springer Publishing Company

H.M. Gloster, Jr. et al., *Absolute Dermatology Review: Mastering Clinical Conditions on the Dermatology Recertification Exam*, DOI 10.1007/978-3-319-03218-4_25, © Springer International Publishing Switzerland 2016

Dermatitis herpetiformis

A. Excoriated papules on extensor surfaces of the arms

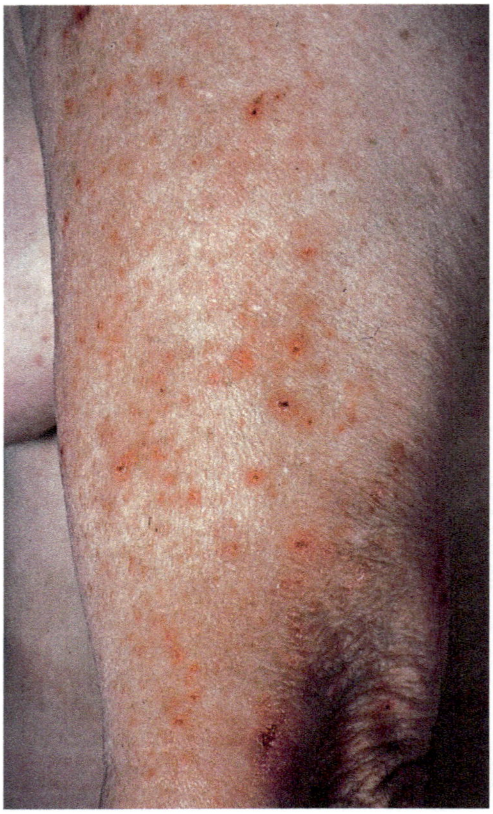

Dermatitis herpetiformis
Photograph courtesy of SpringerImages Database, Springer Publishing Company

Dermatitis herpetiformis

A. Excoriated papules and grouped or herpetiform papules on the buttocks

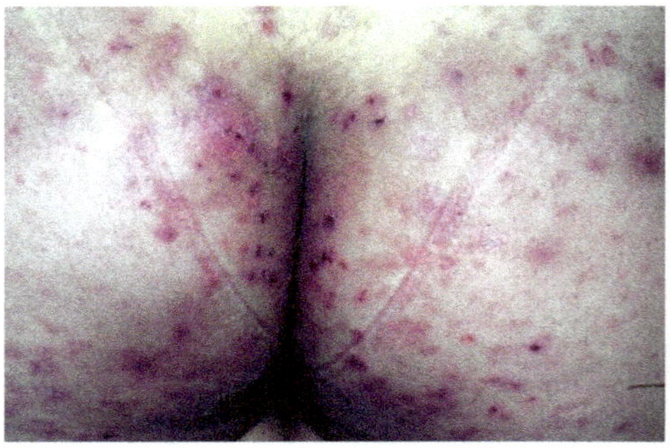

Dermatitis herpetiformis
Photograph courtesy of SpringerImages Database, Springer Publishing Company

Dermatitis herpetiformis

A. Excoriated intensely pruritic papules on the back

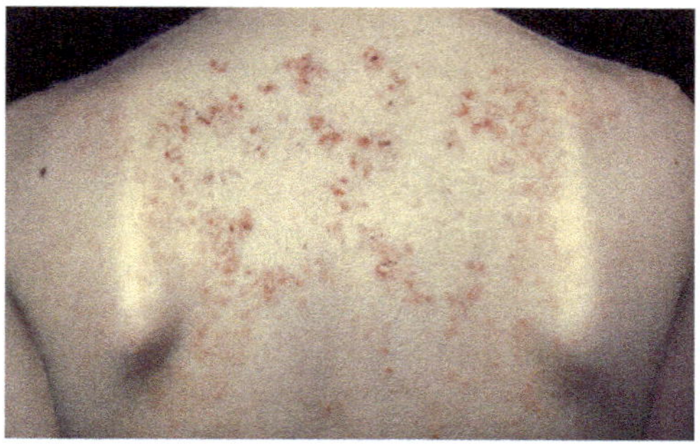

Dermatitis herpetiformis
Photograph courtesy of SpringerImages Database, Springer Publishing Company

Linear IgA Bullous Dermatosis

26

Linear IgA Bullous Dermatosis

A. Occurs in adults and children
B. Linear IgA deposits along basement membrane zone
C. Annular and linear vesicles and tense bullae on an erythematous base ("crown of jewels" or "string of pearls" around central crust)
D. Some patients may present with expanding annular polycyclic plaques
E. In adults, frequently drug induced by vancomycin

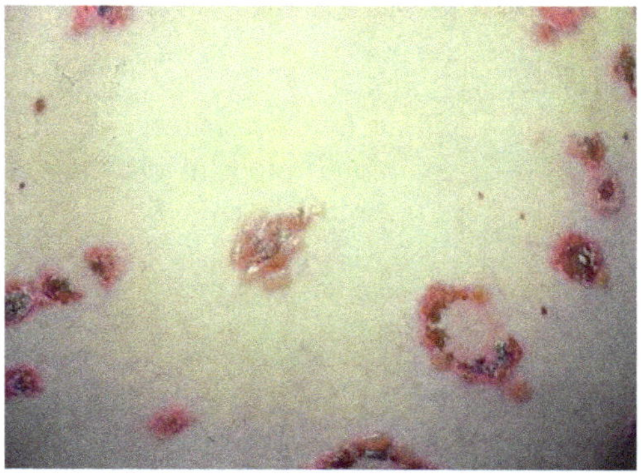

Linear IgA bullous dermatosis
Photograph courtesy of SpringerImages Database, Springer Publishing Company

Linear IgA Bullous Dermatosis

A. Vesiculobullous lesions in an annular and herpetiform arrangement

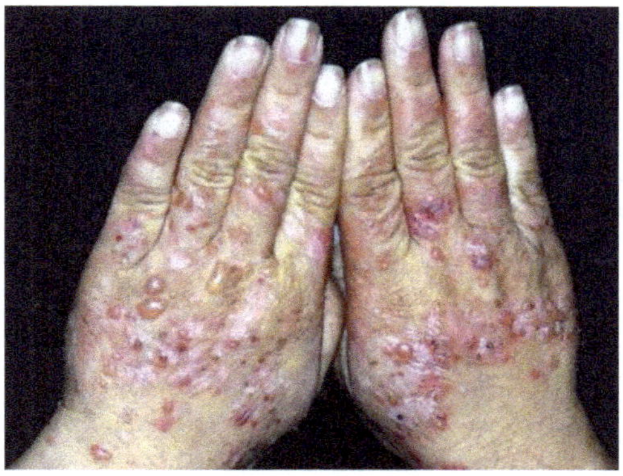

Linear IgA bullous dermatosis
Photograph courtesy of SpringerImages Database, Springer Publishing Company

H.M. Gloster, Jr. et al., *Absolute Dermatology Review: Mastering Clinical Conditions on the Dermatology Recertification Exam*, DOI 10.1007/978-3-319-03218-4_26,

Linear IgA Bullous Dermatosis

A. Childhood disease is known as the chronic bullous disease of childhood
B. Average onset of 5 years, remits by puberty
C. Lesions favor the lower body, 75 % affected in the oral area
D. Vesiculobullous lesions in an annular and herpetiform arrangement

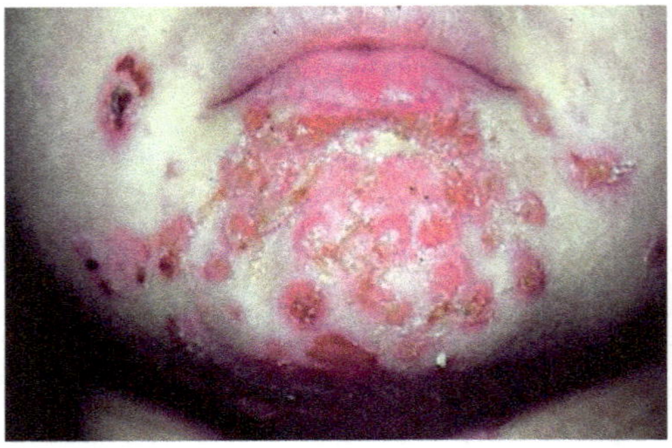

Linear IgA bullous dermatosis
Photograph courtesy of SpringerImages Database, Springer Publishing Company

Linear IgA Bullous Dermatosis (chronic bullous disease of childhood)

A. Vesiculobullous lesions in an annular and herpetiform arrangement
B. Lesions favor the lower body

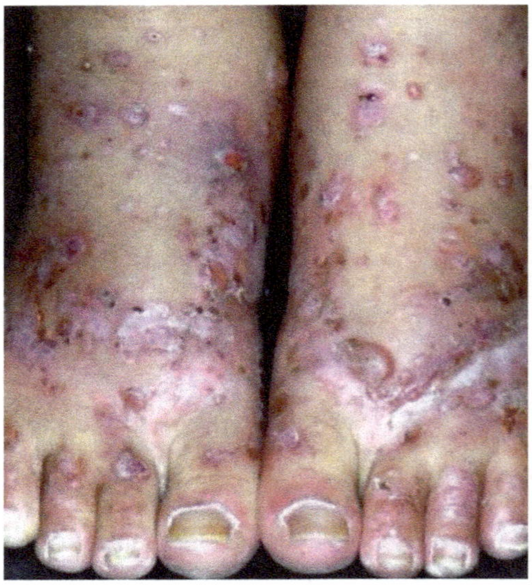

Linear IgA bullous dermatosis
Photograph courtesy of SpringerImages Database, Springer Publishing Company

27 Epidermolysis Bullosa

Epidermolysis bullosa (EB)

A. Congenital blistering disease with a variety of subtypes, classified according to the depth of the blister
B. Mechanically fragile skin (traction on the skin causes shearing), erosions, and blisters
C. Scarring (usually atrophic)
D. Dystrophic or absent nails
E. Milia (tiny firm white papules resembling cysts or pustules)
F. Scarring alopecia of the scalp
G. Extracutaneous features—more common with recessive dystrophic EB (RDEB) and junctional EB (JEB)
   1. Eye (scarring)
   2. Oral cavity
   3. Gastrointestinal (esophageal stricture, dyphagia, growth retardation, poor nutrition, anemia)
   4. Genitourinary (urethral strictures, hematuria, dysuria, sepsis)
   5. Dental enamel hypoplasia with loss of teeth (JEB)
   6. Mitten deformities (RDEB)
   7. Squamous cell carcinoma in sites of chronic scarring and inflammation (RDEB), leading cause of death at or after adolescence

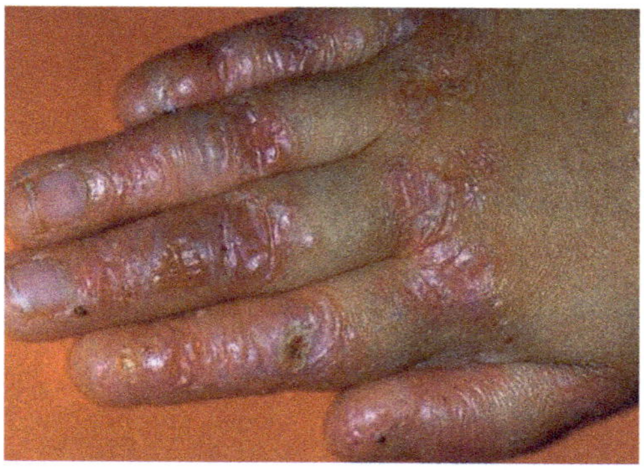

Epidermolysis bullosa
Photograph courtesy of SpringerImages Database, Springer Publishing Company

a. Epidermolysis Bullosa Simplex

Epidermolysis bullosa simplex (EBS)

A. Autostomal dominant, common and mild form of EB, intraepidermal blisters, onset at birth or infancy, normal life expectancy
B. Normal nails, no scarring, no milia
C. EBS-localized (previously Weber-Cockayne) is the most common subtype of EBS
   1. Blisters localized to hands, feet, and knees and other areas of trauma
   2. Palmoplantar bullae, erosions, calluses
   3. Hyperhidrosis

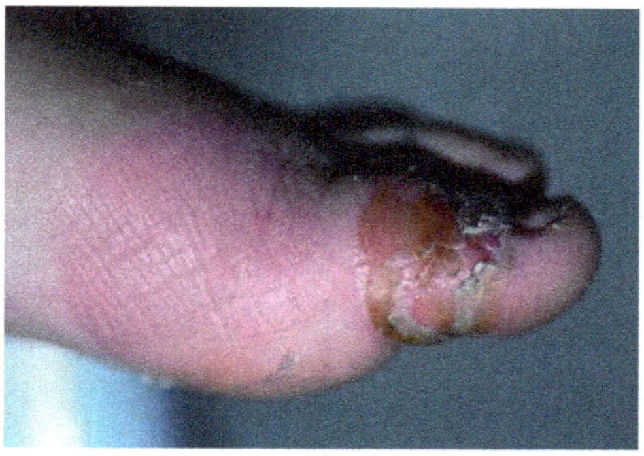

Epidermolysis bullosa simplex
Photograph courtesy of SpringerImages Database, Springer Publishing Company

H.M. Gloster, Jr. et al., *Absolute Dermatology Review: Mastering Clinical Conditions on the Dermatology Recertification Exam*, DOI 10.1007/978-3-319-03218-4_27,

Epidermolysis bullosa simplex (EBS)

A. Dowling-Meara variant
   1. Most severe form of EBS
   2. Mucosal involvement
   3. Grouped herpetiform blisters forming an arcuate or circinate array of blisters
   4. Palmoplantar keratoderma

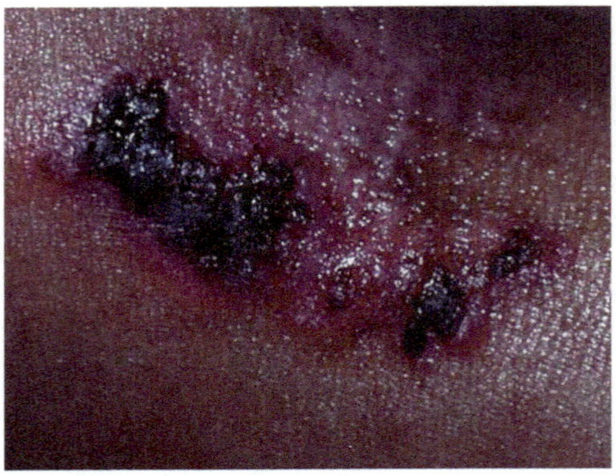

Epidermolysis bullosa simplex
Photograph courtesy of SpringerImages Database, Springer Publishing Company

b. Junctional Epidermolysis Bullosa

Junctional Epidermolysis Bullosa

A. Mechanically induced blistering occurring within the basement membrane at the lamina lucida
B. Mechanically induced erosions and blisters on the hands and feet
C. Characterized by excessive granulation tissue
D. Least common form of EB
E. Poor outcome in infancy

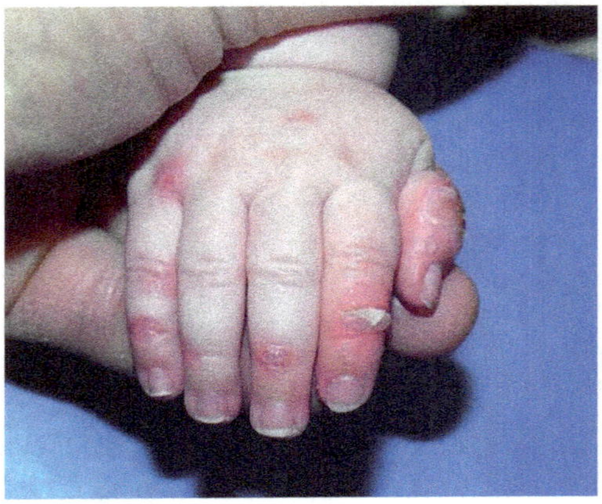

Junctional epidermolysis bullosa
Photograph courtesy of SpringerImages Database, Springer Publishing Company

c. Dominant Dystrophic Epidermolysis Bullosa

Dominant dystrophic epidermolysis bullosa

A. May have generalized blistering at birth similar to other forms of EB
B. Typically more mild course of disease
C. Dystrophic nails
D. Atrophic (or less commonly, hypertrophic) scarring of hands, elbows, knees
E. Milia within scars

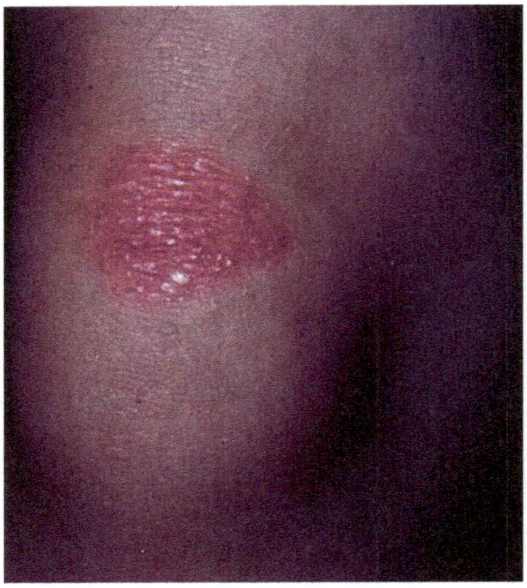

Dominant dystrophic epidermolysis bullosa
Photograph courtesy of SpringerImages Database, Springer Publishing Company

d. Recessive Dystrophic Epidermolysis Bullosa

Recessive dystrophic epidermolysis bullosa

A. Debilitating hand and foot deformities ("mitten deformiites") with pseudosyndactyly are common
B. Generalized erosions and blisters at birth, may have congenital absence of skin
C. Progressive, atrophic mutilating scarring of the skin
D. Corneal blisters or scarring, profound growth retardation, multifactorial anemia, failure to thrive, esophageal strictures

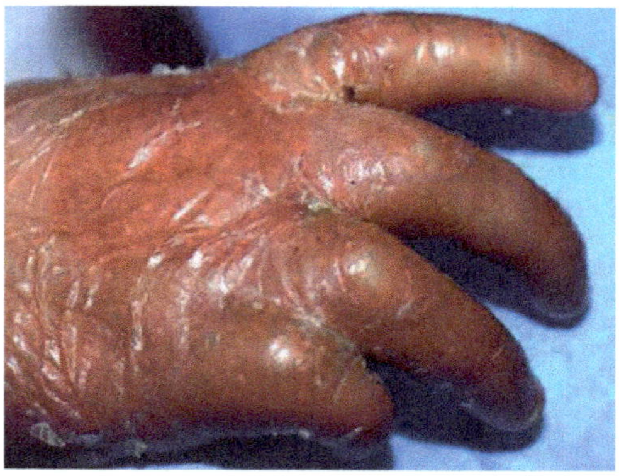

Recessive dystrophic epidermolyis bullosa
Photograph courtesy of SpringerImages Database, Springer Publishing Company

e. Epidermolysis Bullosa Aquisita

Epidermolysis bullosa aquisita

A. Usually occurs in adults, but childhood cases have been reported
B. Acquired mechanobullous disease (autoantibody to type VII collagen)
C. Noninflammatory blisters induced by trauma due to skin fragility followed by erosions that heal with atrophic scarring, milia, and hyperpigmentation and hypopigmentation
D. Lesions occur on trauma-prone surfaces such as the elbows, knees, dorsal hands, feet, and toes

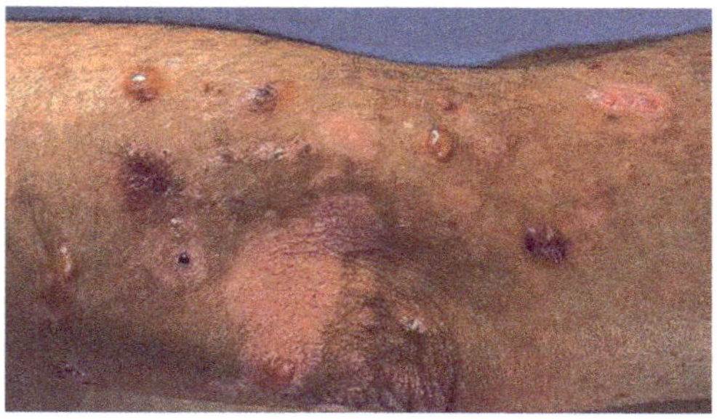

Epidermolysis bullosa aquisita
Photograph courtesy of SpringerImages Database, Springer Publishing Company

Epidermolysis bullosa aquisita

A. Erosions and scarring on the scalp occur in 20 % of patients

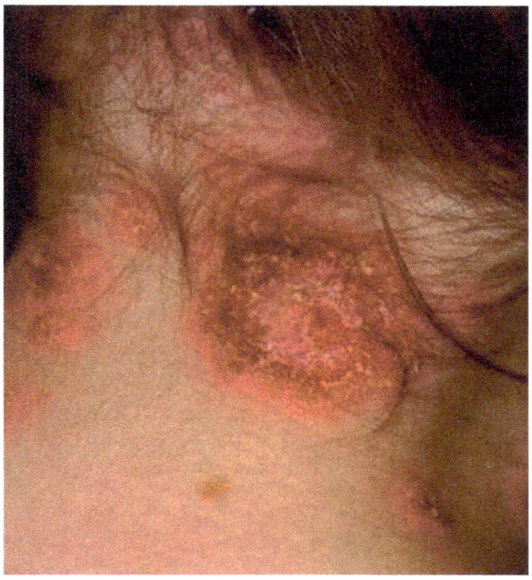

Epidermolysis bullosa aquisita
Photograph courtesy of SpringerImages Database, Springer Publishing Company

28 Erythema Toxicum Neonatorum

Erythema toxicum neonatorum

A. Common (50 % of full-term neonates)
B. Begins 24 to 48 hours after delivery, resolves spontaneously within 1 to 5 days (evanescent—changes rapidly)
C. Asymptomatic tiny erythematous papules, pustules, and vesicles surrounded by blotchy erythematous flare
D. Begins on the face then spreads to proximal extremities, trunk, buttocks (spares palms and soles)
E. Scraping of the lesions reveals sheets of eosinophils.
F. Differential diagnosis
   1. Scabies: burrows on palms and soles (spared in erythema toxicum)
   2. Infantile acropustulosis: occurs later in neonatal period (1–2 years of age); tense pruritic vesicles and pustules on hands and feet
   3. Transient neonatal pustular melanosis: present at birth, pustules on the head and neck that leave a macular hyperpigmentation, uncommon in Caucasians (more common in blacks)

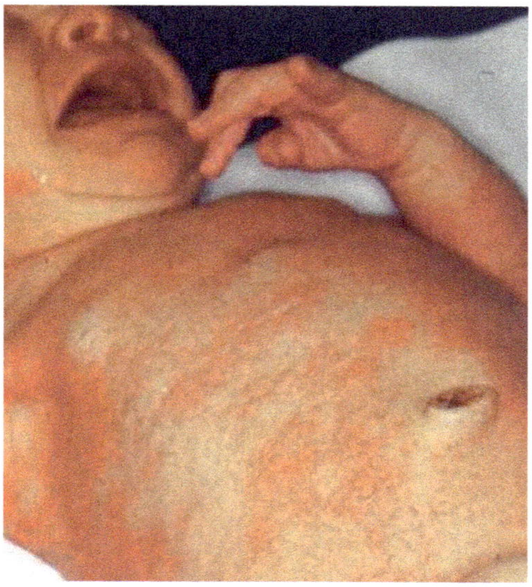

Erythema toxicum neonatorum
Photograph courtesy of SpringerImages Database, Springer Publishing Company

Erythema toxicum neonatorum

A. Lesions may resemble an urticarial flea bite with 1–3 cm red patches with central 1–2 mm papules or pustules

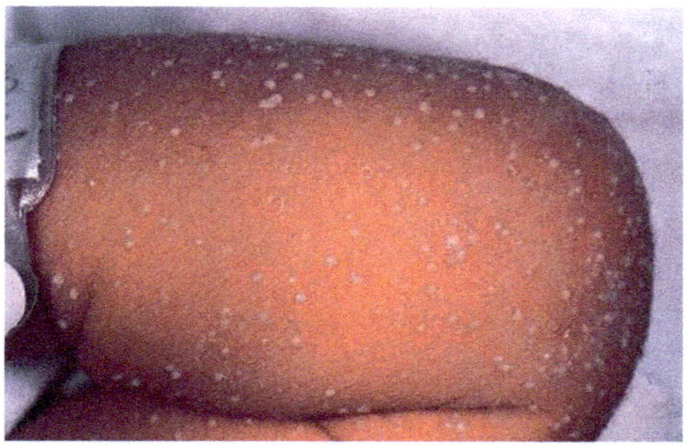

Erythema toxicum neonatorum
Photograph courtesy of SpringerImages Database, Springer Publishing Company

H.M. Gloster, Jr. et al., *Absolute Dermatology Review: Mastering Clinical Conditions on the Dermatology Recertification Exam*, DOI 10.1007/978-3-319-03218-4_28, © Springer International Publishing Switzerland 2016

Chapter IV

Adnexal Diseases

29 Acne Vulgaris

Acne vulgaris

A. Comedones are the hallmark clinical feature of acne: open comedones (black heads) and closed comedones (white heads)
B. No comedones are seen in acne rosacea
C. Lesions occur on the face, ears, chest, back, neck, and upper arms

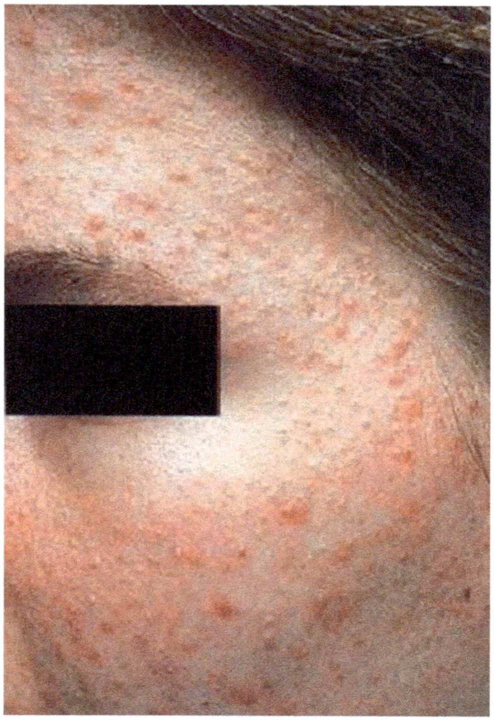

Acne vulgaris
Photograph courtesy of SpringerImages Database, Springer Publishing Company

Acne vulgaris

A. Inflammatory papules, pustules, nodules, and scars may also be seen
B. Lesions are in various stages of formation and resolution

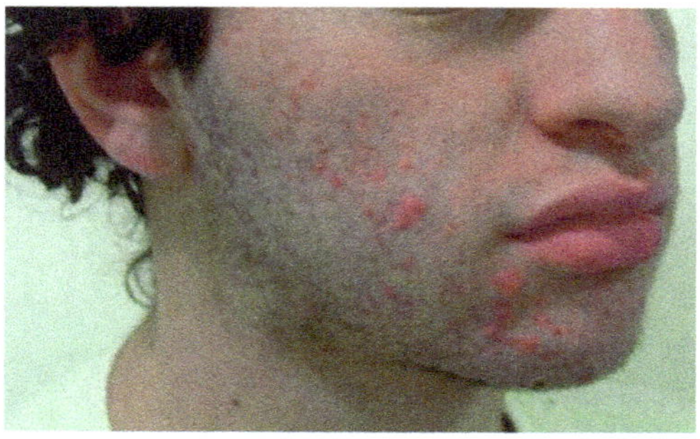

Acne vulgaris
Photograph courtesy of SpringerImages Database, Springer Publishing Company

H.M. Gloster, Jr. et al., *Absolute Dermatology Review: Mastering Clinical Conditions on the Dermatology Recertification Exam*, DOI 10.1007/978-3-319-03218-4_29, © Springer International Publishing Switzerland 2016

30 Acne Rosacea

a. Erythematotelangiectatic Acne Rosacea

Erythematotelangiectatic acne rosacea
   A. Persistent central facial erythema
   B. Flushing
   C. Telangiectasia

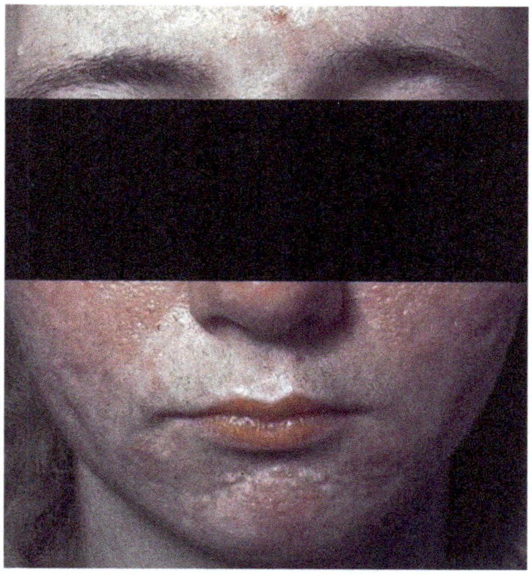

Erythematotelangiectatic acne rosacea
Photograph courtesy of SpringerImages Database, Springer Publishing Company

H.M. Gloster, Jr. et al., *Absolute Dermatology Review: Mastering Clinical Conditions on the Dermatology Recertification Exam*, DOI 10.1007/978-3-319-03218-4_30, © Springer International Publishing Switzerland 2016

Erythematotelangiectatic acne rosacea

A. Persistent central facial erythema, flushing, and telangiectasia

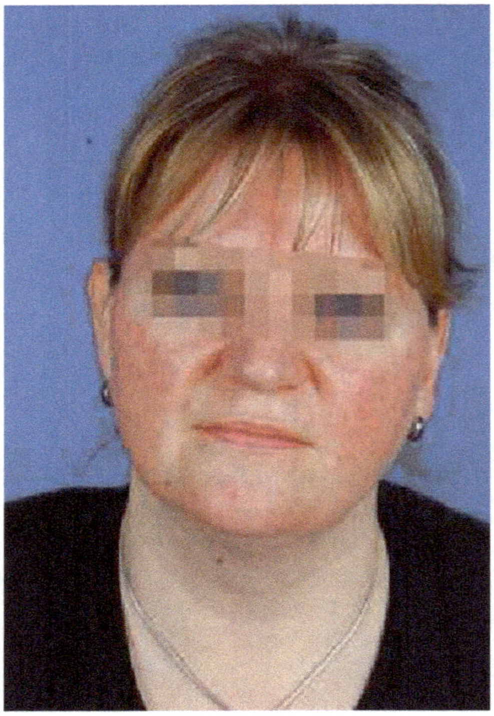

Erythematotelangiectatic acne rosacea
Photograph courtesy of SpringerImages Database, Springer Publishing Company

b. Papulopustular Acne Rosacea

Papulopustular acne rosacea

A. Persistent centrofacial erythema
B. Papules, pustules, and papulopustules of central face
C. Scaling or crust may occur if severe
D. No comedones as with acne vulgaris

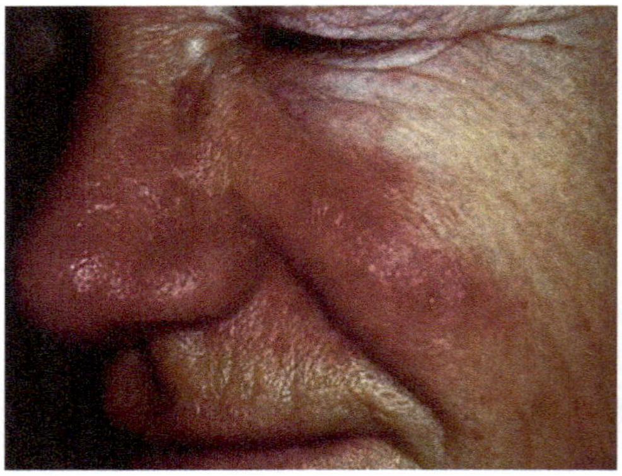

Papulopustular acne rosacea
Photograph courtesy of SpringerImages Database, Springer Publishing Company

Papulopustular acne rosacea

A. Papules, pustules, and papulopustules of central face

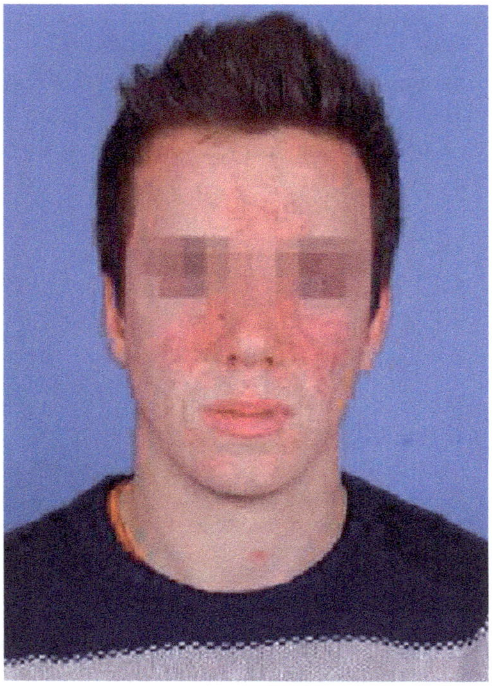

Papulopustular acne rosacea
Photograph courtesy of SpringerImages Database, Springer Publishing Company

c. Phymatous Acne Rosacea

Phymatous acne rosacea

A. Hypertrophy of sebaceous glands of nasal skin
B. Most common in males
C. Telangiectasias of distal nose, dilated pores, hypertrophy of tissue with soft, fleshy, nodular growths

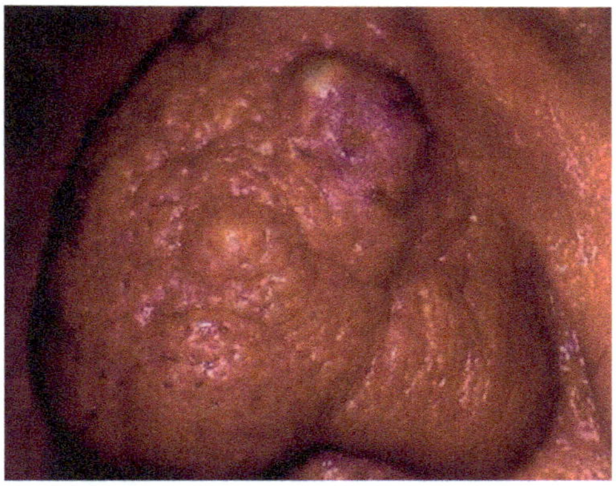

Phymatous acne rosacea
Photograph courtesy of SpringerImages Database, Springer Publishing Company

d. Ocular Acne Rosacea

Ocular acne rosacea

A. Develops in 50 % of patients with erythematotelangiectatic and papulopustular rosacea
B. Itching, tearing, dryness, gritty sensations, crusting of lids
C. Blepharitis—conjunctival injection (red eyes), eyelid swelling, chalazia

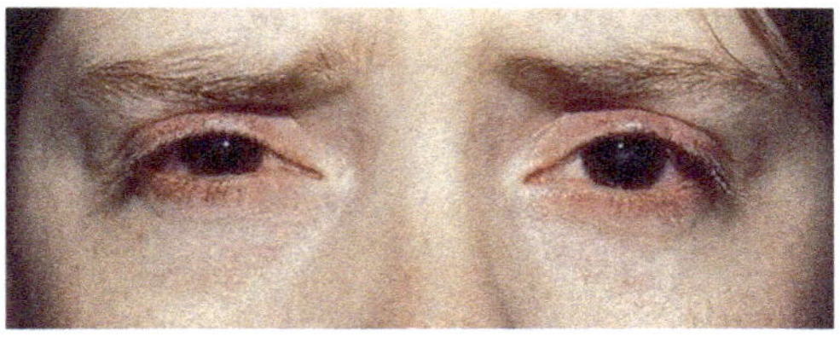

Ocular acne rosacea
Photograph courtesy of SpringerImages Database, Springer Publishing Company

e. Granulomatous Acne Rosacea

Granulomatous acne rosacea

A. Discrete skin-colored to brown facial papules (top figure)
B. Granulomatous inflammation histologically (bottom figure)

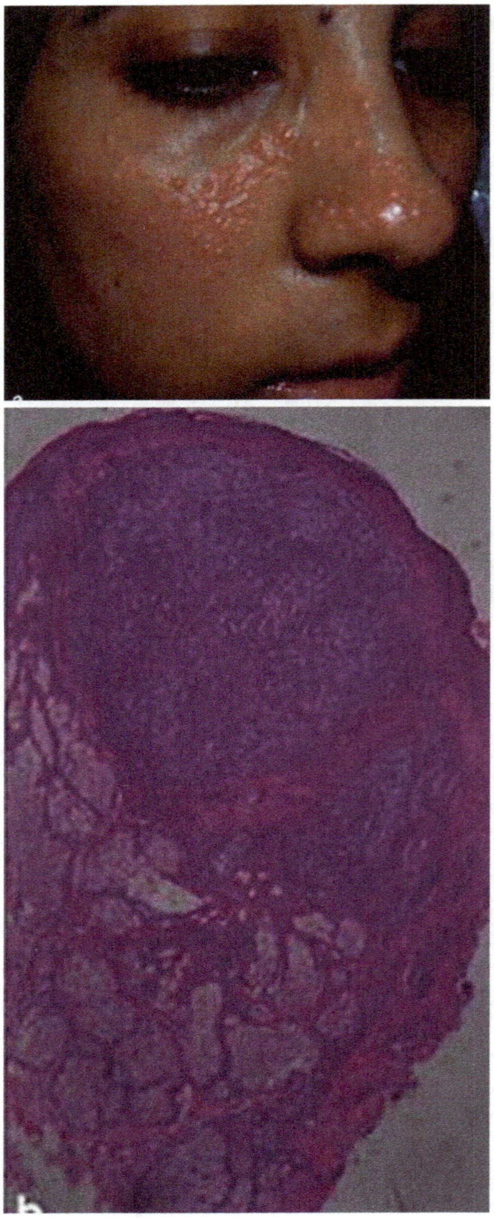

Granulomatous acne rosacea
Photograph courtesy of SpringerImages Database, Springer Publishing Company

f. Rosacea Fulminans

Rosacea Fulminans

A. Cheek plaques studded with pustules

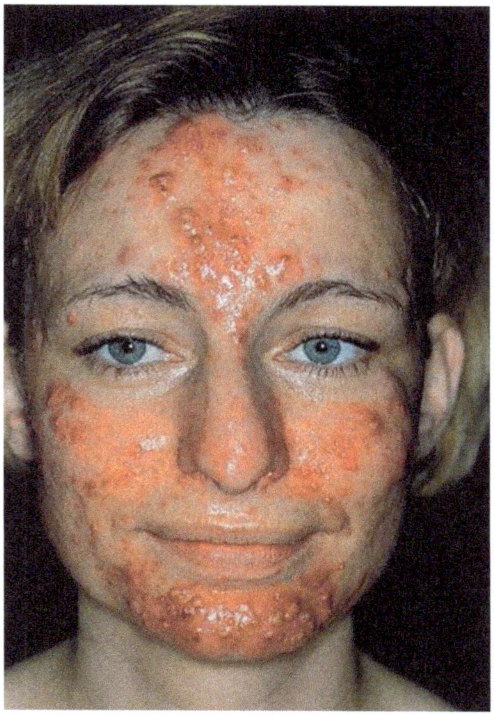

Rosacea fulminans

31 Fox-Fordyce Disease (Apocrine Miliaria)

Fox-Fordyce disease (apocrine miliaria)

A. Monomorphic, dome-shaped, skin-colored follicular papules in axillary, anogenital, and periareolar areas (where apocrine glands are present)
B. May be intensely pruritic
C. Frequently worsens in the summer
D. Most common in women 15–35 years of age
E. Caused by occlusion of apocrine sweat glands, which impedes apocrine sweating in affected areas

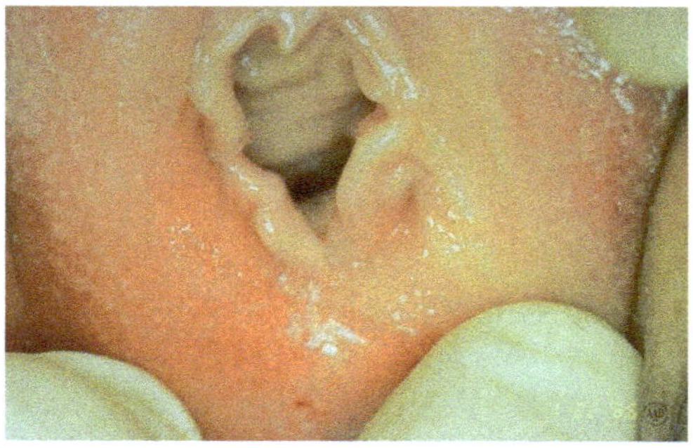

Fox-Fordyce disease (apocrine miliaria)
Photograph courtesy of American Academy of Dermatology

H.M. Gloster, Jr. et al., *Absolute Dermatology Review: Mastering Clinical Conditions on the Dermatology Recertification Exam*, DOI 10.1007/978-3-319-03218-4_31, © Springer International Publishing Switzerland 2016

32 Hidradenitis Suppurativa

Hidradenitis suppurativa

A. Poral occlusion of pilosebaceous units within intertriginous zones (axillary, groin, perianal, inframammary) results in secondary inflammation of apocrine glands, inflamed tender nodules and sterile abscesses, sinus tracts, fistulae, hypertrophic scars, and chronic drainage of serous exudate, blood, pus
B. Begins around puberty
C. More common in females, blacks

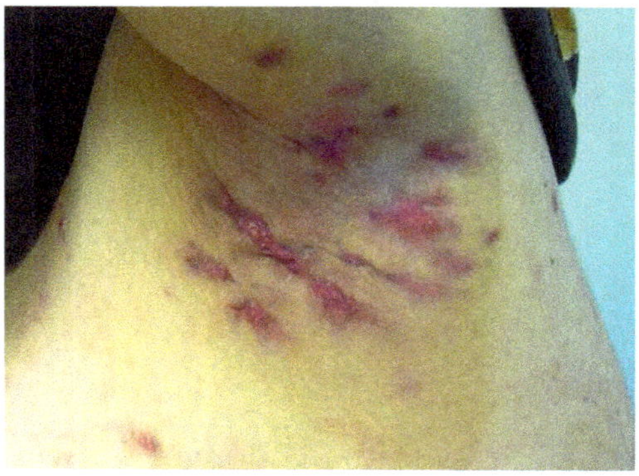

Hidradenitis suppurativa
Photograph courtesy of SpringerImages Database, Springer Publishing Company

Hidradenitis suppurativa

A. Perineal hidradenitis suppurativa with inflamed tender nodules and hypertrophic scars

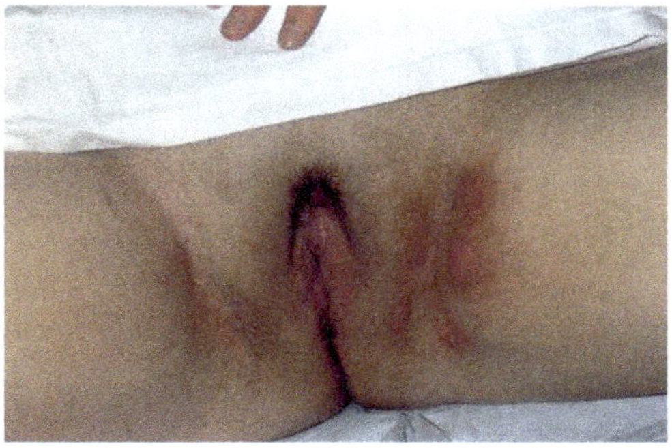

Hidradenitis suppurativa
Photograph courtesy of SpringerImages Database, Springer Publishing Company

H.M. Gloster, Jr. et al., *Absolute Dermatology Review: Mastering Clinical Conditions on the Dermatology Recertification Exam*,
DOI 10.1007/978-3-319-03218-4_32, © Springer International Publishing Switzerland 2016

Hidradenitis suppurativa

A. Hidradenitis suppurativa affecting the inframammary areas with inflamed tender nodules and sterile abscesses

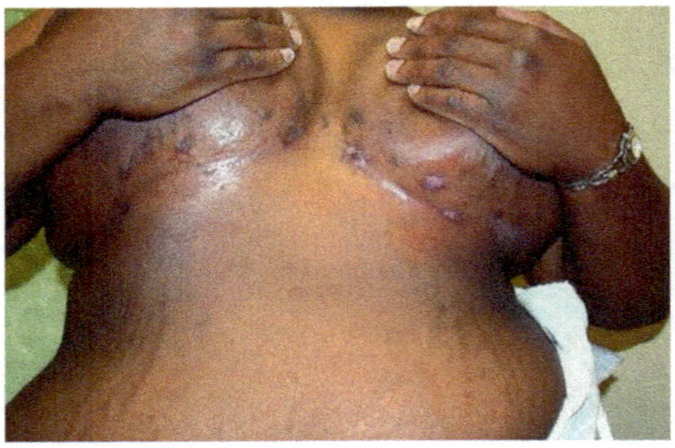

Hidradenitis suppurativa
Photograph Courtesy of SpringerImages Database, Springer Publishing Company

Chapter V

Autoimmune Disorders

Lupus Erythematosus 33

a. Discoid Lupus Erythematosus (Chronic Cutaneous Lupus)

Discoid lupus erythematosus (chronic cutaneous lupus)

A. Most commonly occurs on sun-exposed areas (photosensitive eruption): face, scalp, nose, ears (classically involves the conchal bowl)
B. Erythematous to violaceous plaques with adherent scale, scarring, atrophy, and pigmentary changes
C. Dyspigmentation (hypopigmentation centrally with a peripheral rim of hyperpigmentation) is common
D. Most commonly is localized but may rarely be disseminated (face, thorax, upper extremities)
E. May be hypertrophic

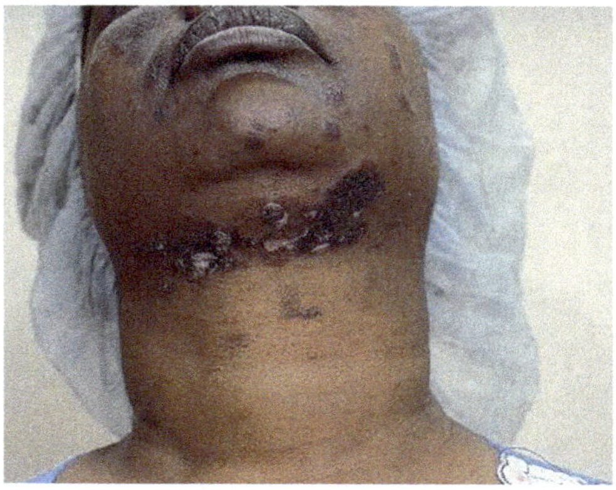

Discoid lupus erythematosus (chronic cutaneous lupus) Photograph courtesy of SpringerImages Database, Springer Publishing Company

Discoid lupus erythematosus (chronic cutaneous lupus)

A. Adnexal involvement is common, and follicular plugs produce "carpet tacking" pattern

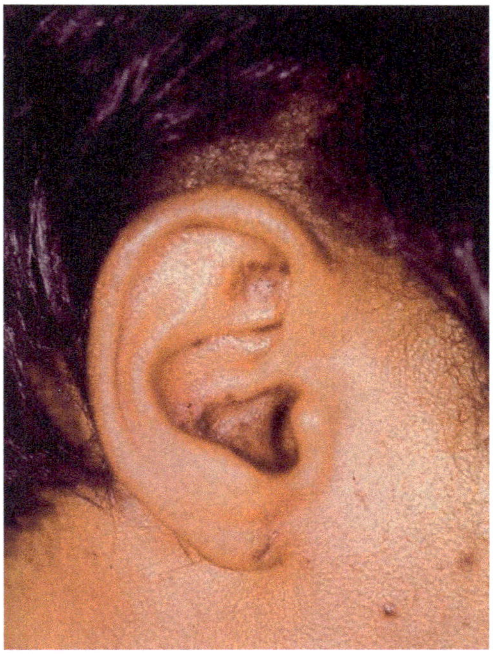

Discoid lupus erythematosus (chronic cutaneous lupus) Photograph courtesy of SpringerImages Database, Springer Publishing Company

H.M. Gloster, Jr. et al., *Absolute Dermatology Review: Mastering Clinical Conditions on the Dermatology Recertification Exam*, DOI 10.1007/978-3-319-03218-4_33, © Springer International Publishing Switzerland 2016

Discoid lupus erythematosus (chronic cutaneous lupus)

A. Extensive scarring, hyperpigmentation, and follicular plugs with a rim of erythema indicating activity

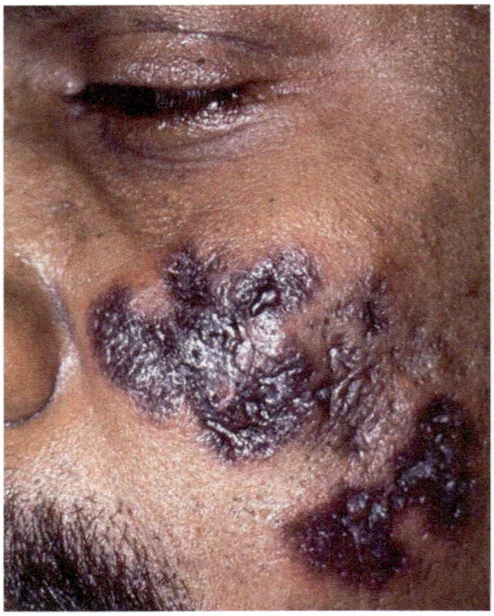

Discoid lupus erythematosus (chronic cutaneous lupus) Photograph courtesy of SpringerImages Database, Springer Publishing Company

Discoid lupus erythematosus (chronic cutaneous lupus)

A. Adnexal involvement is common with scarring alopecia when it involves hair-bearing areas
B. Atrophy, follicular plugs, hyperpigmentation, and hypopigmentation

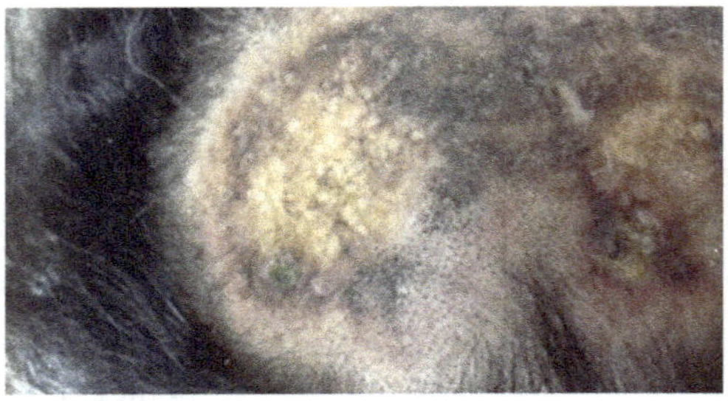

Discoid lupus erythematosus (chronic cutaneous lupus) Photograph courtesy of Hugh Gloster, MD

Discoid lupus erythematosus (chronic cutaneous lupus)

A. Central hypopigmentation and peripheral hyperpigmentation is common in blacks

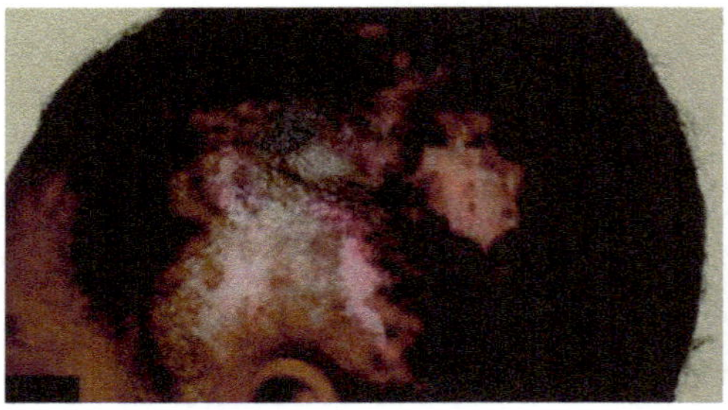

Discoid lupus erythematosus (chronic cutaneous lupus) Photograph courtesy of SpringerImages Database, Springer Publishing Company

b. Subacute Cutaneous Lupus Erythematosus

Subacute cutaneous lupus erythematosus

A. Young to middle-age women
B. Occurs on sun-exposed areas: sides of the face (central face spared), upper trunk (V of the neck, chest, upper back), extensor upper extremities, shoulders
C. Polycyclic annular plaques with red or violaceous raised borders and central clearing on sun-exposed skin
D. Frequently results in dyspigmentation, especially hypopigmentation, but no scarring
E. May be medication induced (e.g., hydrochlorothiazide, terbinafine, calcium channel blocker, nonsteroidal anti-inflammatory drugs, griseofulvin, antihistamines)

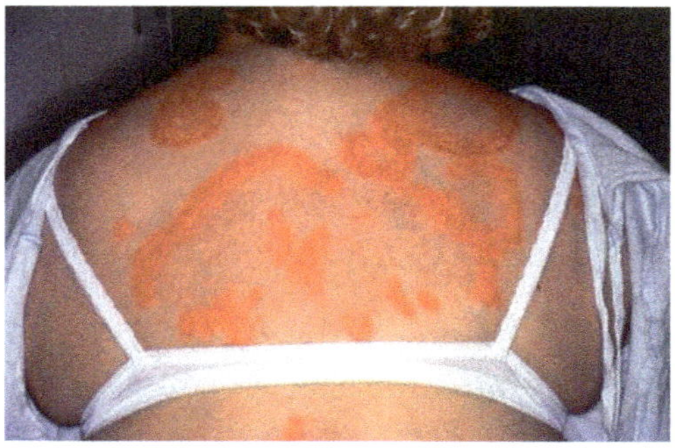

Subacute cutaneous lupus erythematosus
Photograph courtesy of SpringerImages Database, Springer Publishing Company

Subacute cutaneous lupus erythematosus

A. May appear papulosquamous with psoriasiform plaques or be eczematous

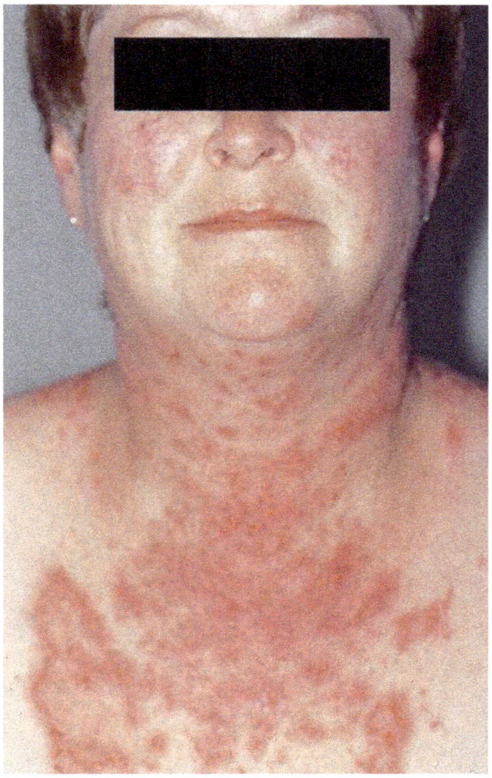

Subacute cutaneous lupus erythematosus
Photograph courtesy of SpringerImages Database, Springer Publishing Company

c. Acute Cutaneous Lupus Erythematosus

Acute cutaneous lupus erythematosus

A. Malar erythema (butterfly rash): highly associated with systemic lupus erythematosus

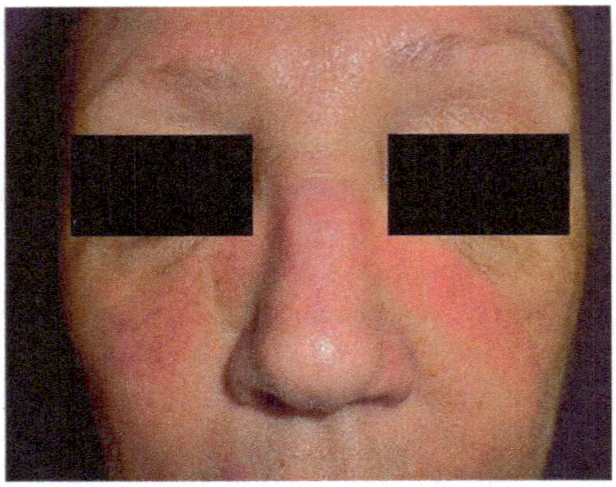

Acute cutaneous lupus erythematosus
Photograph courtesy of SpringerImages Database, Springer Publishing Company

Acute cutaneous lupus erythematosus

A. Malar erythema (butterfly rash) may have poikiloderma (telangiectasia, dyspigmentation, atrophy) and erosions

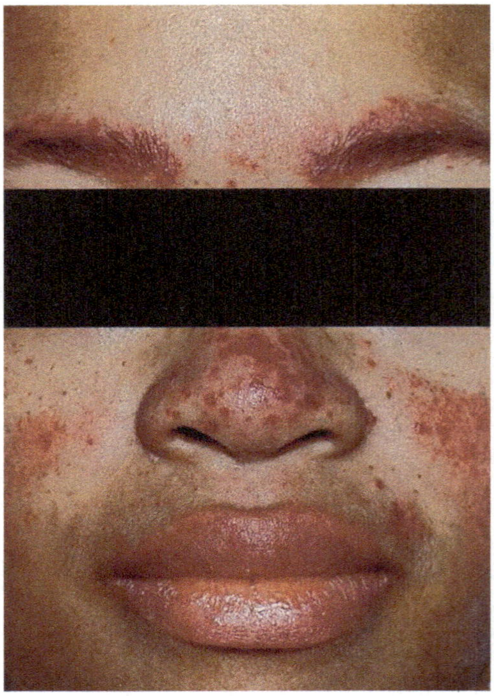

Acute cutaneous lupus erythematosus
Photograph courtesy of SpringerImages Database, Springer Publishing Company

Acute cutaneous lupus erythematosus

A. Malar erythema (butterfly rash) and photodistributed erythematous eruption

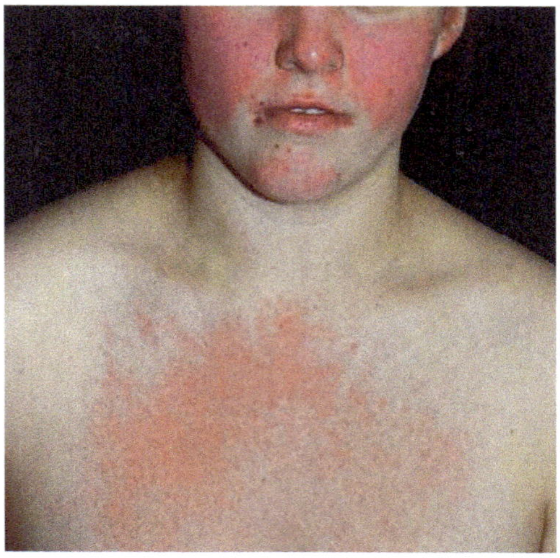

Acute cutaneous lupus erythematosus
Photograph courtesy of SpringerImages Database, Springer Publishing Company

d. Systemic Lupus Erythematosus

Systemic lupus erythematosus

A. Malar rash
   1. "Butterfly" pattern may include sun-exposed areas on the bridge of the nose, malar region, eyebrows, and the tip of the chin
   2. The shaded areas under the eyebrows and nasolabial folds are spared (this characteristic helps differentiate this rash from seborrheic dermatitis)
   3. New malar rashes usually signify increased systemic disease activity
   4. Usually heals without significant scarring, although pigmentary alterations may occur

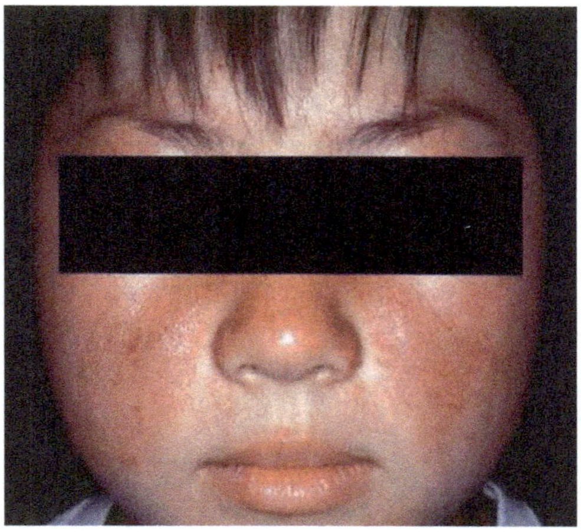

Systemic lupus erythematosus
Photograph courtesy of SpringerImages Database, Springer Publishing Company

Systemic lupus erythematosus

A. Discoid lesions

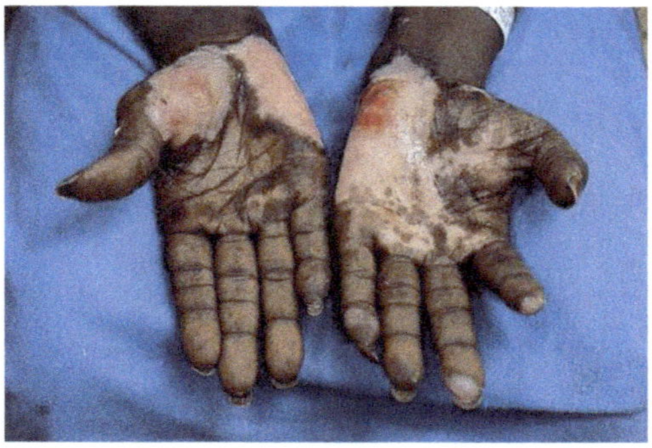

Systemic lupus erythematosus
Photograph courtesy of SpringerImages Database, Springer Publishing Company

Systemic lupus erythematosus

A. Photodistributed erythematous eruption

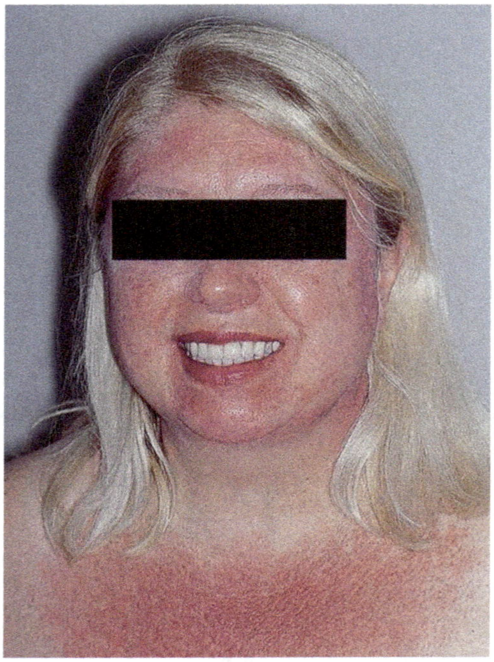

Systemic lupus erythematosus
Photograph courtesy of SpringerImages Database, Springer Publishing Company

Systemic lupus erythematosus

A. Oral ulcers

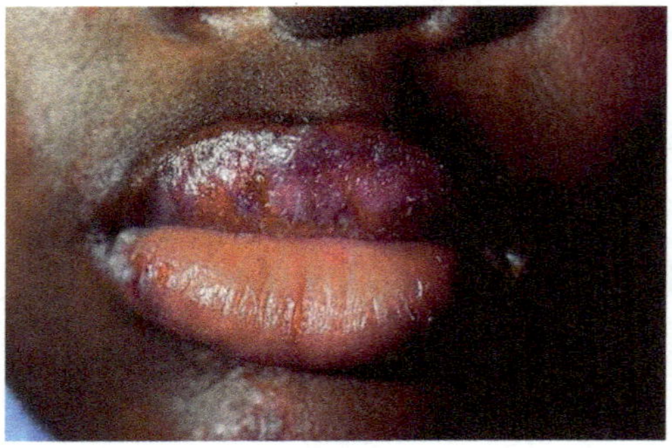

Systemic lupus erythematosus
Photograph courtesy of SpringerImages Database, Springer Publishing Company

e. Bullous Lupus Erythematosus

Bullous lupus erythematosus

A. Vesicles and bullae (filled with neutrophils) may occur in the setting of acute or subacute cutaneous lupus erythematosus or de novo

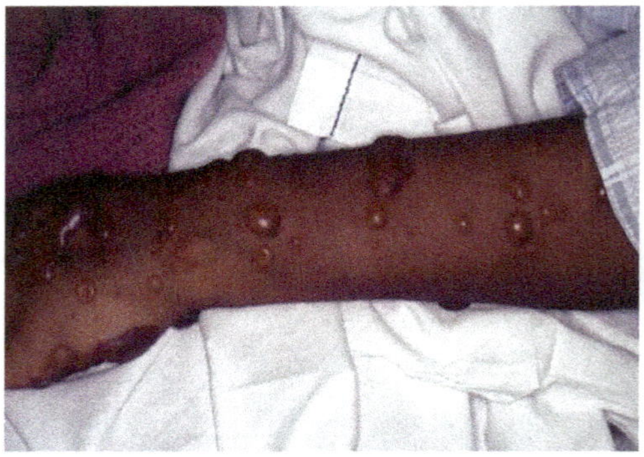

Bullous lupus erythematosus
Photograph courtesy of SpringerImages Database, Springer Publishing Company

f. Tumid Lupus Erythematosus

Tumid lupus erythematosus

A. Involves the dermis, not epidermis
B. Annular indurated pink–violet plaques without epidermal change (no scale or follicular plugging)
C. Most common on the face or trunk

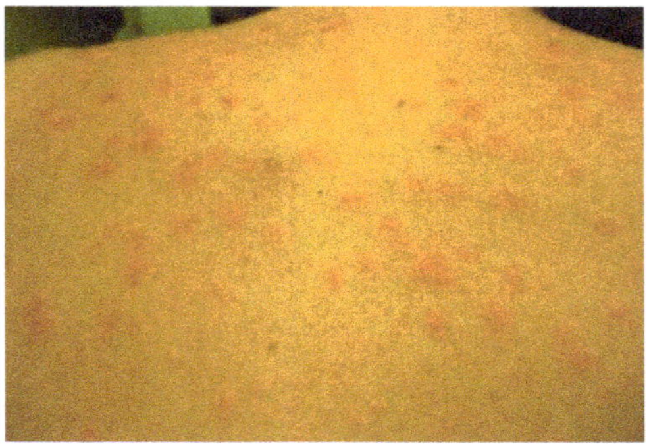

Tumid lupus erythematosus
Photograph courtesy of SpringerImages Database, Springer Publishing Company

Tumid lupus erythematosus

A. Annular indurated pink–violet plaques without epidermal change on the face

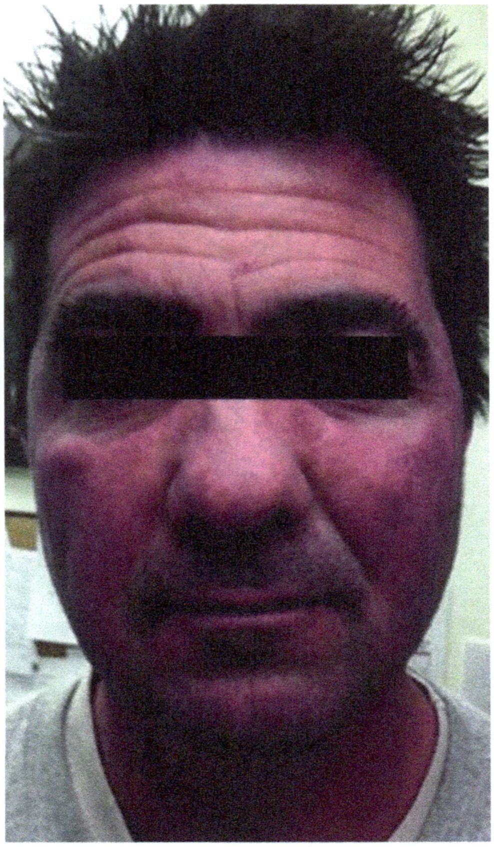

Tumid lupus erythematosus
Photograph courtesy of SpringerImages Database, Springer Publishing Company

g. Lupus Panniculitis

Lupus panniculitis

A. Involves the subcutaneous tissue
B. Indurated depressed plaques and disfiguring scars with lipoatrophy
C. Most commonly on the face, upper arms, upper trunk, breast, buttocks, thighs

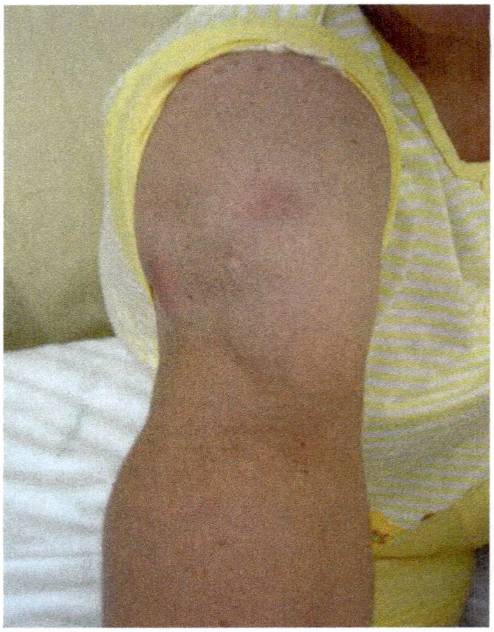

Lupus panniculitis
Photograph courtesy of SpringerImages Database, Springer Publishing Company

Lupus panniculitis

A. Indurated depressed plaques and disfiguring scars with lipoatrophy on the upper arms

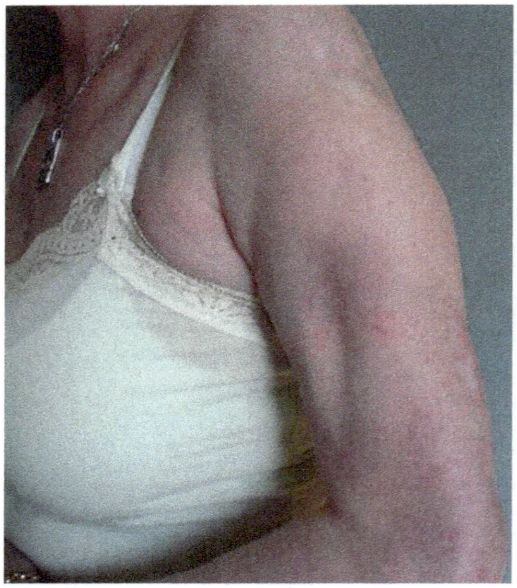

Lupus panniculitis
Photograph courtesy of SpringerImages Database, Springer Publishing Company

h. Chilblain Lupus (Lupus Pernio)

Chilblain lupus (lupus pernio)

A. Red or dusky purple papules and plaques on the toes, fingers, and sometimes the nose, elbows, knees, and lower legs
B. Exacerbated by cold

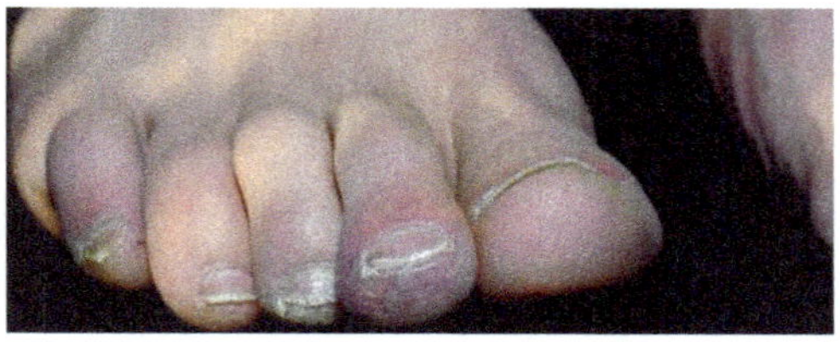

Chilblain lupus (lupus pernio)
Photograph courtesy of SpringerImages Database, Springer Publishing Company

Chilblain lupus (lupus pernio)

A. Red or dusky purple papules and plaques on the toes exacerbated by cold

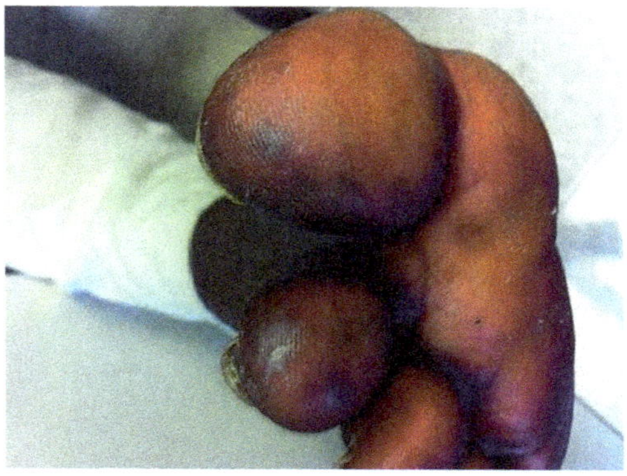

Chilblain lupus (lupus pernio)
Photograph courtesy of SpringerImages Database, Springer Publishing Company

i. Neonatal Lupus Erythematosus

Neonatal lupus erythematosus

A. Infants, usually girls, whose mothers have anti-Ro antibodies (babies also have them)
B. Subacute cutaneous lupus like lesions (annular erythematous scaling plaques) on the scalp, periocular region (raccoon eyes), malar area
C. Photosensitivity is common
D. Lesions are usually not present at birth but develop in first few weeks of life and resolve by 6 months of age as antibodies wane but may leave dyspigmentation and telangiectasias
E. Extracutaneous manifestations
   1. Congenital heart block, third degree, that is permanent in 10–50 %
   2. Cardiomyopathy
   3. Hepatobiliary disease
   4. Thrombocytopenia

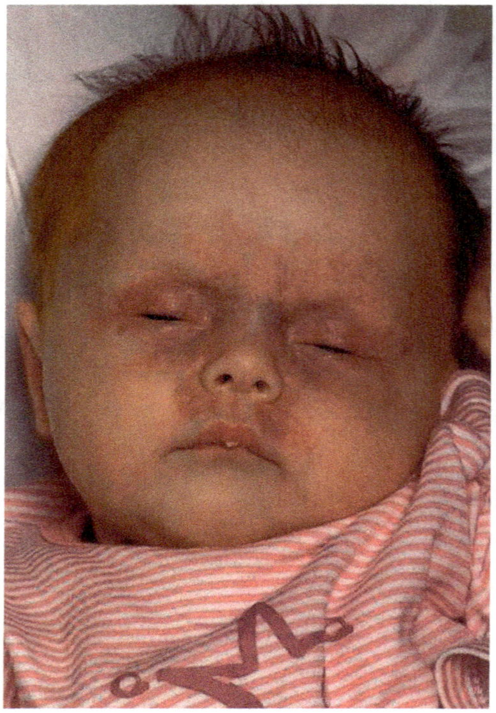

Neonatal lupus erythematosus
Photograph courtesy of SpringerImages Database, Springer Publishing Company

Neonatal lupus erythematosus

A. Annular erythematous scaling plaques on the periocular region (raccoon eyes) and malar area

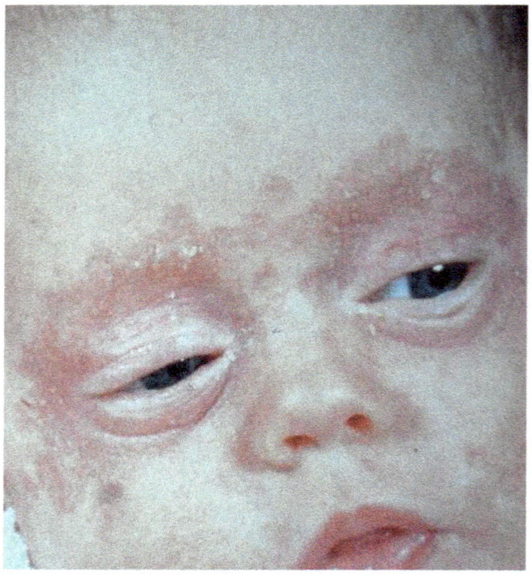

Neonatal lupus erythematosus
Photograph courtesy of SpringerImages Database, Springer Publishing Company

34 Dermatomyositis

Dermatomyositis

A. Photodistributed violaceous papules that coalesce into plaques with overlying scale and may progress to poikilodermatous changes (hyperpigmentation, hypopigmentation, telangiectasia, epidermal atrophy) of the "V" area of the chest and upper back and shoulders producing a "shawl pattern"
B. Facial or malar erythema
C. Poikiloderma, nonscarring alopecia, and pruritus of the scalp
D. Gottron's sign: pink to violaceous papules and plaques on elbows and knees
E. Pruritus
F. Nail fold signs: cuticular dystrophy (ragged cuticles) and proximal nail fold telangiectasias
G. Calcinosis cutis
   1. More common in juvenile dermatomyositis
   2. Hard white papules and nodules that may drain chalky material
   3. Favors sites of trauma (elbows, knees, fingers)

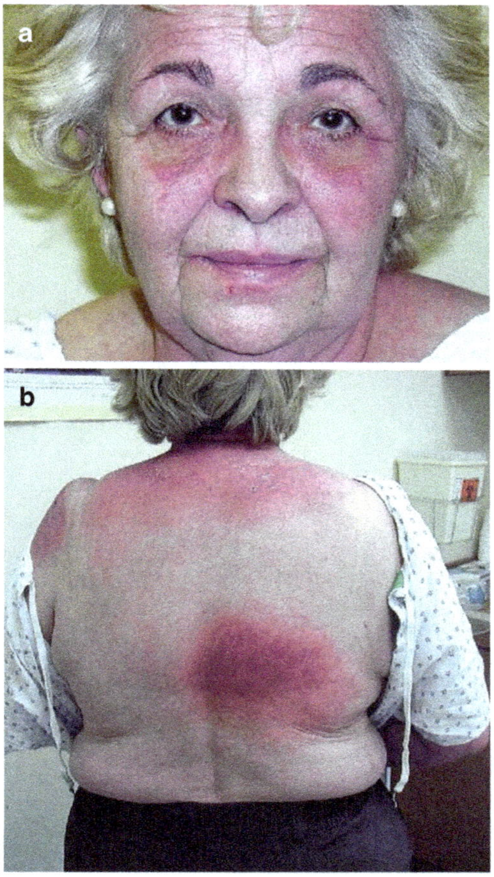

Dermatomyositis
Photograph courtesy of SpringerImages Database, Springer Publishing Company

H.M. Gloster, Jr. et al., *Absolute Dermatology Review: Mastering Clinical Conditions on the Dermatology Recertification Exam*, DOI 10.1007/978-3-319-03218-4_34, © Springer International Publishing Switzerland 2016

Dermatomyositis

A. Heliotrope sign—periocular violaceous to red color with periorbital edema

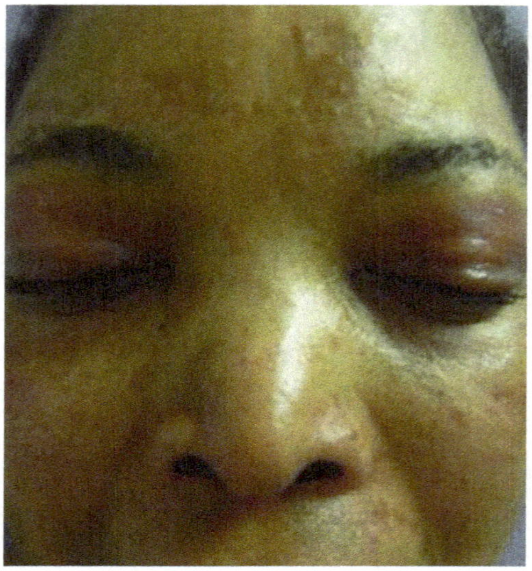

Dermatomyositis
Photograph courtesy of SpringerImages Database, Springer Publishing Company

Dermatomyositis

A. Gottron's papules: flat-topped, pink to violaceous, polygonal lichenoid papules on the knuckles and joints

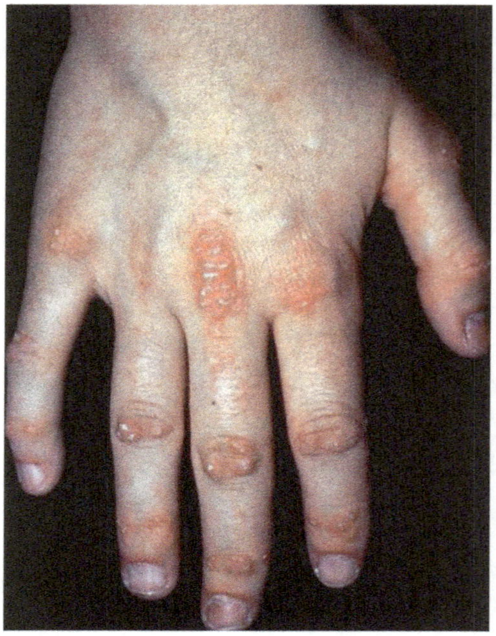

Dermatomyositis
Photograph courtesy of SpringerImages Database, Springer Publishing Company

Dermatomyositis

A. Gottron's papules: flat-topped, pink to violaceous, polygonal lichenoid papules on the knuckles and joints

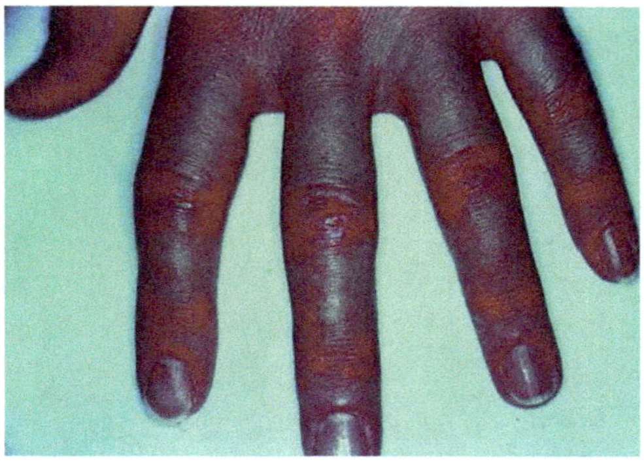

Dermatomyositis
Photograph courtesy of SpringerImages Database, Springer Publishing Company

Dermatomyositis

A. Mechanic's hands: hyperkeratosis, erythema, scaling, fissuring ,and hyperpigmentation on the hands

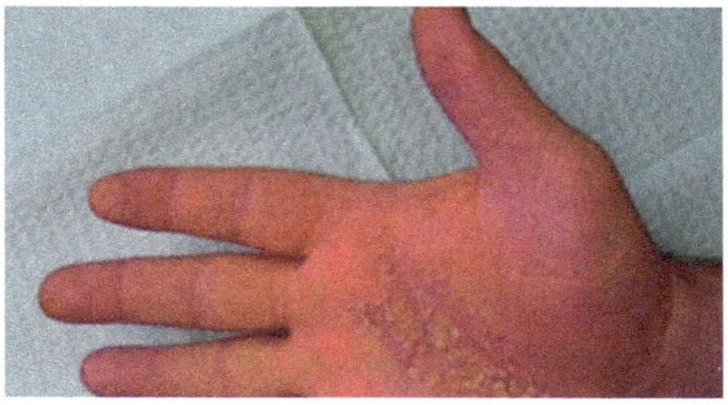

Dermatomyositis
Photograph courtesy of SpringerImages Database, Springer Publishing Company

35 Scleroderma and Sclerodermoid Skin Conditions

a. Scleroderma (Progressive Systemic Sclerosis)

Scleroderma (progressive systemic sclerosis)

A. Early changes consist of symmetric hardening (fibrosis) and thickening of the skin of the fingers, hands, and face that may later generalize to trunk and proximal extremities
B. Face: beaked nose, tight shiny facial skin, microstomia, and radial perioral furrowing resulting in expressionless, mask like facies
C. Systemic involvement may develop in the lungs (leading cause of death), gastrointestinal tract, kidney, heart
D. Two major clinical subtypes
   1. Limited Systemic Sclerosis
      a. Fibrotic skin changes limited to below elbows and knees (hands and fingers) and face
      b. Develop internal involvement later in disease course (sometimes decades)
      c. Includes CREST syndrome: *C*alcinosis (extremities, usually near joints), *R*aynaud's phenomenon, *E*sophageal involvement, *S*clerodactyly (tapering of fingertips), and *T*elangiectasia
   2. Diffuse Systemic Sclerosis
      a. Generalized fibrotic skin changes (distal and proximal extremities, trunk, face)
      b. Associated with internal organ involvement (within 5 years of disease onset) and a worse prognosis

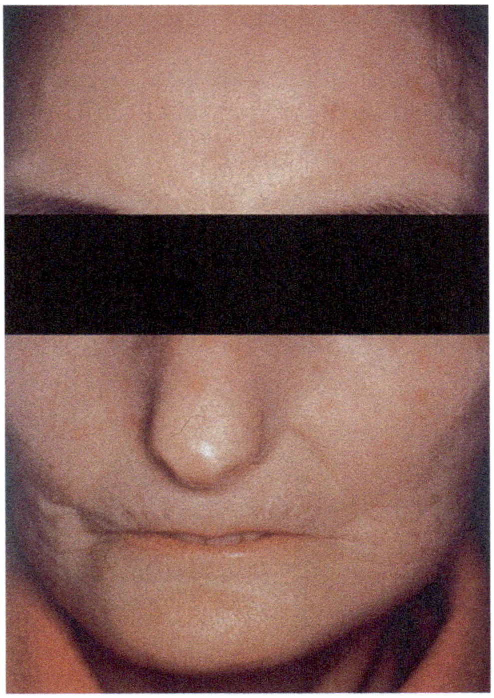

Scleroderma (progressive systemic sclerosis)
Photograph courtesy of SpringerImages Database, Springer Publishing Company

Scleroderma (progressive systemic sclerosis)

A. Sclerodactyly of the fingers and hands
   1. Early edematous phase (pitting edema of the digits)
   2. Indurated phase (fingers harden with taut shiny appearance)
   3. Late atrophic stage (thinning of the skin), distal digital ulceration, scarring or loss of finger pads, flexion contractures (claw-like hands)

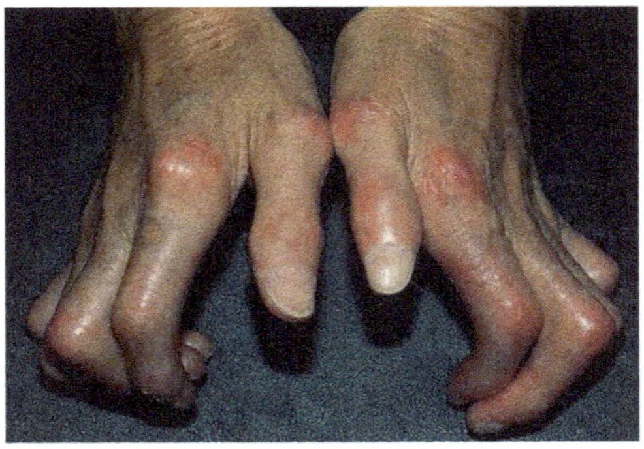

Scleroderma (progressive systemic sclerosis)
Photograph courtesy of SpringerImages Database, Springer Publishing Company

H.M. Gloster, Jr. et al., *Absolute Dermatology Review: Mastering Clinical Conditions on the Dermatology Recertification Exam*, DOI 10.1007/978-3-319-03218-4_35,

Scleroderma (progressive systemic sclerosis)

A. Sclerodactyly of the fingers and hands

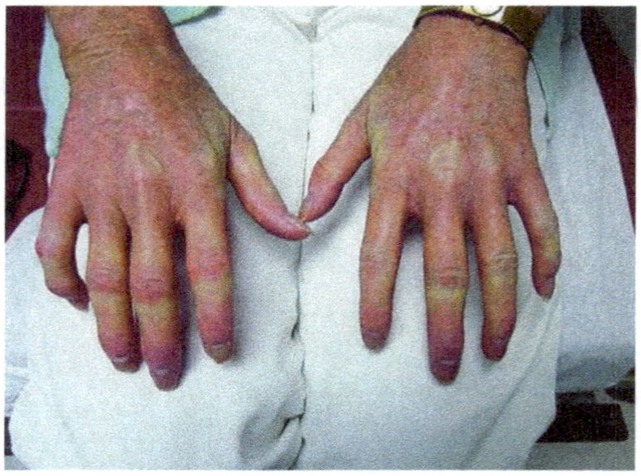

Scleroderma (progressive systemic sclerosis)
Photograph courtesy of SpringerImages Database, Springer Publishing Company

Scleroderma (progressive systemic sclerosis)

A. Raynaud's phenomenon

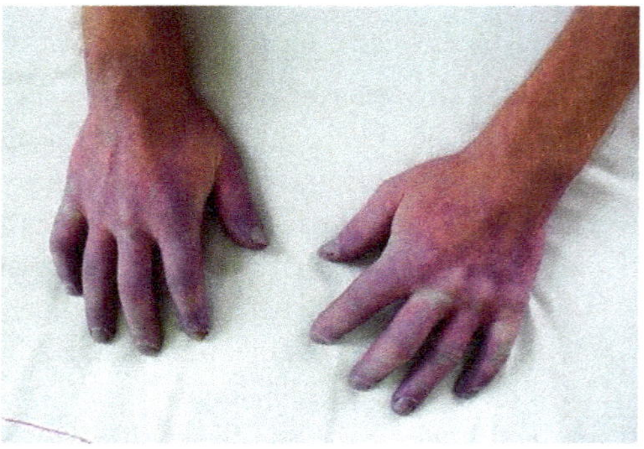

Scleroderma (progressive systemic sclerosis)
Photograph courtesy of SpringerImages Database, Springer Publishing Company

Scleroderma (progressive systemic sclerosis)

A. Telangiectasias in the CREST syndrome

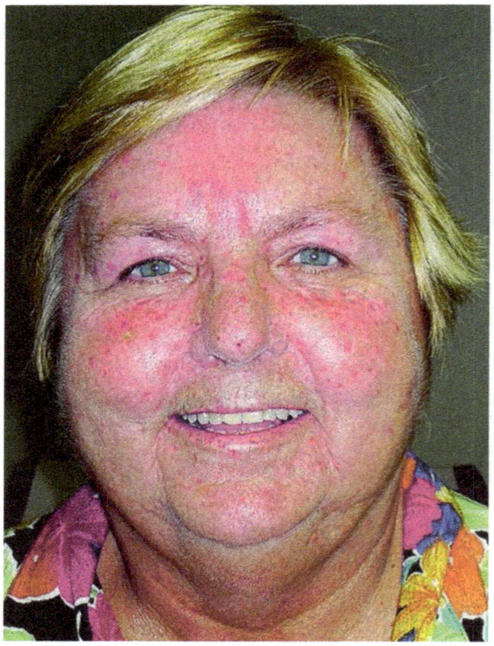

Scleroderma (progressive systemic sclerosis)
Photograph courtesy of SpringerImages Database, Springer Publishing Company

Scleroderma (progressive systemic sclerosis)

A. Diffuse systemic sclerosis with generalized fibrotic skin changes on the distal and proximal extremities, trunk, face

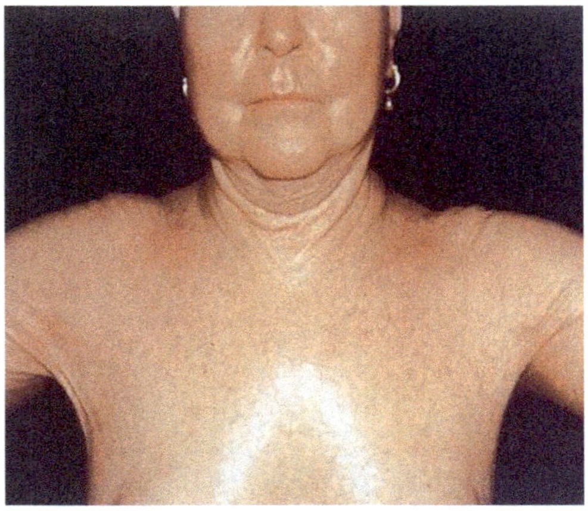

Scleroderma (progressive systemic sclerosis)
Photograph courtesy of SpringerImages Database, Springer Publishing Company

b. Morphea

i. Plaque Morphea

Plaque morphea

A. Early inflammatory stage: insidious onset of asymptomatic red or violaceous edematous plaques with centrifugal expansion
B. Central portion transforms into sclerotic scar-like tissue (skin becomes indurated)
C. Lesions may be 2–15 cm in diameter
D. Typically progresses for 3–5 years then stops and resolves leaving atrophy and hyperpigmentation

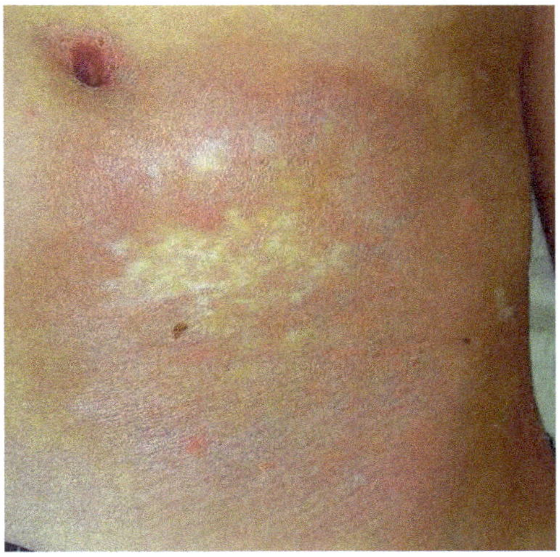

Plaque morphea
Photograph courtesy of SpringerImages Database, Springer Publishing Company

Plaque morphea

A. Active lesions have a lilac, violaceous border with central shiny white color corresponding to areas of bound-down skin

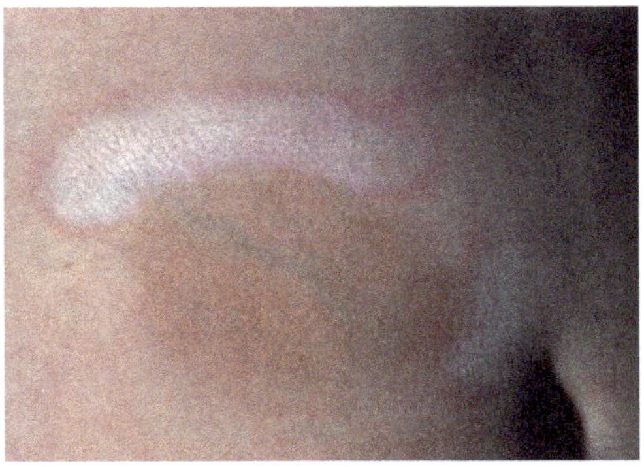

Plaque morphea
Photograph courtesy of SpringerImages Database, Springer Publishing Company

Plaque morphea
 A. Absence of the lilac ring indicates that the progression of the lesion has halted
 B. Inactive lesions may become hyperpigmented

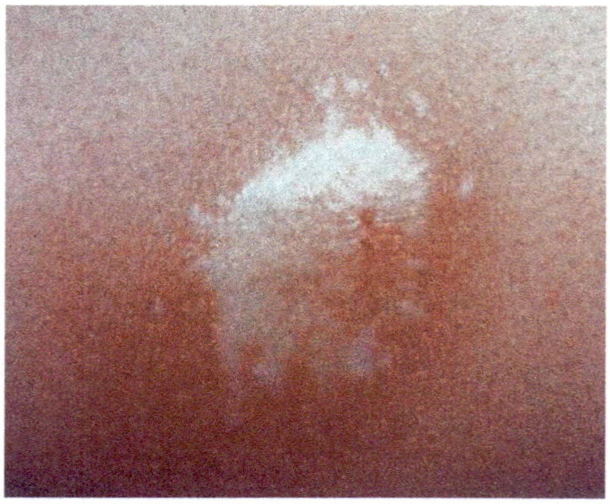

Plaque morphea
Photograph courtesy of SpringerImages Database, Springer Publishing Company

ii. Linear Morphea

Linear morphea
 A. Most commonly occurs in children
 B. Usually begins as a lesion of plaque-like morphea that extends longitudinally as a series of plaques that then joins to form a scar-like band
 C. Sometimes begins as a linear red inflammatory streak
 D. Sclerosis may extend deep into fat or underlying fascia, muscle, bone resulting in severely impaired mobility of the affected limb, especially if it extends over joints
 E. Lesions persist and do not resolve

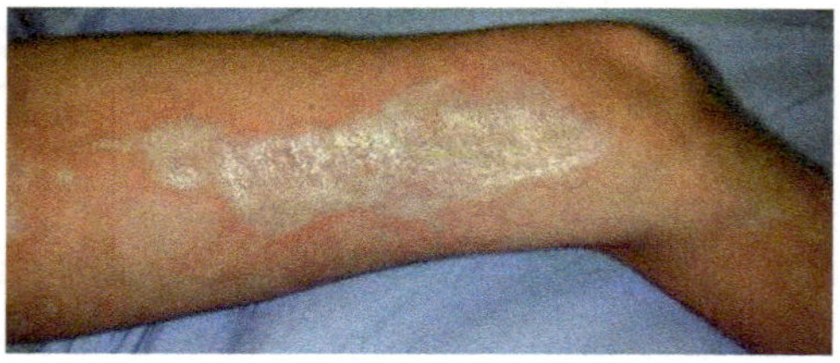

Linear morphea
Photograph courtesy of SpringerImages Database, Springer Publishing Company

Linear morphea
 A. En coup de sabre morphea
  1. Linear morphea of the central forehead or scalp
  2. Leaves a linear hairless crevice that may be sclerotic or atrophic
  3. May extend into the scalp and cross the eye to the nose

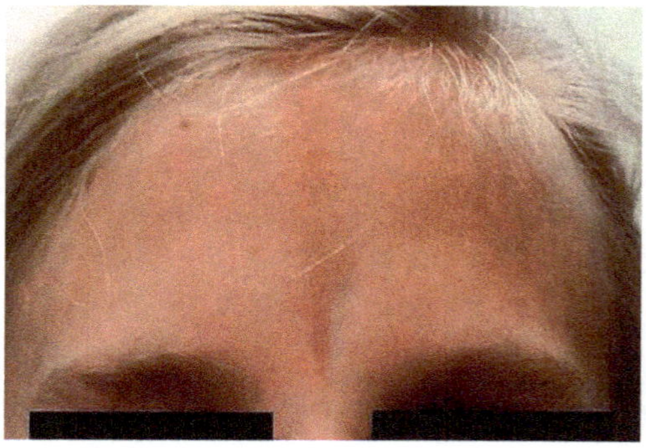

Linear morphea
Photograph courtesy of SpringerImages Database, Springer Publishing Company

iii. Generalized Morphea

Generalized morphea
- A. Rapidly progressive plaque morphea in which multiple enlarging plaques appear at once and coalesce to involve large portions of the trunk and extremities
- B. Sparing of the nipples is a common feature of generalized morphea
- C. May result in disabling restrictions and impaired breathing

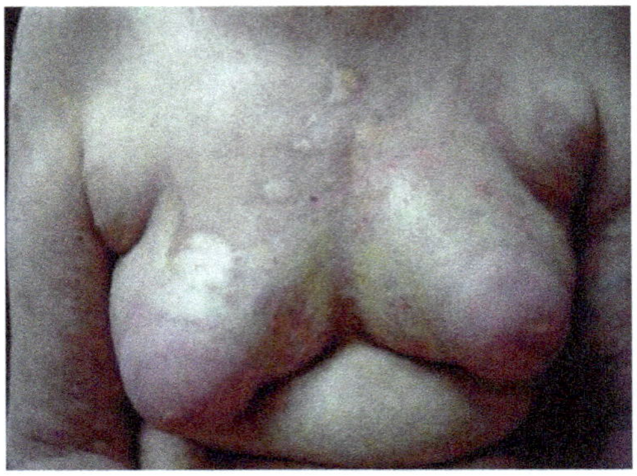

Generalized morphea
Photograph courtesy of SpringerImages Database, Springer Publishing Company

c. Eosinophilic Fasciitis

Eosinophilic fasciitis
- A. History of strenuous activity in 30 % of patients
- B. Acute onset of edema and pain of the involved extremities (symmetric, spares hands and feet), followed by the rapid onset of woody induration (fibrosis) and a dimpled "pseudo-cellulite" appearance with rippling, puckering, and peau d'orange skin
- C. "Groove sign" or "dry river bed sign": linear depressions where veins appear sunken in indurated skin
- D. Peripheral eosinophilia is often present

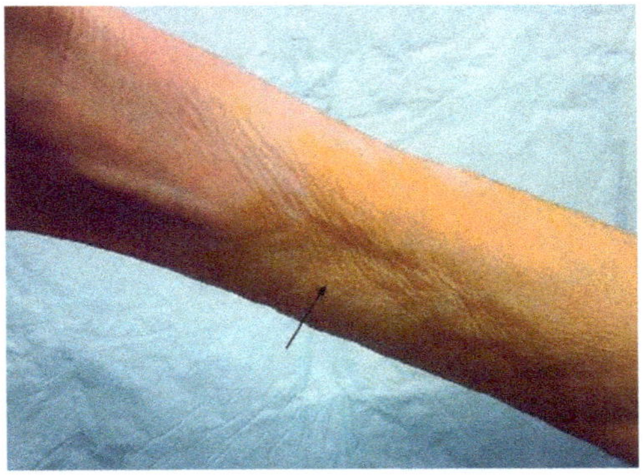

Eosinophilic fasciitis
Photograph courtesy of SpringerImages Database, Springer Publishing Company

d. Lichen Sclerosus et Atrophicus

i. Extragenital lichen sclerosus et atrophicus
- A. More common in women
- B. Bimodal age distribution in prepubertal children and postmenopausal adults
- C. Most commonly affects anogenital skin but may be extragenital
- D. Extragenital lichen sclerosus et atrophicus
  1. Commonly involves the trunk but may also involve the neck, shoulders, flexor wrists, sites of trauma or pressure
  2. Asymptomatic (unlike genital lesions)
  3. Multiple well-defined, sclerotic, ivory white macules and patches with overlying atrophy (shiny wrinkled "cigarette paper" surface) and follicular plugging
  4. Differential diagnosis includes morphea, atrophic lichen planus, and sclerodermoid graft-versus-host disease
  5. Occasionally may form hemorrhagic bullae

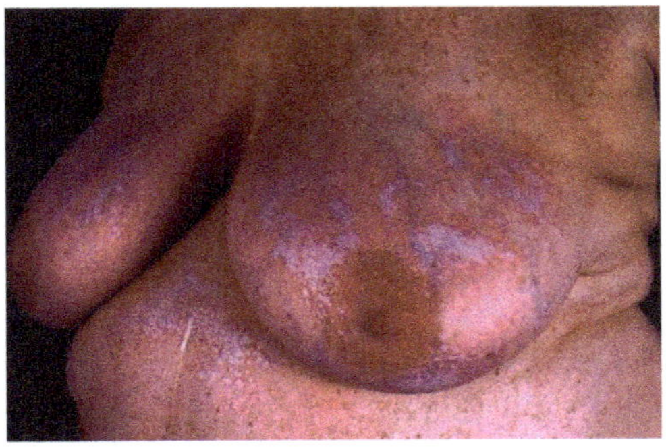

Lichen sclerosus et atrophicus
Photograph courtesy of SpringerImages Database, Springer Publishing Company

ii. Genital Lichen Sclerosus et Atrophicus

Genital lichen sclerosus et atrophicus

A. Genital lichen sclerosus et atrophicus (in women)
   1. Vulva and perianal region often involved in a figure-of-eight formation
   2. Labia most commonly involved
   3. Severe pruritus and soreness results in dysuria, dyspareunia, pain on defecation, and constipation in children
   4. Begins as a sharply demarcated area of erythema which may be eroded
   5. Erythema evolves into well-demarcated, shiny, hypopigmented, sclerotic, atrophic patches
   6. Fissures, ulcerations, and scarring eventually occur with burying of the clitoris, fusion of labia minora and majora, and introital fusion

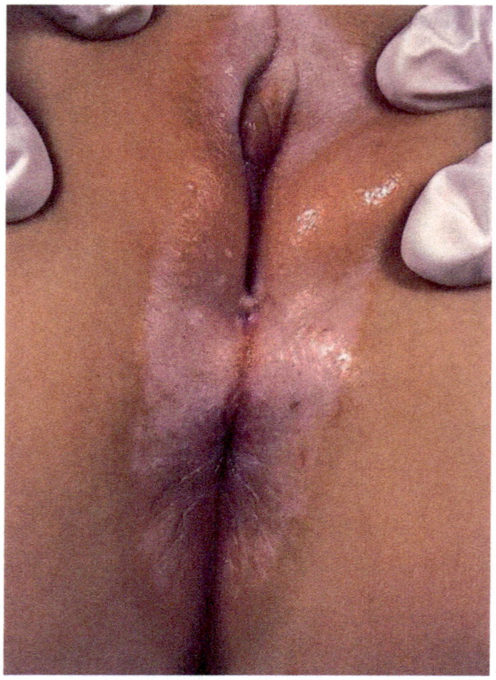

Genital lichen sclerosus et atrophicus
Photograph courtesy of SpringerImages Database, Springer Publishing Company

Genital lichen sclerosus et atrophicus

A. Genital lichen sclerosus et atrophicus (in women): well-demarcated, shiny, hypopigmented, sclerotic, atrophic patches of the labia and vulva

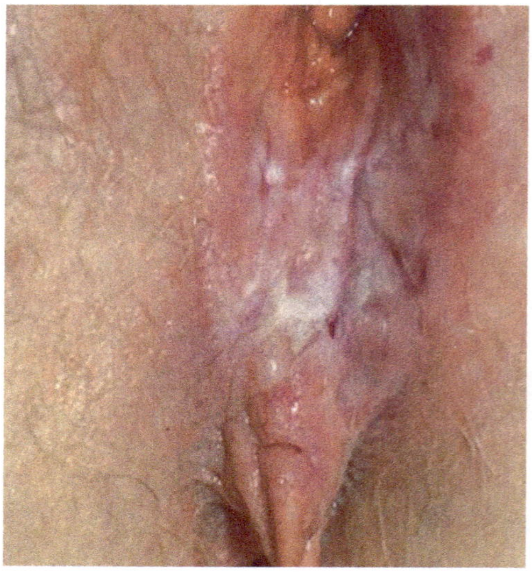

Genital lichen sclerosus et atrophicus
Photograph courtesy of SpringerImages Database, Springer Publishing Company

Genital lichen sclerosus et atrophicus

A. Genital lichen sclerosus et atrophicus (in men)
   1. Painful and pruritic, sharply demarcated blue–red eroded plaques which develop into atrophic white sclerotic patches and plaques
   2. Pain on erection, dysuria, obstruction, phimosis, or paraphimosis
   3. Phimosis (difficulty retracting foreskin) and recurrent balanitis are main presenting features

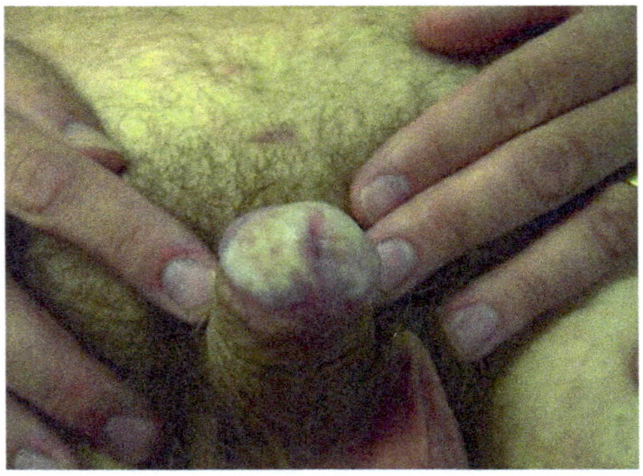

Genital lichen sclerosus et atrophicus
Photograph courtesy of SpringerImages Database, Springer Publishing Company

e. Nephrogenic Systemic Fibrosis

Nephrogenic systemic fibrosis

A. Patterned plaques: red to hyperpigmented (purple–brown) thick indurated "cobblestone" plaques symmetrically on the extremities (lower greater than upper) and trunk
B. Joint contractures and loss of mobility as a result of the confluent arrangement of plaques or thickening and induration of the skin
C. Cobblestone skin: marked woody induration and thickening of the skin with peau d'orange appearance
D. Yellow scleral plaques of the eyes
E. Systemic fibrosis of heart, lungs, skeletal muscle

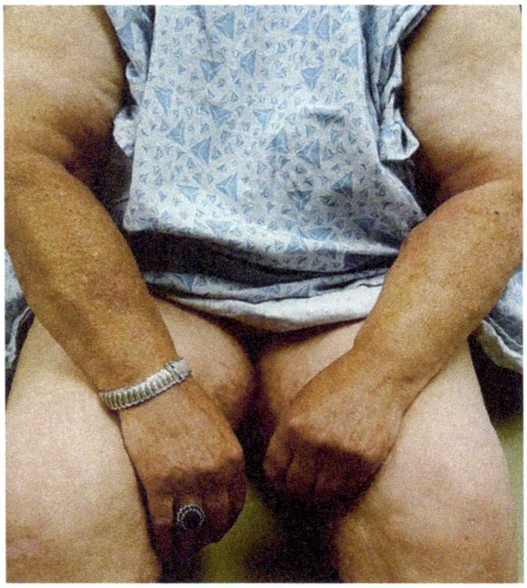

Nephrogenic systemic fibrosis
Photograph courtesy of SpringerImages Database, Springer Publishing Company

Nephrogenic systemic fibrosis

A. Hyperpigmentation, induration, and tethering of the skin and fixed flexion contractures of the fingers and elbows

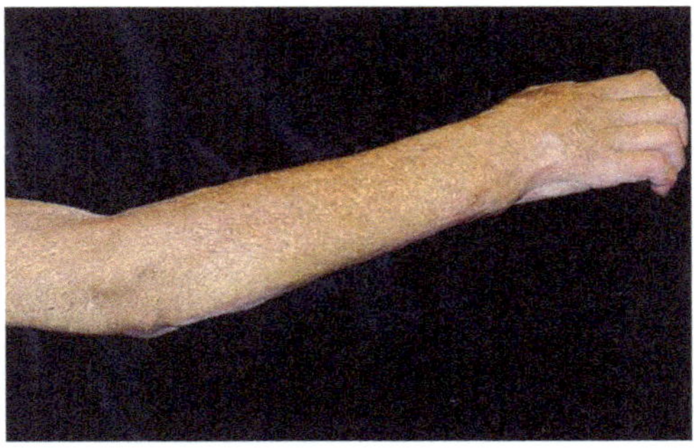

Nephrogenic systemic fibrosis
Photograph courtesy of SpringerImages Database, Springer Publishing Company

Nephrogenic systemic fibrosis

A. Indurated skin with peau d'orange changes and cobblestone appearance and flexion contractures of the knees

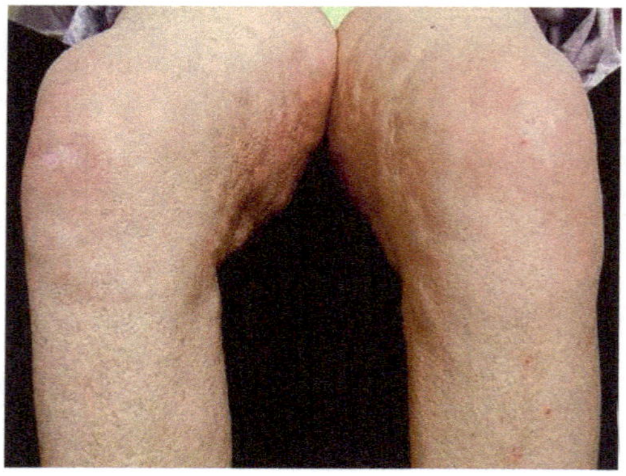

Nephrogenic systemic fibrosis
Photograph courtesy of SpringerImages Database, Springer Publishing Company

Nephrogenic systemic fibrosis

A. Yellow scleral plaques

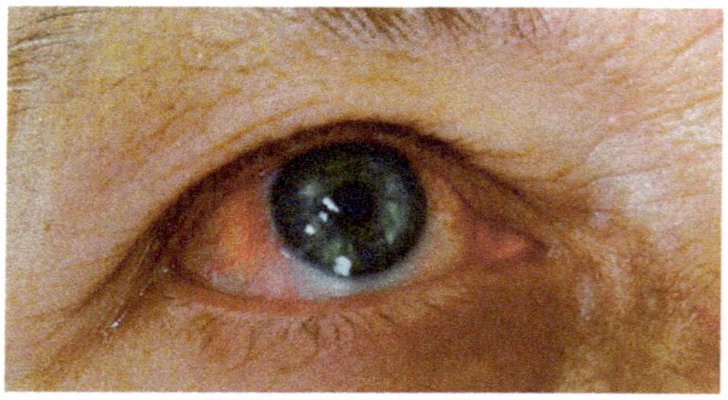

Nephrogenic systemic fibrosis
Photograph courtesy of SpringerImages Database, Springer Publishing Company

f. Lipodermatosclerosis

i. Lipodermatosclerosis (Acute Phase)

Lipodermatosclerosis (acute phase)

A. Favors the medial aspect of lower extremities above the malleolus
B. Develops in the setting of chronic venous insufficiency
C. Acute phase: erythema, warmth, tenderness (looks like cellulitis)

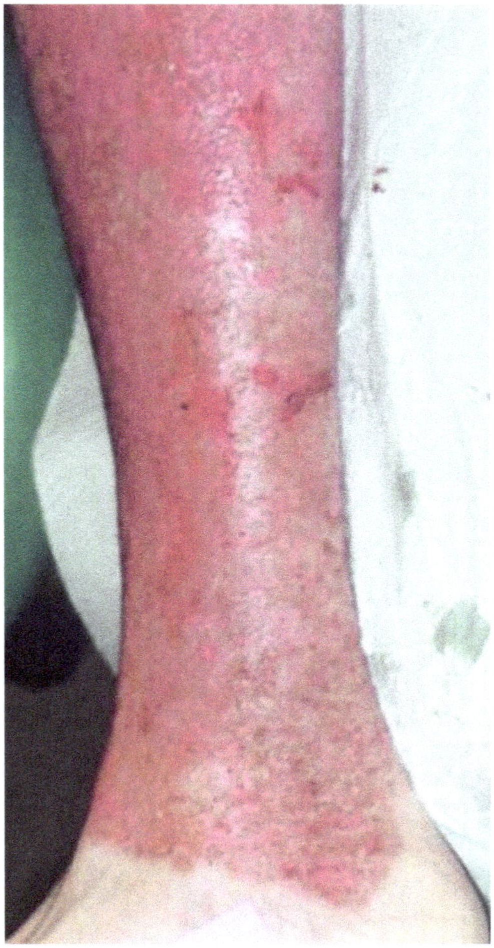

Lipodermatosclerosis (acute phase)
Photograph courtesy of SpringerImages Database, Springer Publishing Company

ii. Lipodermatosclerosis (Chronic Phase)

Lipodermatosclerosis (chronic phase)

A. Induration with woody bound-down skin (due to sclerosis of the dermis and subcutaneous fat)
B. Red, brown, or violet hyperpigmentation
C. Leg looks like *"inverted wine bottle"

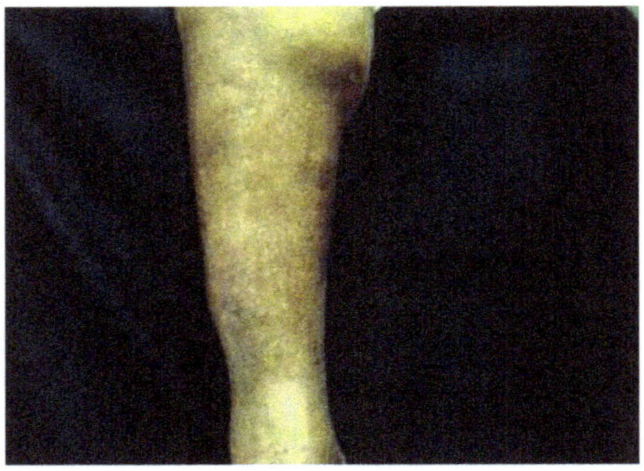

Lipodermatosclerosis (chronic phase)
Photograph courtesy of SpringerImages Database, Springer Publishing Company

36 Graft-Versus-Host Disease

a. Acute Graft-Versus-Host Disease

Acute graft-versus-host disease

A. Gastrointestinal symptoms (nausea, vomiting, diarrhea, abdominal pain), evidence of liver disease (elevated liver function tests and bilirubin)
B. Stage 1
   1. Discrete and coalescing red macules and papules (morbilliform eruption) with follicular or eccrine duct accentuation
   2. Less than 25 % body surface area
   3. Acral predilection initially (palms, soles, ears), then generalizes
   4. Usually appears 4–6 weeks after transplant
C. Stage 2: as in Stage 1 but 25–50 % body surface area
D. Stage 3: as above in Stage 1 but 50 % body surface area to generalized erythroderma
E. Stage 4: generalized erythroderma with bullae resembling toxic epidermal necrolysis

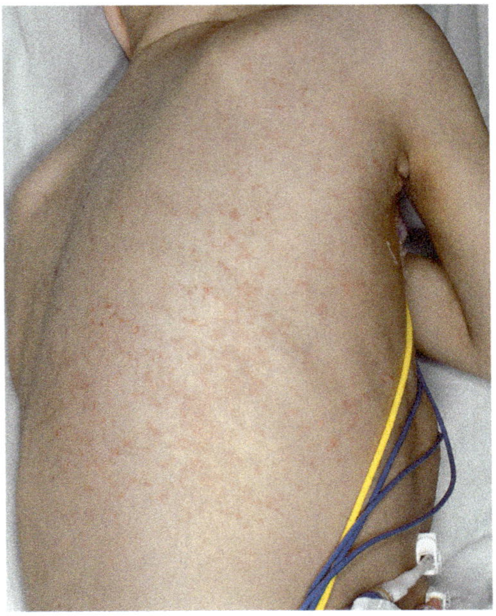

Acute graft-versus-host disease
Photograph courtesy of Dr. Kara Shah, MD, PhD, Cincinnati Children's Hospital, Cincinnati, OH

Acute graft-versus-host disease

A. Stage 4: generalized erythroderma with bullae resembling toxic epidermal necrolysis

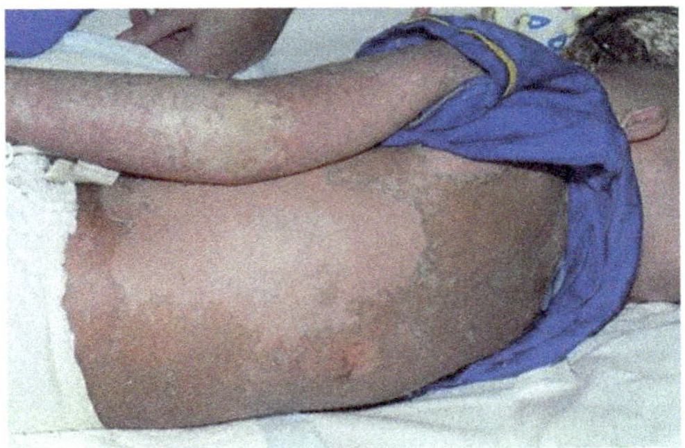

Acute graft-versus-host disease
Photograph courtesy of SpringerImages Database, Springer Publishing Company

H.M. Gloster, Jr. et al., *Absolute Dermatology Review: Mastering Clinical Conditions on the Dermatology Recertification Exam*,
DOI 10.1007/978-3-319-03218-4_36, © Springer International Publishing Switzerland 2016

b. Chronic Graft-Versus-Host Disease

Chronic graft-versus-host disease

A. May appear after or with acute graft-versus-host disease
B. Eruption occurs greater than 100 days after transplant
C. May appear similar to lichen planus (lichenoid)
   1. Reticulate pink to violet papules and plaques with scale
   2. Favors acral sites, trunk, proximal extremities (differs from lichen planus, which favors flexor forearms, mucosa, genitalia)
   3. Most common form of chronic graft-versus-host disease

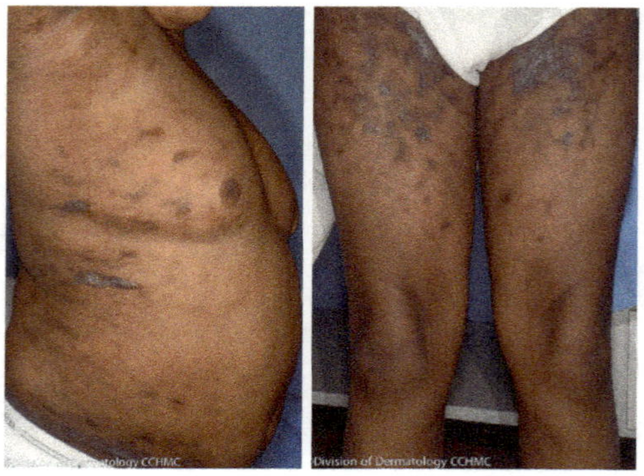

Chronic graft-versus-host disease
Photograph courtesy of Dr. Kara Shah, MD, PhD, Cincinnati Children's Hospital, Cincinnati, OH

Chronic graft-versus-host disease

A. May appear sclerodermoid
   1. Lichen sclerosus–like: shiny wrinkled gray white plaques on the upper back with or without follicular plugging
   2. Morphea-like: shiny sclerotic plaques, especially at sites of prior trauma or friction (e.g., the waist)
   3. Scleroderma-like: patchy and diffuse symmetric induration (no sclerodactyly or pinched facies)

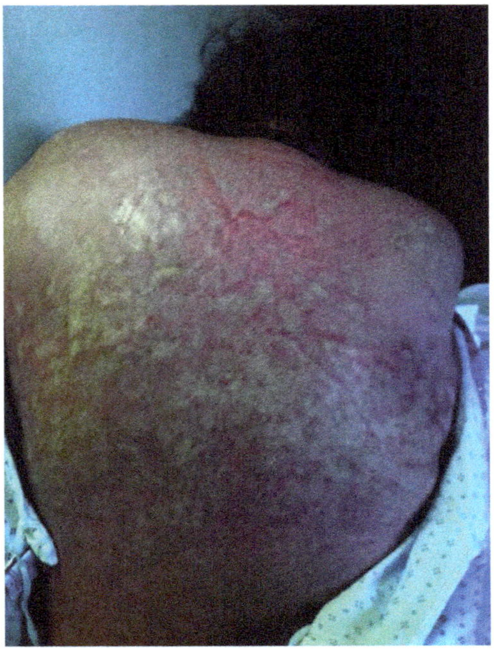

Chronic graft-versus-host disease
Photograph courtesy of SpringerImages Database, Springer Publishing Company

Chronic graft-versus-host disease

A. May appear scleroderma-like with patchy and diffuse symmetric induration

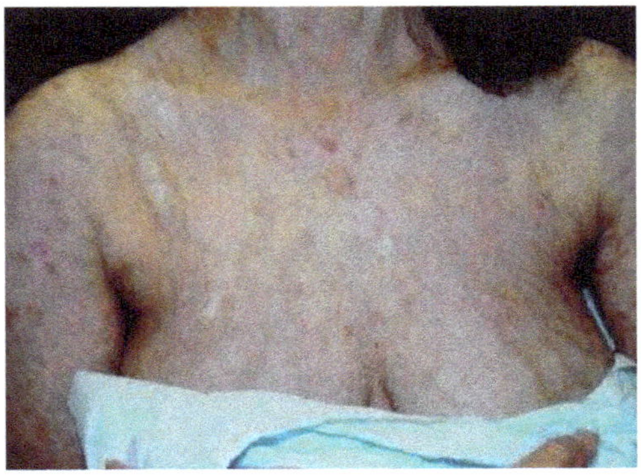

Chronic graft-versus-host disease
Photograph courtesy of SpringerImages Database, Springer Publishing Company

Chapter VI

Metabolic and Deposition Diseases

37 Mucinoses

a. Scleromyxedema

Scleromyxedema (generalized lichen myxedematosus)

A. Numerous minute monomorphic 2–3 mm firm waxy skin-colored to pink close-spaced papules in a widespread symmetrical distribution that coalesce into plaques
B. Most commonly occur on the head and neck, upper trunk, upper extremities (mostly sun-exposed areas)
C. Papules are often arranged in a linear array
D. The skin may be shiny and indurated (sclerodermoid) with erythematous indurated plaques and skin thickening with deep furrows and folds on skin of the trunk
E. Paraproteinemia: IgG monoclonal gammopathy and lambda light chains, less than 10 % develop multiple myeloma
F. Internal manifestations: muscular (proximal muscle weakness), neurological (peripheral neuropathy, carpal tunnel), rheumatologic, pulmonary (restrictive/obstructive lung disease), renal, cardiovascular
G. Localized variants
   1. Localized lichen myxemdematosus
   2. Follicular mucinosis (two types)
      a. Type 1
         1. Children and young adults
         2. Pink plaques composed of grouped follicular papules
         3. Face and scalp (leads to alopecia)
      b. Type 2
         1. Older age group
         2. Larger and more numerous plaques
         3. Associated with atopics and cutaneous T cell lymphoma

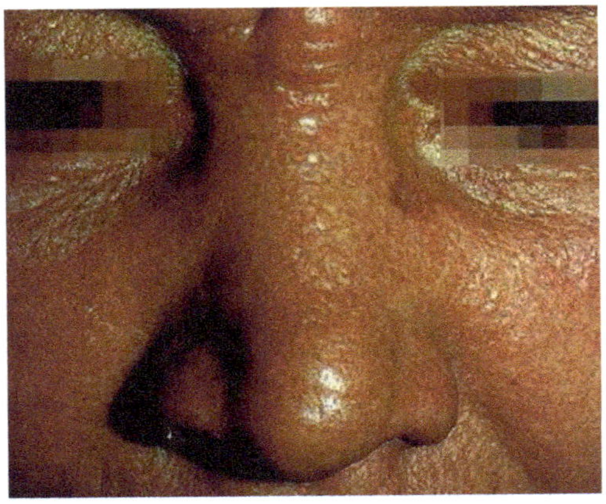

Scleromyxedema
Photograph courtesy of SpringerImages Database, Springer Publishing Company

H.M. Gloster, Jr. et al., *Absolute Dermatology Review: Mastering Clinical Conditions on the Dermatology Recertification Exam*,
DOI 10.1007/978-3-319-03218-4_37,

Scleromyxedema

A. Deep longitudinal furrowing of the glabella resulting in leonine facies

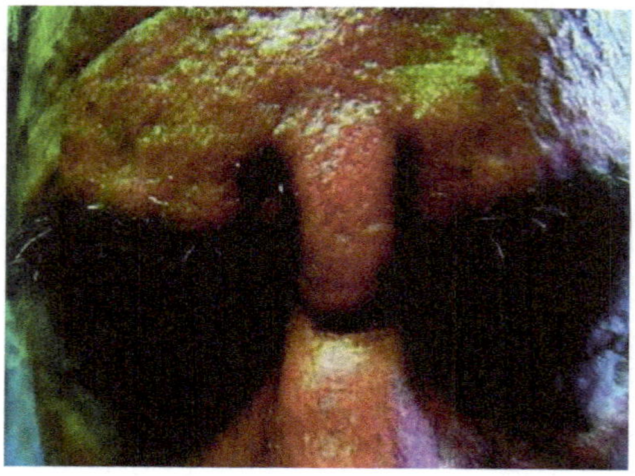

Scleromyxedema
Photograph courtesy of SpringerImages Database, Springer Publishing Company

Scleromyxedema

A. Numerous minute monomorphic 2–3 mm firm waxy skin-colored to pink close-spaced papules
B. Stiffening of the skin and decreased joint mobility of the hands and sclerodactyly
C. Doughnut sign: central depression with elevated rim (due to thick skin) over proximal interphalangeal joints

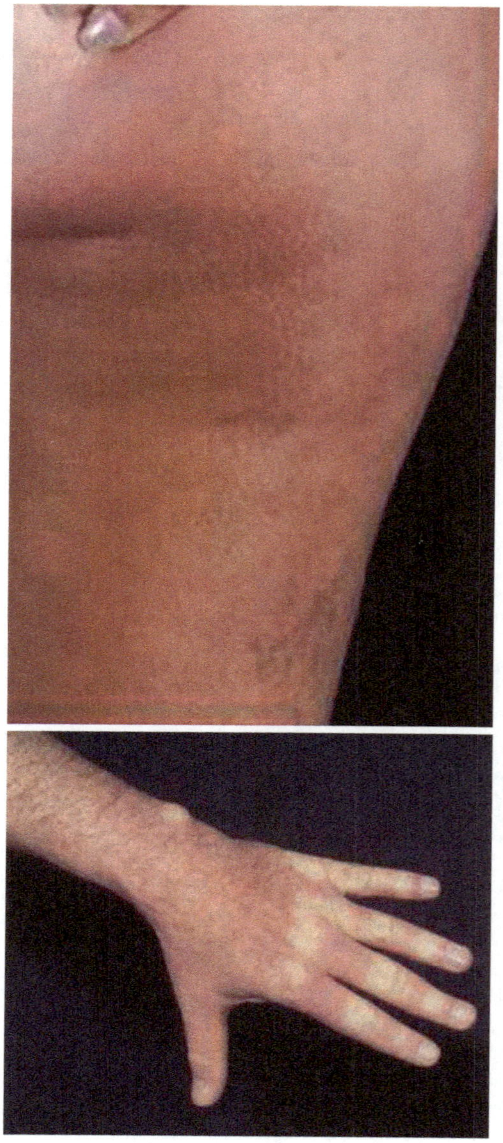

Scleromyxedema
Photograph courtesy of SpringerImages Database, Springer Publishing Company

b. Scleredema

Scleredema

A. Three types characterized by stiffening and hardening of the skin due to mucin deposition
   1. Type 1
      a. Middle-age women and children
      b. Preceded by upper respiratory infection (usually streptococcal) with fever and malaise
      c. Skin of the neck and face suddenly hardens (face is expressionless, opening the mouth and swallowing is difficult), hardening of the skin then extends to trunk and proximal arms
      d. Resolves in a few months
   2. Type 2
      a. Same clinical features as type 1 with more subtle onset, no preceding illness, persists for years
      b. Associated monoclonal gammopathy
   3. Type 3
      a. Obese middle-age men with insulin-dependent diabetes mellitus (scleredema diabeticorum)
      b. Erythema and doughy induration of the posterior neck and back with a sharp step-off and peau d'orange skin
      c. Persists years
B. Systemic manifestations (may be present in all three types): serositis, dysarthria, dysphagia, myositis, parotitis, ocular and cardiac disease

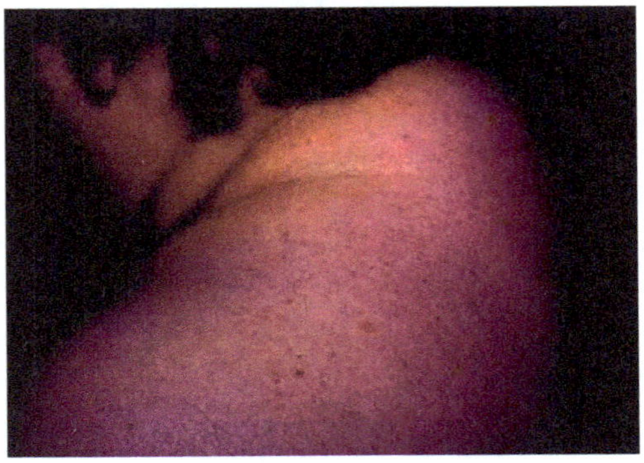

Scleredema
Photograph courtesy of SpringerImages Database, Springer Publishing Company

Scleredema diabeticorum

A. Erythema and doughy induration of the posterior neck and back in an insulin-dependent diabetic

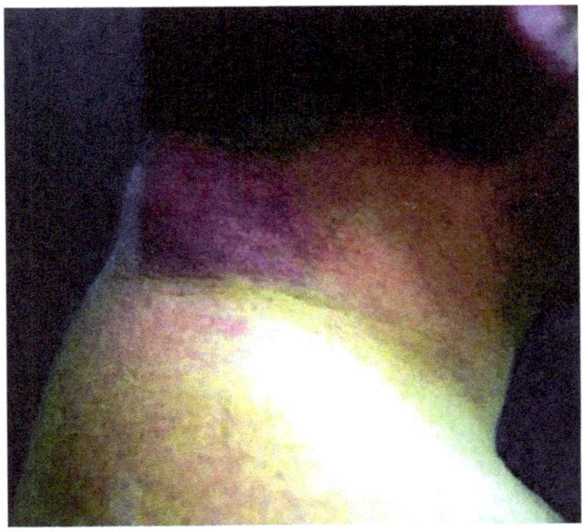

Scleredema
Photograph courtesy of SpringerImages Database, Springer Publishing Company

c. Pretibial Myxedema

Pretibial myxedema

A. Localized mucin deposition leading to cutaneous induration of the shins
B. Most often associated with hyperthyroidism (Grave's disease)
C. Erythematous to skin-colored, purple–brown, or yellow waxy indurated nodules or plaques with a peau d'orange texture (prominent hair follicles) on the anterolateral aspect of lower legs (shins) or feet

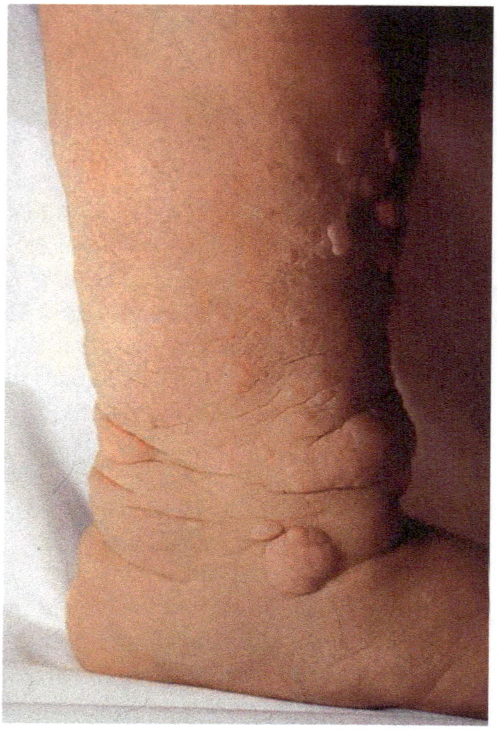

Pretibial myxedema
Photograph courtesy of SpringerImages Database, Springer Publishing Company

Pretibial myxedema

A. Indurated nodules and plaques with a peau d'orange texture (prominent hair follicles) on the anterolateral aspect of lower legs

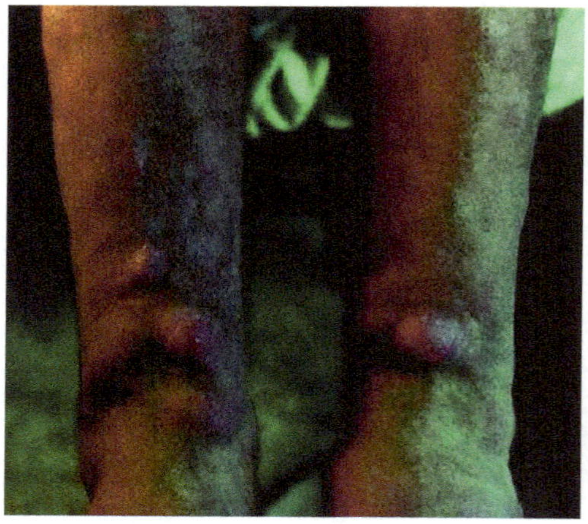

Pretibial myxedema
Photograph courtesy of SpringerImages Database, Springer Publishing Company

Pretibial myxedema
  A. Plaque-type with orange peel appearance on the skin

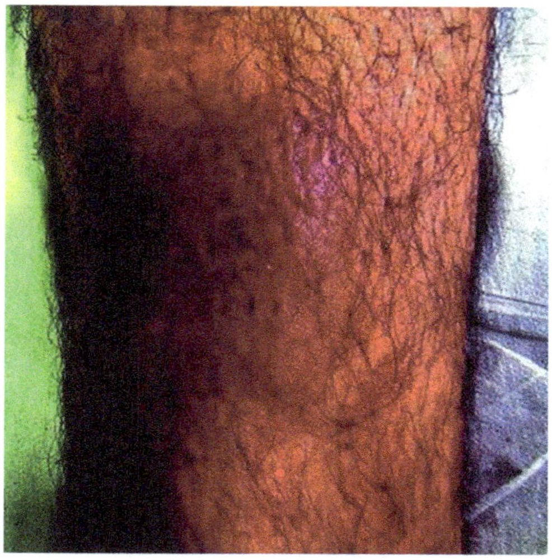

Pretibial myxedema
Photograph courtesy of SpringerImages Database, Springer Publishing Company

d. Follicular Mucinosis

i. Type 1 Follicular Mucinosis

Type 1 follicular mucinosis
  A. Localized variant of scleromyxedema
  B. Most often in children and young adults on the head and neck
  C. Pink plaques composed of grouped follicular papules, when present on face and scalp may lead to alopecia (alopecia mucinosa)
  D. Histologically, folliculotropic infiltrates sparing the epidermis and mucinous degeneration of hair follicles may be present

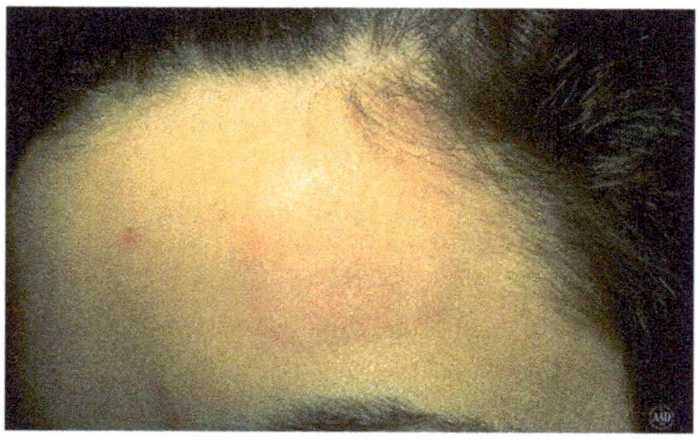

Type 1 follicular mucinosis
Photograph courtesy of SpringerImages Database, Springer Publishing Company

Type 1 follicular mucinosis
  A. Pink plaques composed of grouped follicular papules with hair loss

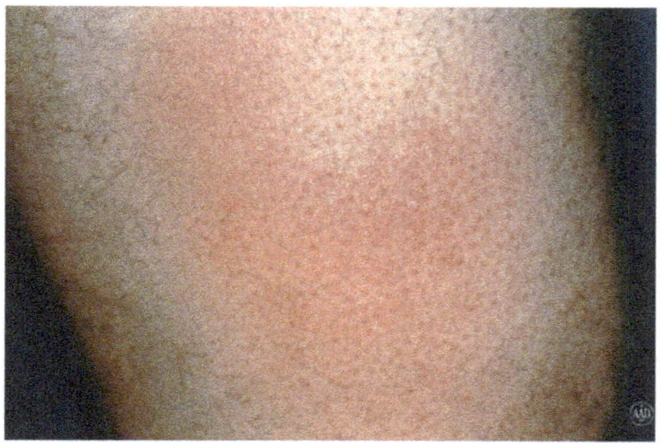

Type 1 follicular mucinosis
Photograph courtesy of the American Academy of Dermatology

Type 1 follicular mucinosis
  A. Pink plaques composed of grouped follicular papules

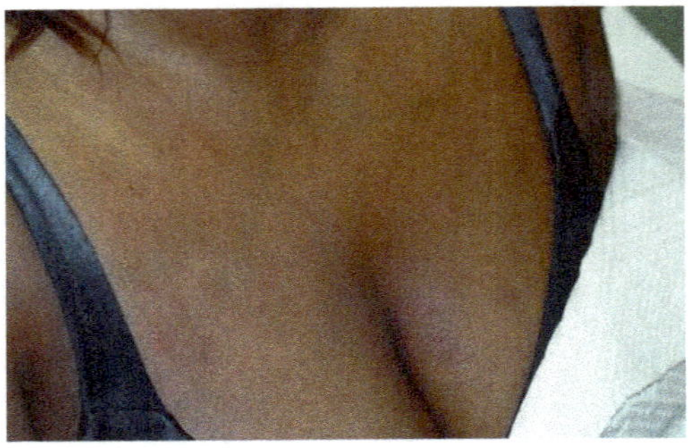

Type 1 follicular mucinosis
Photograph courtesy of SpringerImages Database, Springer Publishing Company

ii. Type 2 Follicular Mucinosis

Type 2 follicular mucinosis
  A. Localized variant of scleromyxedema
  B. Compared to type 1 follicular mucinosis: older age-group, larger and more numerous plaques, may be associated with atopics and cutaneous T cell lymphoma
  C. When present on face and scalp, may lead to alopecia (alopecia mucinosa)
  D. Infiltrated plaques in eyebrow area with alopecia are common

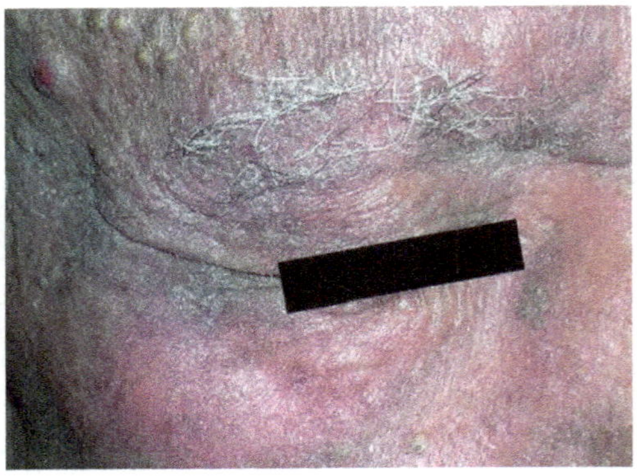

Type 2 follicular mucinosis

38 Amyloidosis

a. Macular Amyloidosis

Macular amyloidosis
  A. Reticulate or rippled macular hyperpigmentation
  B. Usually upper back

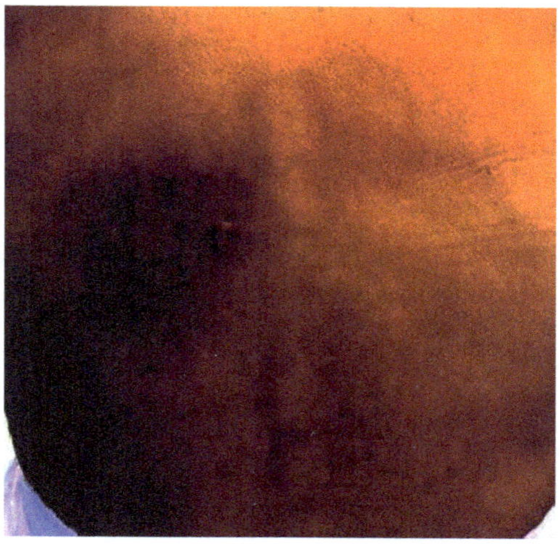

Macular amyloidosis
Photograph courtesy of SpringerImages Database, Springer Publishing Company

b. Lichen Amyloidosis

Lichen amyloidosis
  A. Multiple discrete pruritic hyperpigmented papules that coalesce into rippled or linear plaques
  B. Most commonly arise on the extensor extremities, usually the shins

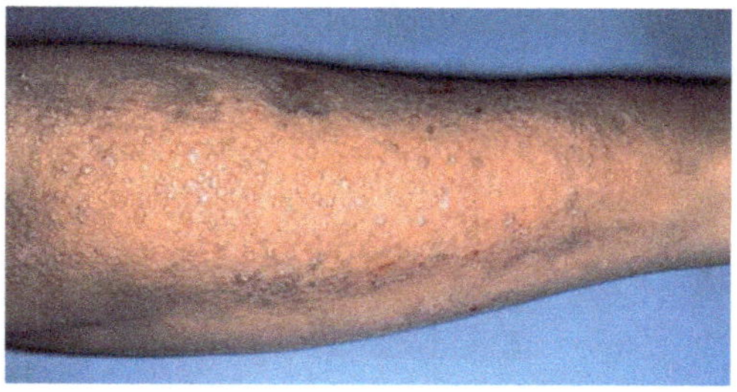

Lichen amyloidosis
Photograph courtesy of SpringerImages Database, Springer Publishing Company

H.M. Gloster, Jr. et al., *Absolute Dermatology Review: Mastering Clinical Conditions on the Dermatology Recertification Exam*, DOI 10.1007/978-3-319-03218-4_38, © Springer International Publishing Switzerland 2016

c. Primary Nodular Cutaneous Amyloidosis

Primary nodular cutaneous amyloidosis

A. Waxy skin-colored to pink firm plaques or nodules

B. Most commonly on the trunk or extremities

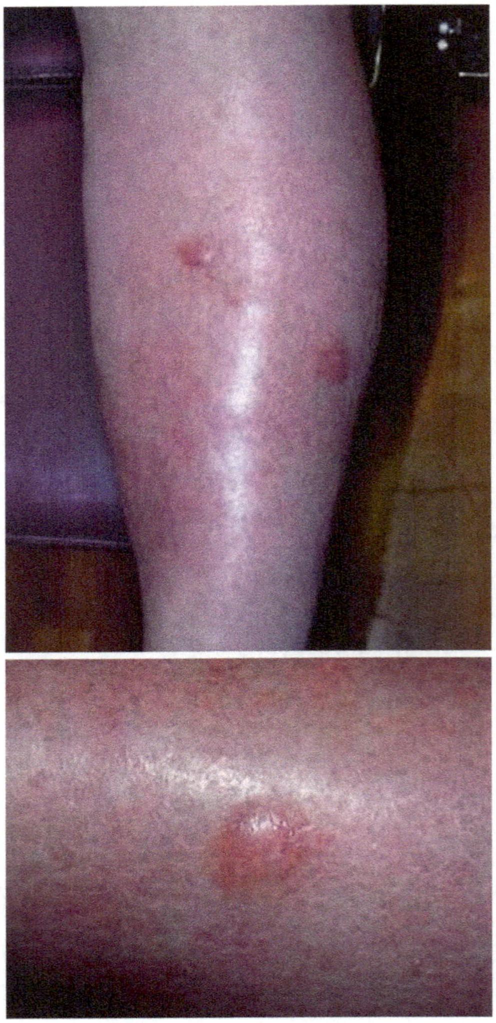

Primary nodular cutaneous amyloidosis
Photograph courtesy of SpringerImages Database, Springer Publishing Company

d. Primary Systemic Amyloidosis

Primary systemic amyloidosis

A. Pinch purpura: hemorrhagic macules (ecchymoses) especially common around the eyes, most common mucocutaneous manifestation of primary systemic amyloidosis

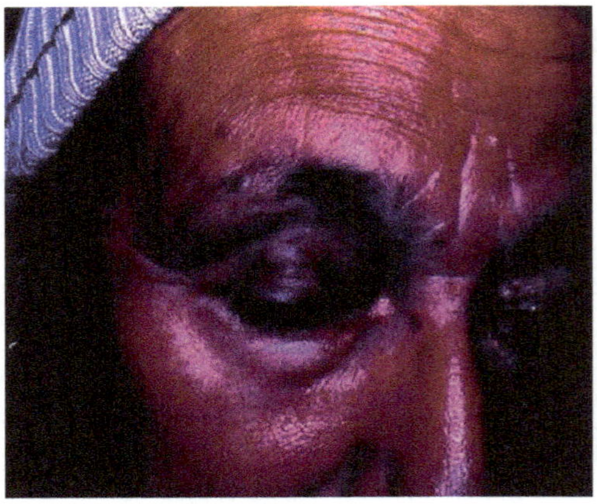

Primary systemic amyloidosis
Photograph courtesy of SpringerImages Database, Springer Publishing Company

Primary systemic amyloidosis
A. Macroglossia

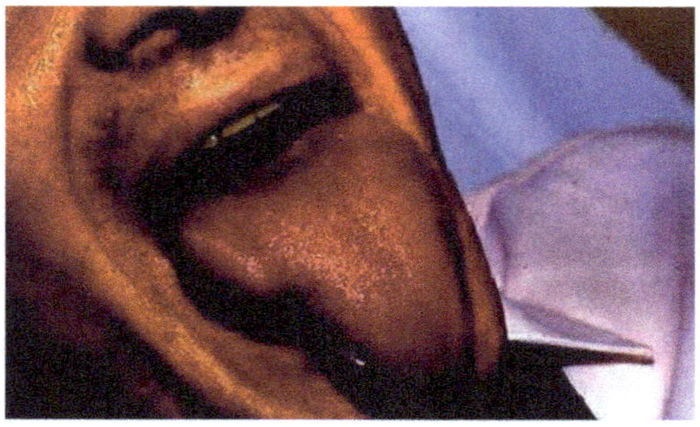

Primary systemic amyloidosis
Photograph courtesy of SpringerImages Database, Springer Publishing Company

Primary systemic amyloidosis
A. Waxy yellow–brown papules, nodules, or plaques
B. Most commonly located on the palms, face (periorbital, perioral), neck, and scalp

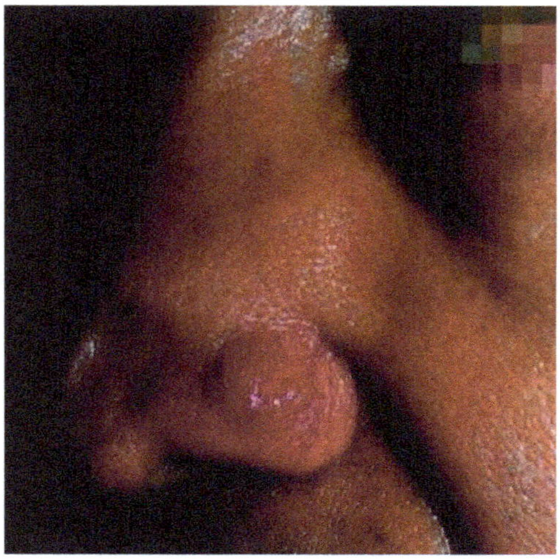

Primary systemic amyloidosis
Photograph courtesy of SpringerImages Database, Springer Publishing Company

39 Porphyria Cutanea Tarda

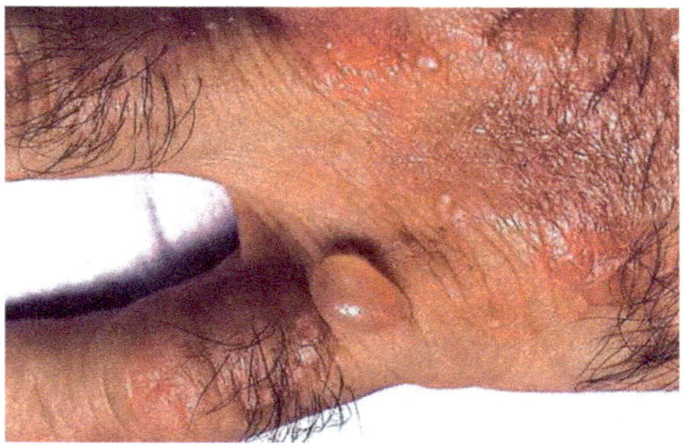

Porphyria cutanea tarda
Photograph courtesy of SpringerImages Database, Springer Publishing Company

Porphyria cutanea tarda

A. Most common type of porphyria
B. Decreased uroporphyrinogen decarboxylase (defect in hemoglobin production) results in accumulation of precursors upstream in the cycle
    1. Urine: increased uroporphyrins, low corproporphyrins (the urine fluoresces coral pink with Woods light)
C. Usually occurs in the third to fourth decade
D. Associations: hepatitis C virus, alcoholism, liver disease, hemochromatosis, HIV
E. Two types
    1. Type 1—acquired, most common, dysfunctional enzyme only in liver
    2. Type II—autosomal dominant inheritance, enzyme defect in all tissues
F. Clinical features
    1. Moderate to severe photosensitivity
    2. Skin fragility, non-inflammatory bullae, vesicles, erosions, and crusts
    3. Bullae resolve with milia, scarring, dyspigmentation
    4. Occurs on sun-exposed skin (especially the dorsal hands but also the face, forearms, and ears)
    5. Hypertrichosis (cheeks and temples)
    6. Diffuse hyperpigmentation of the face, neck, and hands
    7. Scarring alopecia
    8. Morpheaform and sclerodermoid changes with long-standing disease

H.M. Gloster, Jr. et al., *Absolute Dermatology Review: Mastering Clinical Conditions on the Dermatology Recertification Exam*, DOI 10.1007/978-3-319-03218-4_39, © Springer International Publishing Switzerland 2016

Porphyria cutanea tarda

A. Skin fragility, noninflammatory bullae, vesicles, erosions, crusts, milia, scarring, and dyspigmentation on the dorsal hand and fingers

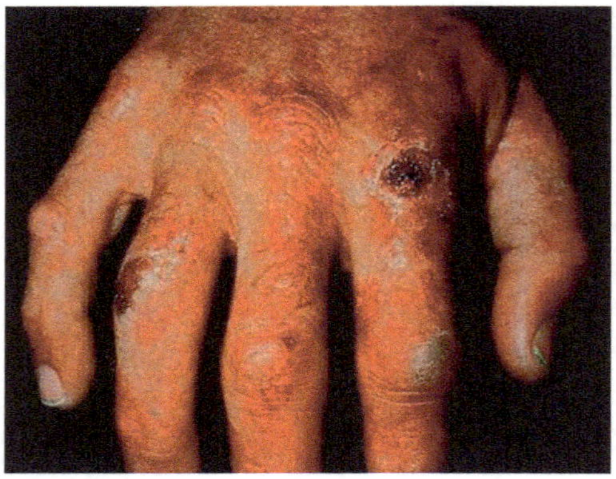

Porphyria cutanea tarda
Photograph courtesy of SpringerImages Database, Springer Publishing Company

Porphyria cutanea tarda

A. Hypertrichosis of the cheeks and temples

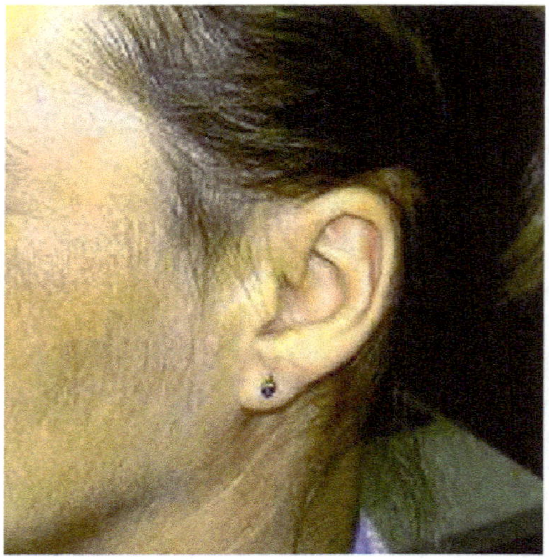

Porphyria cutanea tarda

40 Calcifying Disorders

a. Calcinosis Cutis

Calcinosis cutis

A. Yellowish white subcutaneous nodules that may extrude white chalky material and ulcerate, particularly at sites of trauma (especially on the digits)
B. Most commonly occurs on the hands, upper extremities, and over bony prominences (elbows, knees)

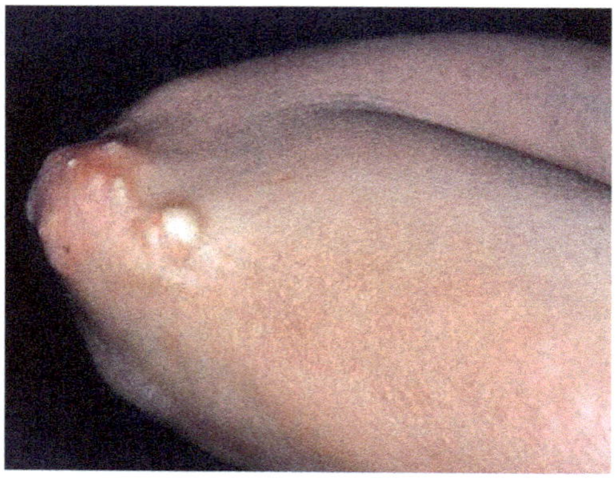

Calcinosis cutis
Photograph courtesy of SpringerImages Database, Springer Publishing Company

Calcinosis cutis

A. Yellowish white subcutaneous nodules on the digits that may extrude white chalky material and ulcerate, particularly at sites of trauma

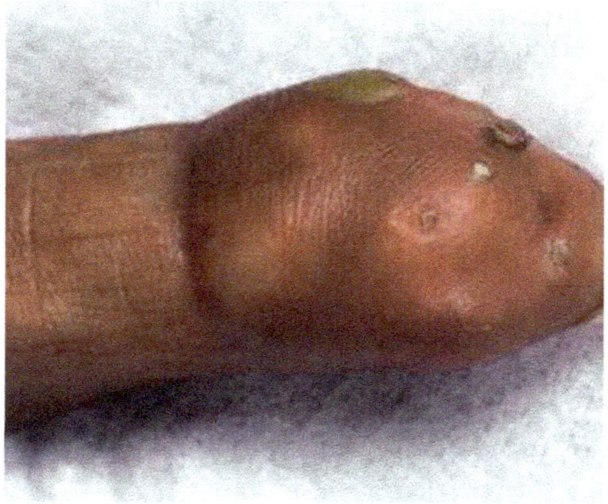

Calcinosis cutis
Photograph courtesy of SpringerImages Database, Springer Publishing Company

H.M. Gloster, Jr. et al., *Absolute Dermatology Review: Mastering Clinical Conditions on the Dermatology Recertification Exam*, DOI 10.1007/978-3-319-03218-4_40, © Springer International Publishing Switzerland 2016

b. Calciphylaxis

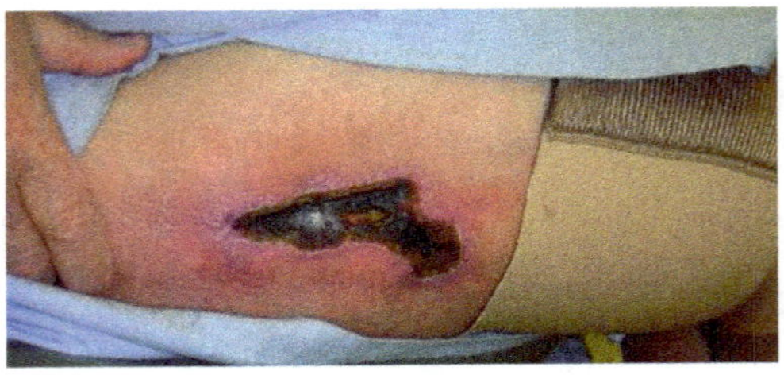

Calciphylaxis
Photograph courtesy of SpringerImages Database, Springer Publishing Company

Calciphylaxis

A. Systemic metabolic disorder resulting in metastatic calcium deposits
B. Chronic renal failure, resulting in increased calcium and phosphate, is the most common cause
C. Progressive vascular calcification of pannicular arterioles results in ischemic necrosis of the skin and soft tissue
D. Clinically characterized by very painful violaceous, reticulated, stellate plaques (retiform purpuric plaques) on the abdomen or lower extremities that soon develop bullae or a gray color heralding imminent necrosis with ulceration and black eschar

41 Nutritional Deficiencies

a. Scurvy

Scurvy

A. Vitamin C (ascorbic acid) deficiency results in impaired collagen synthesis (vitamin C is a necessary cofactor for enzymes in collagen synthesis)
B. Affects tissues with collagen: skin, mucosa, vessels, bones
C. May occur in infants and toddlers, food fads, psychiatric disease, alcoholism, and other causes of malnutrition
D. Clinical features begin 1–3 months after insufficient intake of fresh fruits and vegetables
   1. Skin: corkscrew hairs, hemorrhage (perifollicular, subungual, submucosal, subcutaneous), petechiae, ecchymoses, keratotic follicular plugs (forearms, abdomen, legs)
   2. Mucosal: gingival swelling and hypertrophy with erosions and bleeding, tooth loosening or loss
   3. Bone: periosteal hemorrhage and joint swelling

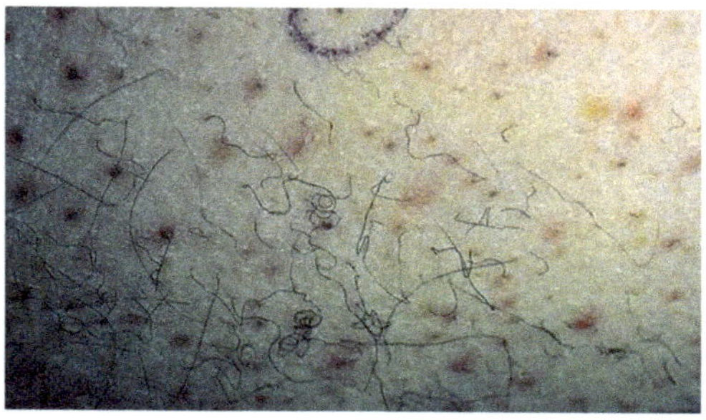

Scurvy
Photograph courtesy of SpringerImages Database, Springer Publishing Company

H.M. Gloster, Jr. et al., *Absolute Dermatology Review: Mastering Clinical Conditions on the Dermatology Recertification Exam*,
DOI 10.1007/978-3-319-03218-4_41, © Springer International Publishing Switzerland 2016

Scurvy

A. Keratotic follicular plugs with perifollicular hemorrhage

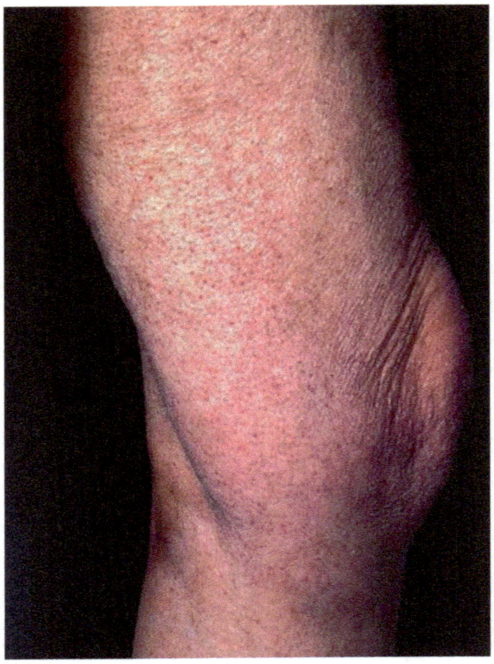

Scurvy
Photograph courtesy of SpringerImages Database, Springer Publishing Company

Scurvy

A. Perifollicular hemorrhage

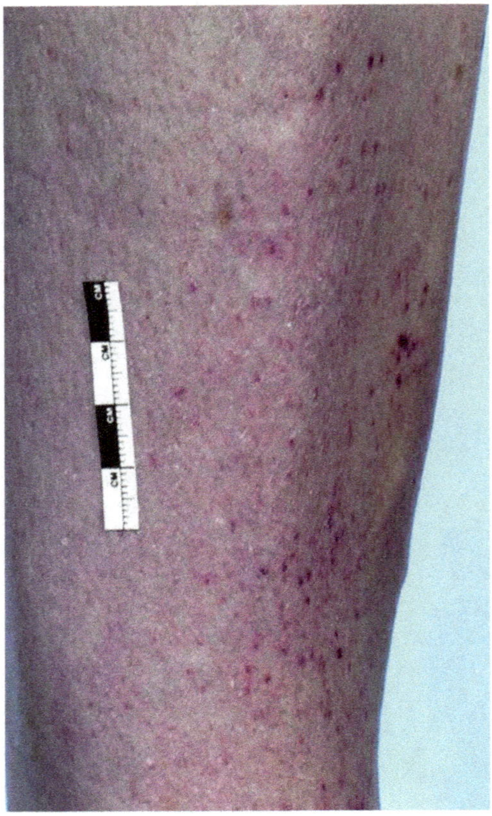

Scurvy
Photograph courtesy of SpringerImages Database, Springer Publishing Company

b. Pellagra

Pellagra

A. Niacin deficiency (nicotinic acid, vitamin B3)
B. Niacin is found in meat (poultry, pork, beef, salmon)
C. Seen in alcoholics, food fads, colitis, malabsorption, carcinoid, diets based predominantly on corn
D. 3 Ds (dementia, dermatitis, diarrhea)
   1. Dementia—Psychiatric problems (depression, anxiety, disorientation)
   2. Diarrhea (gastrointestinal symptoms—diarrhea, abdominal pain)
   3. Dermatitis
      a. Photodistributed erythema that becomes scarlet or hyperpigmented with a scaly, cracked, and brittle surface that has a shiny "shellac" appearance
      b. Commonly occurs on the face, neck (Casal's necklace: well-demarcated band around the neck), and hands and feet (painful fissures of palms and soles and glove-like pigmentation)
      c. Perianal and oral erosions, vaginitis
      d. Glossitis (atrophic, red tongue) and cheilitis

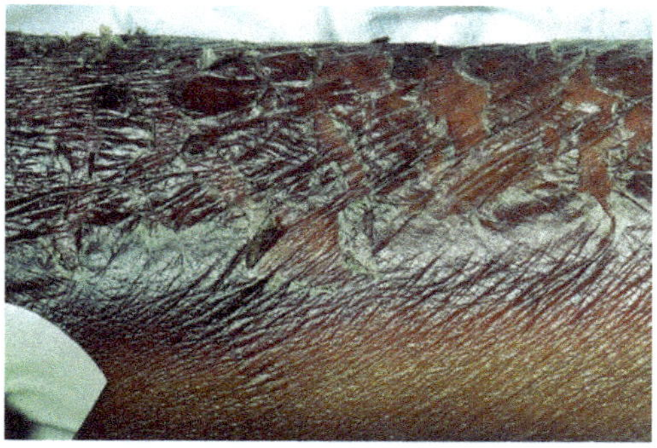

Pellagra
Photograph courtesy of SpringerImages Database, Springer Publishing Company

Pellagra

A. Casal's necklace: photodistributed erythematous to hyperpigmented, well-demarcated band around the neck

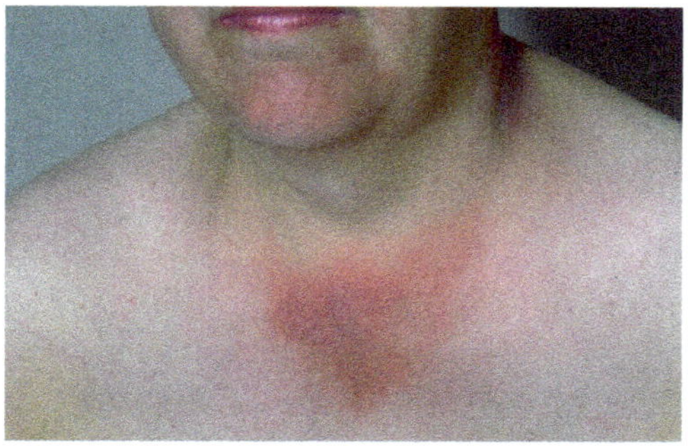

Pellagra
Photograph courtesy of SpringerImages Database, Springer Publishing Company

Pellagra

A. Casal's necklace: photodistributed erythematous to hyperpigmented, well-demarcated band around the neck

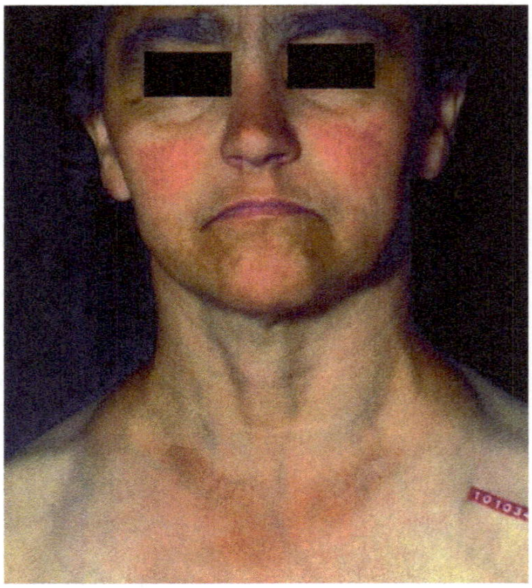

Pellagra
Photograph courtesy of SpringerImages Database, Springer Publishing Company

c. Zinc Deficiency (Acrodermatitis Enteropathica)

Zinc deficiency (acrodermatitis enteropathica)

A. Erythema, scale crusts, and erosions in periorifical and acral areas (perioral, perineum, palms/soles)
B. Occasionally vesicles, bullae, and psoriasiform plaques may occur
C. May be inherited or acquired
   1. Inherited (acrodermatitis enteropathica): autosomal recessive, mutation in the gene coding for zinc transport in the intestines and kidney, symptoms appear after weaning breast milk or after bottle feeding
   2. Acquired: vegan diets, alcoholism, anorexia, AIDS, malabsorptive syndromes, sickle-cell disease, chronic renal and hepatic disease

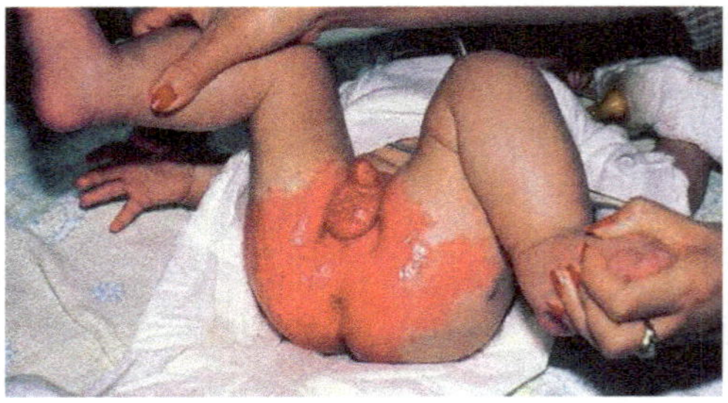

Zinc deficiency (acrodermatitis enteropathica)
Photograph courtesy of SpringerImages Database, Springer Publishing Company

Acrodermatitis enteropathica

A. Perioral erythema, scale crusts, and erosions

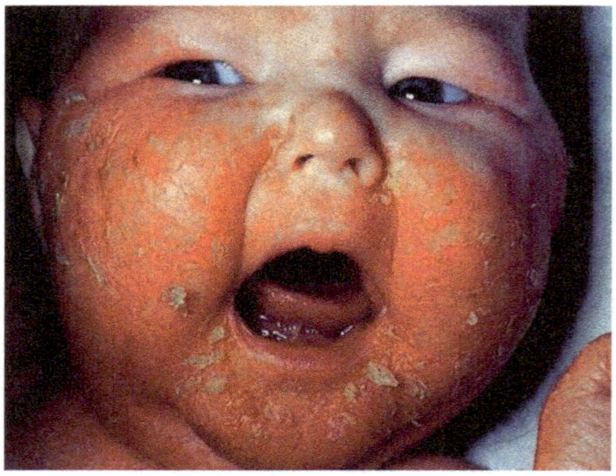

Zinc deficiency (acrodermatitis enteropathica)
Photograph courtesy of SpringerImages Database, Springer Publishing Company

Ochronosis

42

a. Exogenous Ochronosis

Exogenous ochronosis

A. History of hydroquinone application to areas of hyperpigmentation, may also occur after the use of other lightening agents (phenol, resorcinol, mercury, picric acid, benzene)
B. Small caviar-like papules may be superimposed on hyperpigmentation
C. Common on the face (especially the malar region), neck, and ears
D. Sites of involvement correspond to sites of application of lightening cream

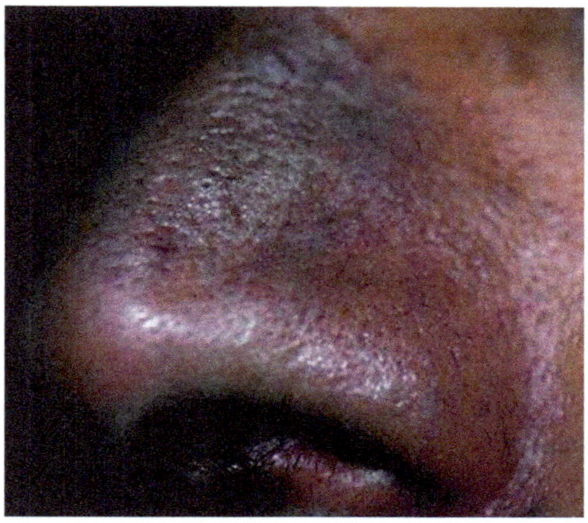

Exogenous ochronosis
Photograph courtesy of SpringerImages Database, Springer Publishing Company

b. Endogenous Ochronosis (Alkaptonuria)

Endogenous ochronosis (Alkaptonuria)

A. Autosomal recessive deficiency of homogentisate dioxygenase in liver and kidneys with accumulation of homogentisic acid in tissues
B. Oxidation of homogentisic acid forms benzoquinones that form melanin-like polymers that result in hyperpigmentation
C. Dark urine (turns black when left standing) and dark sweat (dark skin around sweat glands)
E. Cartilaginous tissues are involved at first then hyperpigmentation generalizes to involve the fingers, ears, genital regions, axillae, and buccal mucosa.
F. Dark skin most commonly involves sun-exposed areas (especially the ears and nose)
G. Valvular heart disease, joint disease, and kidney disease may occur

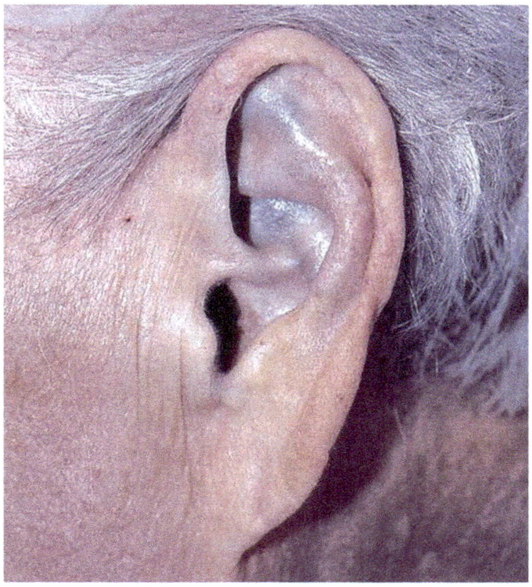

Endogenous ochronosis (alkaptonuria)
Photograph courtesy of SpringerImages Database, Springer Publishing Company

H.M. Gloster, Jr. et al., *Absolute Dermatology Review: Mastering Clinical Conditions on the Dermatology Recertification Exam*,
DOI 10.1007/978-3-319-03218-4_42, © Springer International Publishing Switzerland 2016

Endogenous ochronosis (Alkaptonuria)
A. Hyperpigmentation of the sclera

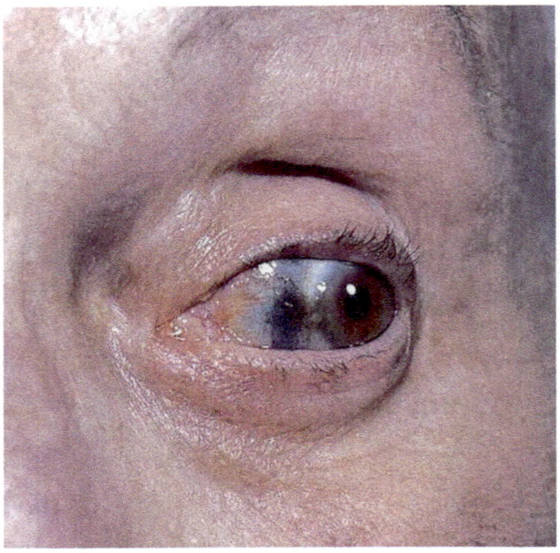

Endogenous ochronosis (alkaptonuria)
Photograph courtesy of SpringerImages Database, Springer Publishing Company

Endogenous ochronosis (Alkaptonuria)
A. Hyperpigmentation of the fingers

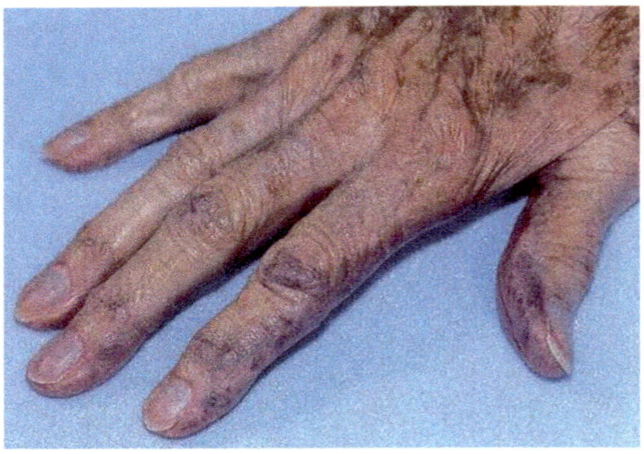

Endogenous ochronosis (alkaptonuria)
Photograph courtesy of SpringerImages Database, Springer Publishing Company

Chapter VII

Cutaneous Manifestations of Systemic Diseases

Cutaneous Manifestations of Rheumatoid Arthritis

43

Rheumatoid arthritis

A. Rheumatoid nodules: subcutaneous nodules on the third and fifth distal interphalangeal joints
B. Bywater's lesions: purpuric papules on the ulnar aspect of the fourth and fifth digits due to small vessel vasculitis

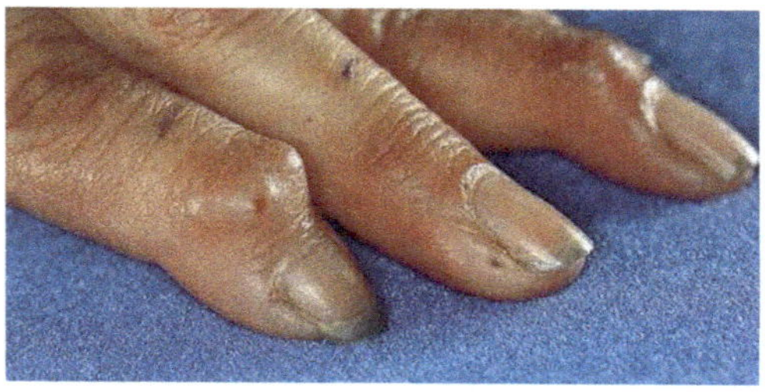

Rheumatoid arthritis
Photograph courtesy of SpringerImages Database, Springer Publishing Company

Rheumatoid arthritis

A. Rheumatoid nodule: subcutaneous nodule along the extensor surface of the forearm

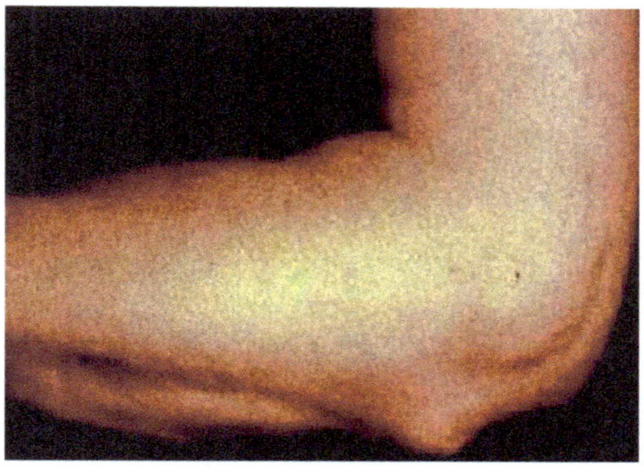

Rheumatoid arthritis
Photograph courtesy of SpringerImages Database, Springer Publishing Company

H.M. Gloster, Jr. et al., *Absolute Dermatology Review: Mastering Clinical Conditions on the Dermatology Recertification Exam*,
DOI 10.1007/978-3-319-03218-4_43,

44 Cutaneous Manifestations of Diabetes Mellitus

a. Necrobiosis Lipoidica Diabeticorum

Necrobiosis lipoidica diabeticorum

A. Well-demarcated, waxy plaques with violaceous to red–brown, palpable peripheral rims and yellow–brown atrophic centers with telangiectasias
B. Plaques may be multiple and bilateral and may ulcerate with trauma
C. The shins are the most common site
D. 15–65 % have diabetes
E. Most common in young to middle-age adults, women more frequently than men

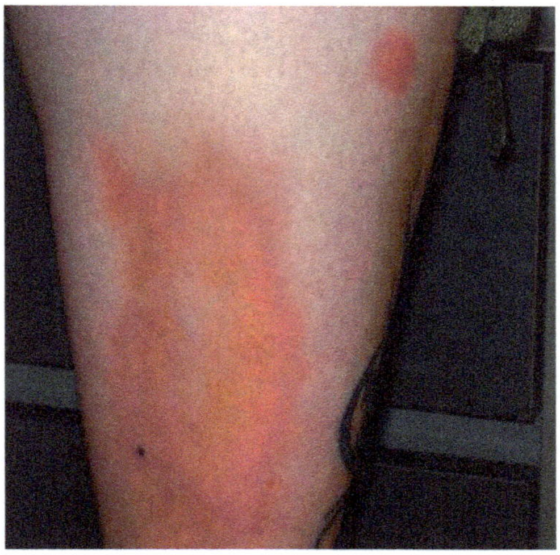

Necrobiosis lipoidica diabeticorum
Photograph courtesy of SpringerImages Database, Springer Publishing Company

H.M. Gloster, Jr. et al., *Absolute Dermatology Review: Mastering Clinical Conditions on the Dermatology Recertification Exam*,
DOI 10.1007/978-3-319-03218-4_44, © Springer International Publishing Switzerland 2016

Necrobiosis lipoidica diabeticorum

A. Well-demarcated, waxy plaques on the shins with violaceous to red–brown, palpable peripheral rims and yellow–brown atrophic centers with telangiectasias

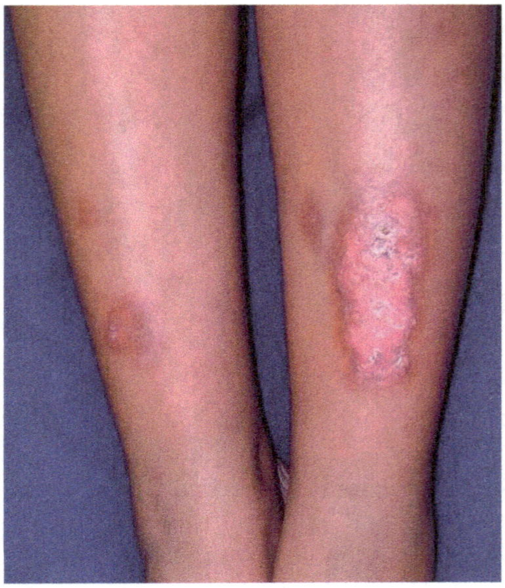

Necrobiosis lipoidica diabeticorum
Photograph courtesy of SpringerImages Database, Springer Publishing Company

b. Acanthosis Nigricans

Acanthosis nigricans

A. Velvety hyperpigmentation of flexural surfaces (neck, axilla, groin) most commonly and less often extensor surfaces (elbows, knees, knuckles)
B. Usually symmetric and bilateral
C. May be associated with insulin resistance
D. Insidious onset, also associated with obesity, more common in Hispanics and blacks

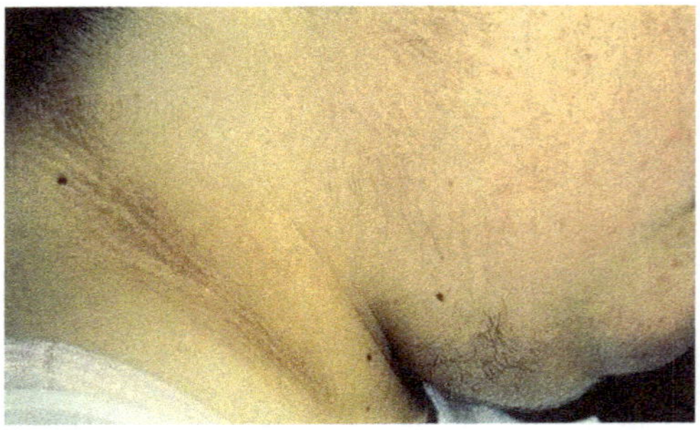

Acanthosis nigricans
Photograph courtesy of SpringerImages Database, Springer Publishing Company

c. Bullous Diabeticorum

Bullous diabeticorum

A. Non-inflammatory bullae on lower extremity in patient with diabetes

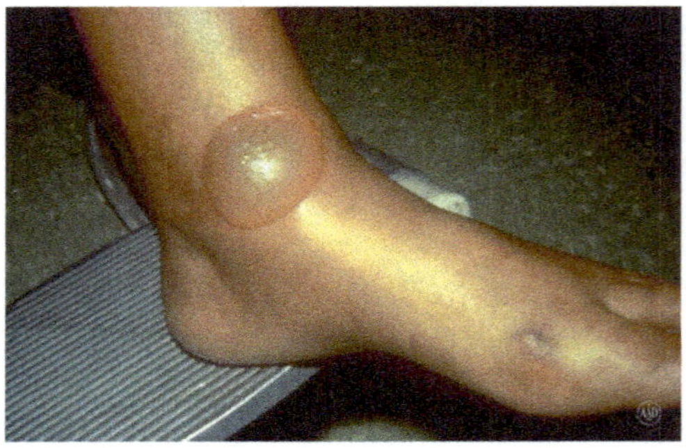

Bullous diabeticorum
Photograph courtesy of the American Academy of Dermatology

d. Diabetic Dermopathy

Diabetic dermopathy
A. Brown atrophic macules and patches on the shins

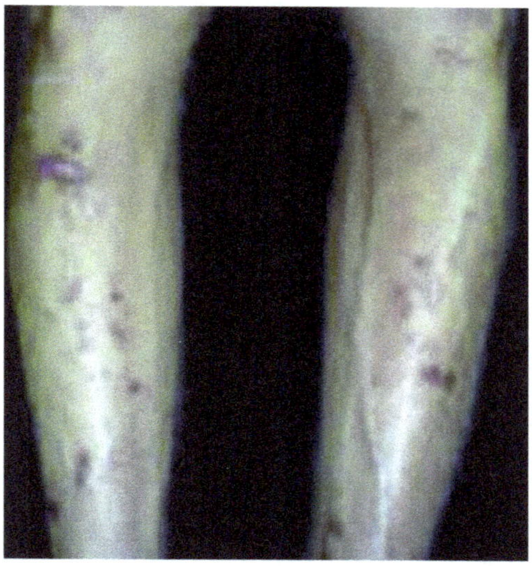

Diabetic dermopathy
Photograph courtesy of SpringerImages Database, Springer Publishing Company

e. Neuropathic Ulcers

Neuropathic ulcers
A. Nontender ulcers with a keratotic rim at pressure points (usually the foot)
B. Seen in diabetic neuropathy

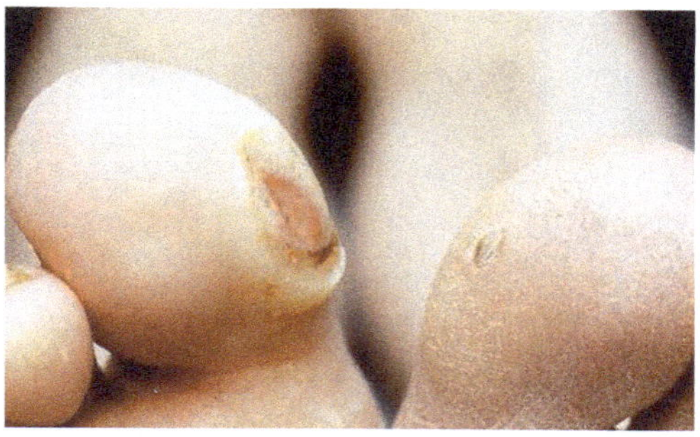

Neuropathic ulcers
Photograph courtesy of SpringerImages Database, Springer Publishing Company

Neuropathic ulcers
A. Nontender ulcer with a keratotic rim on the foot in a patient with diabetic neuropathy

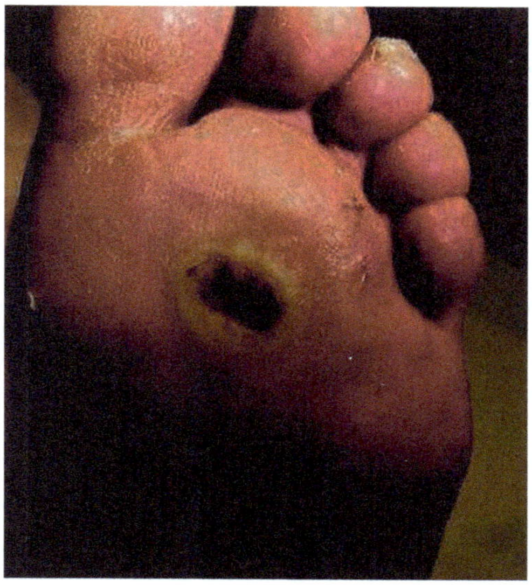

Neuropathic ulcers
Photograph courtesy of SpringerImages Database, Springer Publishing Company

f. Scleredema Diabeticorum

Scleredema diabeticorum

A. Seen in obese middle-age men with diabetes
B. Erythema and doughy induration of the posterior neck and back with a sharp step-off resulting in a peau d'orange quality of the skin

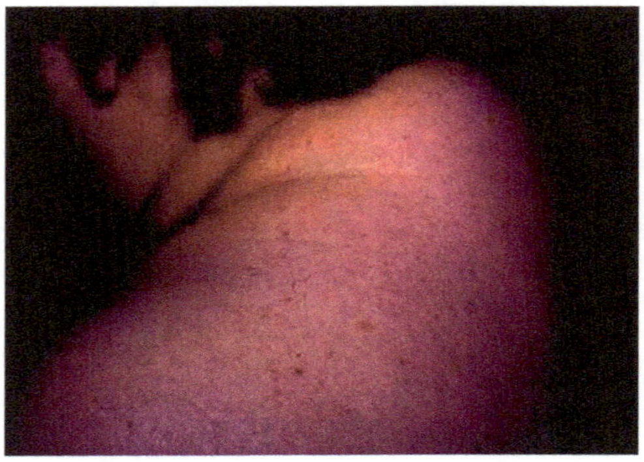

Scleredema diabeticorum
Photograph courtesy of SpringerImages Database, Springer Publishing Company

g. Eruptive Xanthomas

Eruptive xanthomas

A. Small yellow or reddish orange papules extensor extremities (especially the knees), buttocks, and thorax

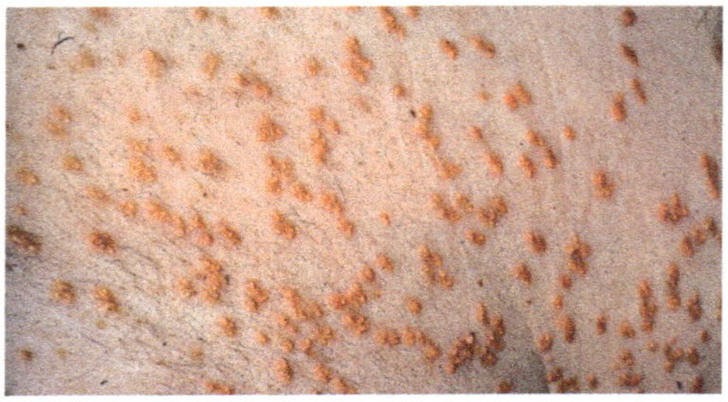

Eruptive xanthomas
Photograph courtesy of SpringerImages Database, Springer Publishing Company

Eruptive xanthomas

A. Small yellow or reddish orange papules on the knee

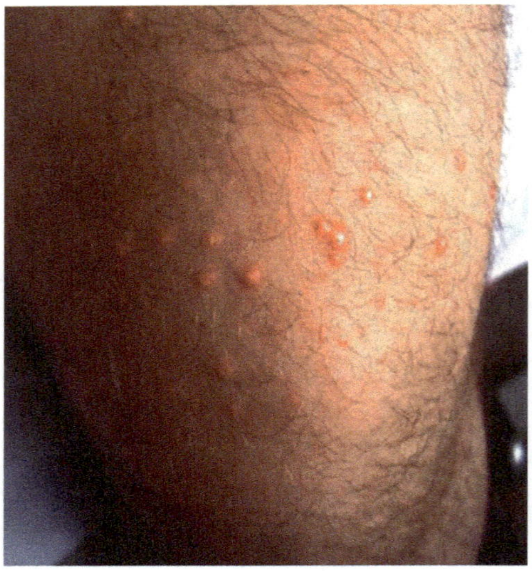

Eruptive xanthomas
Photograph courtesy of SpringerImages Database, Springer Publishing Company

45 Cutaneous Manifestations of Thyroid Disease

a. Pretibial Myxedema

Pretibial myxedema (also see Chap. 6, section 37c)

A. Localized mucin deposition leading to cutaneous induration of the shins
B. Most often associated with hyperthyroidism (Grave's disease)
C. Erythematous to skin-colored, purple–brown, or yellow waxy indurated nodules or plaques with a peau d'orange texture (prominent hair follicles) on the anterolateral aspect of lower legs (shins) or feet

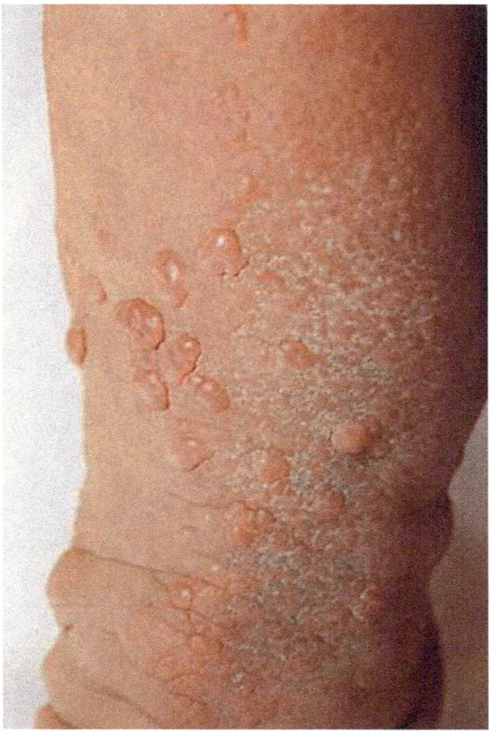

Pretibial myxedema
Photograph courtesy of SpringerImages Database, Springer Publishing Company

H.M. Gloster, Jr. et al., *Absolute Dermatology Review: Mastering Clinical Conditions on the Dermatology Recertification Exam*,
DOI 10.1007/978-3-319-03218-4_45,

Pretibial myxedema

A. Erythematous to skin-colored, purple–brown, or yellow waxy indurated nodules or plaques on the anterolateral aspect of lower legs

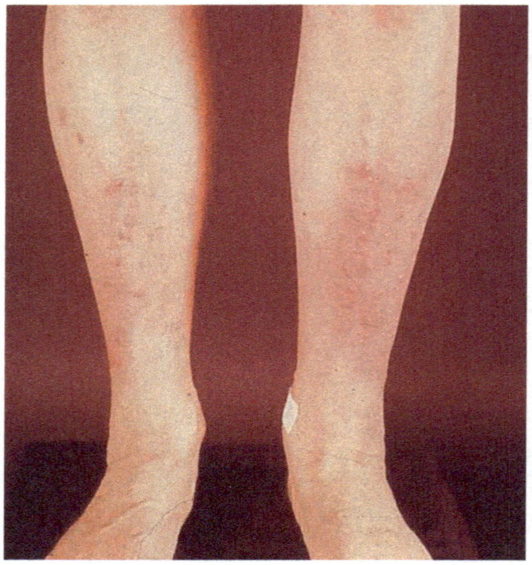

Pretibial myxedema
Photograph courtesy of SpringerImages Database, Springer Publishing Company

b. Generalized Myxedema

Generalized myxedema

A. May be associated with hypothyrodism
B. Typical facies: enlarged and protruding lips, macroglossia, and a broad nose.
C. Boggy and edematous skin

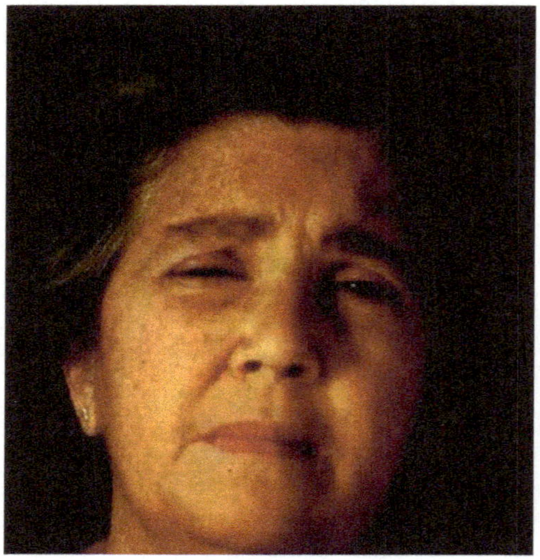

Generalized myxedema
Photograph courtesy of SpringerImages Database, Springer Publishing Company

c. Acquired Ichthyosis

Acquired Ichthyosis
  A. Associated with hypopthyoidism

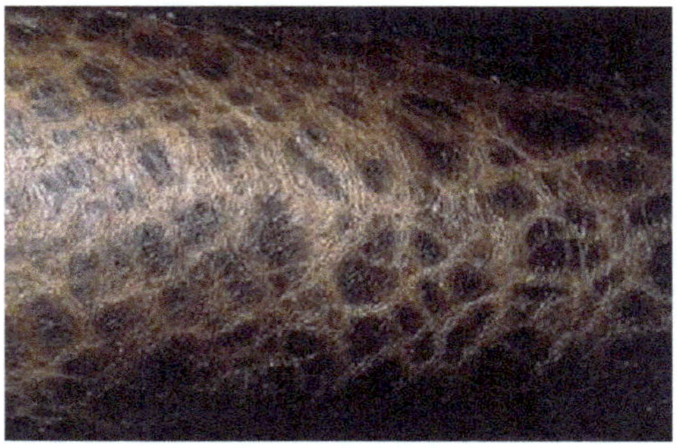

Acquired ichthyosis
Photograph courtesy of SpringerImages Database, Springer Publishing Company

d. Alopecia

Alopecia
  A. Nonscarring alopecia of the scalp, groin, and lateral eyebrows may be associated with hypothyroidism

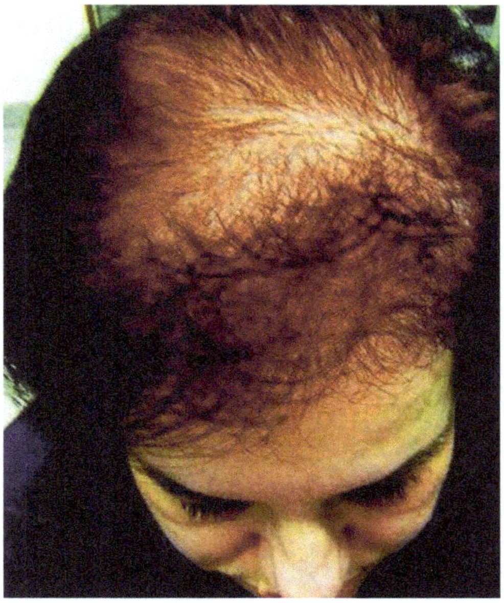

Alopecia
Photograph courtesy of SpringerImages Database, Springer Publishing Company

Cutaneous Manifestations of Cushing's Syndrome

46

Cushing's syndrome

A. Excess glucocorticoid activity
B. Altered subcutaneous fat: dorsal cervical vertebral fat (buffalo hump), moon facies, and increased truncal fat, decreased arm and leg fat
C. Acne, hirsutism

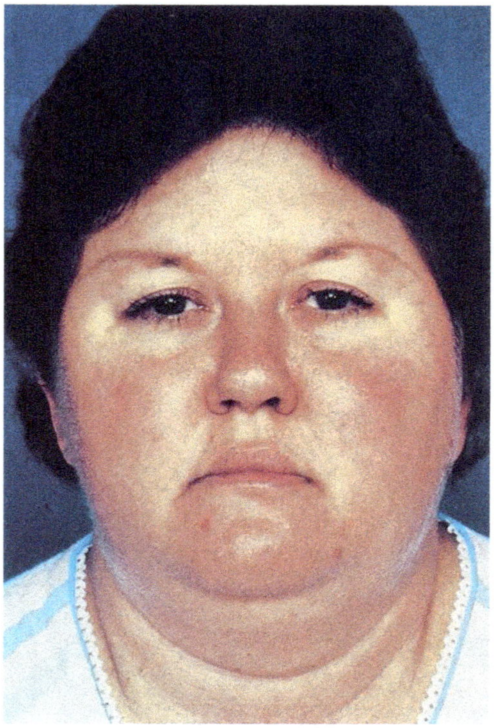

Cushing's syndrome
Photograph courtesy of SpringerImages Database, Springer Publishing Company

H.M. Gloster, Jr. et al., *Absolute Dermatology Review: Mastering Clinical Conditions on the Dermatology Recertification Exam*, DOI 10.1007/978-3-319-03218-4_46, © Springer International Publishing Switzerland 2016

Cushing's syndrome

A. Buffalo hump, full supraclavicular fat pads, and moon facies

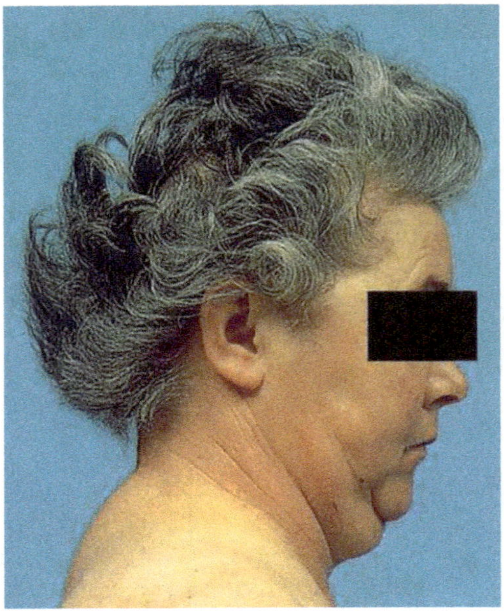

Cushing's syndrome
Photograph courtesy of SpringerImages Database, Springer Publishing Company

Cushing's syndrome

A. Skin atrophy: striae and global atrophy, leading to purpura and fragility

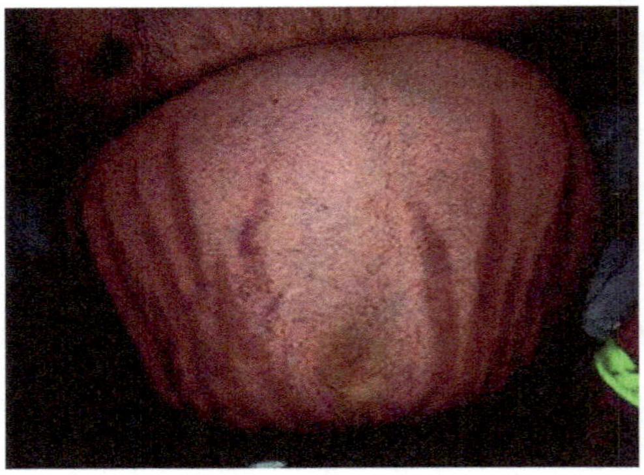

Cushing's syndrome
Photograph courtesy of SpringerImages Database, Springer Publishing Company

47 Cutaneous Manifestations of Addison's Disease

Addison's disease

A. Insufficient glucocorticoid activity
B. Diffuse hyperpigmentation

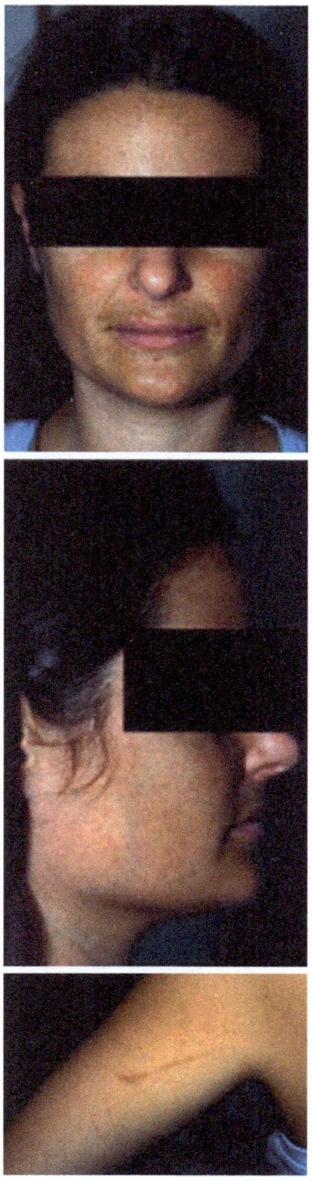

Addison's disease
Photograph courtesy of SpringerImages Database, Springer Publishing Company

H.M. Gloster, Jr. et al., *Absolute Dermatology Review: Mastering Clinical Conditions on the Dermatology Recertification Exam*,
DOI 10.1007/978-3-319-03218-4_47, © Springer International Publishing Switzerland 2016

48 Cutaneous Manifestations of Gastrointestinal Disease

a. Cutaneous Manifestations of Inflammatory Bowel Disease

i. Erythema Nodosum

Erythema nodosum (also see Chap. 21, section 124)

A. Bilateral tender red subcutaneous nodules symmetrically on the pretibial areas which develop into a bruise like appearance in later stages
B. Nodules do not ulcerate and usually resolve within a few days or weeks but may recur
C. Patients may develop fever, malaise, and arthralgias
D. Most cases occur in young women

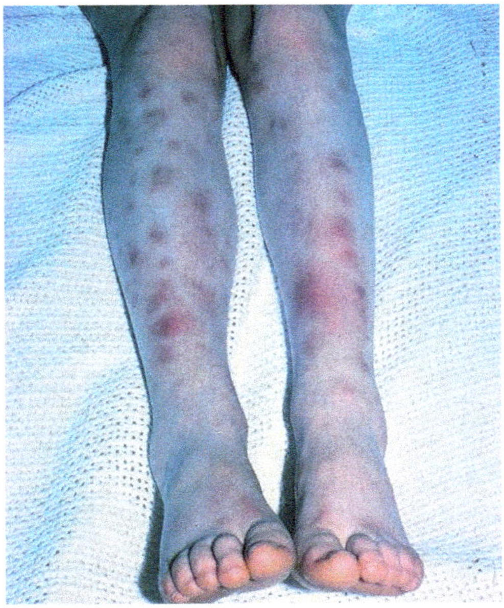

Erythema nodosum
Photograph courtesy of SpringerImages Database, Springer Publishing Company

H.M. Gloster, Jr. et al., *Absolute Dermatology Review: Mastering Clinical Conditions on the Dermatology Recertification Exam*, DOI 10.1007/978-3-319-03218-4_48,

Erythema nodosum

A. Tender red subcutaneous nodules on the pretibial area

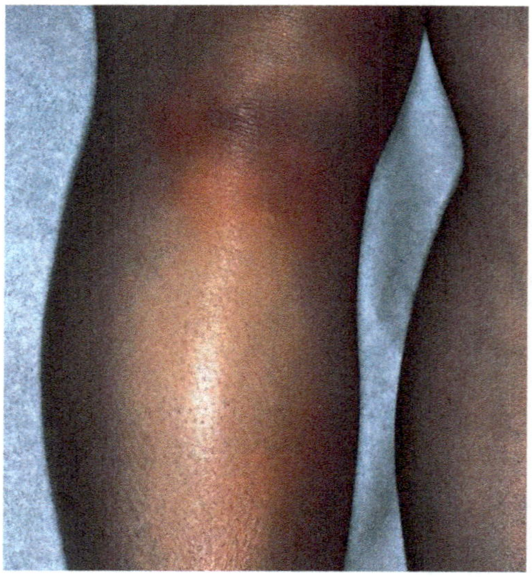

Erythema nodosum
Photograph courtesy of SpringerImages Database, Springer Publishing Company

ii. Leukocytoclastic Vasculitis

Leukocytoclastic vasculitis (also see Chap. 2, section 12)

A. Palpable or macular purpura most commonly on the lower extremities

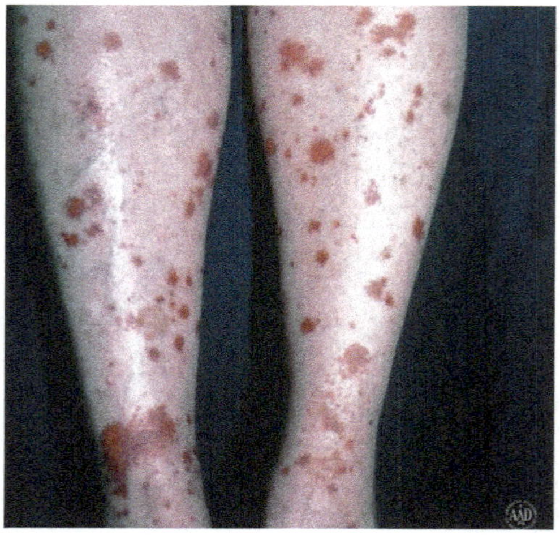

Leukocytoclastic vasculitis
Photograph courtesy of the American Academy of Dermatology

iii. Sweet's Syndrome

Sweet's syndrome (also see Chap. 18, section 111)

A. Upper respiratory tract infection or flu like symptoms with fever and malaise frequently precedes the syndrome
B. Tender, edematous, erythematous papules and plaques; vesicles, bullae, or pustules may develop within the plaques
C. May be associated with inflammatory bowel disease

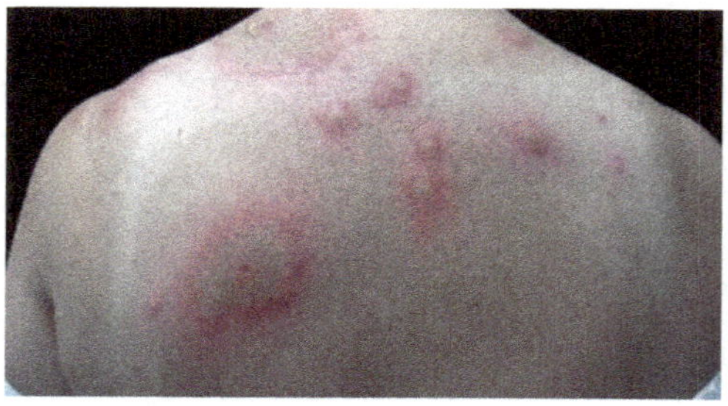

Sweet's syndrome
Photograph courtesy of SpringerImages Database, Springer Publishing Company

Sweet's syndrome

A. Favors the head, neck, and extremities (especially the dorsal hand) but may be widespread in malignancy associated cases
B. Pathergy is common
C. Resolves spontaneously in 5–12 weeks, recurs in 30 %

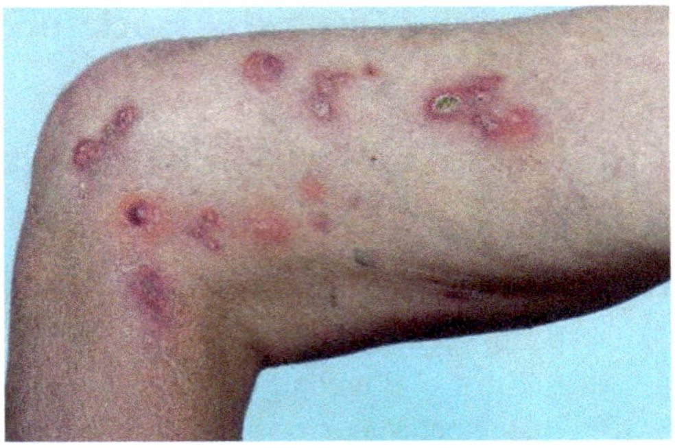

Sweet's syndrome
Photograph courtesy of SpringerImages Database, Springer Publishing Company

iv. Pyoderma Gangrenosum

Pyoderma gangenosum (also see Chap. 18, section 110)

A. Associated with inflammatory bowel disease in 20–30 % of cases
B. Ulcer with irregular, necrotic undermined and overhanging borders
C. The edge of ulcer is undermined and often has a violet-gray gun metal color and inflammatory rim with a purulent or vegetative base
D. The lower extremities, especially the pretibial area, are most commonly affected, but lesions may be anywhere

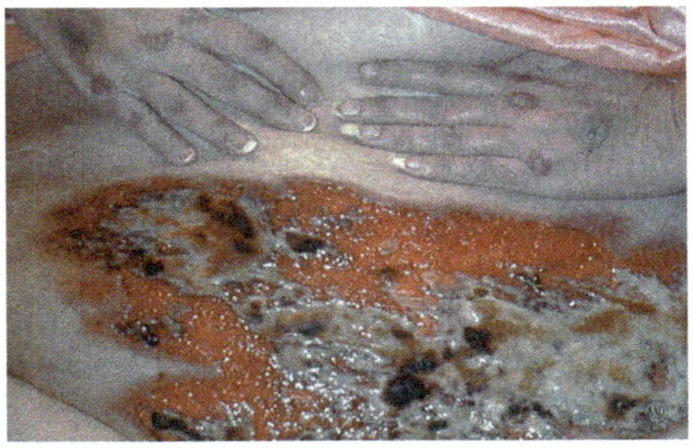

Pyoderma gangenosum
Photograph courtesy of the American Academy of Dermatology

b. Cutaneoous Diseases Associated with Gastrointestinal Bleeding

i. Hereditary Hemorrhagic Telangiectasia (Osler Weber Rendu)

Hereditary hemorrhagic telangiectasia (Osler Weber Rendu, also see Chap. 16, section 106a (iv))

A. Autosomal dominant
B. Telangiectasias on oral mucosa, facial, and acral skin
C. May be associated with upper gastrointestinal hemorrhage, epistaxis, and arteriovenous malformations

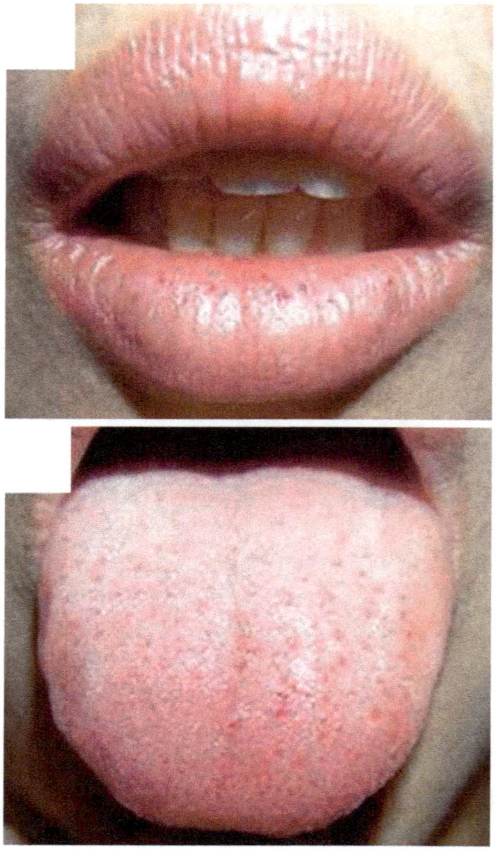

Hereditary hemorrhagic telangiectasia (Osler Weber Rendu)
Photograph courtesy of SpringerImages Database, Springer Publishing Company

Hereditary hemorrhagic telangiectasia (Osler Weber Rendu)

A. Telangiectasia on oral mucosa, facial, and acral skin

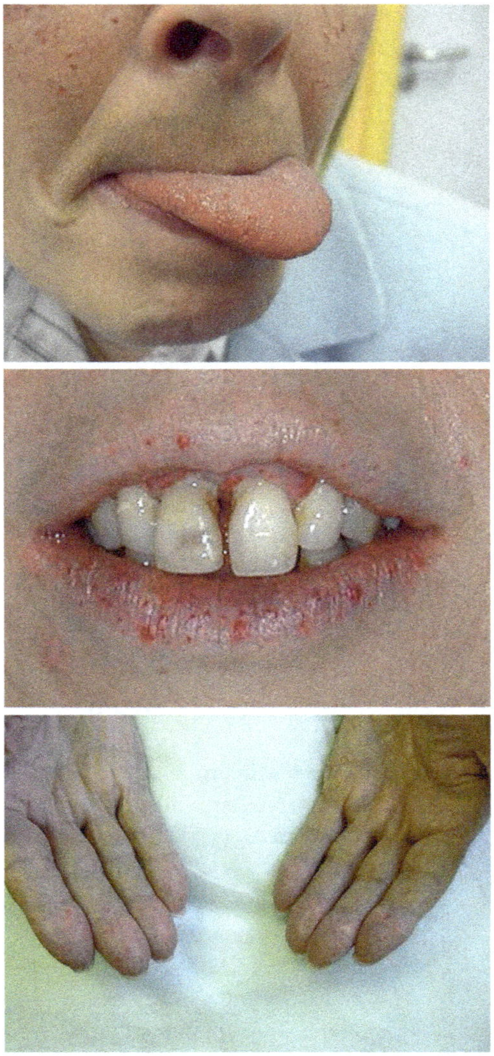

Hereditary hemorrhagic telangiectasia (Osler Weber Rendu)
Photograph courtesy of SpringerImages Database, Springer Publishing Company

ii. Blue Rubber Bleb Nevus Syndrome

Blue rubber bleb nevus syndrome

A. Usually occurs sporadically, though autosomal dominant forms have been reported
B. Blue-purple, soft, rubbery, compressible subcutaneous nodules (venous malformations) which refill after being compressed or fill with dependency
C. Gastrointestinal and central nervous system vascular malformations may also occur

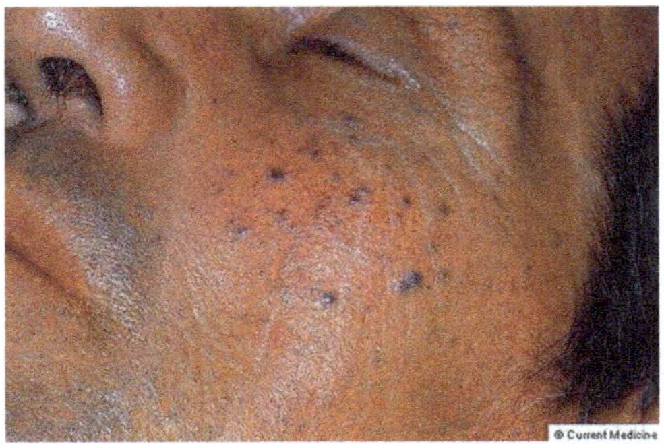

Blue rubber bleb nevus syndrome
Photograph courtesy of SpringerImages Database, Springer Publishing Company

Blue rubber bleb nevus syndrome

A. Blue-purple, soft, rubbery, compressible subcutaneous nodules

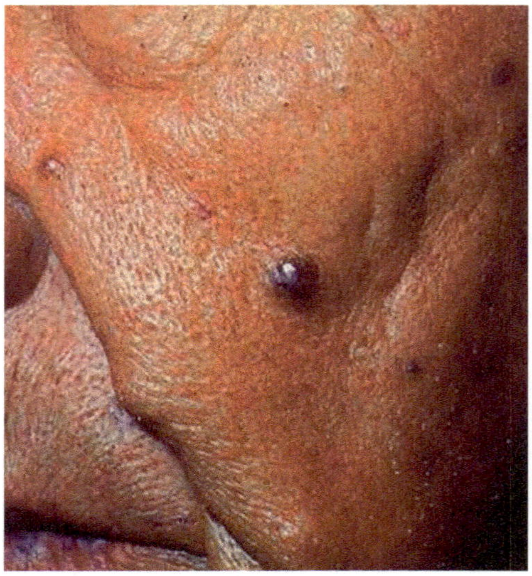

Blue rubber bleb nevus syndrome
Photograph courtesy of SpringerImages Database, Springer Publishing Company

iii. Pseudoxanthoma Elasticum

Pseudoxanthoma elasticum (also see Chap. 8, section 51j)

A. Autosomal recessive disorder characterized by clumped and distorted calcified elastic fibers in the skin, eyes, and cardiovascular system
B. Yellow papules which coalesce cobblestone plaques resembling plucked chicken skin
C. The lateral neck is usually affected first, then flexural areas
D. May be associated with gastrointestinal hemorrhage due to calcification of elastic fibers in medium size arteries and luminal narrowing

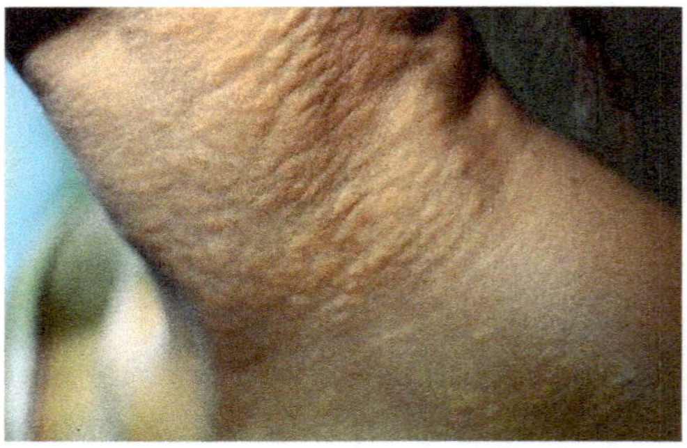

Pseudoxanthoma elasticum
Photograph courtesy of SpringerImages Database, Springer Publishing Company

c. Cutaneous Manifestations of Cirrhosis of the Liver

i. Telangiectasias

Telangiectasia

A. Cutaneous manifestation of cirrhosis of the liver

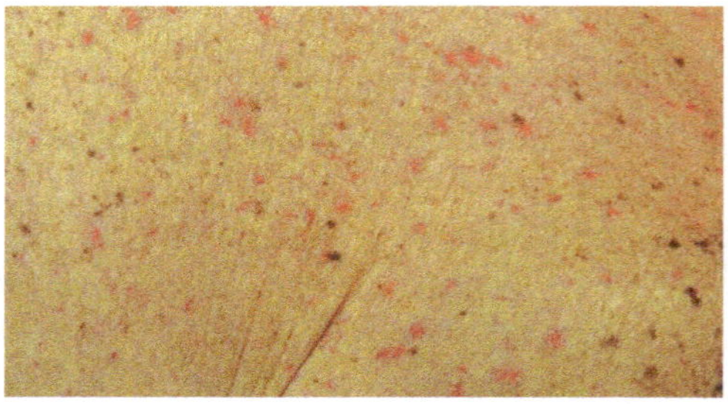

Telangiectasia
Photograph courtesy of SpringerImages Database, Springer Publishing Company

ii. Spider Angiomas

Spider angiomas
  A. Cutaneous manifestation of cirrhosis of the liver

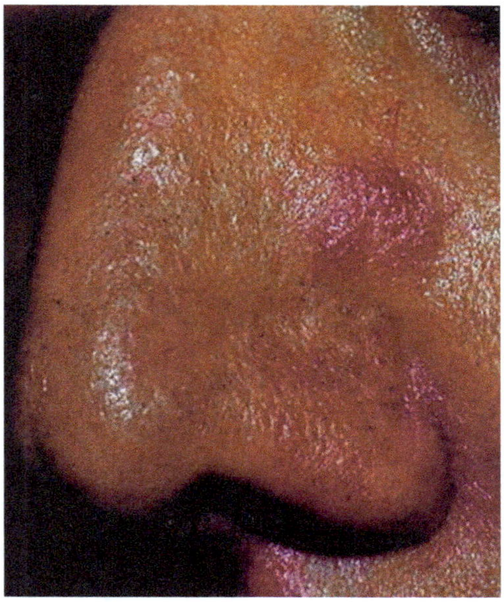

Spider angiomas
Photograph courtesy of SpringerImages Database, Springer Publishing Company

iii. Palmar Erythema

Palmar erythema
  A. Cutaneous manifestation of cirrhosis of the liver

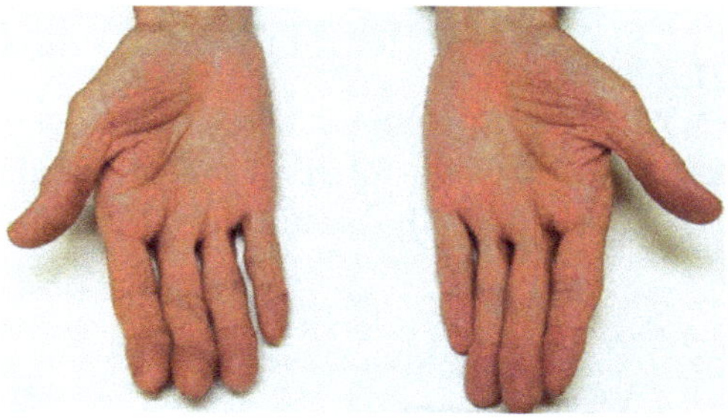

Palmar erythema
Photograph courtesy of SpringerImages Database, Springer Publishing Company

iv. Terry's Nails

Terry's nails

A. Cutaneous manifestation of cirrhosis of the liver
B. Proximal 2/3 of nail bed of all fingernails is white, which obscures the lunulae
C. Distal 1–2 mm of the nail bed is pink
D. Present in up to 82 % of patients with cirrhosis

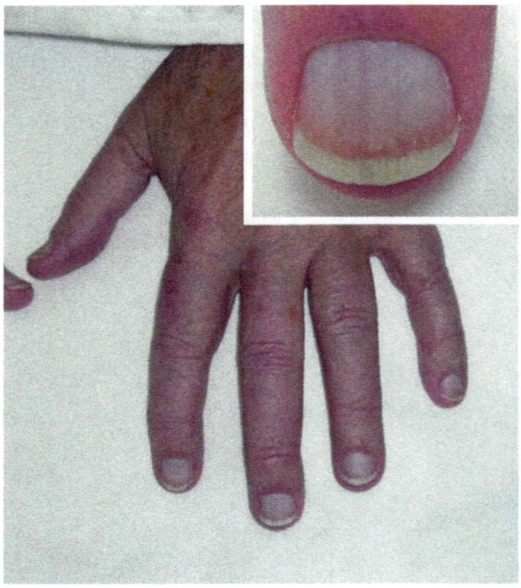

Terry's nails
Photograph courtesy of SpringerImages Database, Springer Publishing Company

v. Hemochromatosis

Hemochromatosis

A. Generalized bronze hyperpigmentation (due to melanin, not iron)
B. Accumulation of iron stores may lead to cirrhosis of the liver, diabetes, cardiac dysfunction

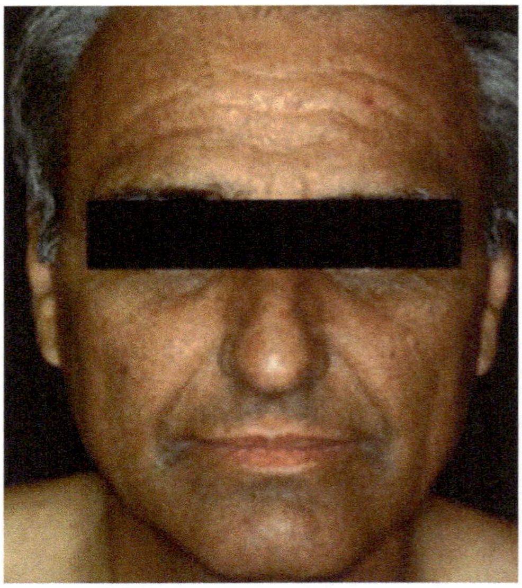

Hemochromatosis
Photograph courtesy of SpringerImages Database, Springer Publishing Company

Hemochromatosis
  A. Diffuse hyperpigmentation

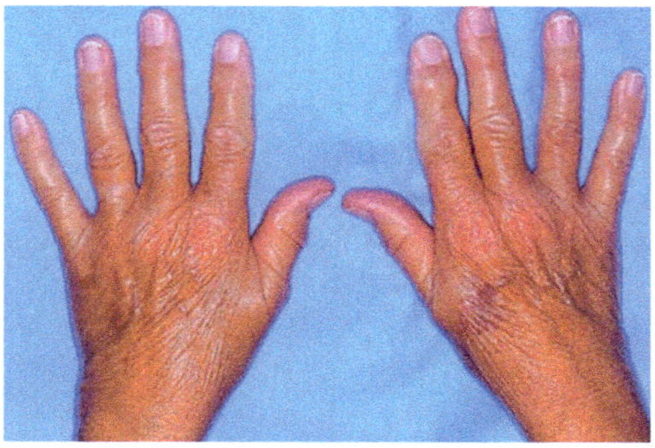

Hemochromatosis
Photograph courtesy of SpringerImages Database, Springer Publishing Company

vi. Wilson's Disease

Wilson's disease
  A. Autosomal recessive disorder of copper metabolism leading to accumulation of copper within internal organs (especially liver, cornea, and brain)
  B. Hepatic damage may result in cirrhosis
  C. Kayser-Fleisher ring – gold brown or green circle of copper in Descemet's membrane at periphery of the cornea
  D. Pretibial hyperpigmentation
  E. Neurologic symptoms
  F. Blue lunulae

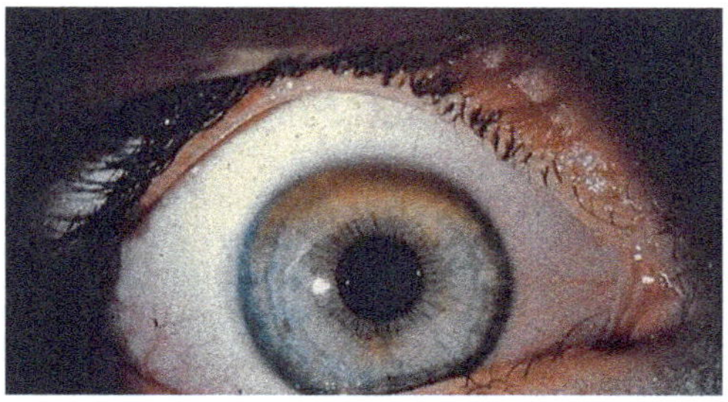

Wilson's disease
Photograph courtesy of SpringerImages Database, Springer Publishing Company

Wilson's disease
  A. Blue lunulae

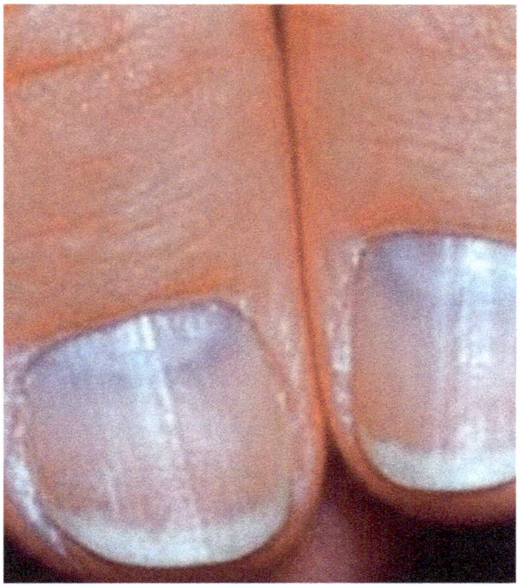

Wilson's disease
Photograph courtesy of SpringerImages Database, Springer Publishing Company

49 Cutaneous Manifestations Renal Disease

a. Nephrogenic Systemic Fibrosis

Nephrogenic systemic fibrosis

A. Patterned plaques: red to hyperpigmented (purple–brown) thick indurated "cobblestone" plaques symmetrically on the extremities (lower greater than upper) and trunk
B. Joint contractures and loss of mobility as a result of the confluent arrangement of plaques or thickening and induration of the skin
C. Cobblestone skin: marked woody induration and thickening of the skin with peau d'orange appearance
D. Yellow scleral plaques
E. Systemic fibrosis of heart, lungs, skeletal muscle

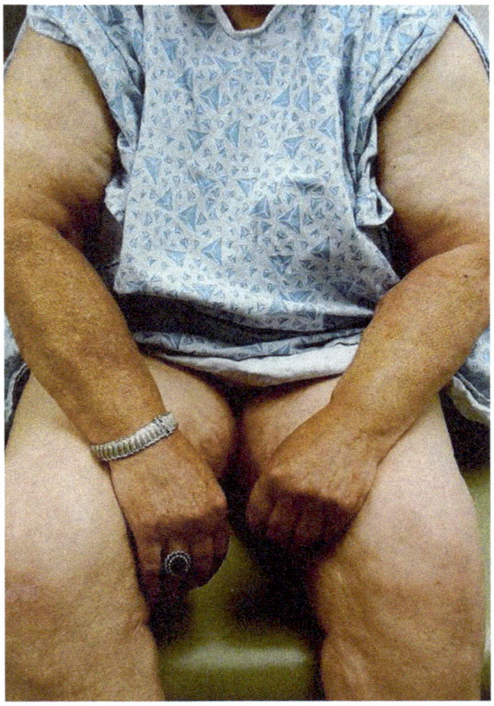

Nephrogenic systemic fibrosis
Photograph courtesy of SpringerImages Database, Springer Publishing Company

H.M. Gloster, Jr. et al., *Absolute Dermatology Review: Mastering Clinical Conditions on the Dermatology Recertification Exam*, DOI 10.1007/978-3-319-03218-4_49,

Nephrogenic systemic fibrosis

A. Hyperpigmentation, induration, and tethering of the skin and fixed flexion contractures of the fingers and elbows

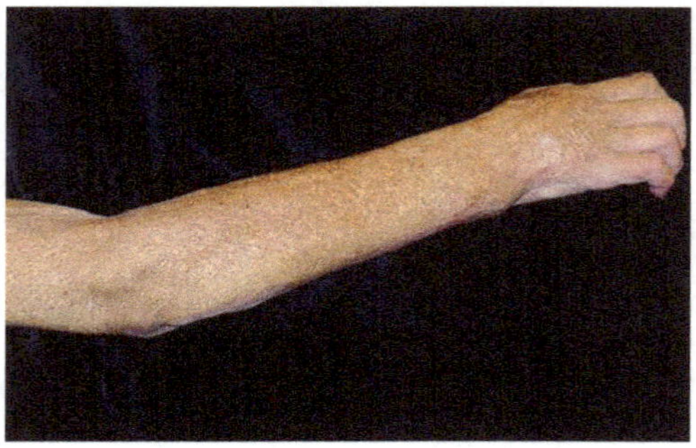

Nephrogenic systemic fibrosis
Photograph courtesy of SpringerImages Database, Springer Publishing Company

Nephrogenic systemic fibrosis

A. Indurated skin with peau d'orange changes and cobblestone appearance and flexion contractures of the knees

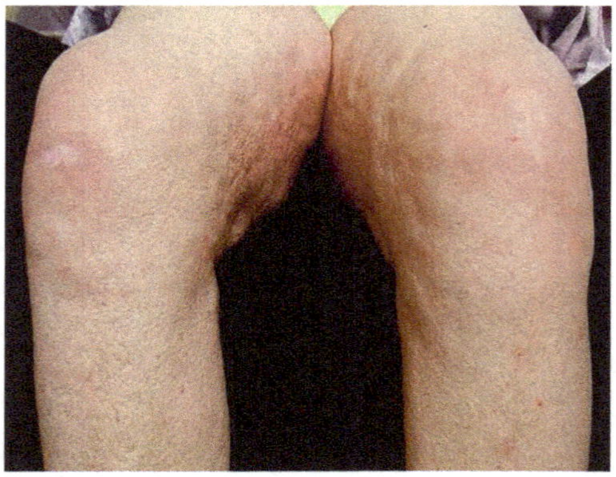

Nephrogenic systemic fibrosis
Photograph courtesy of SpringerImages Database, Springer Publishing Company

Nephrogenic systemic fibrosis

A. Yellow scleral plaques

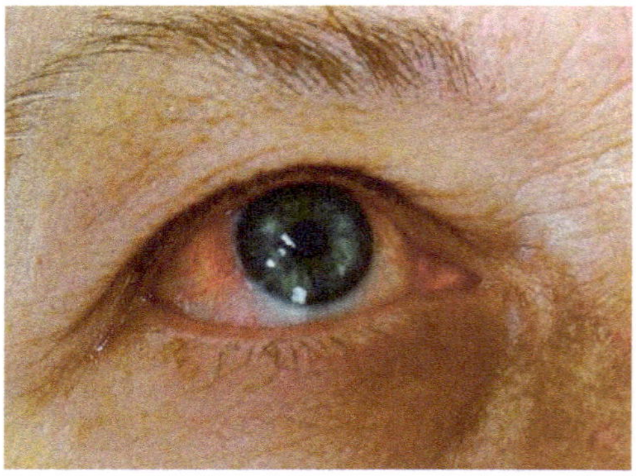

Nephrogenic systemic fibrosis
Photograph courtesy of SpringerImages Database, Springer Publishing Company

b. Acquired Perforating Dermatosis (Kyrle's Disease)

Acquired perforating dermatosis (Kyrle's disease, also see Chap. 21, section 123a)

A. Associated with diabetes (most patients with diabetes have nephropathy) or pruritus of renal failure (most patients have chronic renal failure and are on dialysis)
B. Most commonly on the lower extremities of adults
C. Pruritic papules and nodules with a central keratotic core
D. Late lesions are often excoriated papules with central crusted craters or depressed, atrophic, hyperpigmented scars

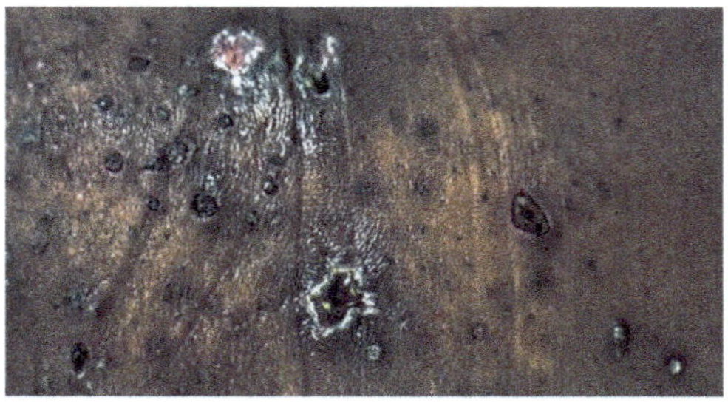

Acquired perforating dermatosis (Kyrle's disease) Photograph courtesy of SpringerImages Database, Springer Publishing Company

Cutaneous Manifestations of Internal Malignancy

50

a. Acanthosis Nigricans

Acanthosis nigricans

A. Velvety hyperpigmentation of flexural surfaces of the neck, axilla, and groin most commonly and less often on extensor surfaces (elbows, knees, knuckles)
B. Usually symmetrical and bilateral
C. May be associated with adenocarcinoma of the stomach (less commonly other gastrointestinal or genitourinary sites), usually in the setting of a rapid onset of acanthosis nigricans and skin tags, tripe palms (ridged, wrinkled, velvety lesions on palms), and multiple seborrheic keratoses (sign of Leser-Trelat: the sudden appearance or rapid increase in size of seborrheic keratoses in association with cancer of the gastrointestinal tract)

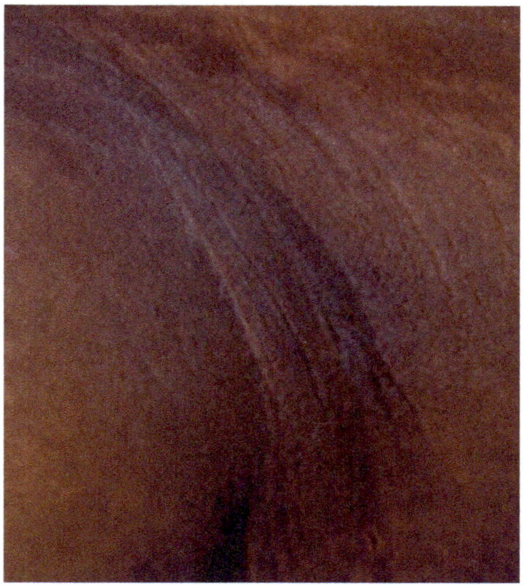

Acanthosis nigricans
Photograph courtesy of SpringerImages Database, Springer Publishing Company

b. Bazex Syndrome (Acrokeratosis Neoplastica)

Bazex's syndrome (acrokeratosis neoplastica)

A. Psoriasiform, violaceous plaques on acral areas (hands and feet, keratoderma may develop with time) and face (especially nose, helices, and cheeks)
B. Nail dystrophy in 75 % (longitudinal and horizontal nail ridging)
C. Associated with carcinoma of upper aerodigestive tract (pharynx, larynx, esophagus)

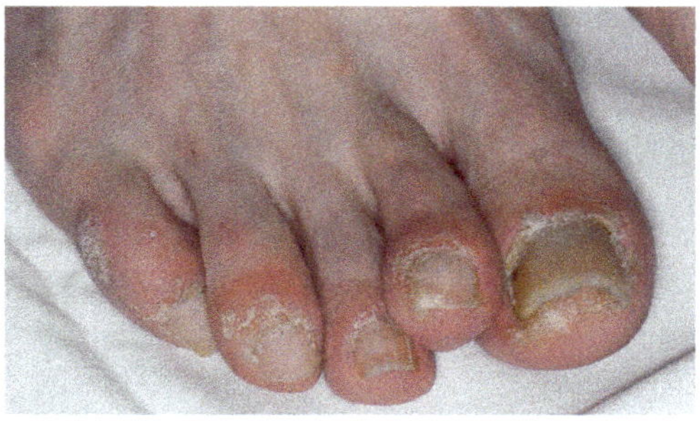

Bazex syndrome (acrokeratosis neoplastica)
Photograph courtesy of the Mayo Clinic Department of Dermatology, Rochester, MN

H.M. Gloster, Jr. et al., *Absolute Dermatology Review: Mastering Clinical Conditions on the Dermatology Recertification Exam*,
DOI 10.1007/978-3-319-03218-4_50, © Springer International Publishing Switzerland 2016

Bazex's syndrome (acrokeratosis neoplastica)

A. Psoriasiform plaques on the feet

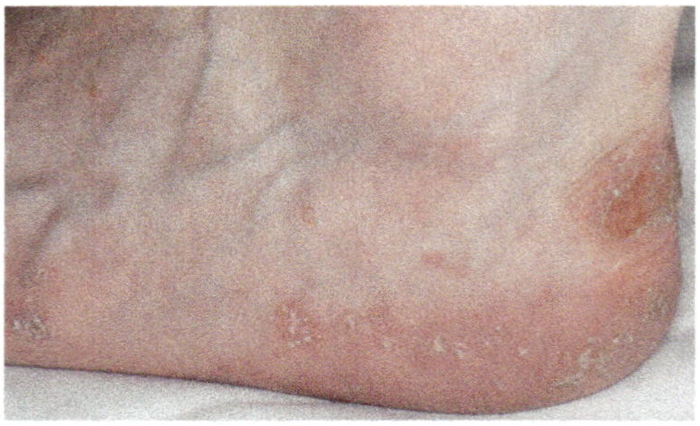

Bazex syndrome (acrokeratosis neoplastica)
Photograph courtesy of the Mayo Clinic Department of Dermatology, Rochester, MN

Bazex's syndrome (acrokeratosis neoplastica)

A. Psoriasiform plaques on the palm

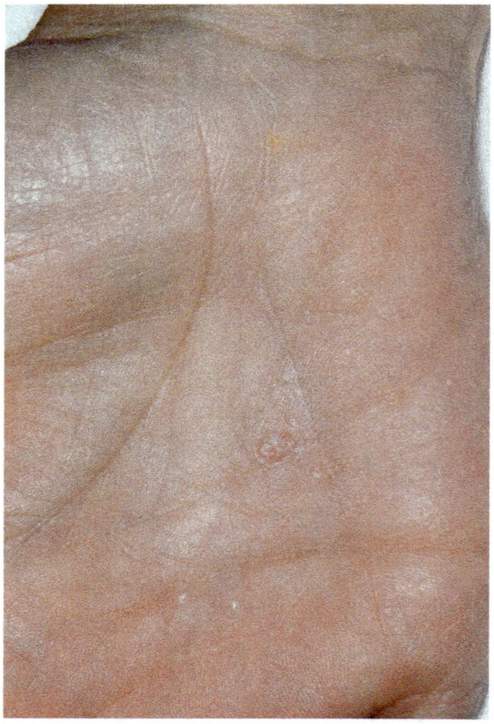

Bazex syndrome (acrokeratosis neoplastica)
Photograph courtesy of the Mayo Clinic Department of Dermatology, Rochester, MN

c. Erythema Gyratum Repens

Erythema gyratum repens

A. Concentric, migratory, gyrate erythematous scaly plaques giving the appearance of grain of wood
B. Plaques spread rapidly, advancing up to 1 cm/day
C. Most common underlying malignancy is lung cancer (also breast, esophagus, and stomach)
D. Resolves when neoplasm is treated

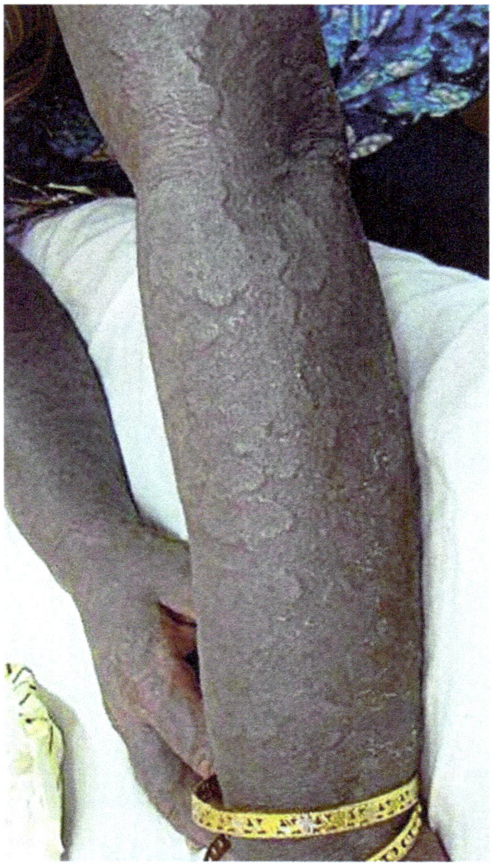

Erythema gyratum repens
Photograph courtesy of SpringerImages Database, Springer Publishing Company

d. Necrolytic Migratory Erythema

Necrolytic migratory erythema

A. Cutaneous manifestation of glucagonoma syndrome—glucagon-secreting islet cell pancreatic tumor and less commonly other liver or other gastrointestinal disorders
B. Superficial epidermal necrosis occurs, leading to flaccid bullae and crusted erythematous eroded patches and plaques, which may have a circinate, polycyclic, or annular appearance
C. Distribution: flexural folds and intertriginous areas (perineum, groin, axilla, buttocks, thighs), distal extremities (red shiny erosive finger-tips), periorificial
D. May resemble intertrigo or seborrheic dermatitis

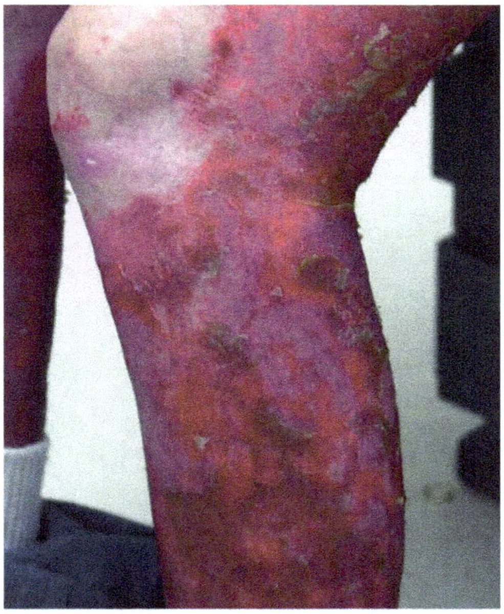

Necrolytic migratory erythema
Photograph courtesy of SpringerImages Database, Springer Publishing Company

Necrolytic migratory erythema

A. Plaques may have a circinate, polycyclic, or annular appearance

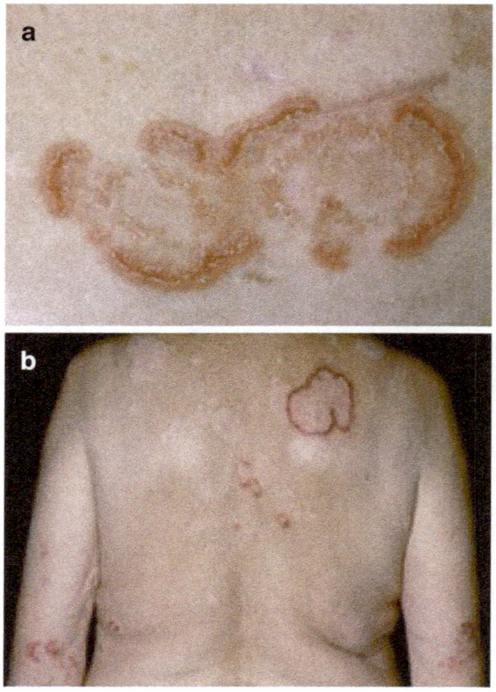

Necrolytic migratory erythema
Photograph courtesy of SpringerImages Database, Springer Publishing Company

Necrolytic migratory erythema

A. Periorificial lesions are common with angular cheilitis and glossitis

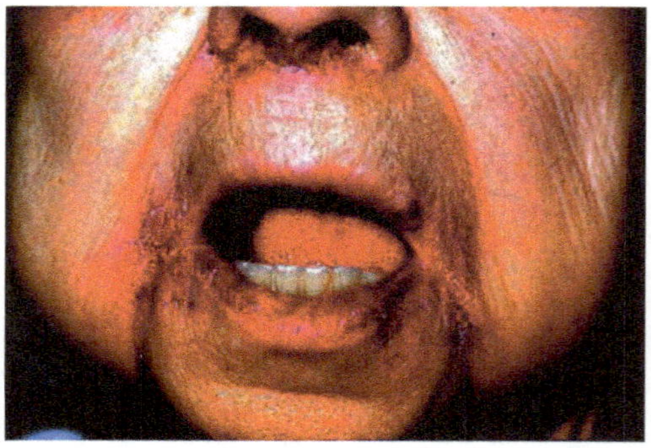

Necrolytic migratory erythema
Photograph courtesy of SpringerImages Database, Springer Publishing Company

e. Acquired Hypertrichosis Lagunosa

Acquired hypertrichosis lanuginosa (malignant down)

A. Growth of silky, nonpigmented lanugo hairs on the face or a generalized distribution, usually comes before the tumor
B. Angular cheilitis or glossitis may be associated
C. Associated with lung, colon, breast cancer

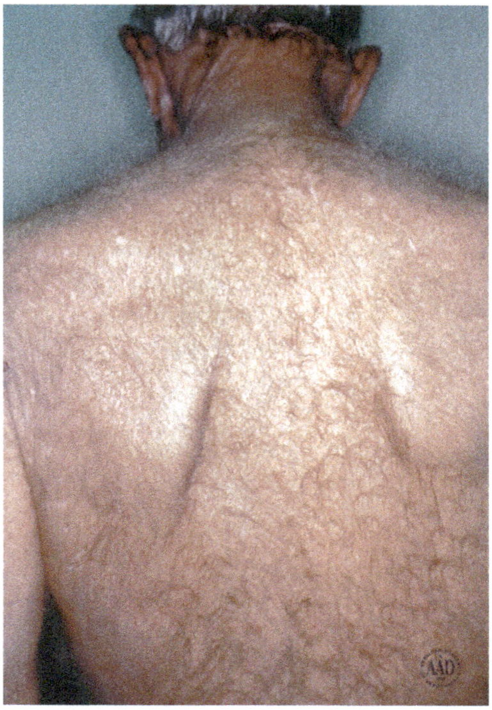

Acquired hypertrichosis lagunosa
Photograph courtesy of the American Academy of Dermatology

f. Paraneoplastic Pemphigus

Paraneoplastic pemphigus (also see Chap. 3, section 24)

A. Intractable stomatitis most commonly associated with non-Hodgkin lymphoma and chronic lymphocytic leukemia

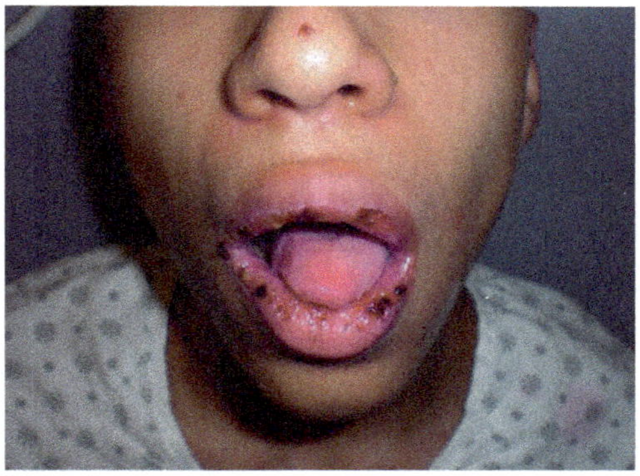

Paraneoplastic pemphigus
Photograph courtesy of SpringerImages Database, Springer Publishing Company

g. Peutz-Jeghers Syndrome

Peutz-Jeghers syndrome

A. Autosomal dominant
B. Melanotic mucocutaneous macules on the lips and around the eyes, nostrils, buccal mucosa, acral skin, and perianal area
C. Gastrointestinal polyps, which may hemorrhage
D. Increased risk of gastrointestinal, breast, and ovarian cancer

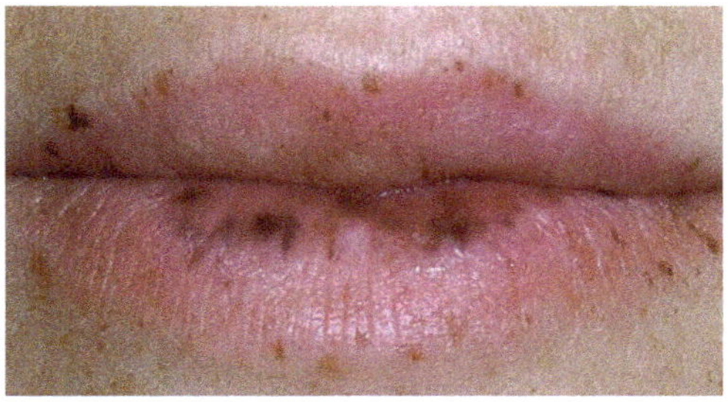

Peutz-Jeghers syndrome
Photograph courtesy of SpringerImages Database, Springer Publishing Company

h. Muir-Torre Syndrome

Muir-Torre syndrome

A. Autosomal dominant
B. Sebaceous neoplasms
   1. Sebaceous hyperplasia (top figure)—small, waxy, firm, usually multiple yellow papules typically on the face
   2. Sebaceous adenoma (bottom figure)—solitary, smooth, firm, waxy yellow, superficial epidermal nodule in older patients
   3. Sebaceous carcinoma
C. Associated with gastrointestinal malignancies, especially colonic adenocarcinoma

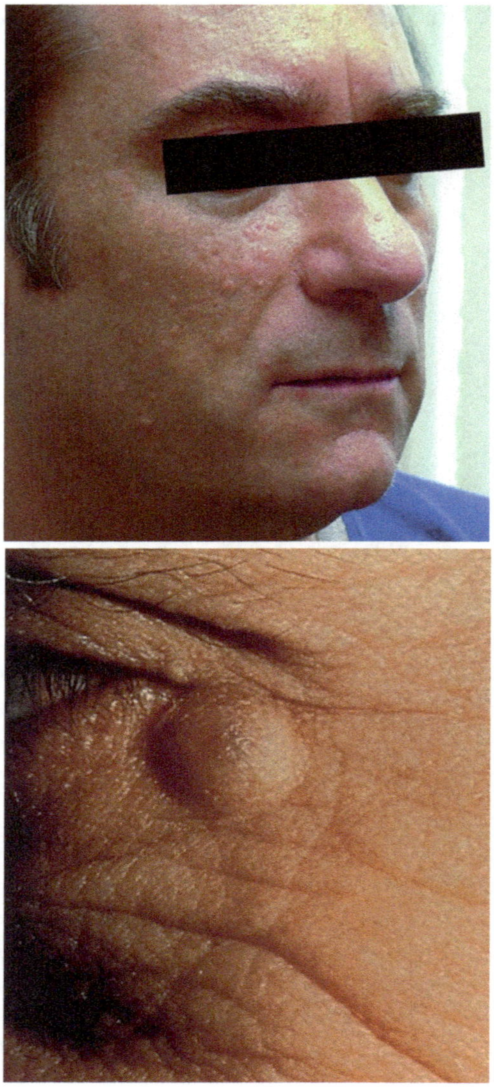

Muir-Torre syndrome
Photograph courtesy of SpringerImages Database, Springer Publishing Company

Muir-Torre Syndrome

A. Multiple keratoacanthomas
   1. Rapidly enlarging dome-shaped pink or skin-colored nodule with rolled shouldered border and central crater filled with a keratotic core
   2. Usually occurs on sun-exposed skin of white middle-aged to elderly adults
   3. Characteristically undergoes spontaneous regression within weeks to several months

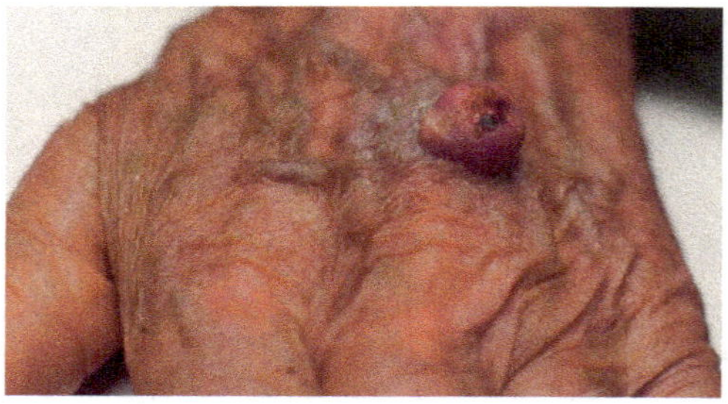

Muir-Torre syndrome
Photograph courtesy of SpringerImages Database, Springer Publishing Company

Chapter VIII

Genodermatoses and Developmental Anomalies

51 Genodermatoses

a. Darier's Disease

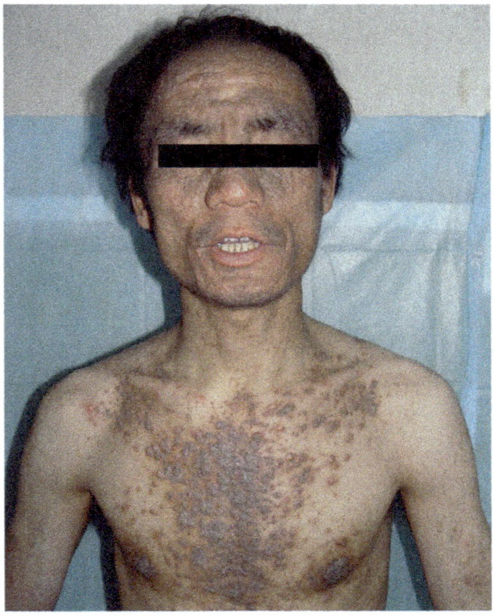

Darier's disease
Photograph courtesy of SpringerImages Database, Springer Publishing Company

Darier's disease

A. Autosomal dominant disorder, peak onset childhood or adolescence
B. Hyperkeratotic crusted greasy red–brown to yellow, pruritic papules and plaques
C. Lesions favor seborrheic areas (central chest, upper back, scalp margins, face), lateral neck, intertriginous areas (axilla, groin, inframammary), and extensor surfaces of the extremities

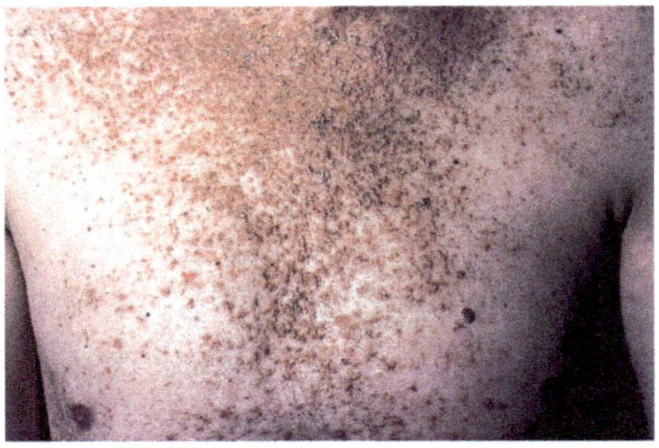

Darier's disease
Photograph courtesy of SpringerImages Database, Springer Publishing Company

Darier's disease

A. Hyperkeratotic crusted greasy red–brown to yellow, pruritic papules and plaques on the chest

H.M. Gloster, Jr. et al., *Absolute Dermatology Review: Mastering Clinical Conditions on the Dermatology Recertification Exam*,
DOI 10.1007/978-3-319-03218-4_51,

Darier's disease

A. Acral keratoses
   1. Flat-top papules on dorsal hands and feet
   2. Keratotic palmar and plantar papules

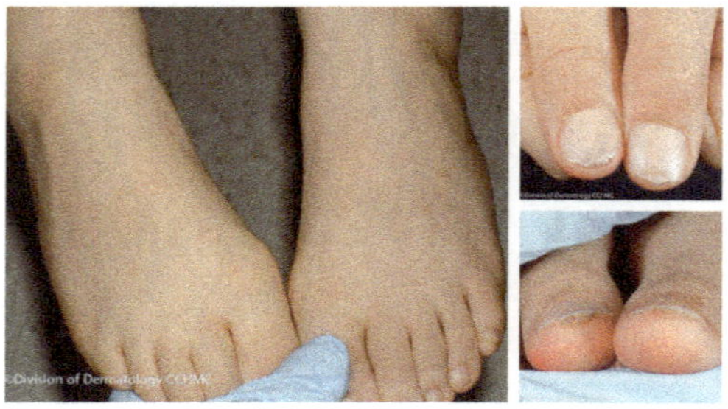

Darier's disease
Photograph courtesy of Kara Shah, M.D, PhD, CCHMC (Cincinnati, OH), Department of Dermatology

Darier's disease

A. Cobblestone mucosal papules: white oral mucosal papules in a cobblestone pattern most commonly on the hard palate (also seen in Cowden's syndrome)

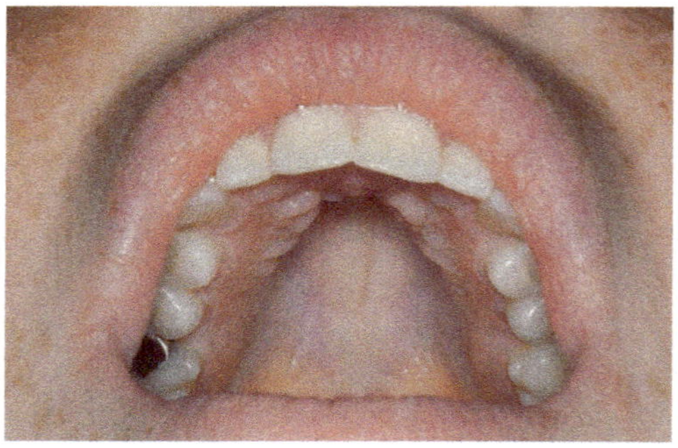

Darier's disease
Photograph courtesy of Mayo Clinic, Department of Dermatology, Rochester MN

Darier's disease

A. Cobblestone mucosal papules of Darier's: white oral mucosal papules in a cobblestone pattern on the hard palate

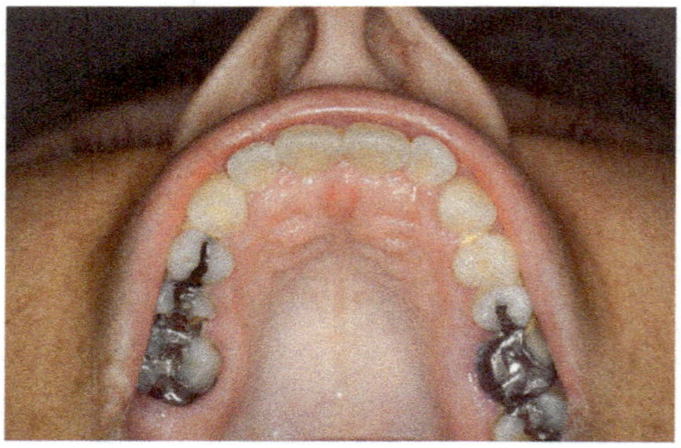

Darier's disease
Photograph courtesy of Mayo Clinic, Department of Dermatology, Rochester MN

Darier's disease

A. Nail findings
   1. Alternating longitudinal red or white lines and brittle nails that break distally resulting in v-shaped notches of the distal margin of the nails
   2. Longitudinal ridges and thickening and wedge-shaped subungual hyperkeratosis may also be seen

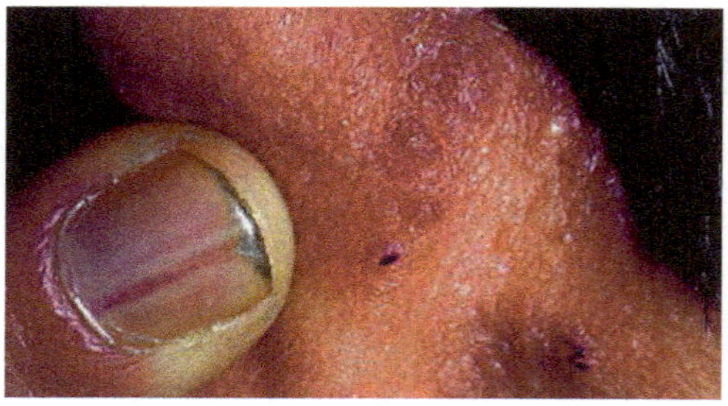

Darier's disease
Photograph courtesy of SpringerImages Database, Springer Publishing Company

b. Ichthyosis

i. Ichthyosis Vulgaris

Ichthyosis vulgaris

A. Autosomal dominant, onset in infancy or childhood, improves with age
B. Fine, adherent white scales ("fish like scales") mainly on the extensor extremities and trunk sparing moist areas such as flexures and the groin
C. Larger plate-like scales are characteristic on the lower legs
D. Hyperlinear palms and soles, furrowed heels

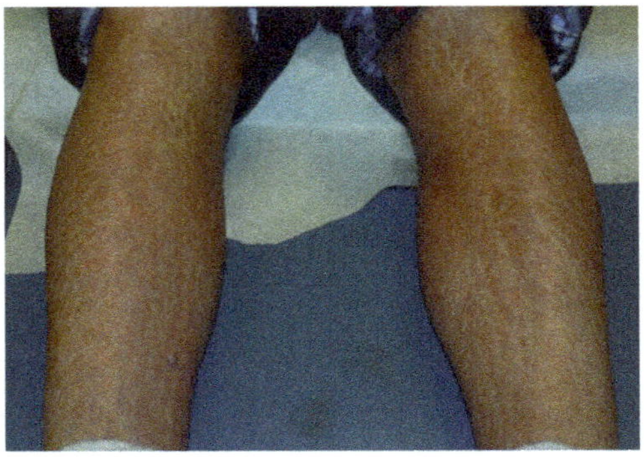

Ichthyosis vulgaris
Photograph courtesy of SpringerImages Database, Springer Publishing Company

ii. Lamellar Ichthyosis

Lamellar ichthyosis

A. Autosomal recessive, onset at birth, persists throughout life, severe form of ichthyosis
B. A collodion membrane at birth is replaced after a few weeks by large, thick, plate-like brown scales that form a mosaic bark-like pattern
C. Prominent on the trunk and forehead, the cheeks may be spared
D. Associated with heat intolerance (due to constriction of sweat ducts), scarring alopecia, ectropion, and eclabium (due to tautness of facial skin)

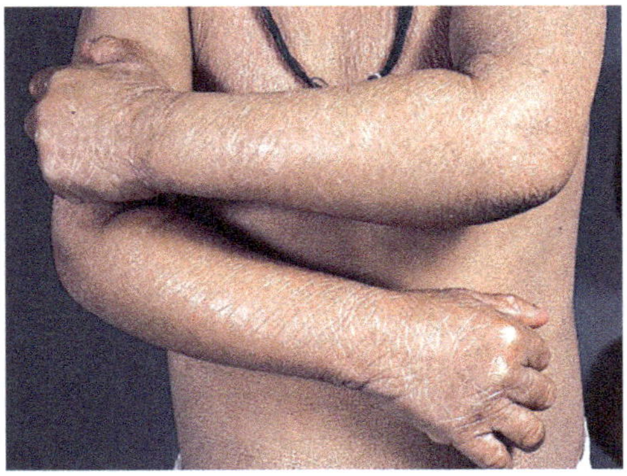

Lamellar ichthyosis
Photograph courtesy of SpringerImages Database, Springer Publishing Company

Lamellar ichthyosis

A. Large, thick, plate-like brown scales that form a mosaic bark-like pattern

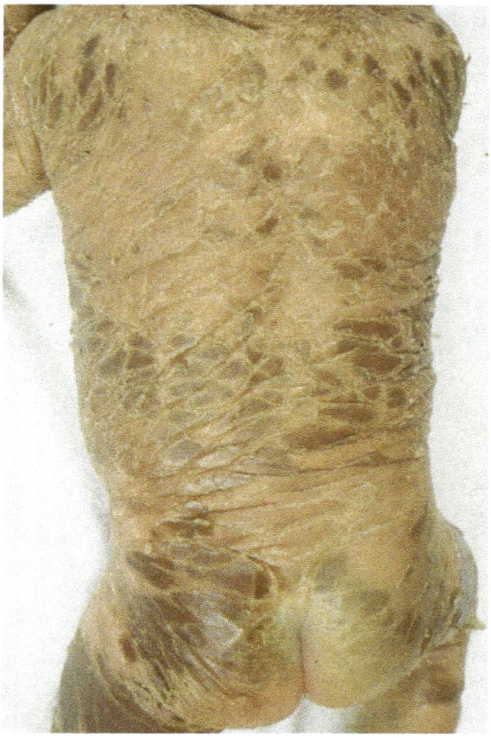

Lamellar ichthyosis
Photograph courtesy of SpringerImages Database, Springer Publishing Company

iii. X Linked Ichthyosis

X-linked ichthyosis

A. Steroid sulfatase deficiency results in increased cholesterol 3-sulfate in epidermis
B. X-linked recessive inheritance (transmitted by asymptomatic female carriers, males only are affected), onset infancy
C. Fine to large, polygonal, dark adherent scales on the extremities, trunk, lateral face, and neck ("dirty neck disease")—sparing of the face except the preauricular area is a pathognomonic feature
D. Spares palms and soles

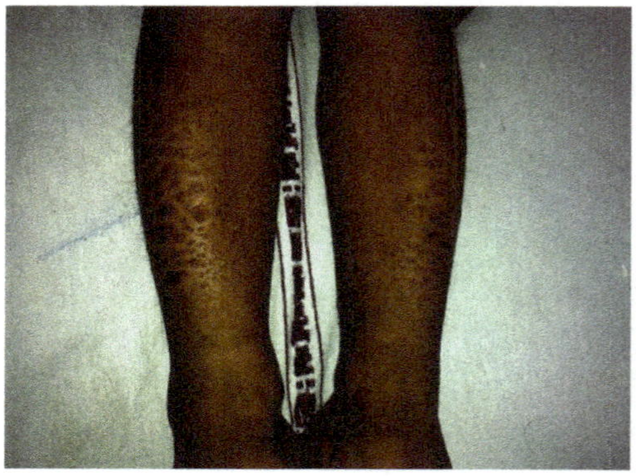

X linked ichthyosis
Photograph courtesy of SpringerImages Database, Springer Publishing Company

X-linked ichthyosis

A. "Dirty" hyperpigmented scale on the extensor surface of the upper extremities

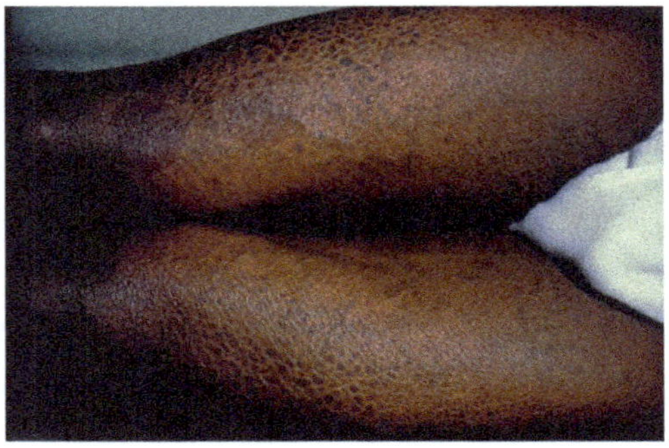

X linked ichthyosis
Photograph courtesy of SpringerImages Database, Springer Publishing Company

iv. Bullous Congenital Ichthyosiform Erythroderma

Bullous congenital ichthyosiform erythroderma (Epidermolytic hyperkeratosis)

A. Autosomal dominant disorder with onset at birth
B. At birth, congenital erythroderma with blisters and erosions with widespread areas of denuded skin
C. Later in life:
   1. Skin fragility, blistering, and erythema decrease whereas severe hyperkeratosis increases
   2. Hyperkeratosis with cobblestone pattern, most prominent over joints
   3. Ridging of flexures (corrugated scale with prominence at flexures)
   4. Variable erythroderma, palmoplantar involvement, blistering
   5. Associated with skin infections, odor, gait and posture abnormalities, severe quality of life, and social problems due to disfigurement and malodor

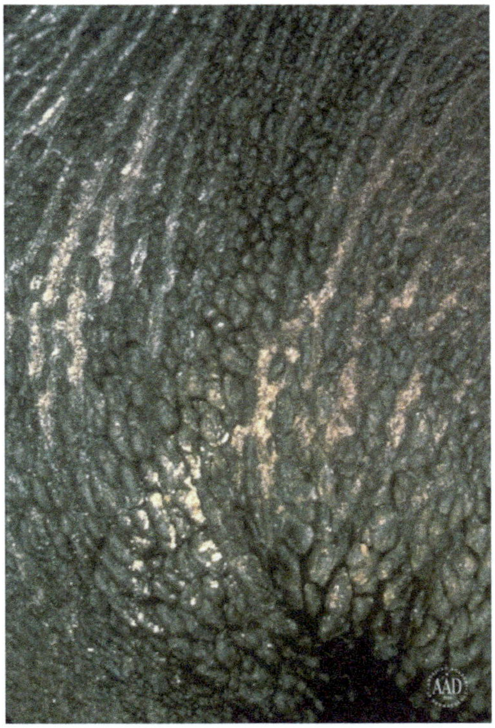

Bullous congenital ichthyosiform erythroderma
Photograph courtesy of the American Academy of Dermatology

Bullous congenital ichthyosiform erythroderma (Epidermolytic hyperkeratosis)

A. Ridging of flexures (corrugated scale with prominence at flexures)

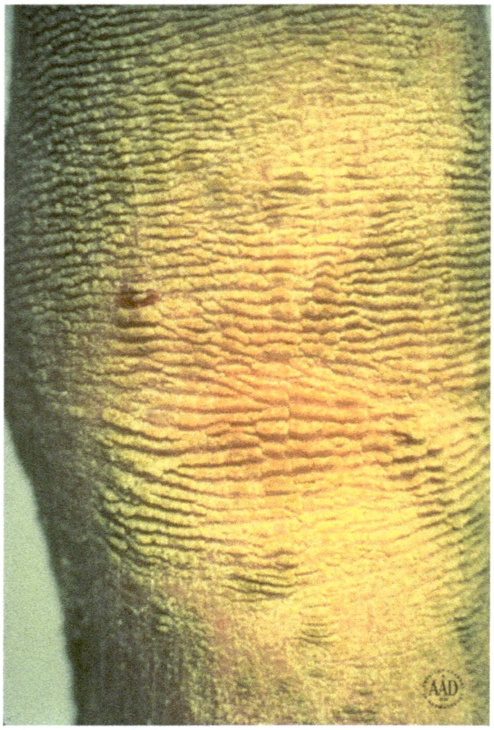

Bullous congenital ichthyosiform erythroderma
Photograph courtesy of the American Academy of Dermatology

v. Netherton's Syndrome

Netherton's syndrome

A. Congenital (autosomal recessive) erythroderma with scaling (figures A, B, and C)
B. Patients may also have atopic dermatitis (figure D)
C. Trichorrhexis invaginata (bamboo hair)—ball and socket appearance of the hair shaft (figure E) resulting in partial alopecia with short, fragile, thin, spiky, and broken hair (figure F)
D. Ichthyosis linearis circumflexa—serpiginous and migratory red plaques bordered by double-edge scale (figure G)

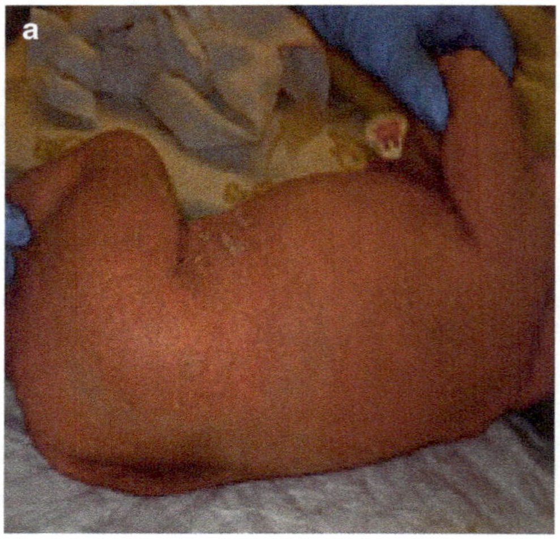

Netherton's syndrome
Photograph courtesy of SpringerImages Database, Springer Publishing Company

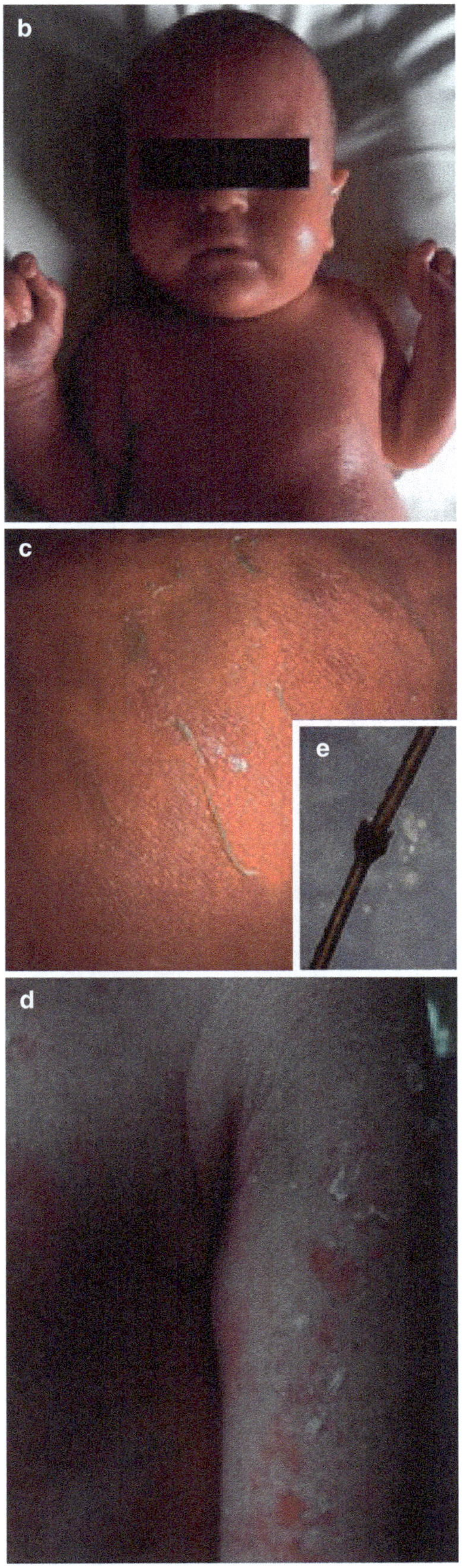

Netherton's syndrome (continued)

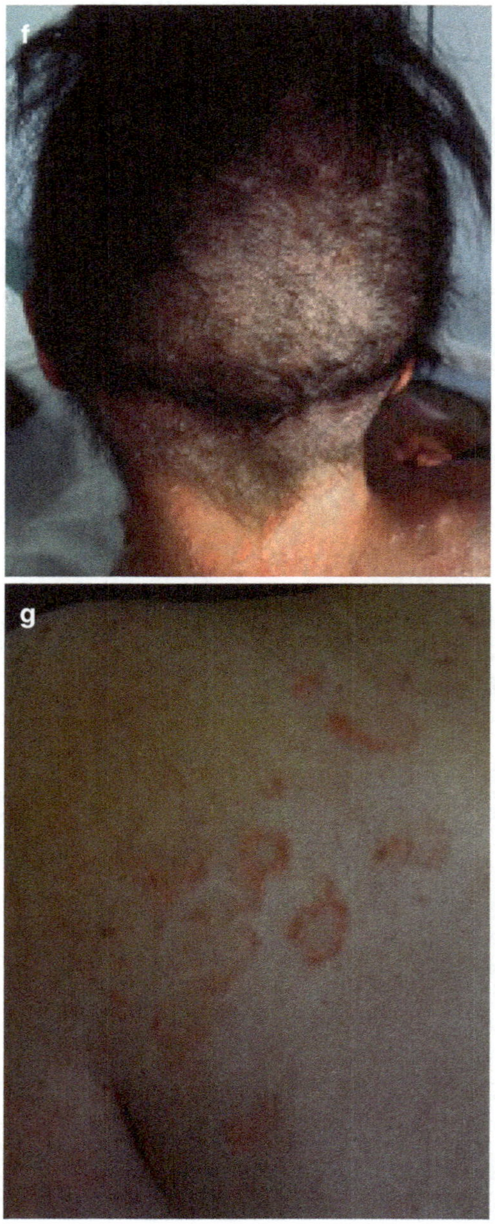

Netherton's syndrome (continued)

c. Neurofibromatosis Type 1

Neurofibromatosis (NF) Type 1

A. Neurofibromas

1. Soft skin-colored to pink-tan dome-shaped or polypoid papules and nodules
2. A diagnostic criteria for NF: greater than or equal to two neurofibromas of any type or one plexiform neurofibroma
3. Develop around pubery
4. Invaginate with pressure: "button hole sign"

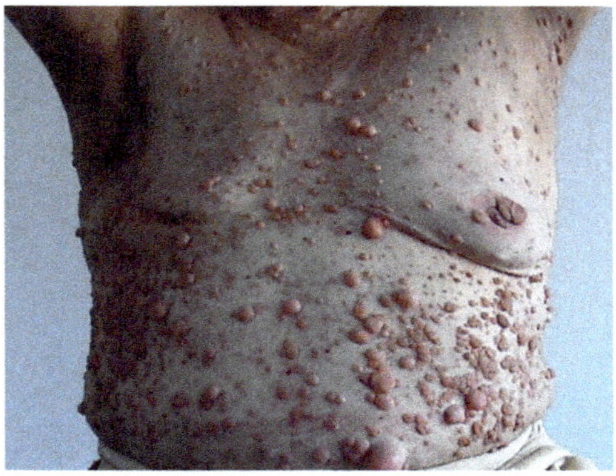

Neurofibromatosis type 1
Photograph courtesy of SpringerImages Database, Springer Publishing Company

Neurofibromatosis Type 1

A. Plexiform neurofibroma

1. May track along nerves to create tender firm subcutaneous nodules resembling a "bag of worms" on palpation
2. May present as a hyperpigmented plaque with hypertrichosis resembling a congenital nevus a sharply demarcated red brown plaque, or a poorly defined sagging pink mass
3. May transform into neurofibrosarcomas

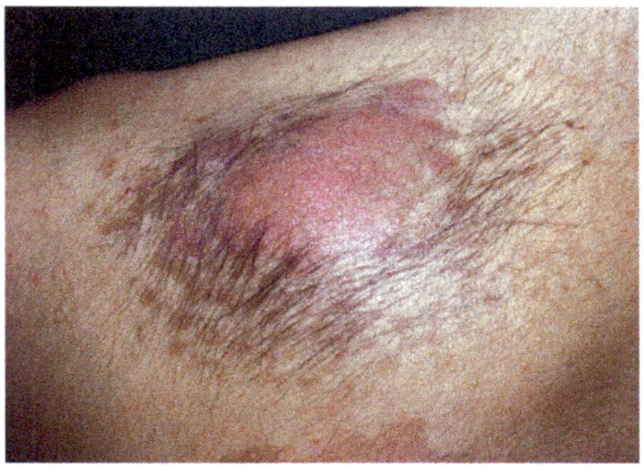

Neurofibromatosis type 1
Photograph courtesy of SpringerImages Database, Springer Publishing Company

Neurofibromatosis Type 1

A. Café au lait macules

1. Oval light to medium brown patches with regular borders and uniform pigment
2. A diagnostic criteria for NF: greater than or equal to six café au lait macules over 5 mm in diameter before puberty and over 15 mm in postpubertal individuals
3. Not often present at birth, apparent during the first year of life

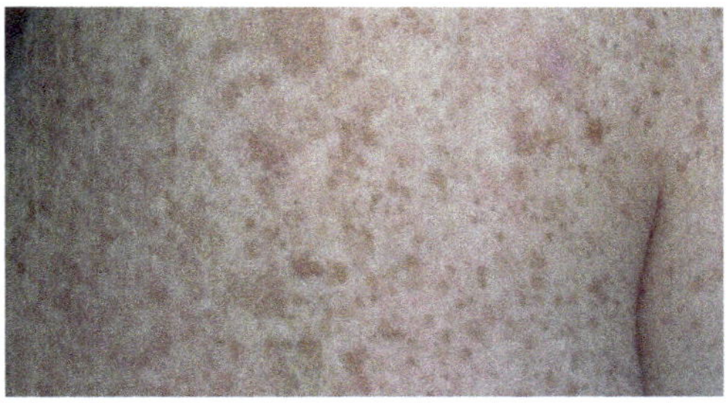

Neurofibromatosis type 1
Photograph courtesy of SpringerImages Database, Springer Publishing Company

Neurofibromatosis Type 1

A. Axillary freckling (Crowe's sign)
   1. A diagnostic criteria for NF: numerous 1–3 mm macules which develop at 4–6 years of age
   2. A flesh-colored neurofibroma, numerous café-au-lait macule, and axillary freckling are illustrated in this figure

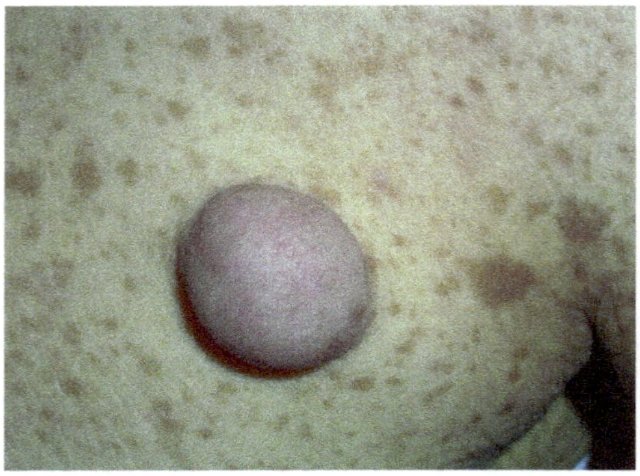

Neurofibromatosis type 1
Photograph courtesy of SpringerImages Database, Springer Publishing Company

Neurofibromatosis Type 1

A. Lisch nodules (iris hamartomas)
   1. A diagnostic criteria for NF: greater than or equal to two 1–2 mm yellow brown papules of the iris
   2. Appear by the age of 5–6 years

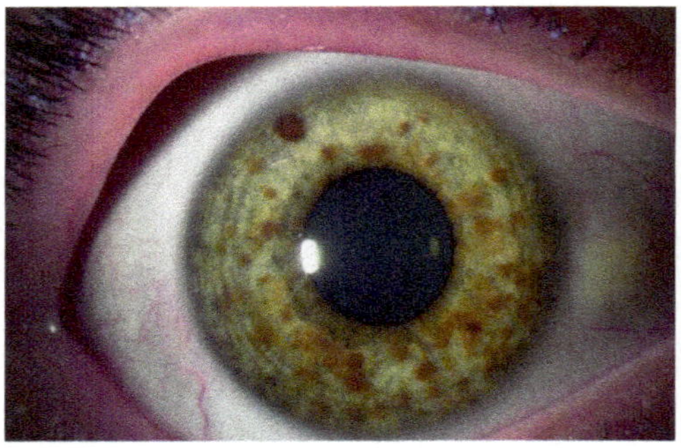

Neurofibromatosis type 1
Photograph courtesy of SpringerImages Database, Springer Publishing Company

d. Tuberous Sclerosis

Tuberous sclerosis

A. Ash leaf spots
   1. Present in 90–100 % of patients
   2. May be diagnosed with Wood's light
   3. Occur at birth or first few months of life
   4. Typically polygonal and lance-ovate-shaped (rounded at one end and tapered at other end) hypopigmented macules
   5. Extracutaneous features of Tuberous sclerosis
      a. Oral—gingival fibromas, dental enamel pits
      b. Neurological—seizures, mental retardation, neuropsychiatric disturbances, multiple calcified subependymal nodules along ventricular surface (CT scan)
      c. Hamartomas—retinal, internal organs (brain, heart, kidney, lungs)

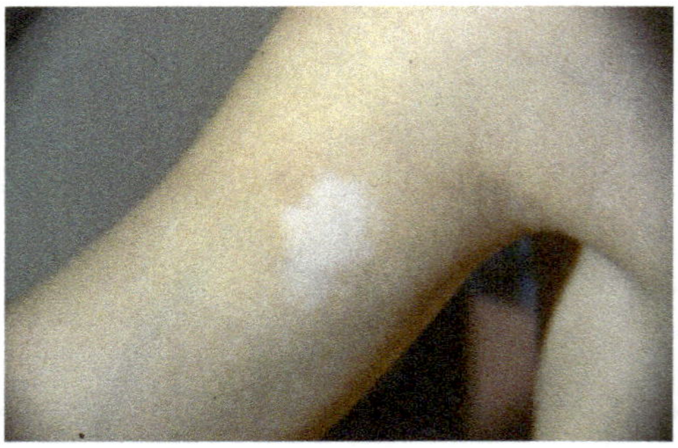

Tuberous sclerosis
Photograph courtesy of SpringerImages Database, Springer Publishing Company

Tuberous sclerosis

A. Angiofibromas
   1. Most common on the central face
   2. Present in 80 % of patients
   3. Occur in the first 2 years of life
   4. Fibrous plaque of the forehead is a large variant of angiofibroma seen in 20 % of patients

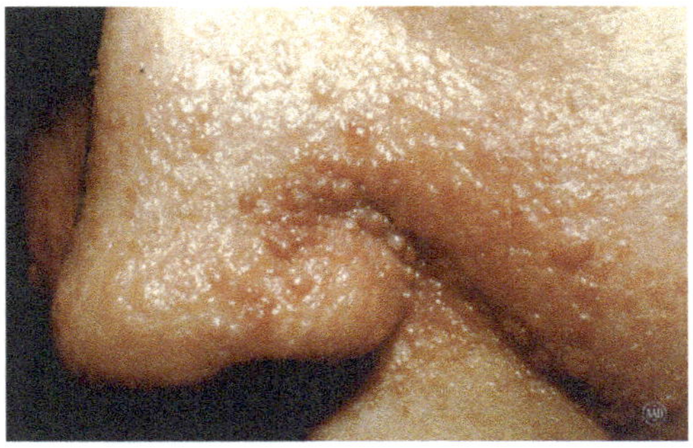

Tuberous sclerosis
Photograph courtesy of SpringerImages Database, Springer Publishing Company

Tuberous sclerosis

A. Angiofibromas: firm papules most common on the central face

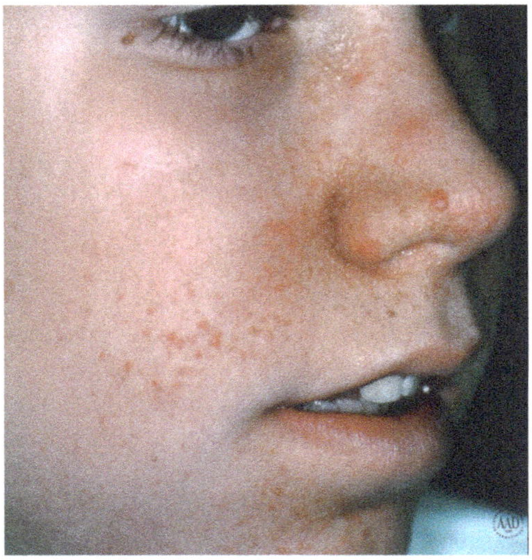

Tuberous sclerosis
Photograph courtesy of SpringerImages Database, Springer Publishing Company

Tuberous sclerosis

A. Shagreen patch
   1. Skin-colored, hyperpigmented, or occasionally hypopigmented plaques with a surface like leather or pigskin on the trunk or limbs
   2. Connective tissue nevus
   3. Present in 40–59 % of patients
   4. Usually occurs at 2 years of age

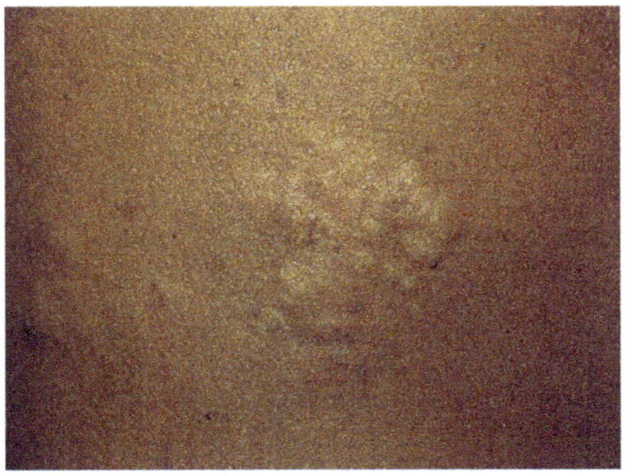

Tuberous sclerosis
Photograph courtesy of SpringerImages Database, Springer Publishing Company

Tuberous sclerosis

A. Periungual fibromas (Koenen's tumor)
   1. Present in 30–60 % of patients
   2. Begin in late childhood
   3. Most common on the periungual area around the fingernails and toenails

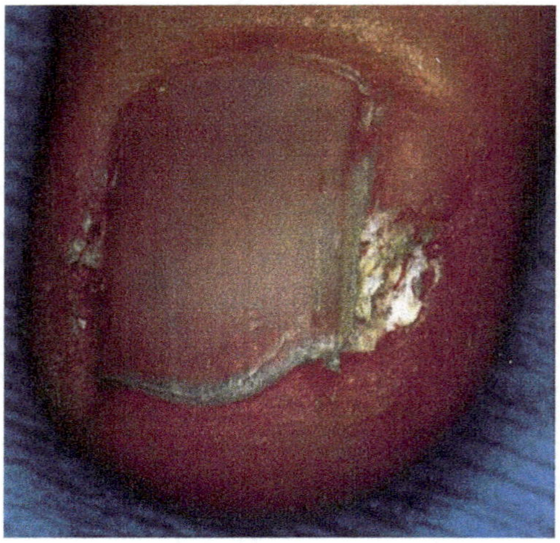

Tuberous sclerosis
Photograph courtesy of SpringerImages Database, Springer Publishing Company

e. Incontinentia Pigmenti

Incontinentia Pigmenti

A. Inflammatory vesicular stage
   1. Linear erythema and blisters present at birth or first 2 weeks of life
   2. Most common on extremities and scalp
   3. Waxes and wanes, then resolves within several months
   4. X-linked dominant inheritance (females only), skin lesions follow Blashko's lines
   5. Extracutaneous manifestations of incontinentia pigmenti: ocular involvement (retinopathy, keratitis), early tooth loss, conical teeth, patchy scarring alopecia, breast hypoplasia, seizures, mental retardation

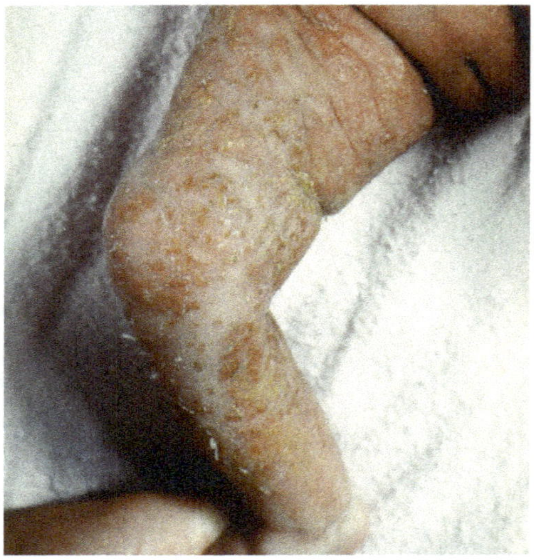

Incontinentia pigmenti
Photograph courtesy of SpringerImages Database, Springer Publishing Company

Incontinentia pigmenti

A. Inflammatory vesicular stage: linear erythema and blisters that favor the extremities and present at birth or first 2 weeks of life

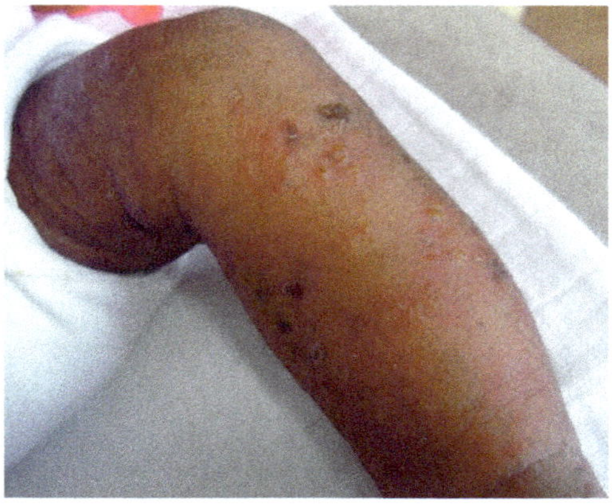

Incontinentia pigmenti
Photograph courtesy of SpringerImages Database, Springer Publishing Company

Incontinentia Pigmenti

A. Verrucous hyperkeratotic stage: verrucous linear plaques that favor the extremities and disappear later in infancy (may last several years)

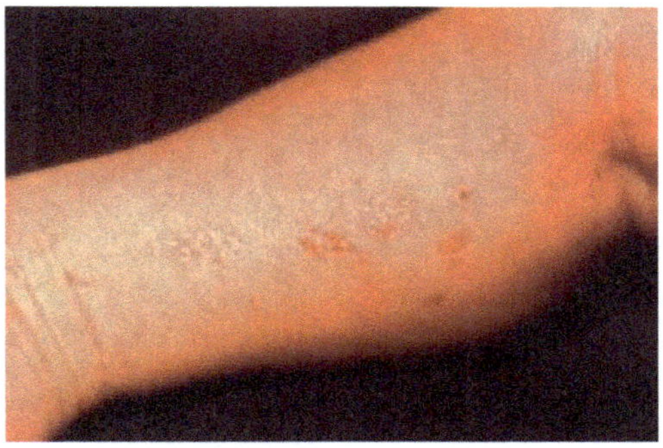

Incontinentia pigmenti
Photograph courtesy of SpringerImages Database, Springer Publishing Company

Incontinentia pigmenti

A. Hyperpigmented stage
   1. Streaks and swirls of reticulate gray–brown hyperpigmentation with scalloped edges ("marble-cake appearance")
   2. Trunk and intertriginous sites
   3. Progresses in first few months of life, then stable, then fades by adolescence (may last for years)

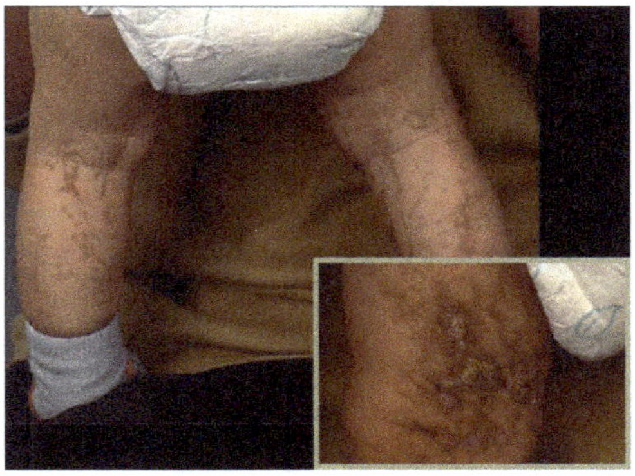

Incontinentia pigmenti
Photograph courtesy of SpringerImages Database, Springer Publishing Company

f. Cowden's Syndrome

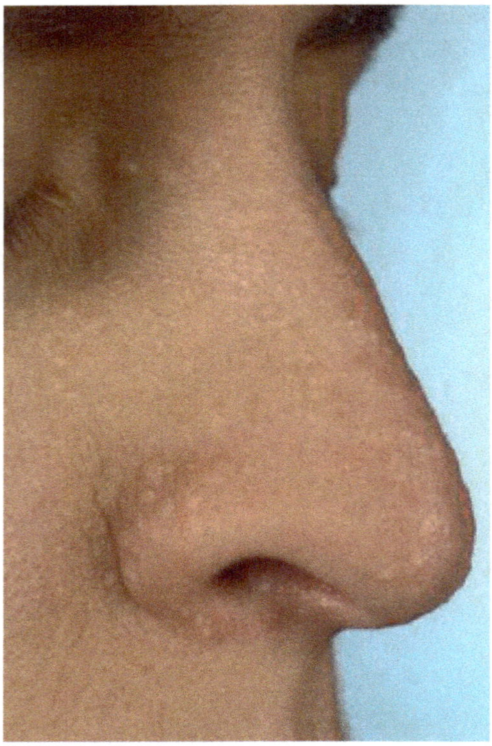

Cowden's syndrome
Photograph courtesy of SpringerImages Database, Springer Publishing Company

Cowden's syndrome

A. Trichilemmomas
   1. Multiple facial or perioral papules (trichilemmomas): skin-colored papules, especially on the nose
   2. Autosomal dominant, begins 20–30 years old
   3. Other signs of Cowden's syndrome
      a. Pigmented macules of penis, perioral lentigines
      b. Liipomas, sclerotic fibromas, hemangiomas
      c. Craniomegaly
      d. Breast disease (fibrocystic disease and cancer) in ¾ of women, thyroid tumors including cancer in 2/3 of patients, endometrial cancer in 5–10 % of patients

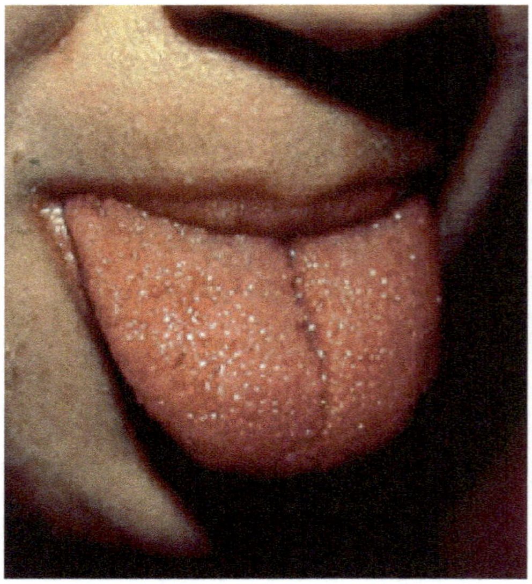

Cowden's syndrome
Photograph courtesy of SpringerImages Database, Springer Publishing Company

Cowden's syndrome

A. Cobblestoning of oral mucosa
   1. Oral papillomas (1–3 mm smooth white papules) of the tongue, palate, gingiva, or lips
   2. Also seen in Darier's disease
   3. Present in 80 % of patients

Cowden's syndrome

A. Cobblestoning of oral mucosa: multiple, pink papillary gingival lesions throughout the oral cavity

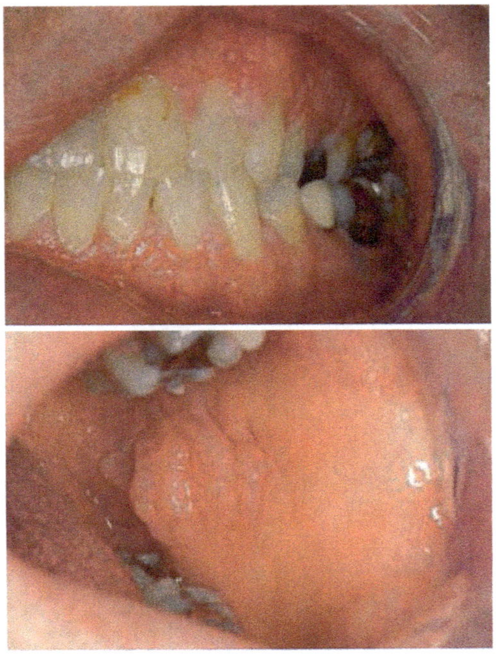

Cobblestoning of oral mucosa (Cowden's syndrome)
Photograph courtesy of SpringerImages Database, Springer Publishing Company

Cowden's syndrome

A. Acral keratotic palmar papules keratotic papules on palms and soles present in 60 % of patients

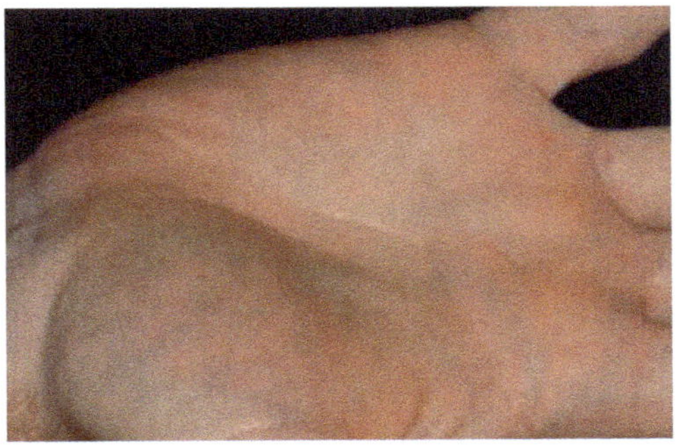

Cowden's syndrome
Photograph courtesy of SpringerImages Database, Springer Publishing Company

g. Cutis Laxa

Cutis laxa

A. Group of conditions characterized by sparse and fragmented elastic fibers
B. Elastolysis leads to loose sagging redundant skin with reduced elasticity and resilience
C. Loose redundant facial skin results in an aged facial appearance with deep wrinkling (bloodhound-like facies: pendulous skin folds of the eyelids, cheeks, and neck)
D. Joints are not hyperextensible as in Ehlers Danlos
E. Extracutaneous features
   1. emphysema
   2. hernias
   3. gastrointestinal and genitourinary diverticula

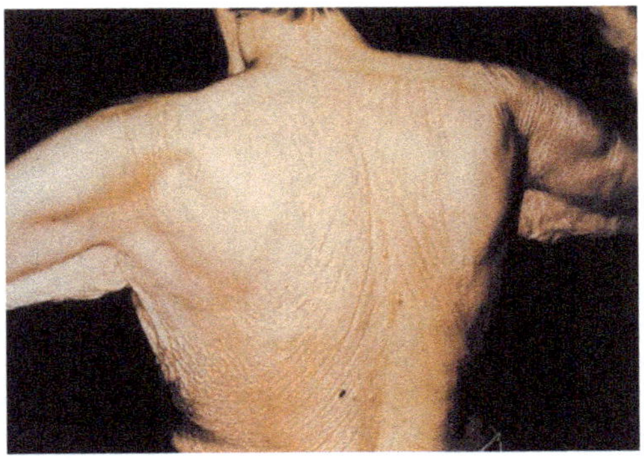

Cutis laxa
Photograph courtesy of SpringerImages Database, Springer Publishing Company

Cutis laxa

A. Loose redundant facial skin results in an aged facial appearance with deep wrinkling

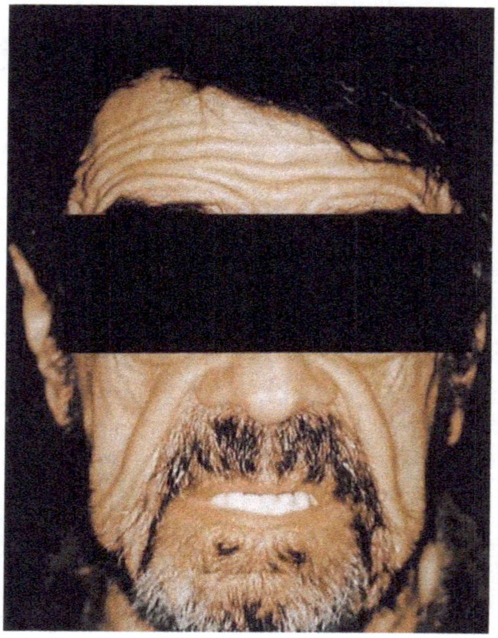

Cutis laxa
Photograph courtesy of SpringerImages Database, Springer Publishing Company

h. Ehlers Danlos Syndrome

Ehlers-Danlos Syndrome

A. Genetic disorder of collagen (not elastic tissue as with cutis laxa)
B. Autosomal dominant and autosomal recessive inheritance pattern
C. Hyperextensible skin: collagen is abnormal (elastic tissue is normal), so skin is not lax and returns to normal position after stretching (unlike in cutis laxa)
D. Hyperextensible joints
E. Subcutaneous spheroids: multiple small hard nodules over bony prominences (calcified fat globules)
F. Gorlin's sign—ability to touch tip of nose with tongue (seen in 50 % of Ehlers-Danlos patients compared to 10 % of general population)
G. Elastosis perforans serpiginosa
H. Piezogenic papules: herniations of fat on the hands and feet due to a collagen defect
I. Extracutaneous features: scoliosis, hernias, spontaneous arterial/intestinal/uterine rupture

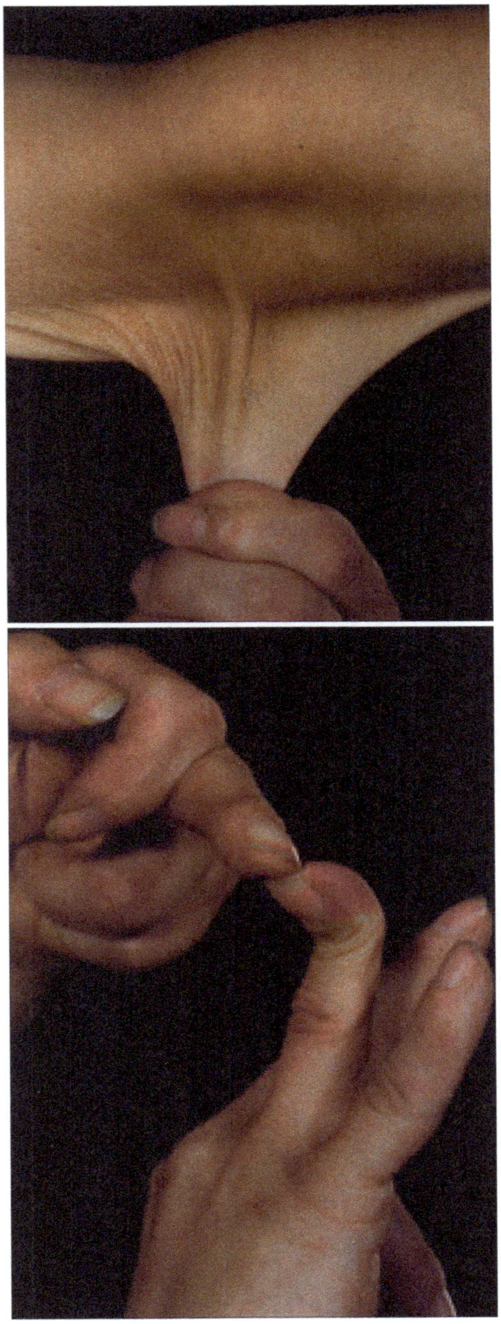

Ehlers Danlos syndrome
Photograph courtesy of SpringerImages Database, Springer Publishing Company

Ehlers-Danlos syndrome

A. Fragile skin: skin splits as a result of trauma resulting in gaping fish mouth wounds and wide atrophic scars with "cigarette paper" atrophy, poor wound healing, dehiscence, easy bruising due to fragile small blood vessels

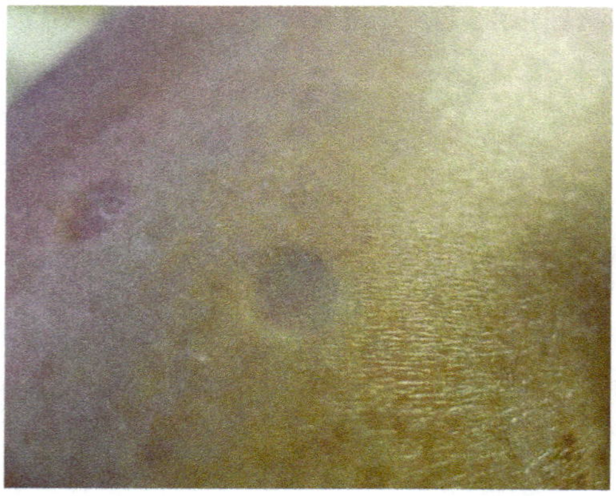

Ehlers Danlos syndrome
Photograph courtesy of SpringerImages Database, Springer Publishing Company

Ehlers Danlos Syndrome

A. Extensive bruising and scars with cigarette paper atrophy

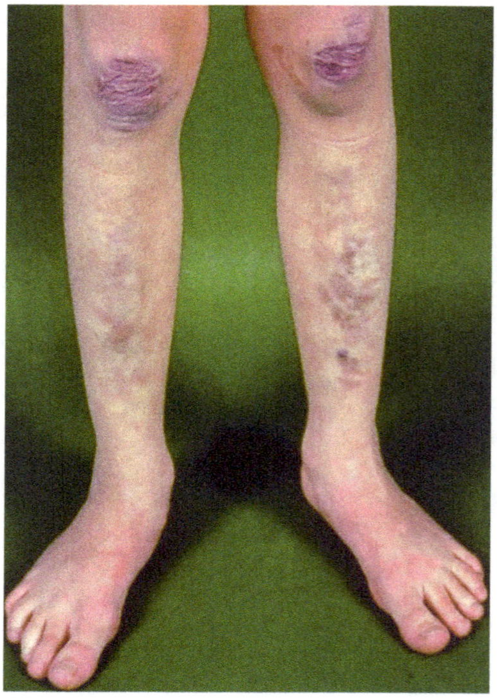

Ehlers Danlos syndrome
Photograph courtesy of SpringerImages Database, Springer Publishing Company

i. Pachyonychia Congenita

Pachonychia congenita

A. Autosomal dominant, nonepidermolytic palmoplantar keratoderma
B. Painful palmoplantar keratoderma (mainly plantar) with blistering and callosities that usually arise at sites of friction, pressure, or trauma
C. Hypertrophic nail dystrophy (thickened fingernails and toenails), wedge-shaped subungual hyperkeratosis resulting in elevation of nail plate and pincer nail effect
D. Premature dentition
E. Two types of pachyonychia congenita
    1. Type 1—Oral leukokeratosis
    2. Type 2—Pilosebaceous cysts (steatocystoma multiplex, eruptive vellus hair cysts, epidermal or pilar cysts)

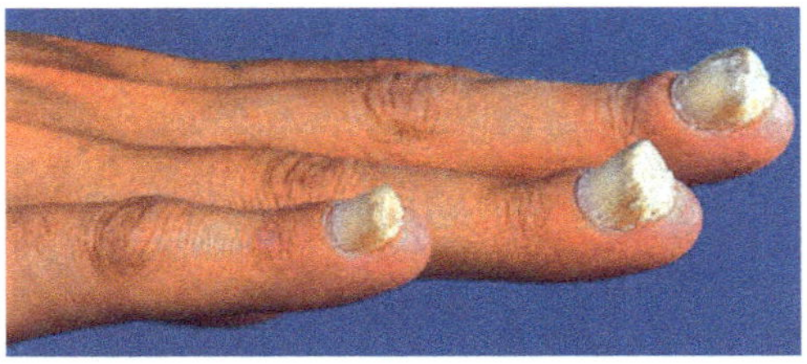

Pachyonychia congenita
Photograph courtesy of SpringerImages Database, Springer Publishing Company

Pachonychia congenita

A. Oral leukokeratosis and premature dentition

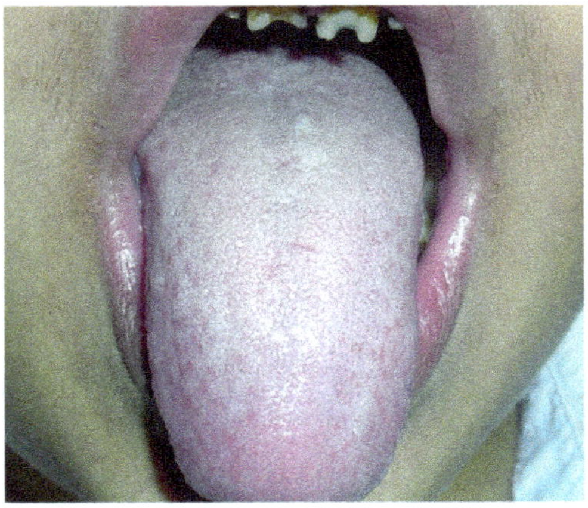

Pachyonychia congenita
Photograph courtesy of SpringerImages Database, Springer Publishing Company

Pachonychia congenita

A. Hypertrophic nail dystrophy (thickened fingernails)

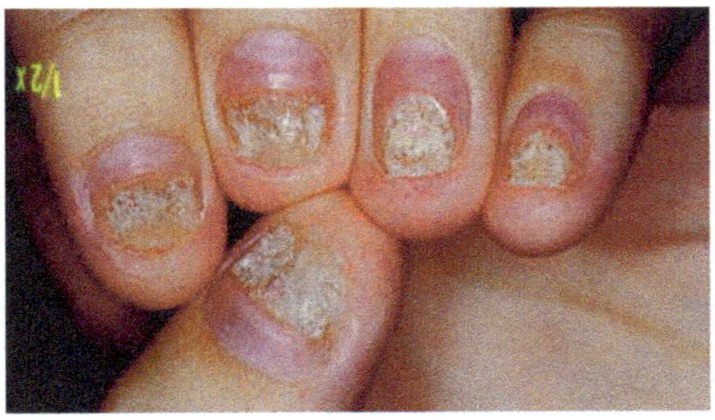

Pachyonychia congenita
Photograph courtesy of SpringerImages Database, Springer Publishing Company

j. Pseudoxanthoma Elasticum

Pseudoxanthoma elasticum (also see Chap. 7, section 48b (iii))

A. Autosomal recessive disorder characterized by clumped and distorted calcified elastic fibers in the skin, eyes, and cardiovascular system
B. Yellow papules most commonly, which coalesce into cobblestone plaques resembling plucked chicken skin
   1. Appear first decade
   2. The lateral neck is usually affected first, then flexural areas
C. Firm papules or plaques (dermal calcium)
D. Yellow papules on the lower lip
E. Cardiovascular: claudication, renal hypertension, angina, myocardial infarction, gastrointestinal hemorrhage (due to calcification of elastic fibers in medium-size arteries and luminal narrowing)
F. Eyes: angioid streaks (breaks in the calcified elastic lamina of Bruch's membrane) and a peau d'orange mottling of retinal pigment epithelium (most prevalent eye finding)

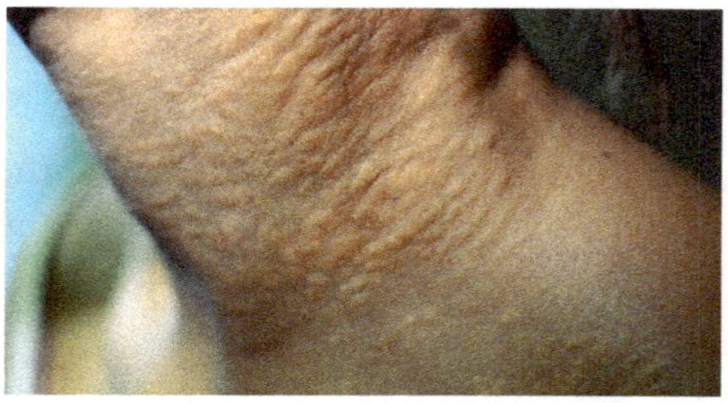

Pseudoxanthoma elasticum
Photograph courtesy of SpringerImages Database, Springer Publishing Company

Pseudoxanthoma elasticum

A. Yellow papules most commonly, which coalesce into cobblestone plaques resembling plucked chicken skin

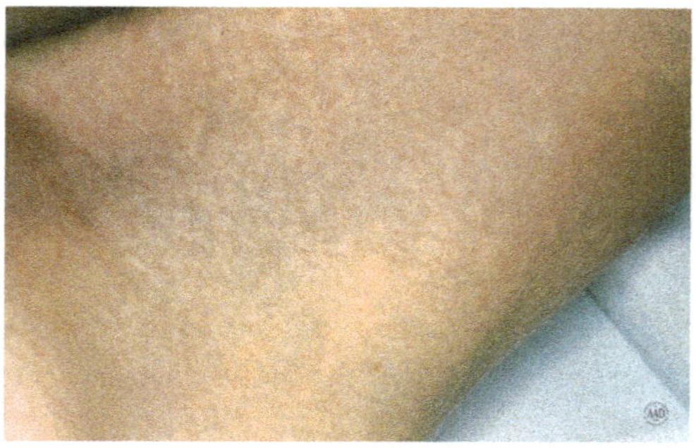

Pseudoxanthoma elasticum
Photograph courtesy of the American Academy of Dermatology

Pseudoxanthoma elasticum

A. Yellow papules most commonly, which coalesce into cobblestone plaques resembling plucked chicken skin

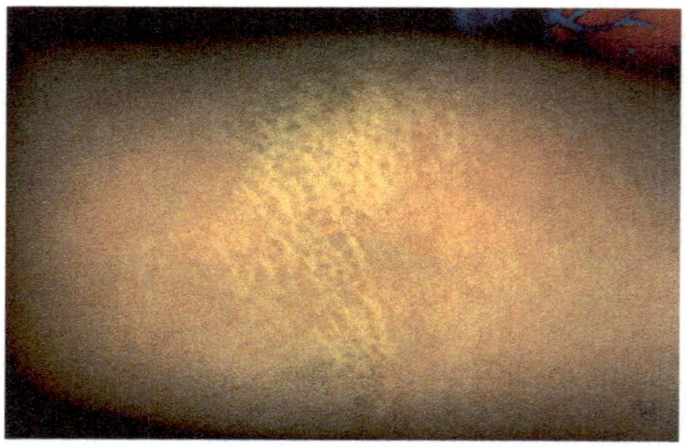

Pseudoxanthoma elasticum
Photograph courtesy of the American Academy of Dermatology

Pseudoxanthoma elasticum

A. Yellow papules on the lower lip

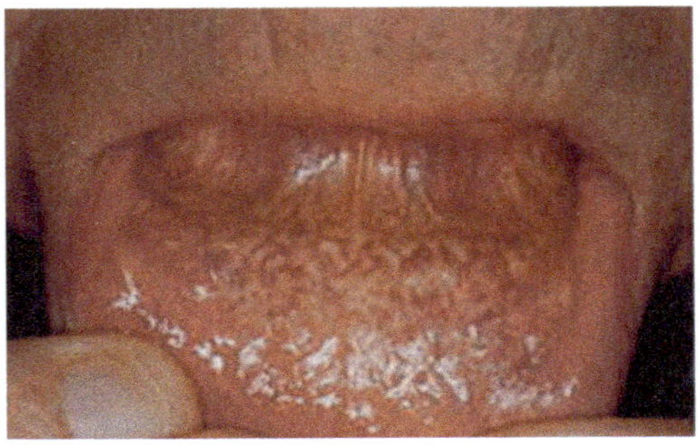

Pseudoxanthoma elasticum
Photograph courtesy of SpringerImages Database, Springer Publishing Company

Developmental Anomalies

52

a. Aplasia Cutis Congenita

Aplasia cutis congenita

A. Localized areas of skin are absent or scarred at birth (localized defect of the epidermis, dermis, and sometimes subcutaneous fat)
B. Most commonly occurs on the scalp (especially at or near the vertex)
C. Scalp lesions involve the underlying skull in 20–30 % of cases
D. Most defects are 1–2 cm in diameter
E. 25 % may have greater than one lesion
F. Most small lesions heal within first few months leaving a scar

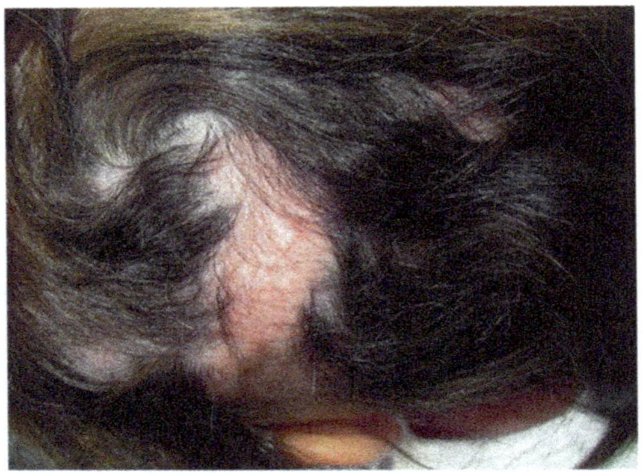

Aplasia cutis congenita
Photograph courtesy of SpringerImages Database, Springer Publishing Company

Aplasia cutis congenita

A. May appear as an erosion or ulcer

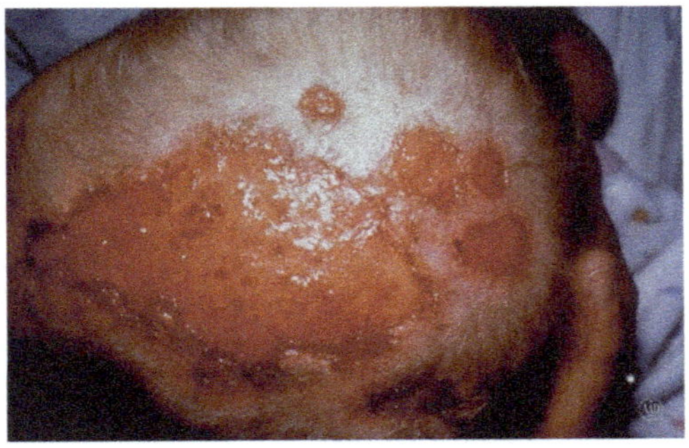

Aplasia cutis congenita
Photograph courtesy of the American Academy of Dermatology

H.M. Gloster, Jr. et al., *Absolute Dermatology Review: Mastering Clinical Conditions on the Dermatology Recertification Exam*, DOI 10.1007/978-3-319-03218-4_52, © Springer International Publishing Switzerland 2016

Aplasia cutis congenita

A. May appear as a stellate hemorrhagic plaque

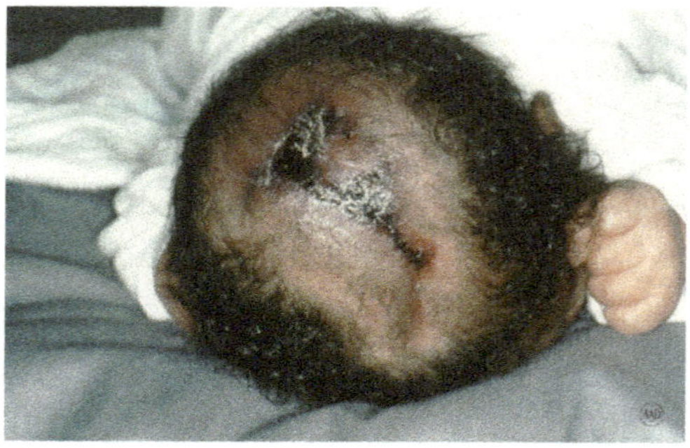

Aplasia cutis congenita
Photograph courtesy of the American Academy of Dermatology

Aplasia cutis congenita

A. May appear as a well-formed scar (often presents as a hairless, round, scarred plaque when on the scalp)

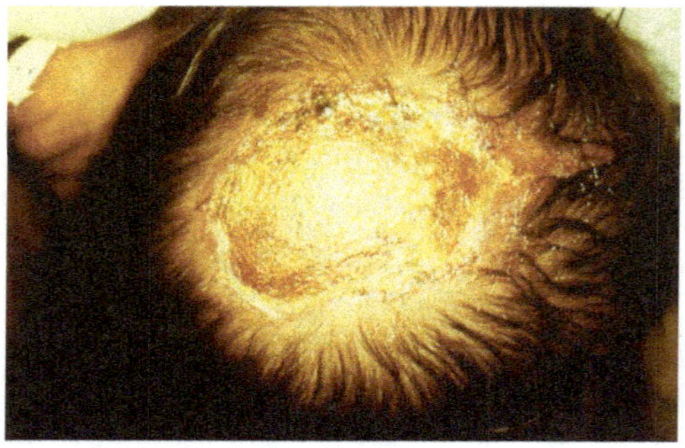

Aplasia cutis congenita
Photograph courtesy of SpringerImages Database, Springer Publishing Company

Aplasia cutis congenita

A. May appear as a discrete ovoid defect covered by a membranous vesicle or bullae
B. Most common form of aplasia cutis congenita
C. Usually occurs on the scalp, especially the vertex
D. Presents at birth as sharply demarcated punched-out oval round 1–2 cm defect covered by a thin translucent membrane
E. Usually circular but may be irregular, elongated, or stellate
F. Usually single but may be multiple
G. May be surrounded by hair collar (if surrounded by a hair collar, there may be underlying heterotropic brain tissue or meninges)

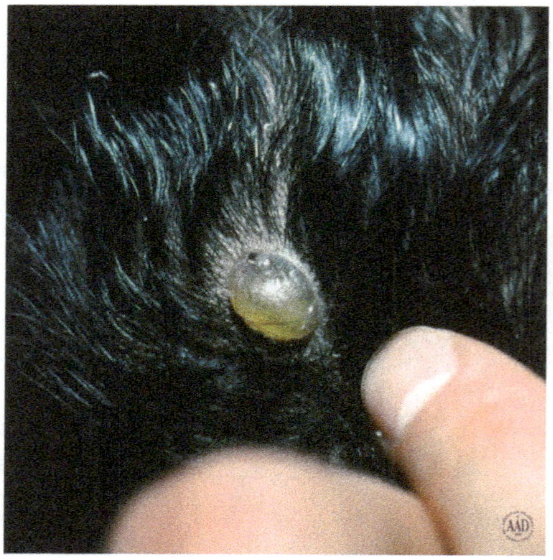

Aplasia cutis congenita
Photograph courtesy of the American Academy of Dermatology

b. Hair Collar Sign

Hair Collar Sign

A. Ring of long, dark, coarse hair surrounding a congenital scalp nodule or lesion of aplasia cutis congenita
B. Most commonly occurs with the membranous subtype of aplasia cutis (represents forme fruste of a neural tube defect)
C. May be isolated and benign or may be a specific marker for ectopic neural tissue—can be associated with a connection to the central nervous system structural central nervous system abnormalities, or cerebrovascular anomalies
D. Imaging should be done in more severe cases and all patients with hair collar sign, vascular stain, or underlying mass to rule out underlying encephalocele and menigocele

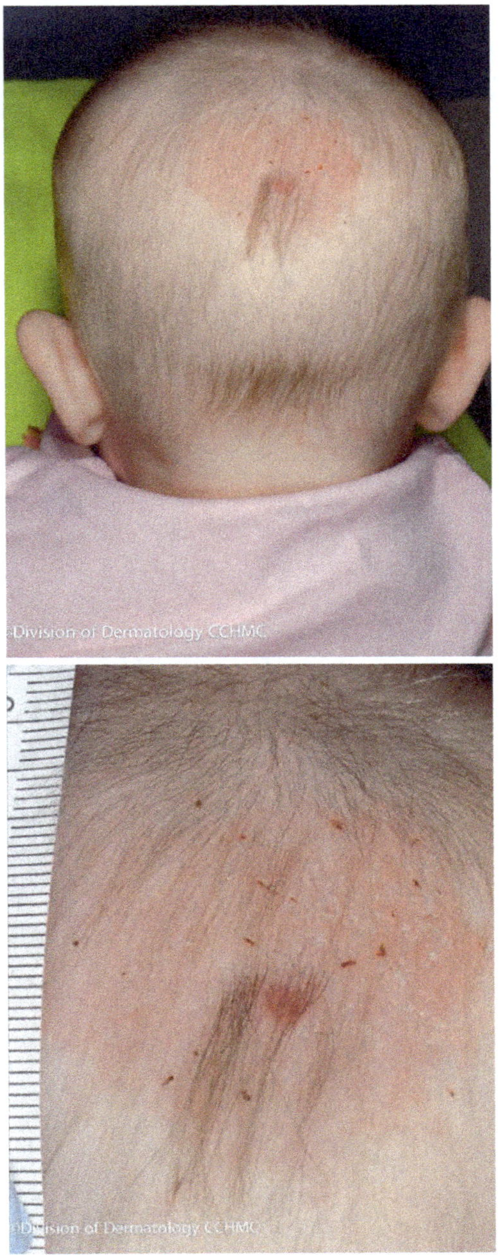

Hair collar sign
Photograph courtesy of Kara Shah, M.D, PhD, CCHMC (Cincinnati, OH), Department of Dermatology

Chapter IX

Infections

Viral Infections 53

a. Condyloma Acuminata (Anogenital Warts)

Condyloma acuminata (anogenital warts)

A. Occur on the external genitalia, perineum, perianal, mons pubis, inguinal fold
B. May extend into the vagina, urethra, or anal canal
C. Discrete, sessile, exophytic, cauliflower papillomas or verrucous papules which may be skin colored, brown, or white
D. May be several centimeters in diameter and form confluent hyperpigmented plaques
E. Caused by HPV 6 or HPV 11 in 90 % of cases
F. Often transmitted sexually, so when present search for other sexually transmitted diseases

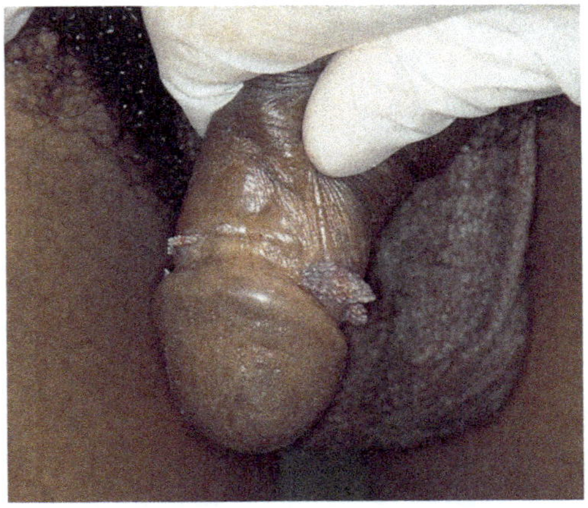

Condyloma acuminata (anogenital warts)
Photograph courtesy of SpringerImages Database, Springer Publishing Company

Condylomata acuminata

A. Discrete sessile exophytic cauliflower papillomas or verrucous papules on the anogenital area which may be skin colored, brown, or white

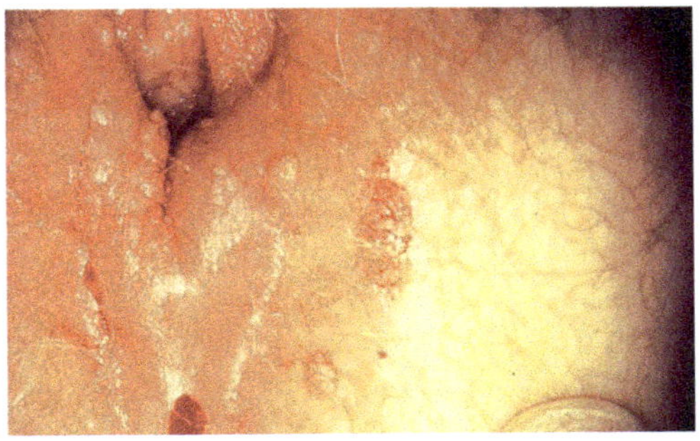

Condyloma acuminata (anogenital warts)
Photograph courtesy of SpringerImages Database, Springer Publishing Company

H.M. Gloster, Jr. et al., *Absolute Dermatology Review: Mastering Clinical Conditions on the Dermatology Recertification Exam*, DOI 10.1007/978-3-319-03218-4_53, © Springer International Publishing Switzerland 2016

b. Bowenoid Papulosis

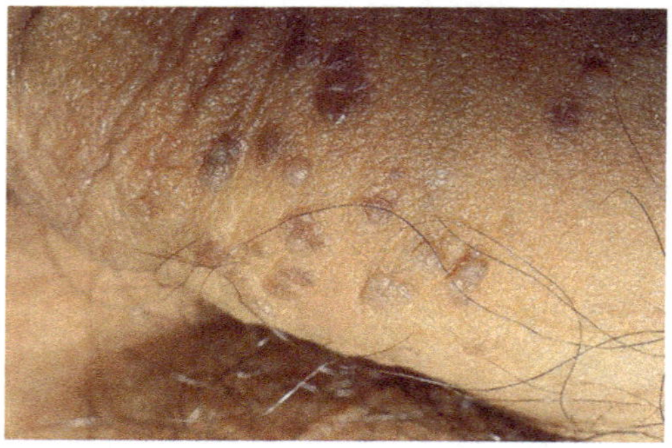

Bowenoid papulosis
Photograph courtesy of SpringerImages Database, Springer Publishing Company

Bowenoid papulosis

A. Multiple red brown papules or nonconfluent plaques on external genitalia, anal area, perineum
B. Young adults
C. Squamous cell carcinoma in situ histologically
D. May be associated with HPV 16

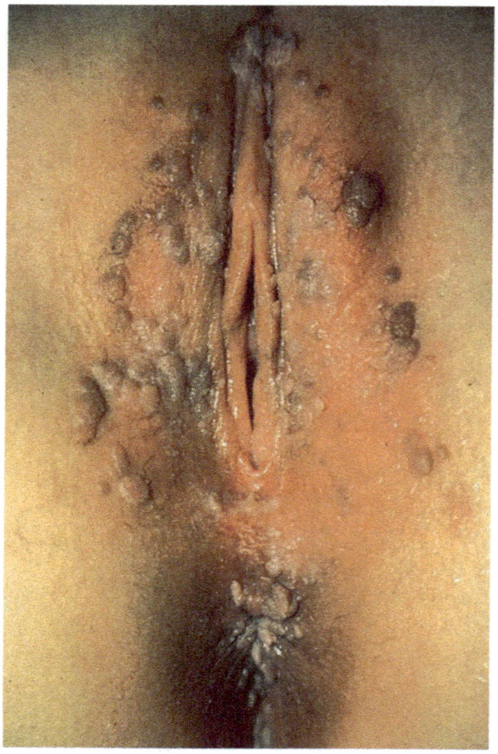

Bowenoid papulosis
Photograph courtesy of SpringerImages Database, Springer Publishing Company

Bowenoid papulosis

A. Multiple red brown papules or nonconfluent plaques on external genitalia

c. Verruca Vulgaris (Common Wart)

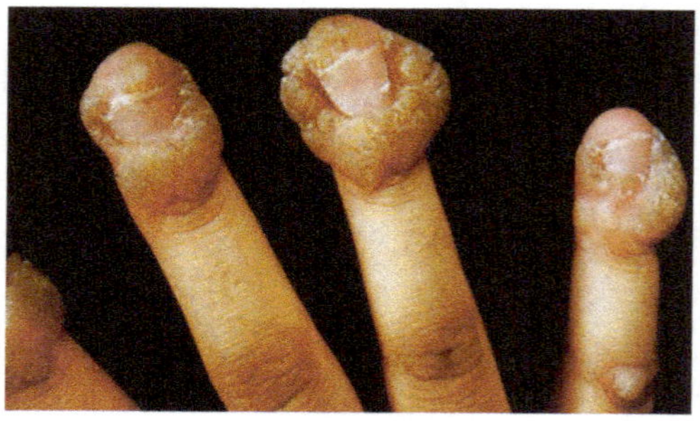

Verruca vulgaris (common wart)
Photograph courtesy of SpringerImages Database, Springer Publishing Company

Verruca vulgaris (common wart)

A. Caused by the human papillomavirus (HPV)
B. Hyperkeratotic, exophytic, papillomatous dome-shaped papules or plaques with punctate black dots (thrombosed capillaries) that bleed after shaving the hyperkeratotic surface
C. Usually occur on the hands (fingers or periungual) or other sites prone to trauma like knees or elbows

d. Palmar and Plantar Warts

Palmar and plantar warts

A. Thick endophytic papules on palms, soles, lateral hands, and feet
B. May be painful on the soles of the feet
C. Plantar warts can coalesce into large plaques called mosaic warts
D. In contrast to calluses, plantar warts often result in discontinuation of normal skin lines and have punctate dark brown dots, which represent vessel thrombosis in the superficial dermis

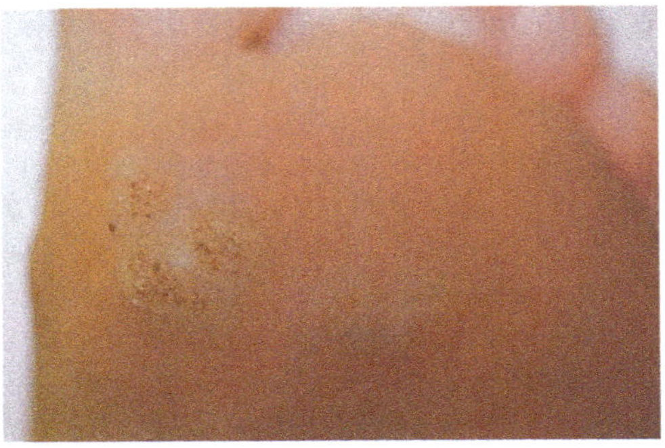

Palmar and plantar warts
Photograph courtesy of SpringerImages Database, Springer Publishing Company

e. Flat Warts

Flat warts

A. Skin-colored pink brown smooth-surfaced flat-top papules
B. Dorsal hand, arms, face
C. Often linear array

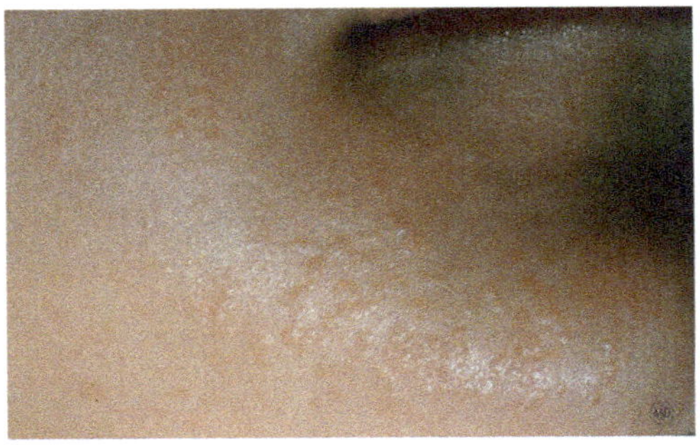

Flat warts
Photograph courtesy of the American Academy of Dermatology

f. Epidermodysplasia Verruciformis

Epidermodysplasia verruciformis

A. Autosomal recessive condition with a particular susceptibility to HPV that does not normally occur in adults
B. Widespread scaly papules and plaques resembling flat warts (skin-colored pink brown smooth-surfaced flat-top papules) appear in childhood or patients may present with generalized pink to red macules and plaques resembling tinea versicolor
C. Actinic keratoses may arise after age 30 and transform into squamous cell carcinomas which develop on sun-exposed areas

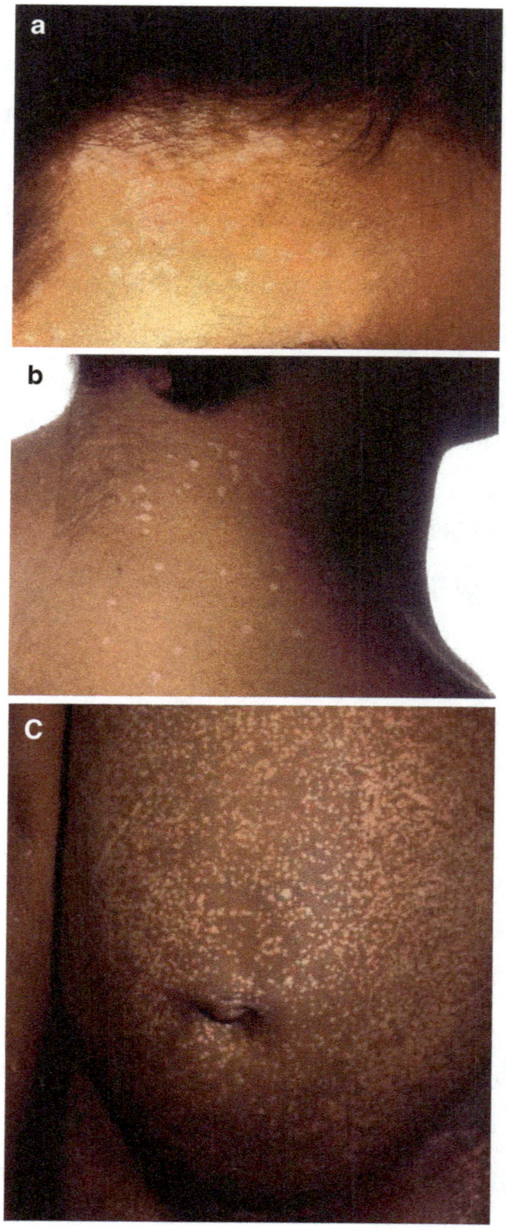

Epidermodysplasia verruciformis
Photograph courtesy of SpringerImages Database, Springer Publishing Company

g. Erythema Infectiosum (Fifth Disease)

Erythema infectiosum (Fifth Disease)

A. Seasonal pattern (winter and spring), most common in school-age children 4–11 years of age
B. Parvovirus B19, the etiological agent, has tropism for erythrocytes and may cause anemia, reticulocytopenia (transient aplastic anemic crisis can occur in the setting of hemoglobinopathies and those on chemotherapy)
C. Mild prodrome (fever, myalgia, headache) 7–10 days followed by bright red macular erythema of the cheeks ("slapped cheeks") with sparing of nasal bridge and mouth region

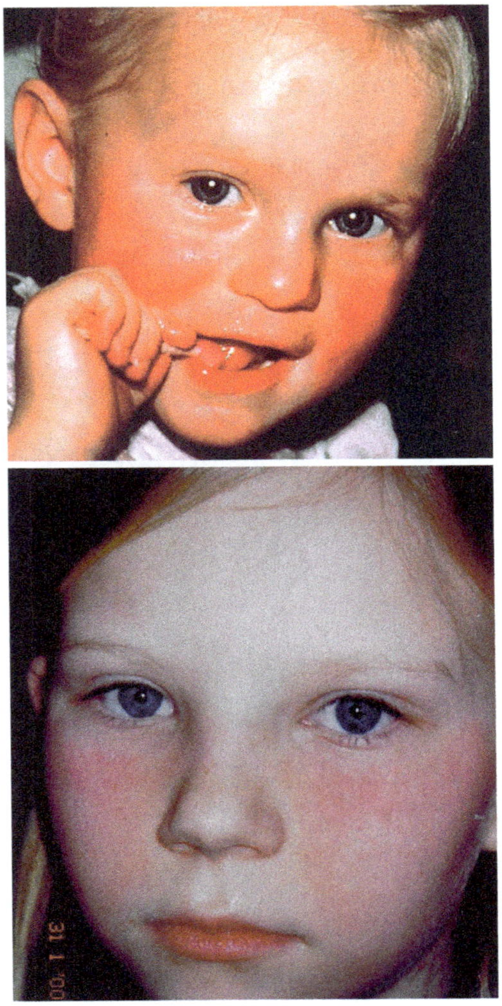

Erythema infectiosum (fifth disease)
Photograph courtesy of SpringerImages Database, Springer Publishing Company

Erythema infectiosum (Fifth Disease)

A. One to four days after the appearance of macular erythema of the cheeks, lacy reticulated red macules and papules appear mainly on the extesor extremities, lasts 1–3 weeks and frequently fluctuates
B. Arthritis and arthralgia in 10 %, most often on the hands and feet, usually resolves
C. Fetal infection ranges from self-limited anemia, fetal hydrops, spontaneous miscarriage, and still birth
D. Most fetal losses occur when nonimmune pregnant female 20–28 weeks gestation is infected (10 % fetal demise in nonimmune females with acute infection)

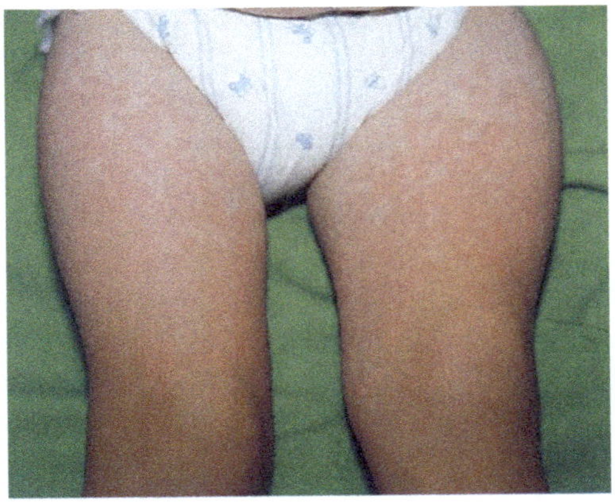

Erythema infectiosum (fifth disease)
Photograph courtesy of SpringerImages Database, Springer Publishing Company

Erythema infectiosum (Fifth Disease)

A. Papular purpuric gloves and socks syndrome: painful edema, erythema, petechiae, and purpura involving palms and soles

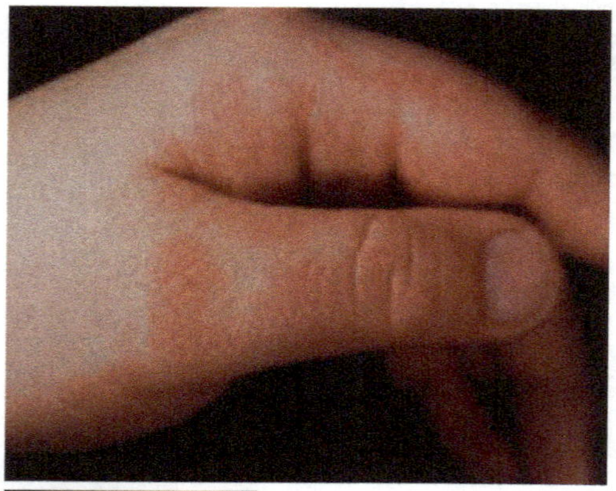

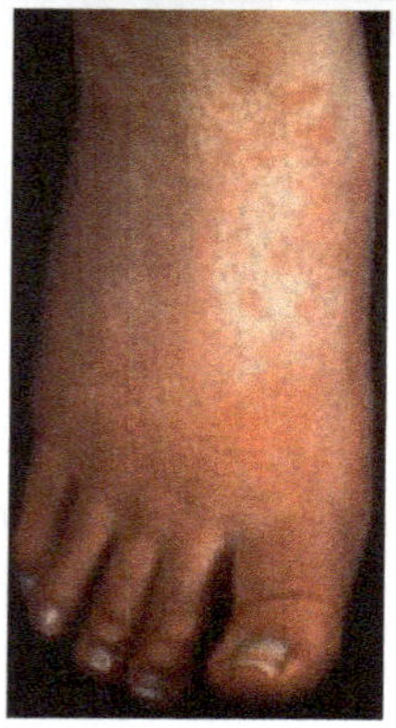

Erythema infectiosum (fifth disease)
Photograph courtesy of SpringerImages Database, Springer Publishing Company

h. Hand-Foot-Mouth Disease

Hand-foot-mouth disease

A. Enterovirus (coxackie A 16 virus infection)
B. Most common in children ages 2–10 years in the late summer and fall
C. Prodrome of fever, malaise, mouth pain, headache, abdominal pain, diarrhea
D. Red papules initially evolve into oval gray vesicles on the palms, soles, buttocks, and perineum
E. Vesicles may run parallel to skin surface lines
F. Oral vesicles rupture leaving painful erosions and ulcers on an erythematous base, the buccal mucosa and tongue are most commonly affected (90 % have oral involvement)
G. Rash fades in about a week

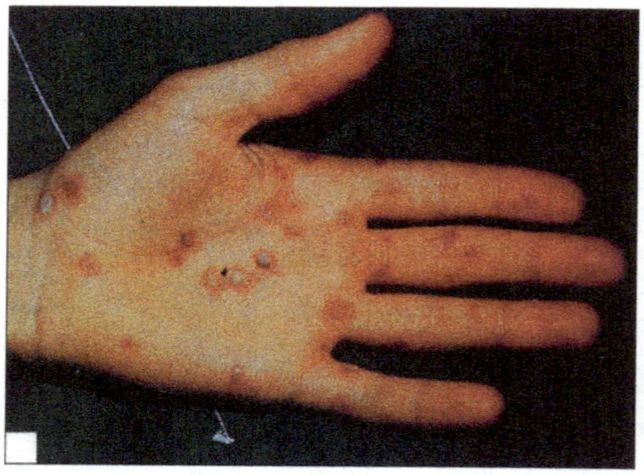

Hand-foot-mouth disease
Photograph courtesy of SpringerImages Database, Springer Publishing Company

Hand-foot-mouth syndrome

A. Multiple shallow minor aphthous-like ulcers of the posterior soft palate and uvula with associated erythema

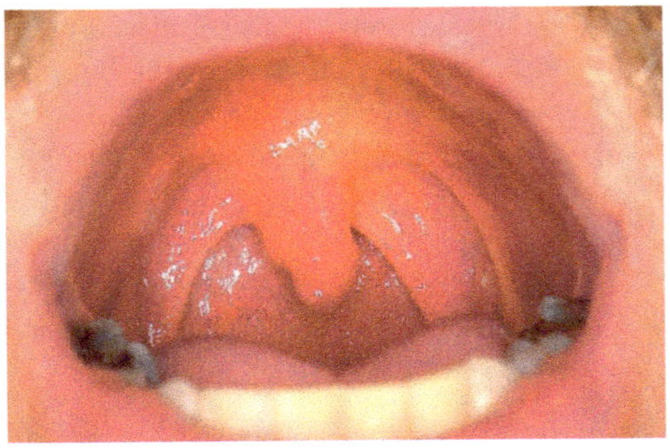

Hand-foot-mouth disease
Photograph courtesy of SpringerImages Database, Springer Publishing Company

i. Herpes Simplex Virus

Herpes simplex virus (HSV)

A. Prodrome of burning, tingling, tenderness
B. Typical lesions consist of grouped painful vesicles on an erythematous base which may form pustules, erosions, or ulcerations with scalloped borders

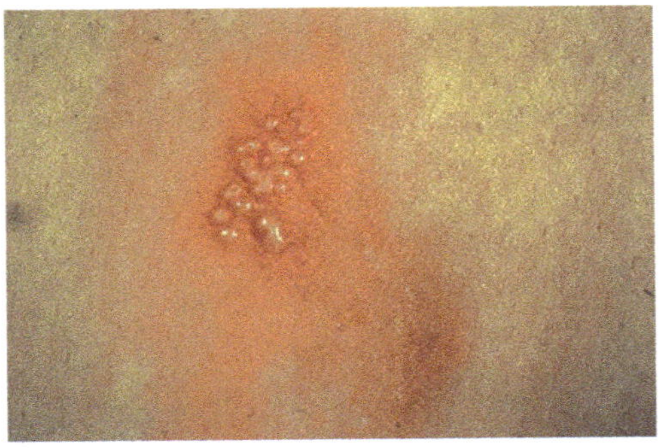

Herpes simplex virus
Photograph courtesy of SpringerImages Database, Springer Publishing Company

i. Oral-labial Herpes Simplex Virus-1

Orolabial herpes simplex virus-1 infection

A. Lips and mouth most common
B. Pathognomonic fever blisters characteristically involve the vermilion border of the lip in recurrent outbreaks

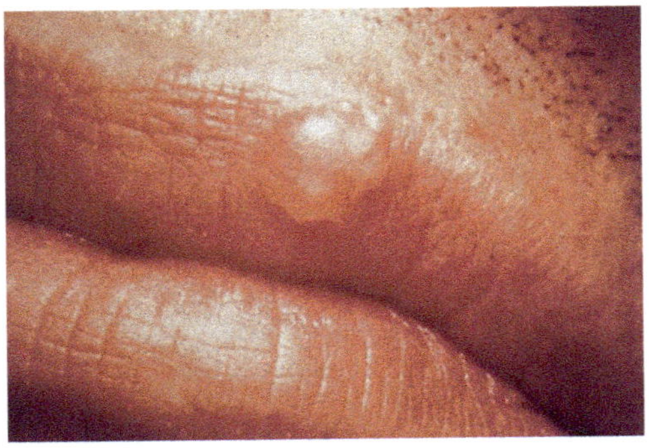

Oral-labial herpes simplex virus-1
Photograph courtesy of SpringerImages Database, Springer Publishing Company

Orolabial herpes simplex virus-1 infection (primary infection)

A. Vesicles and ulceration of the buccal mucosa and gingiva are most common in primary infection
B. Primary infections are usually asymptomatic, but symptomatic infections may present as gingivostomatitis in children or pharyngitis in young adults

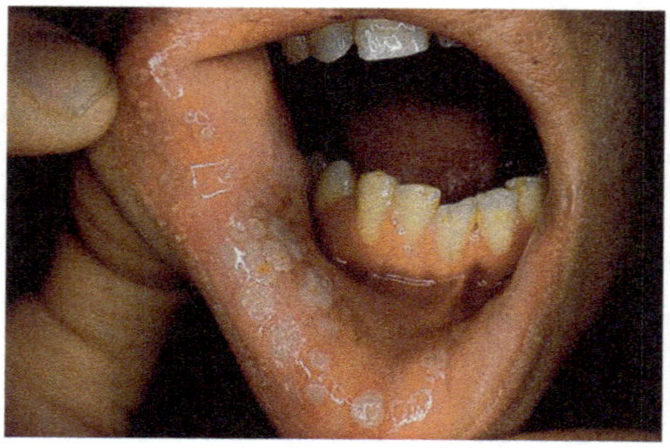

Oral-labial herpes simplex virus-1
Photograph courtesy of SpringerImages Database, Springer Publishing Company

ii. Genital Herpes Simplex Virus-2

Genital herpes simplex virus-2 infection

A. Primary
    1. Women: cervix, buttocks, perineum, vagina, vulva
    2. Men: glans or shaft
B. Recurrent
    1. Usually mild, may appear on the buttocks in women, penis in men

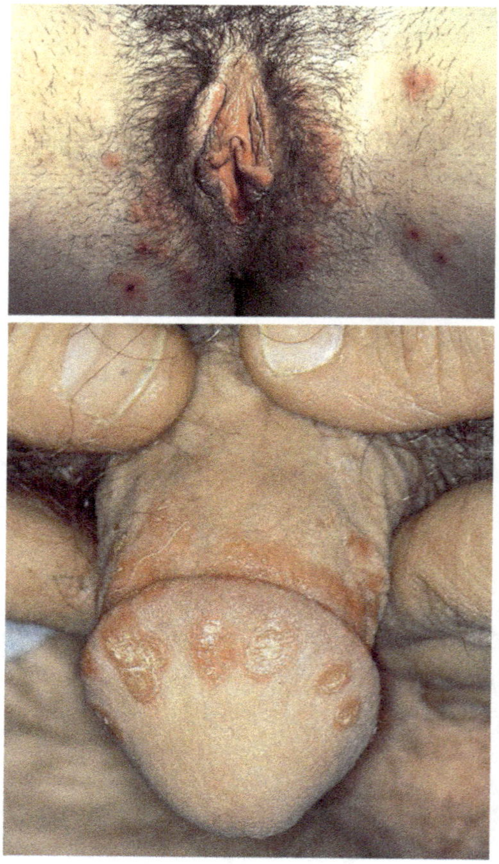

Genital herpes simplex virus-2
Photograph courtesy of SpringerImages Database, Springer Publishing Company

iii. Eczema Herpeticum (Kaposi's Varicelliform Eruption)

Eczema herpeitcum (Kaposi's varicelliform eruption)

A. Rapid, widespread HSV dissemination in areas of dermatitis or skin barrier disruption
B. Most often occurs in children and adults with atopic dermatitis
C. Can also occur in patients with burns, pemphigus vulgaris and foliaceous, Darier's disease, Hailey-Hailey disease, mycosis fungodes, sezary syndrome, ichthyoses
D. Monomorphic discrete punched-out erosions with scalloped border and hemorrhagic crust
E. May be complicated by secondary bacterial infection or disseminated HSV

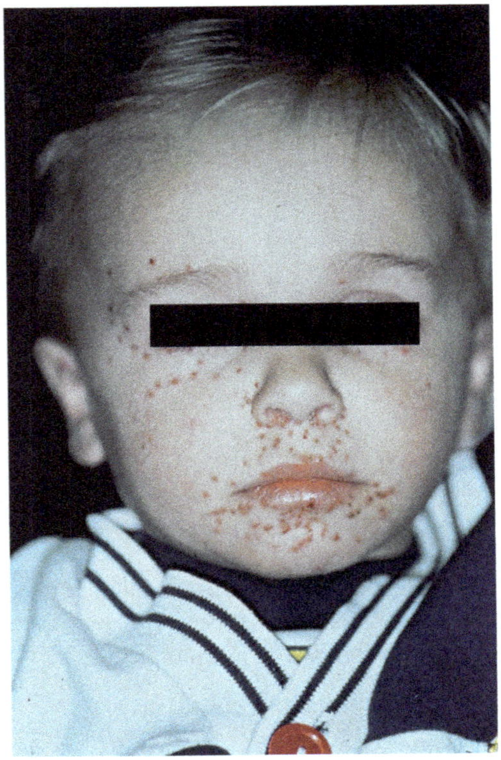

Eczema herpeticum (Kaposi's varicelliform eruption) Photograph courtesy of SpringerImages Database, Springer Publishing Company

Eczema herpeitcum (Kaposi's varicelliform eruption)

A. Vesicles, superficial ulcers, and crusts in the antecubital fossa of this toddler with atopic dermatitis

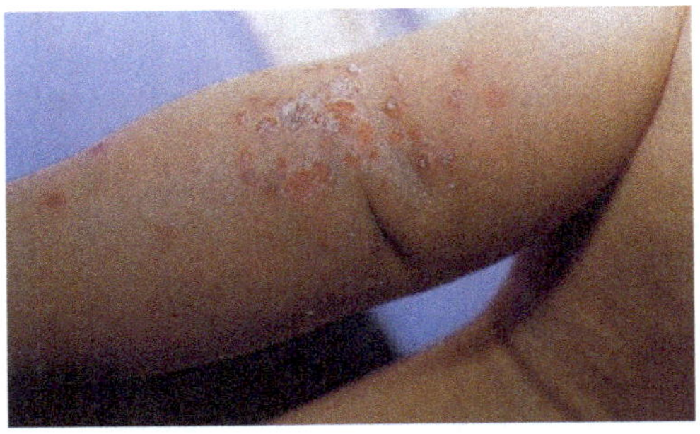

Eczema herpeticum (Kaposi's varicelliform eruption) Photograph courtesy of SpringerImages Database, Springer Publishing Company

Eczema herpeitcum (Kaposi's varicelliform eruption)

A. Monomorphic discrete punched-out erosions with scalloped borders and hemorrhagic crusts in an adult with eczema

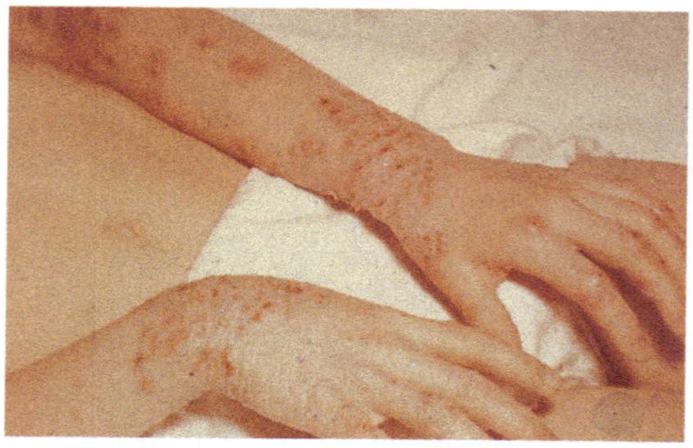

Eczema herpeticum (Kaposi's varicelliform eruption)
Photograph courtesy of SpringerImages Database, Springer Publishing Company

iv. Herpetic Whitlow

Herpetic whitlow

A. Herpes simplex virus infection of the digits resulting in pain, swelling, and vesicular lesions
B. Most often seen in children

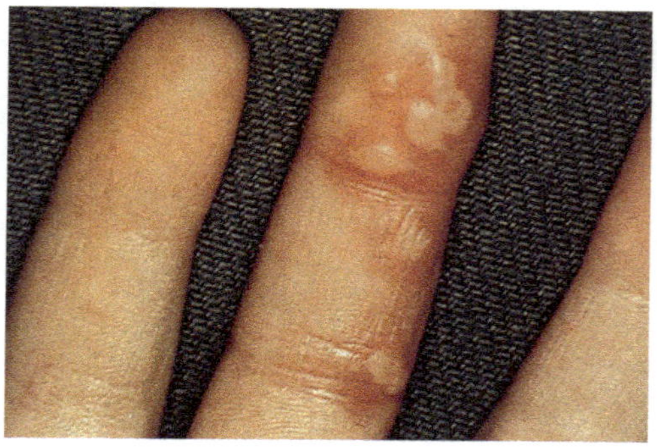

Herpetic whitlow
Photograph courtesy of SpringerImages Database, Springer Publishing Company

v. Neonatal Herpes Simplex Virus Infection

Neonatal herpes simplex virus infection

A. Usually due to exposure to HSV during vaginal delivery
B. Onset from birth to 2 weeks, usually greater than 5 days post partum
C. Vesiculopustular lesions may coalesce to form bullae, and erosions may develop
D. Lesions may be localized (usually to the scalp and trunk) or disseminated
E. May involve the oral mucosa, eye, central nervous system, and multiple internal organs

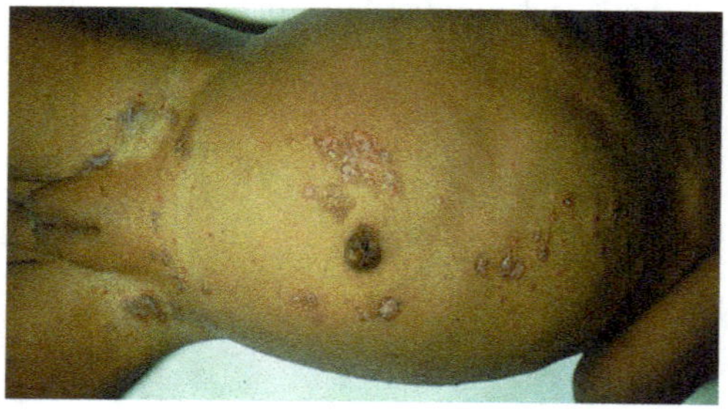

Neonatal herpes simplex virus infection
Photograph courtesy of SpringerImages Database, Springer Publishing Company

j. Herpes Zoster

Herpes Zoster

A. Reactivation of latent virus that persisted following an earlier attack of varicella
B. Usually occurs in older patients, greater risk in immunocompromised patients
C. Prodrome of burning, tingling, tenderness, hyperesthesia, intense pain
D. Painful grouped vesicles (may be preceded by red papules and plaques) on red base in a unilateral dermatomal distribution , vesicles may progress to pustules and bullae
E. Complications are more severe with increasing age and in immunocompromised patients:
   1. Postherpetic neuralgia
   2. Granulomatous and pseudolymphomatous lesions may develop within the site of zoster
   3. Secondary bacterial infection, scarring, encephalitis, pneumonitis, hepatitis
   4. Disseminated cutaneous lesions that cross midline and involve multiple dermatomes may occur in 10 % of immunocompromised patients

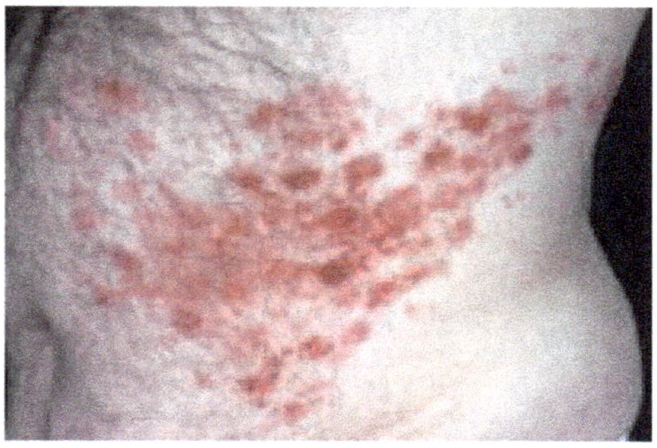

Herpes zoster
Photograph courtesy of SpringerImages Database, Springer Publishing Company

i. Disseminated Herpes Zoster

Disseminated herpes zoster

A. Disseminated cutaneous lesions resembling the widespread vesicular skin eruptions of chicken pox may occur in 10 % of immunocompromised patients
B. Lesions cross midline and involve multiple dermatomes
C. Patients with disseminated skin lesions should be evaluated for visceral involvement especially if immunocompromised

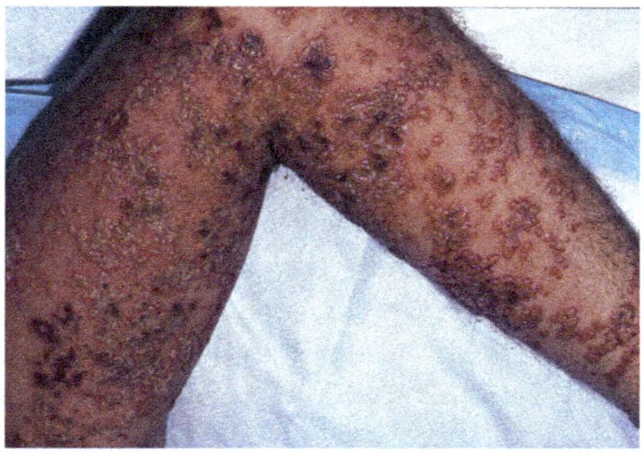

Disseminated herpes zoster
Photograph courtesy of SpringerImages Database, Springer Publishing Company

ii. Acute Herpes Zoster Ophthalmicus

Acute herpes zoster ophthalmicus

A. Vesicular lesions over the distribution of the ophthalmic branch of the trigeminal nerve
B. Hutchinson's sign: Zoster of the nasal tip suggests involvement of the nasociliary nerve, which also supplies the cornea and can be a sign of ocular disease

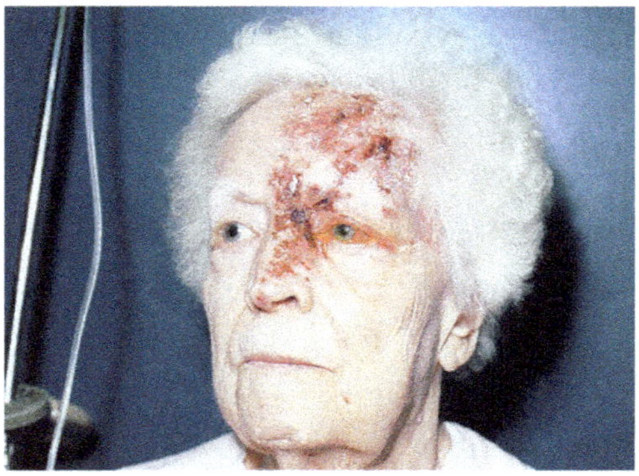

Acute herpes zoster ophthalmicus
Photograph courtesy of SpringerImages Database, Springer Publishing Company

iii. Ramsay Hunt Syndrome

Ramsay Hunt syndrome

A. Zoster affecting the external auditory canal and conchal bowl may involve cranial nerve 7 and 8 resulting in ipsilateral facial paralysis (Bell's palsy),tinnitus, hearing loss, and vertigo

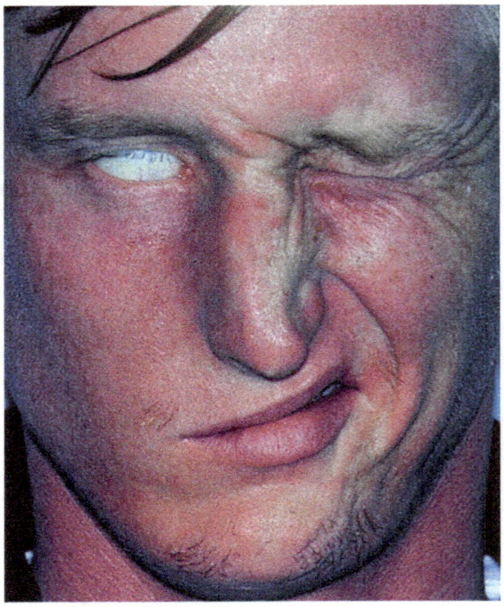

Ramsay hunt syndrome
Photograph courtesy of SpringerImages Database, Springer Publishing Company

k. Varicella (Chicken Pox)

Varicella (chicken pox)

A. Primary infection by varicella zoster virus
B. Pruritic red macules and papules starting on the scalp and face, then spreading to the trunk and extremities (distal and lower extremities are frequently spared)
C. Over the next 12 hours, macular and papular lesions become clear vesicles surrounded by a red halo ("dew drops on rose petal")
D. Vesicles often develop central umbilication
E. Oral mucosa may be involved
F. New lesions continue to erupt for 3–5 days
G. Older lesions form pustules and crusts, heal in 7–10 days, and may heal with scarring
H. Hallmark: lesions in all stages of development (macules, papules, vesicles surrounded by a red halo, pustules and crusts)
I. Usually mild and self-limited in children, may be more severe in adults with increased skin lesions, pneumonitis, encephalitis

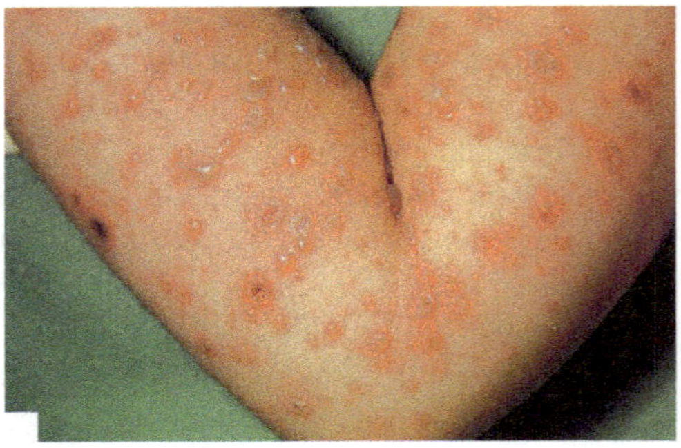

Varicella (chicken pox)
Photograph courtesy of SpringerImages Database, Springer Publishing Company

I. Molluscum Contagiosum

Molluscum contagiosum
  A. Caused by a poxvirus
  B. Common in children, usually a sexually transmitted disease in adults
  C. Increased in immunocompromised hosts (e.g., HIV)
  D. Transmission by skin contact
  E. Firm dome-shaped flesh-colored to pink pearly 2–8 mm papules with waxy surface and central dell (umbilication) often with central white core
  F. Molluscum dermatitis (papule surrounded by eczematous dermatitis) can occur in children with atopic dermatitis

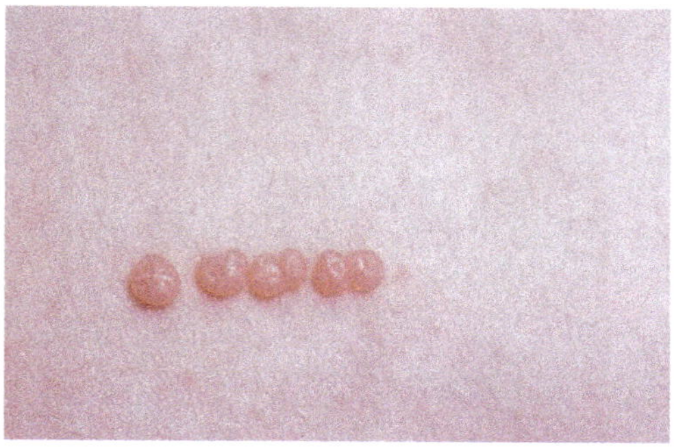

Molluscum contagiosum
Photograph courtesy of SpringerImages Database, Springer Publishing Company

Molluscum contagiosum
  A. 1–5 mm, solitary, dome-shaped, umbilicated firm pearly pink papules on a child's face (top figure)
  B. Large umbilicated papules on the face of an immunocompromised patient (bottom figure)

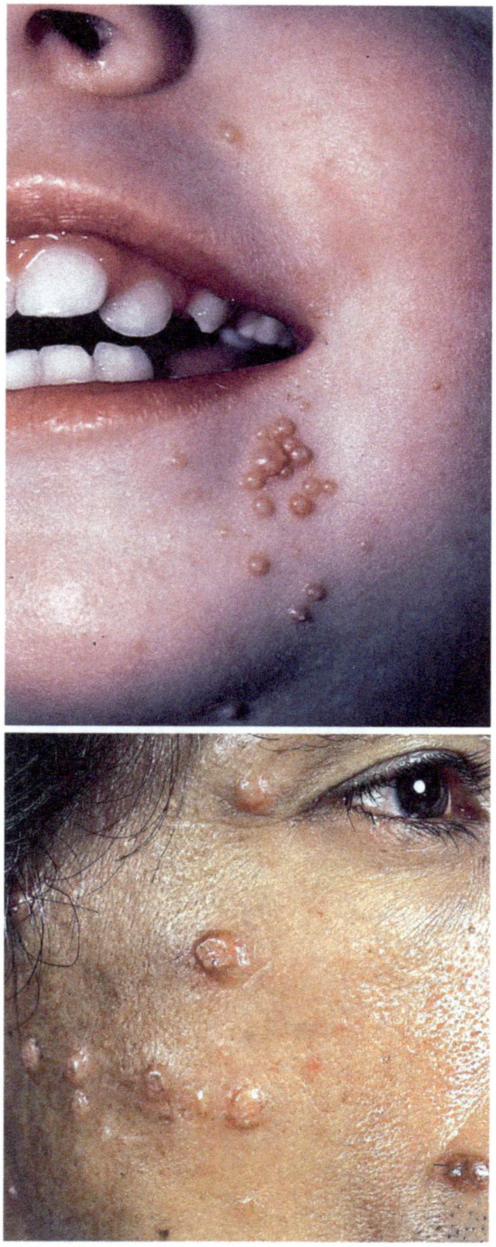

Molluscum contagiosum
Photograph courtesy of SpringerImages Database, Springer Publishing Company

54 Fungal Infections

a. Deep Fungal Infections

i. Blastomycosis

Blastomycosis

A. The soil is the most important source of infection
B. The lungs are usually the first site of infection by inhalation with subsequent spread to the skin, primary cutaneous disease is rare
C. Papulopustules and well-demarcated verrucous plaques with scale crust are characteristic
   1. Small microabscesses may be found at the periphery of lesions
   2. Plaques may develop an annular appearance and ulcerate centrally, resembling pyoderma gangrenosum
D. The extremities (especially the legs) and face (especially the nose) are common sites
E. Mucous membrane involvement is possible

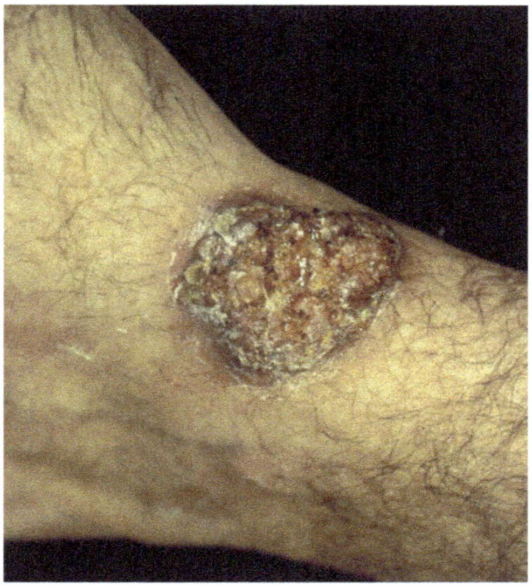

Blastomycosis
Photograph courtesy of SpringerImages Database, Springer Publishing Company

Blastomycosis

A. Well-demarcated annular verrucous plaque with scale crust and central ulceration on the leg

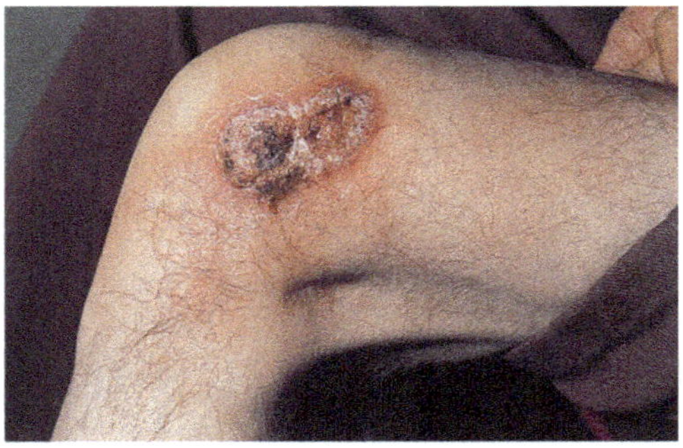

Blastomycosis
Photograph courtesy of SpringerImages Database, Springer Publishing Company

H.M. Gloster, Jr. et al., *Absolute Dermatology Review: Mastering Clinical Conditions on the Dermatology Recertification Exam*,
DOI 10.1007/978-3-319-03218-4_54,

ii. Sporotrichosis

Sporotrichosis

A. The most common clinical presentation is lymphocutaneous
B. A papule or nodule, usually on the hand or other extremity, appears several weeks after inoculation and eventually becomes eroded or ulcerated, drains purulent material, and spreads along the lymphatics in an ulcerated nodular pattern forming a linear arrangement of dermal or subcutaneous nodules following lymphatic drainage (sporotrichoid spread)
C. Usually seen in gardners (acquired through thorns or wood)
D. Sporotrichoid lymphangitic spread may be seen in Sporotrichosis, Leishmaniasis, Atypical mycobacteria (M. marinum), Nocardia, and Blastomyces

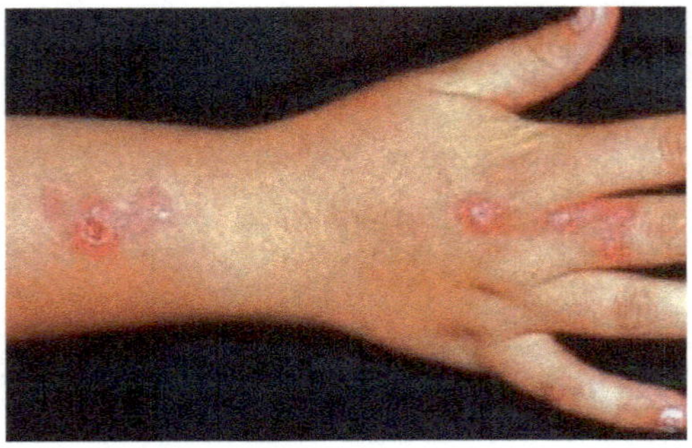

Sporotrichosis
Photograph courtesy of SpringerImages Database, Springer Publishing Company

Sporotrichosis

A. Eroded, ulcerated nodules draining purulent material that spread along the lymphatics in a linear arrangement

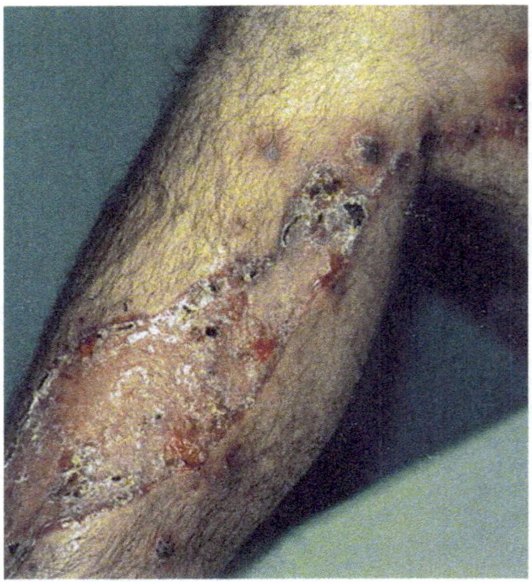

Sporotrichosis
Photograph courtesy of SpringerImages Database, Springer Publishing Company

iii. Coccidioidomycosis

Coccidiodomycosis

A. Spores are inhaled resulting in pulmonary infection (asymptomatic in 60 %, flu-like symptoms in 40 %) which then may disseminate to skin (primary inoculation is rare)
B. Usually presents as a verrucous plaque with pustules on the face

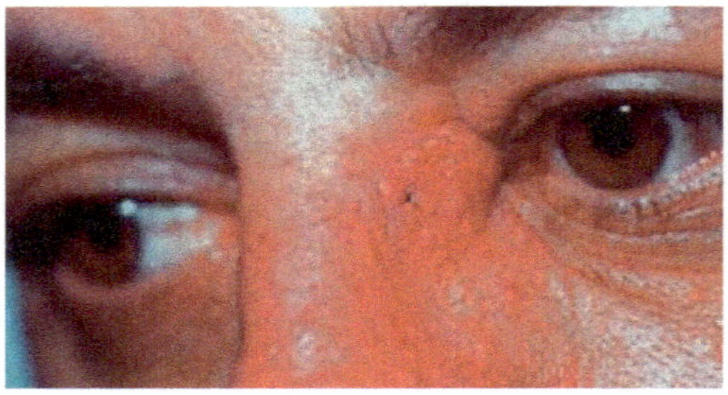

Coccidioidomycosis
Photograph courtesy of SpringerImages Database, Springer Publishing Company

Coccidiodomycosis

A. Verrucous plaque with pustules on the eyelid

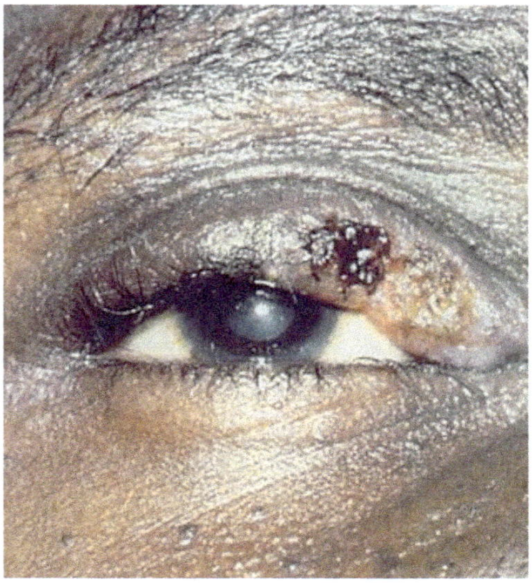

Coccidioidomycosis
Photograph courtesy of SpringerImages Database, Springer Publishing Company

iv. Cryptococcosis

Cryptococcosis

A. Papulonodules with umbilication, resembling molluscum (common presentation in AIDS patients)
B. Ulcers
C. Cellulitis-like lesions

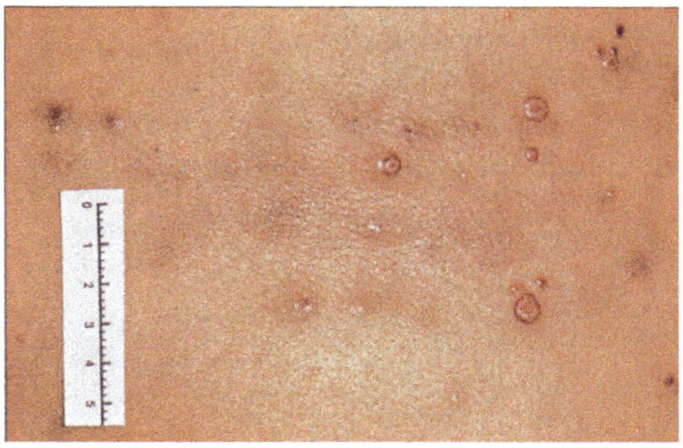

Cryptococcosis
Photograph courtesy of SpringerImages Database, Springer Publishing Company

Cryptococcosis

A. Papulonodules with umbilication, resembling molluscum in an AIDS patient

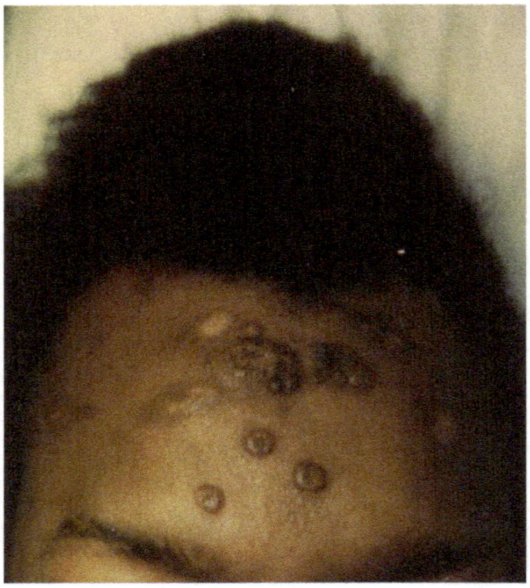

Cryptococcosis
Photograph courtesy of SpringerImages Database, Springer Publishing Company

Cryptococcosis

A. Cellulitis-like lesions on the arm at a venipuncture site in a patient with chronic lymphocytic leukemia

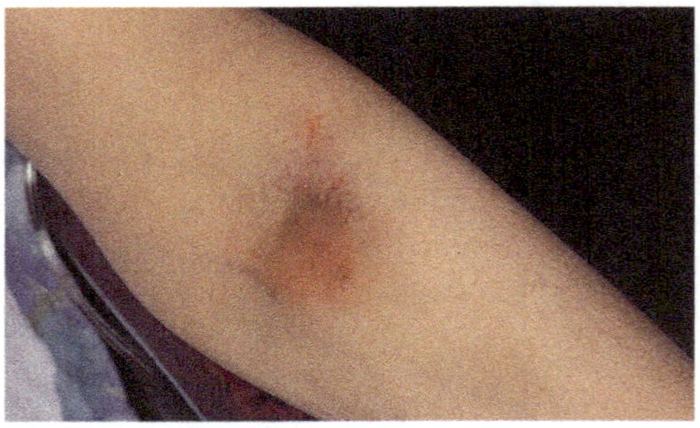

Cryptococcosis
Photograph courtesy of SpringerImages Database, Springer Publishing Company

b. Fungal Folliculitis

i. Malassezia (Pityrosporum) Folliculitis

Malassezia (pityrosporum) folliculitis

A. Young adults with aggravating factors (warm weather, occlusion, excess sebum, antibiotic therapy—especially tetracycline, immunosuppression)
B. Pruritic follicular papules with central white-yellow color which is keratin, not pus
C. Most common on the back, chest, and shoulders

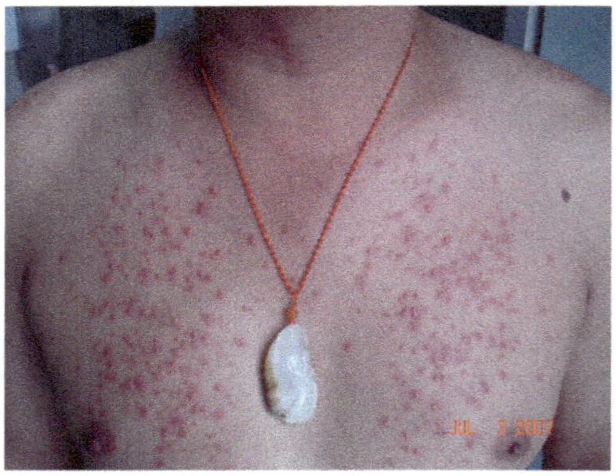

Malassezia (pityrosporum) folliculitis
Photograph courtesy of SpringerImages Database, Springer Publishing Company

Malassezia (pityrosporum) folliculitis
A. Pruritic follicular papules with central white-yellow color

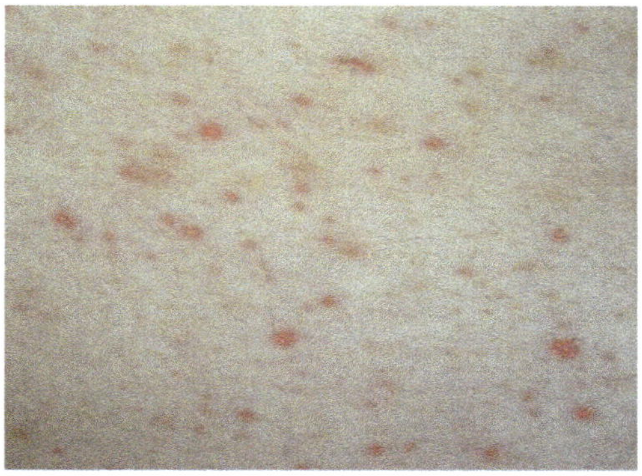

Malassezia (pityrosporum) folliculitis
Photograph courtesy of SpringerImages Database, Springer Publishing Company

c. Onychomycosis

Onychomycosis
A. 90% are caused by dermatophytes, Tinea rubrum is the most common cause
B. Toenails more commonly involved than fingernails, single or multiple nails (more common) may be involved
C. Three patterns exist based on the point of fungal entry into the skin:
1. Distal/lateral subungual (most common pattern)—invasion of the hyponichium resulting in subungual hyperkeratosis of the nail bed, yellowing and thickening of the nail plate, and onycholysis of the distal nail plate
2. Superficial white—direct penetration into the dorsal surface of the nail plate resulting in discrete white patches or transverse striate bands
3. Proximal subungual—invasion under the proximal nail fold, usually occurs in immunocompromised patients

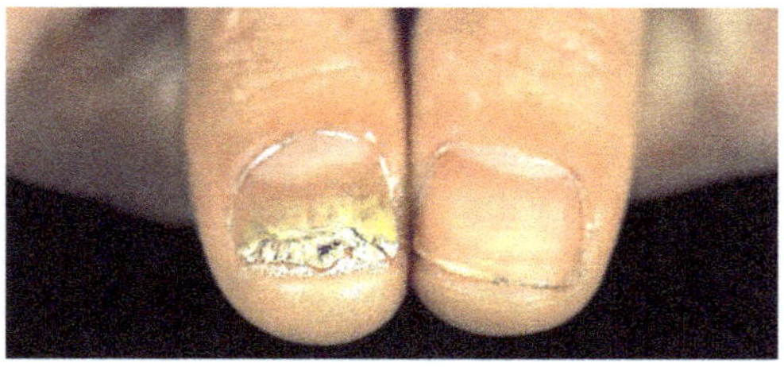

Onychomycosis (distal lateral subungual)
Photograph courtesy of SpringerImages Database, Springer Publishing Company

ii. Superficial white onychomycosis
A. Direct penetration into the dorsal surface of the nail plate resulting in discrete white patches or transverse striate bands

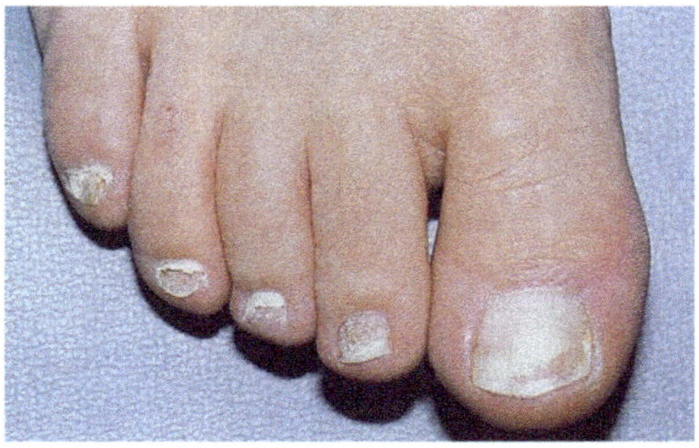

Onychomycosis (superficial white)
Photograph courtesy of SpringerImages Database, Springer Publishing Company

iii. Proximal subungual onychomycosis
   A. Invasion under the proximal nail fold, usually occurs in immunocompromised patients

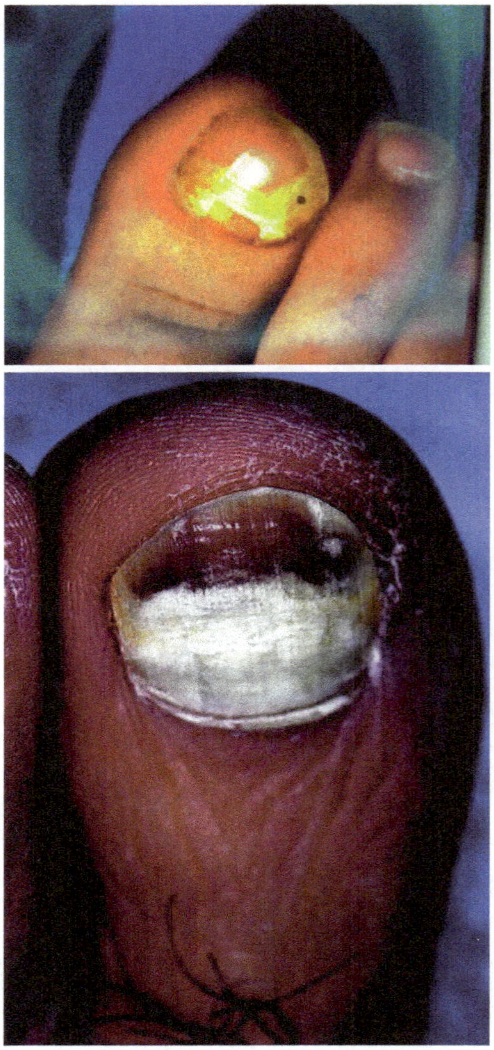

Onychomycosis (proximal subungual)
Photograph courtesy of SpringerImages Database, Springer Publishing Company

d. Dermatophyte (Tinea) Infections

i. Tinea Pedis

Tinea pedis
   A. Dermatophyte infection of the soles and interdigital web spaces
   B. Associated with onychomycosis
   C. Most common location for dermatophyte infections
   D. Four clinical types: moccasin, interdigital, vesiculobullous, ulcerative

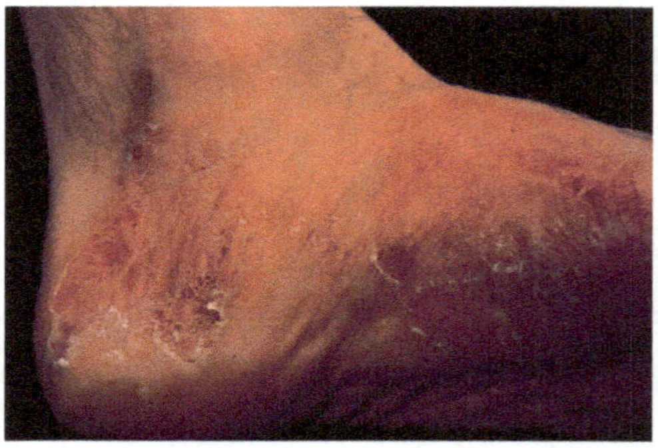

Mocassin tinea pedis
Photograph courtesy of SpringerImages Database, Springer Publishing Company

1. Moccasin Tinea Pedis

Moccasin tinea pedis

A. Erythema and scale on the soles and lateral aspects of one or both feet in a slipper or moccasin distribution

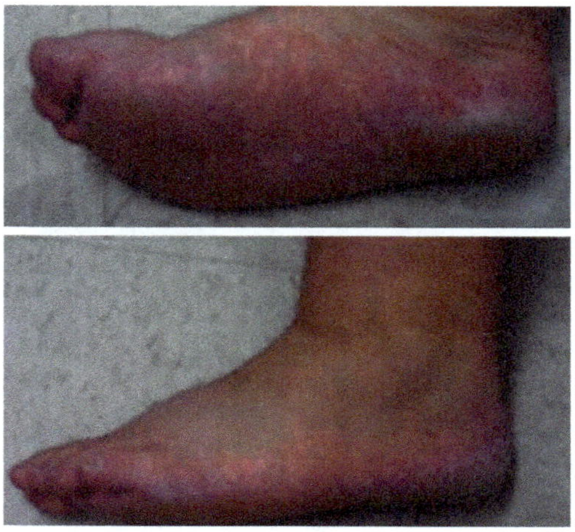

Mocassin tinea pedis
Photograph courtesy of SpringerImages Database, Springer Publishing Company

2. Interdigital Tinea Pedis

Interdigital tinea pedis

A. Most common type of tinea pedis
B. Maceration and scaling in the toe web spaces (most commonly between the fourth and fifth web space)
C. May be associated with itching, burning, malodor
D. High moisture and occlusion predispose to toe web tinea infections

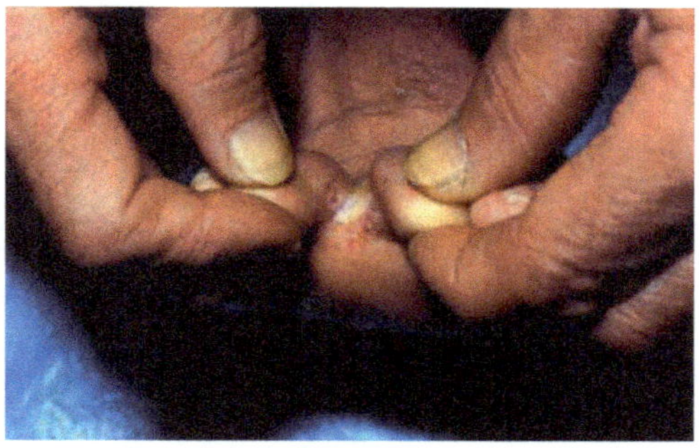

Interdigital tinea pedis
Photograph courtesy of SpringerImages Database, Springer Publishing Company

Moccasin and interdigital tinea pedis

A. Erythema and scale on the soles and lateral aspects of both feet in a slipper or moccasin distribution (figure a)
B. Maceration and scaling in the toe web spaces (figure b)

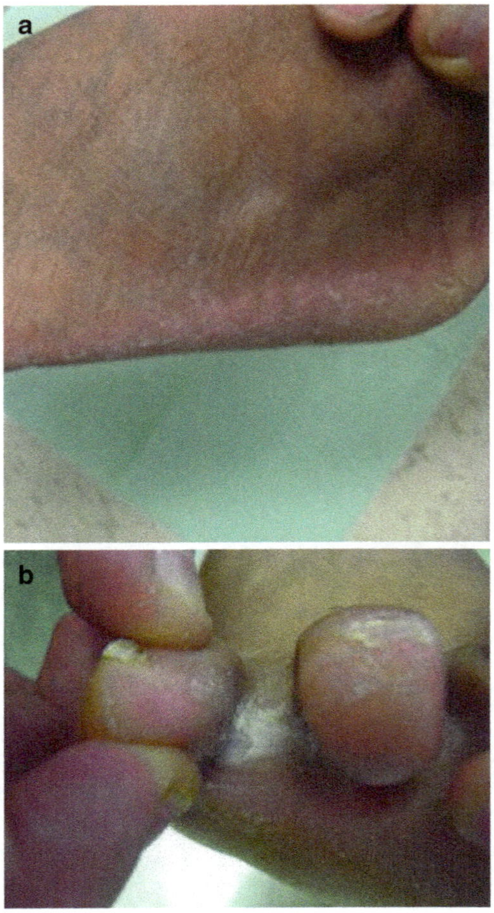

Mocassin and interdigital tinea pedis
Photograph courtesy of SpringerImages Database, Springer Publishing Company

3. Vesiculobullous Tinea Pedis

Vesiculobullous tinea pedis

A. Pustules, vesicles, and bullae on the medial foot (arches, sides of feet)
B. Type most often associated with dermatophytid reaction

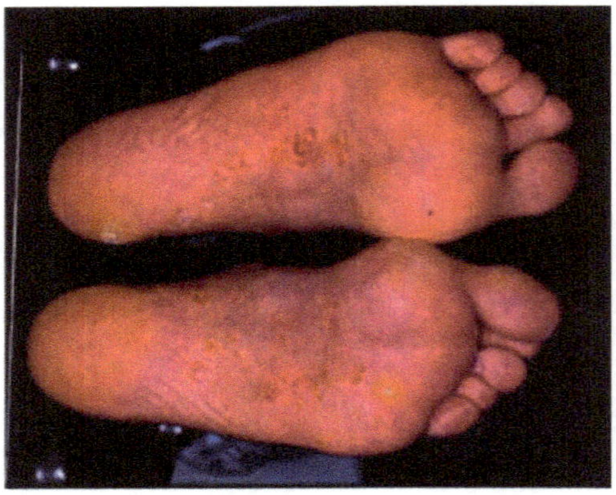

Vesiculobullous tinea pedis
Photograph courtesy of SpringerImages Database, Springer Publishing Company

ii. Tinea Manuum

Tinea Manuum
A. Usually noninflammatory and often unilateral (two feet and one hand syndrome)
B. Diffuse scaling with accentuation in the creases on the palms or an annular plaque on dorsal surface of the hand

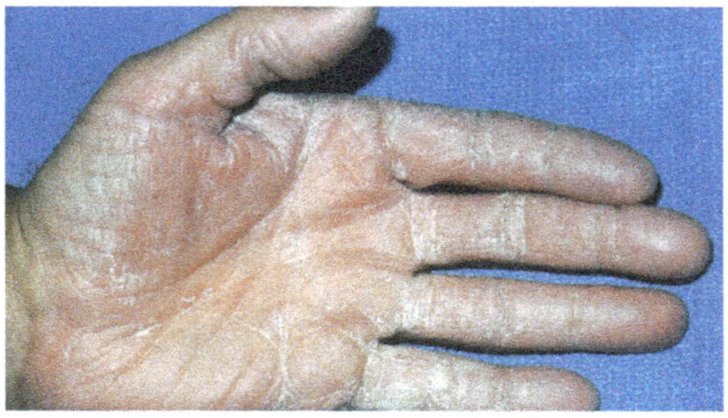

Tinea manuum
Photograph courtesy of the American Academy of Dermatology

Tinea Manuum
A. Diffuse scaling with accentuation in the creases on the palms

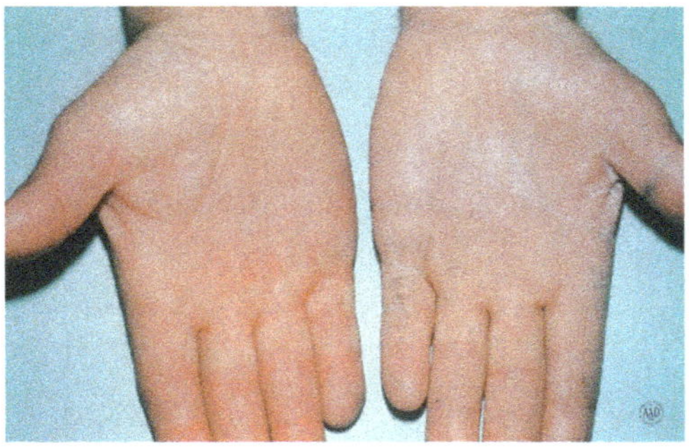

Tinea manuum
Photograph courtesy of the American Academy of Dermatology

iii. Tinea Corporis

Tinea corporis
A. Dermatophyte (T. rubrum most common) infection of the stratum corneum on trunk and extremities
B. Multiple clinical presentations
   1. Annular scaly plaques with central clearing and scale most prominent at the leading edge (centrifugal spread with central clearing, see figure), pustules and vesicles may be within the active border
   2. Concentric rings (arcuate, circinate)
   3. Majocchi's granuloma
      a. Perifollicular papules and pustules (T. rubrum)
      b. Most common in women with tinea pedis or onychomycosis who shave their legs
      c. Deep fungal folliculitis in which wall of follicle is disrupted

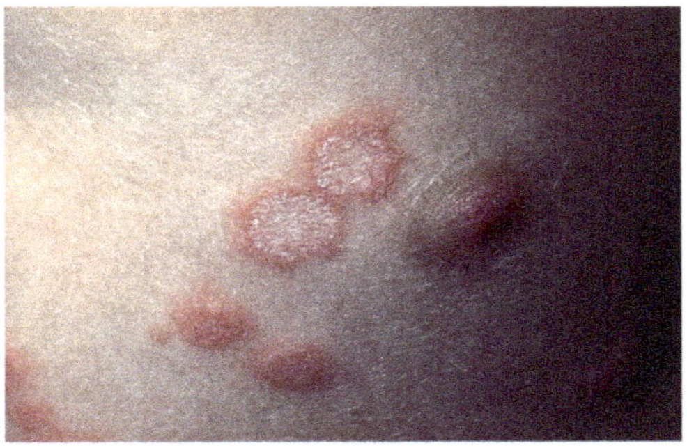

Tinea corporis
Photograph courtesy of SpringerImages Database, Springer Publishing Company

Tinea corporis

A. Annular scaly plaques with central clearing and scale most prominent at the leading edge (centrifugal spread with central clearing)

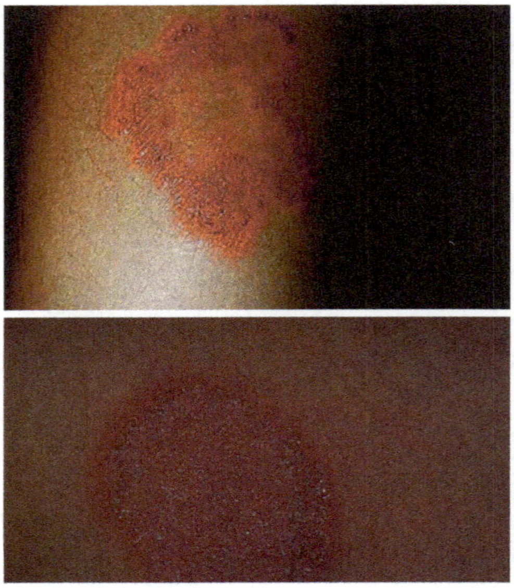

Tinea corporis
Photograph courtesy of SpringerImages Database, Springer Publishing Company

Tinea Corporis

A. Annular scaling plaques forming concentric rings

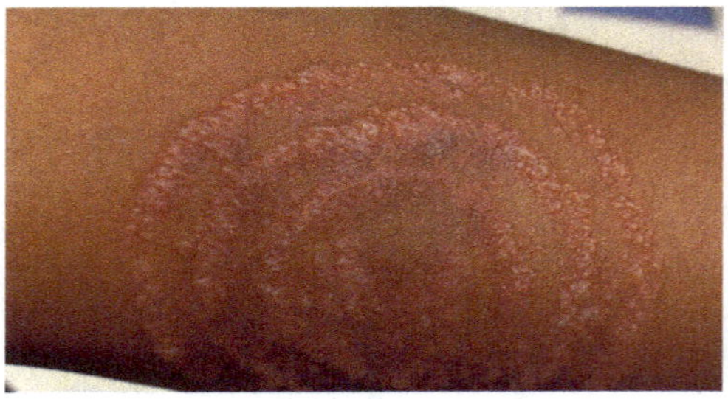

Tinea corporis
Photograph courtesy of Hugh Gloster, MD

iv. Majocchi's Granuloma

Majocchi's granuloma

A. Deep fungal folliculitis in which the wall of the follicle is disrupted resulting in perifollicular papules, pustules, and nodules or pustules at the edge of tinea cruris or corporis
B. Most common in women with tinea pedis or onychomycosis who shave their legs

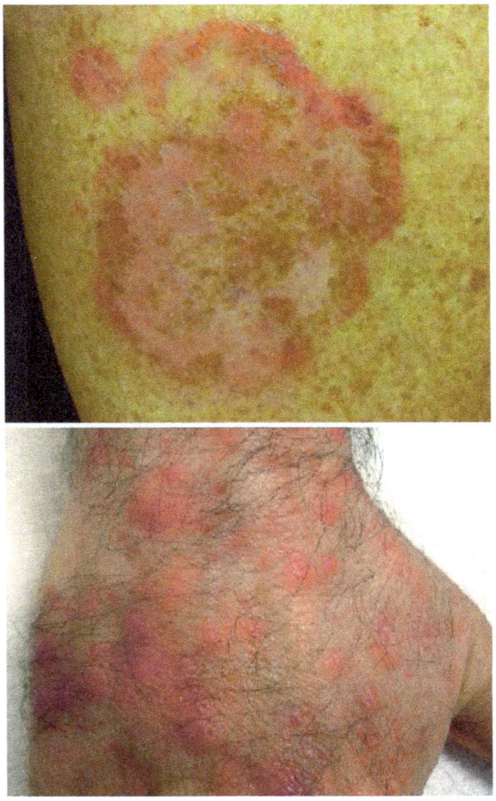

Majocchi's granuloma
Photograph courtesy of SpringerImages Database, Springer Publishing Company

v. Tinea Faciei

Tinea faciei

A. Most frequently misdiagnosed fungal infection, thus high clinical suspicion is necessary
B. May be photosensitive, many patients are misdiagnosed as having photosensitivity disorder
C. Most often presents in children and adolescents
D. Most have classic features of dermatophyte infection (annular configuration, scale, pustules at the border), yet some may be more difficult to diagnose

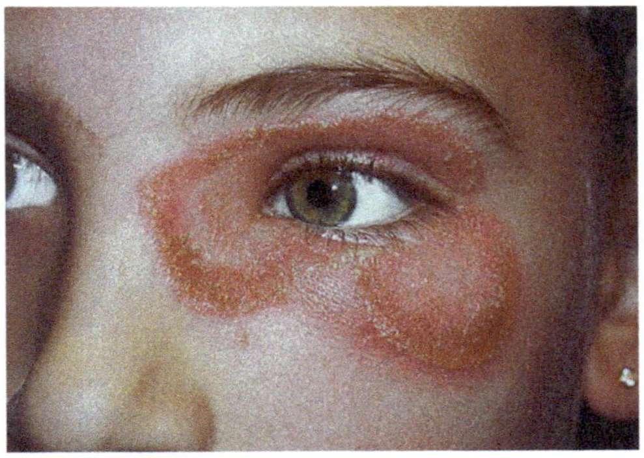

Tinea faciei
Photograph courtesy of SpringerImages Database, Springer Publishing Company

Tinea faciei

A. Annular, erythematous scaly plaque

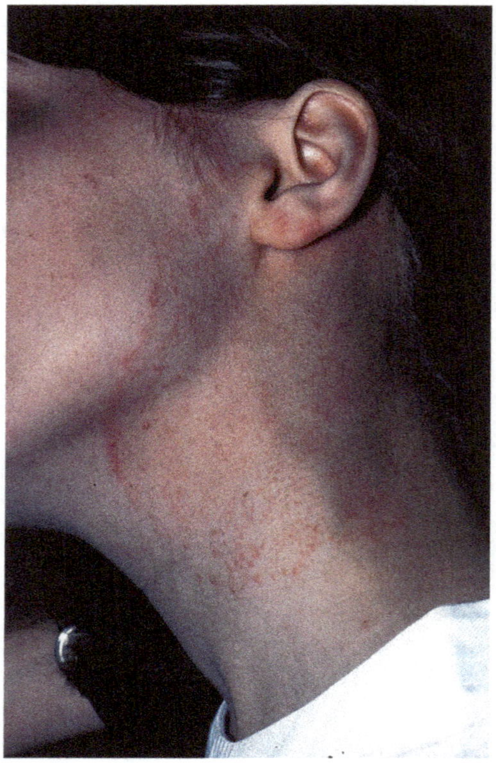

Tinea faciei
Photograph courtesy of SpringerImages Database, Springer Publishing Company

vi. Tinea Barbae

Tinea barbae

A. Inflammatory papules and pustules involving the bearded area of the face and neck in men, abscesses and sinus tracts may develop

B. Often acquired from animals, seen in male farm workers

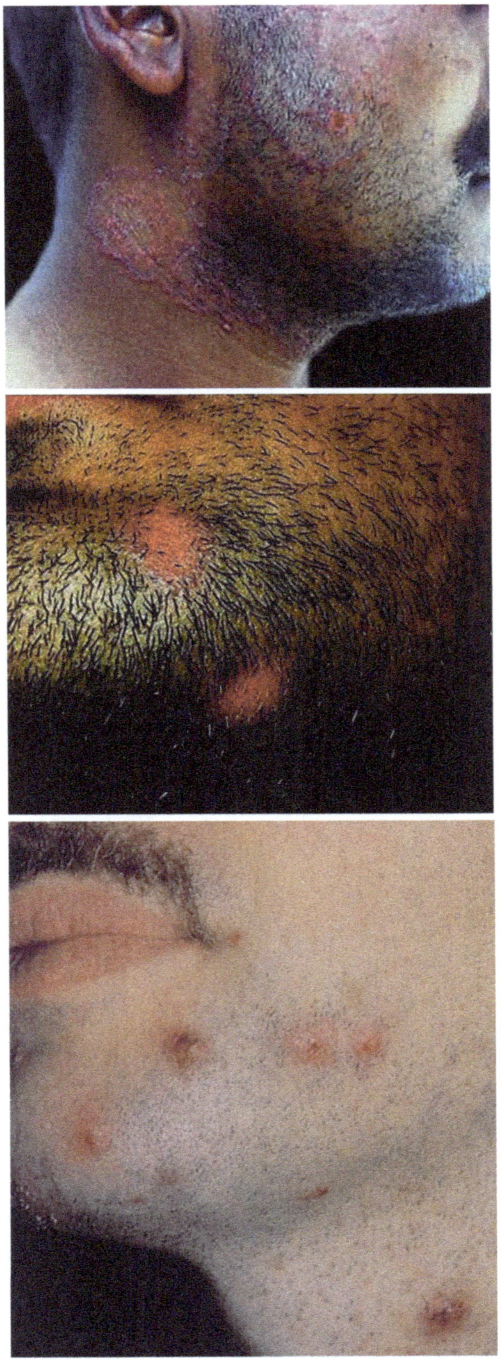

Tinea barbae
Photograph courtesy of the American Academy of Dermatology

vii. Tinea Capitis

Tinea capitis

A. Common dermatophyte infection in children (rare in adults), Trichophyton tonsurans most common
B. Most common presentation is alopecia with or without scale
C. May have cervical or postauricular adenopathy

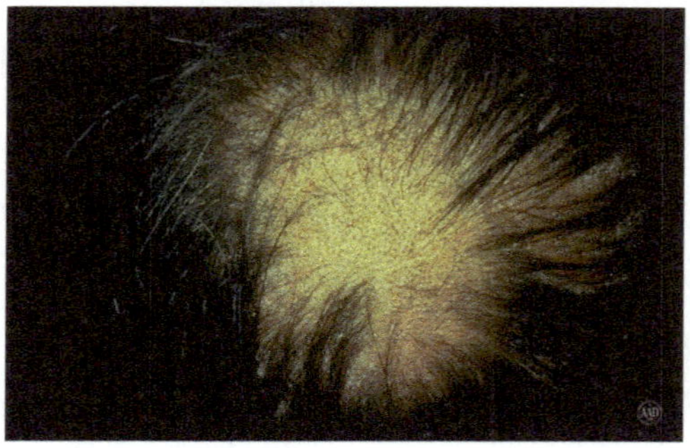

Tinea capitis
Photograph courtesy of the American Academy of Dermatology

Tinea capitis

A. Dry scaly patches of alopecia with little inflammation which may mimic alopecia areata (gray patch tinea capitis), frequently caused by microsporum species

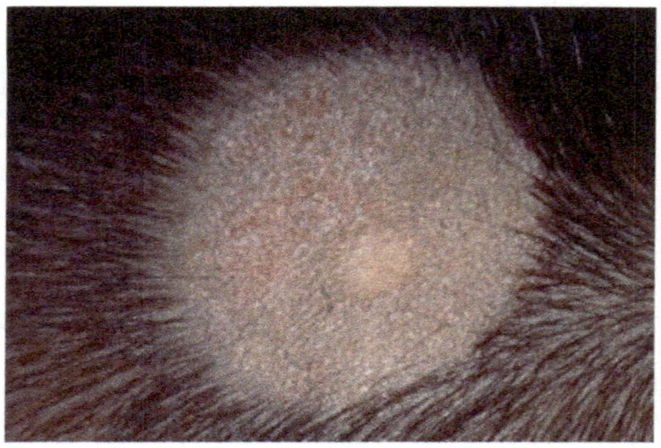

Tinea capitis
Photograph courtesy of SpringerImages Database, Springer Publishing Company

1. Black Dot Tinea Capitis

Black dot tinea capitis

A. Patchy alopecia with black dots (hair breakage near scalp) that may occur in discrete patches or involve the entire scalp

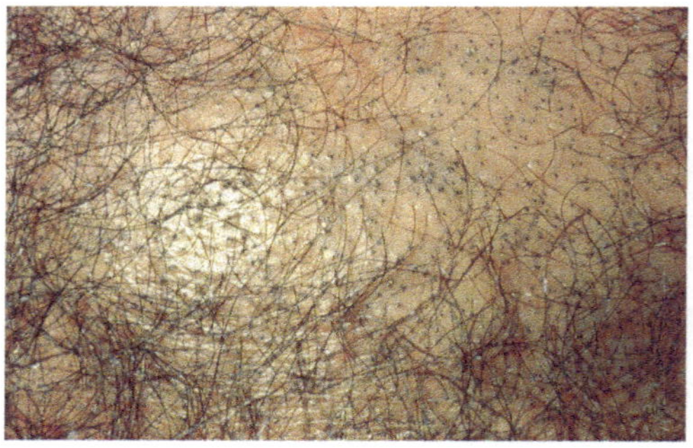

Black dot tinea capitis
Photograph courtesy of the American Academy of Dermatology

2. Kerion

Tinea capitis (kerion)

A. Boggy purulent plaques with abscess formation and alopecia

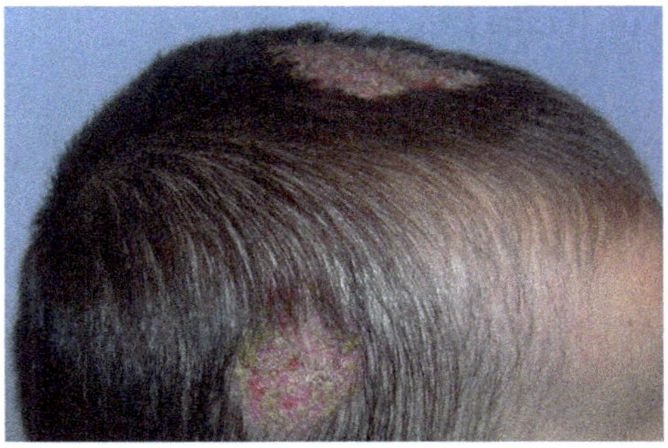

Kerion
Photograph courtesy of SpringerImages Database, Springer Publishing Company

Tinea capitis (kerion)

A. Boggy purulent plaques with abscess formation and alopecia

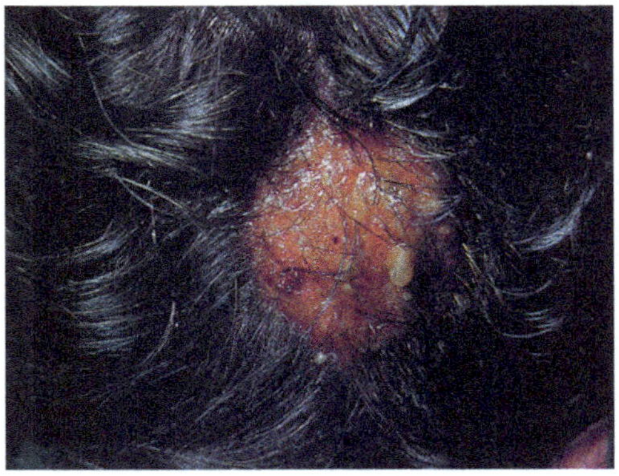

Kerion
Photograph courtesy of SpringerImages Database, Springer Publishing Company

3. Favus

Favus

A. Most severe form of dermatophyte hair infection
B. Caused by Trychophyton schoenleinii
C. Wood's light: blue white fluorescence
D. Thick yellow crusts composed of hyphae and skin debris (keratin) called scutula, leads to scarring alopecia

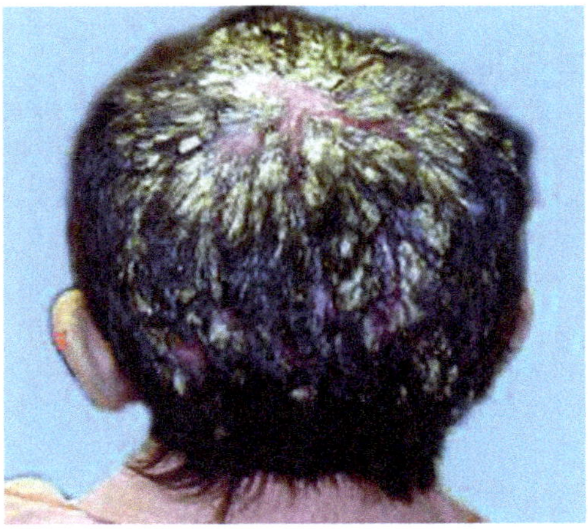

Favus
Photograph courtesy of SpringerImages Database, Springer Publishing Company

viii. Tinea Cruris

Tinea cruris

A. Dermatophyte infection of inguinal area, especially the inner upper thighs, with occasional extension to buttocks and abdomen
B. Sharply demarcated raised red plaque with scaly advancing border that may contain pustules, may initially be arcuate, then become serpiginous
C. Scrotum is spared (consider candidiasis if scrotum involved or if there are erosions or satellite pustules with collarettes of scale)

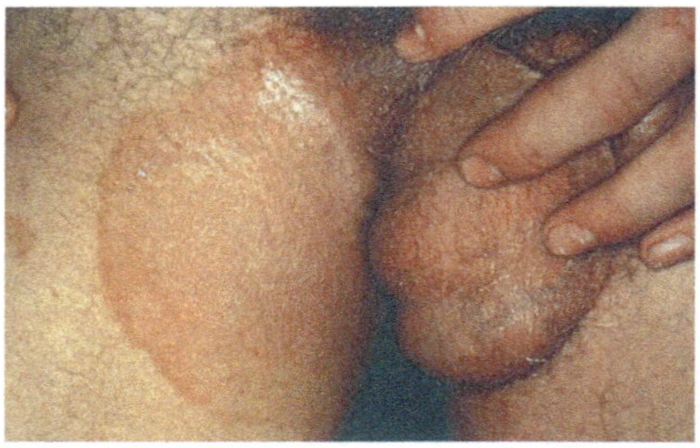

Tinea cruris
Photograph courtesy of SpringerImages Database, Springer Publishing Company

Tinea cruris

A. A sharply demarcated raised red plaque with scaly advancing border on the inner upper thighs

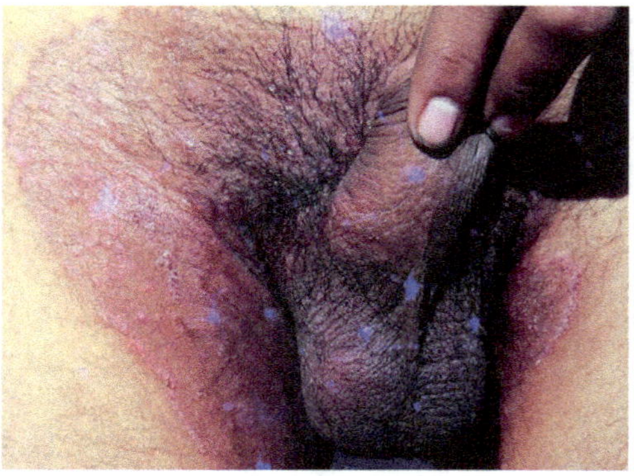

Tinea cruris
Photograph courtesy of SpringerImages Database, Springer Publishing Company

ix. Tinea Incognito

Tinea incognito

A. Scale is decreased or absent due to application of topical steroids, resulting in the loss of the characteristic features of tinea

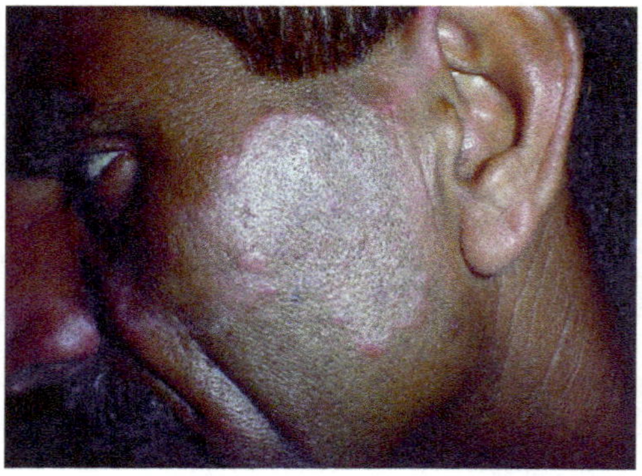

Tinea incognito
Photograph courtesy of SpringerImages Database, Springer Publishing Company

ix. Tinea Incognito

Tinea incognito

A. The application of topical steroids results in the loss of characteristic features of tinea (no scale, no tendency to central clearing, and indistinct borders)

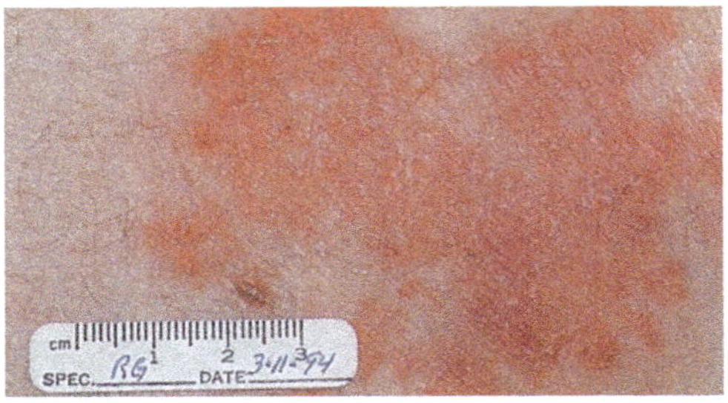

Tinea incognito
Photograph courtesy of SpringerImages Database, Springer Publishing Company

x. Tinea Versicolor

Tinea versicolor

A. Multiple brown, tan, or hypopigmented oval to round, patches or thin plaques with mild fine scale on the seborrheic regions of the neck, upper trunk, and shoulders
B. KOH (potassium hydroxide) prep shows hyphae resembling "spaghetti and meatballs" (malassezia furfur)
C. Demonstration of scale may require scratching or stretching the skin surface
D. Inverse tinea versicolor: occurs in flexural areas (groin, submammary, antecubital fossa)

Tinea versicolor
Photograph courtesy of SpringerImages Database, Springer Publishing Company

Tinea versicolor

A. The fine, branny scaling is not readily evident until lesions are gently scraped with the end of a glass microscope slide

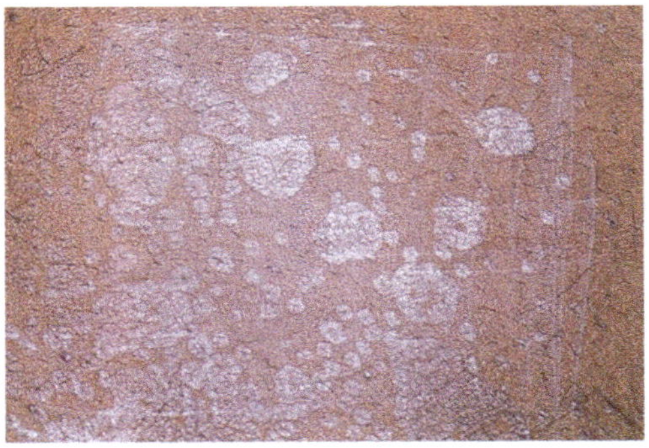

Tinea versicolor
Photograph courtesy of SpringerImages Database, Springer Publishing Company

Tinea versicolor

A. In black skin, tinea versicolor is often hypopigmented and may affect the face

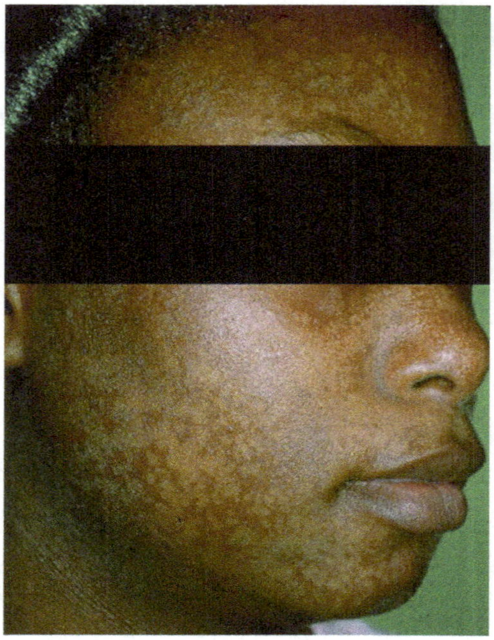

Tinea versicolor
Photograph courtesy of SpringerImages Database, Springer Publishing Company

Tinea versicolor

A. Hyperpigmented tinea versicolor with perifollicular round, hyperpigmented barely palpable patches and plaques with fine, branny scaling

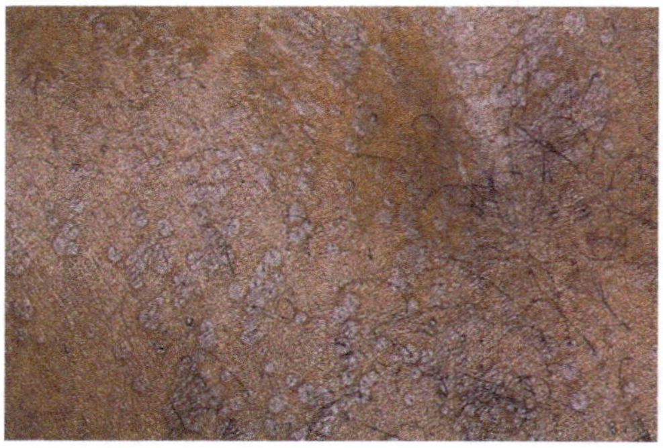

Tinea versicolor
Photograph courtesy of SpringerImages Database, Springer Publishing Company

Bacterial Infections 55

a. Cellulitis

Cellulitis

A. Infection of the deep dermis and subcutaneous tissue characterized by poorly defined erythema with nonpalpable borders, swelling, warmth, and tenderness
B. Borders are not as sharply demarcated as in erysipelas
C. Preceded by fever, chills, malaise
D. Vesicles, bullae, pustules, necrosis, adenopathy, and ascending lymphangitis may be seen in severe infections
E. Bullae and petechiae are more common on the lower extremities
F. Presents more commonly on the head and neck in children and the extremities in adults
G. Most commonly caused by Group A streptococci or staphylococcus
H. Usually initiated by a break in skin barrier, on the leg tinea pedis is the most common portal of entry

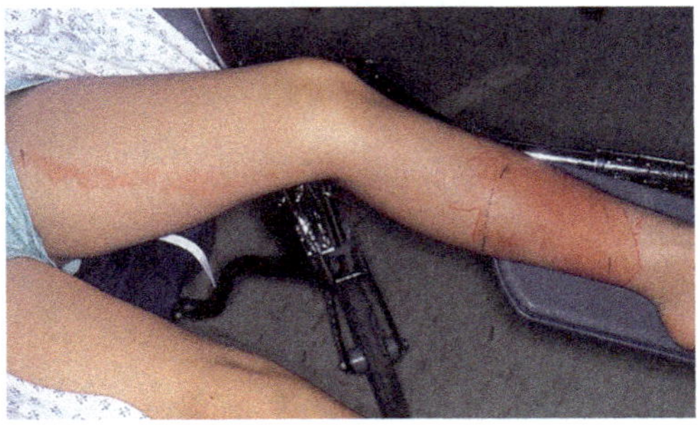

Cellulitis
Photograph courtesy of SpringerImages Database, Springer Publishing Company

H.M. Gloster, Jr. et al., *Absolute Dermatology Review: Mastering Clinical Conditions on the Dermatology Recertification Exam*,
DOI 10.1007/978-3-319-03218-4_55,

b. Perianal Streptococcal Cellulitis

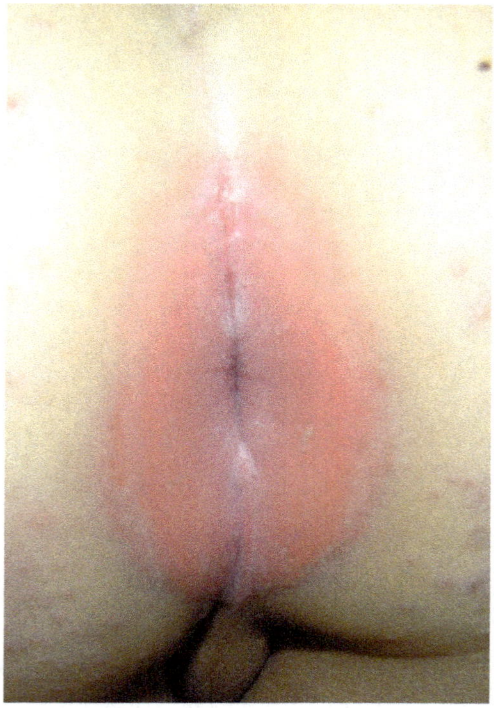

Perianal streptococcal cellulitis
Photograph courtesy of SpringerImages Database, Springer Publishing Company

Perianal streptococcal cellulitis.

A. Caused by Streptococcus pyogenes
B. Occurs most commonly in children, especially boys less than 4 years old
C. Characterized by sharply demarcated, bright red, beefy erythema extending 2–3 cm around the anus
D. Painful fissures and pain on defacation may occur

c. Erythrasma

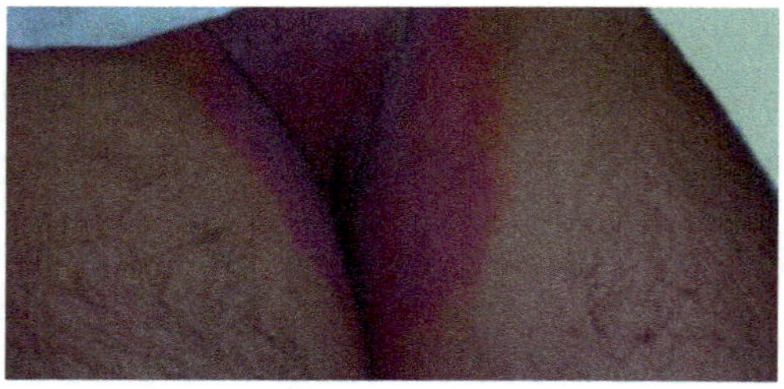

Erythrasma
Photograph courtesy of SpringerImages Database, Springer Publishing Company

Erythrasma

A. Caused by excessive proliferation of corynebacterium minutissimum within the stratum corneum of moist intertriginous areas (groin, axillae, intergluteal fold, inframmmary, abdominal fat folds, umbilicus, toe web spaces)
B. Pink to brown, sharply defined patches with scant scaling; with time, red patches fade to brown; mildly pruritic or asymptomatic
C. Interdigital erythrasma, which presents with maceration and scaling of the toe web spaces, is the most common bacterial infection of the foot and most common form of erythrasma
D. Coral red fluorescence by Wood's light (bacteria produces porphyrin)

Erythrasma
  A. Coral red fluorescence by Wood's light

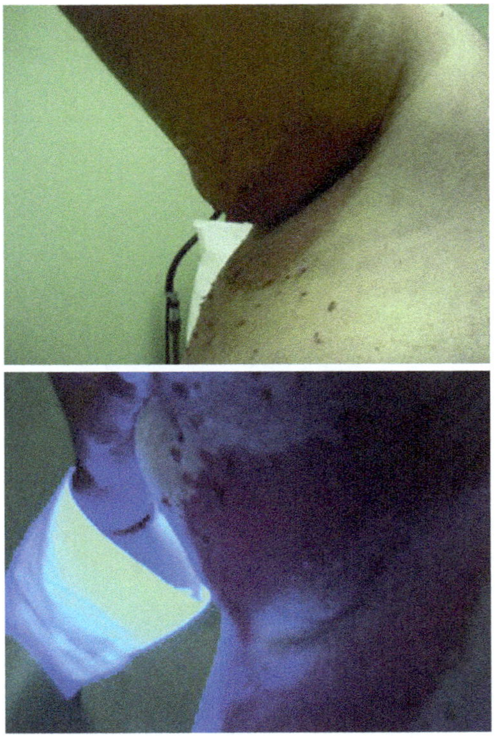

Erythrasma
Photograph courtesy of SpringerImages Database, Springer Publishing Company

d. Folliculitis

i. Bacterial Folliculitis

1. Staphylococcal Folliculitis

Staphylococcal Folliculitis
  A. Follicular pustules and papules on an erythematous base
  B. Neck, axillae, groin, buttocks most common
  C. Caused by Staphylococcus aureus

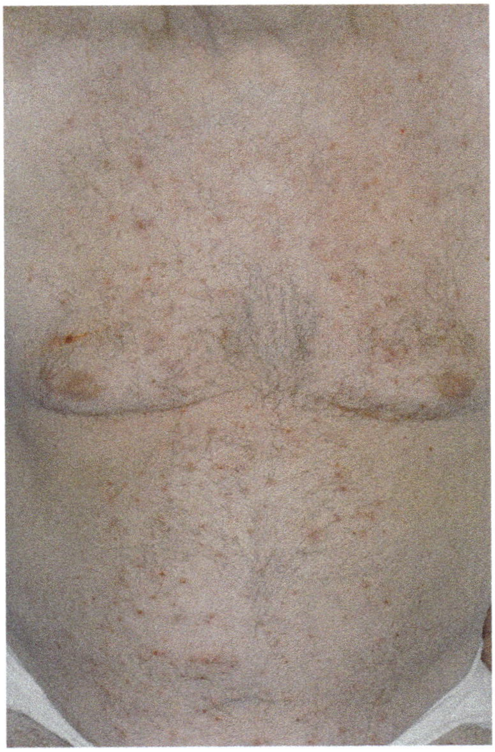

Staphylococcal folliculitis
Photograph courtesy of SpringerImages Database, Springer Publishing Company

Staphylococcal Folliculitis

A. Follicular pustules and papules on an erythematous base

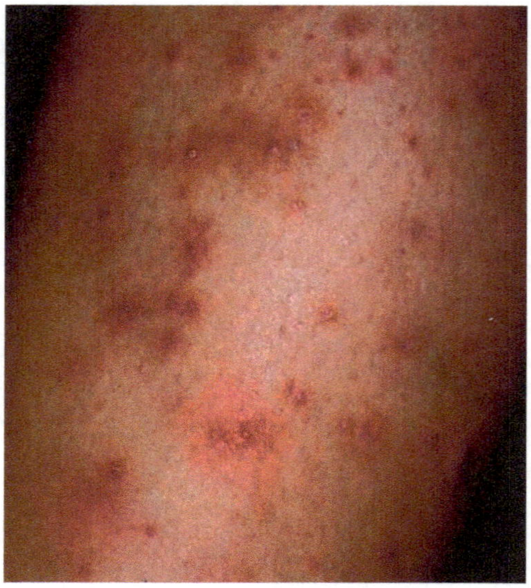

Staphylococcal folliculitis
Photograph courtesy of SpringerImages Database, Springer Publishing Company

Staphylococcal folliculitis

A. Follicular pustules and papules on an erythematous base

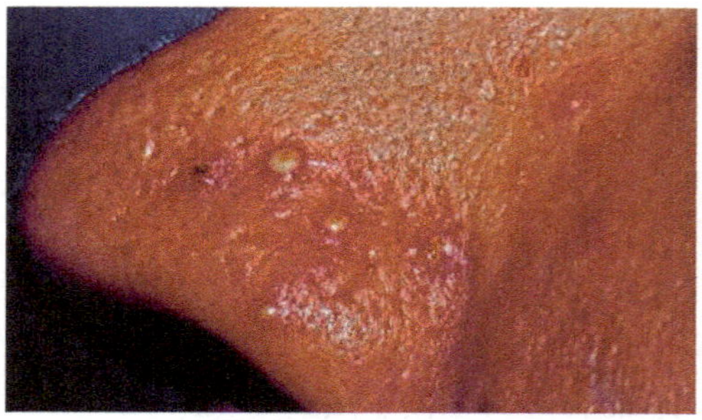

Staphylococcal folliculitis
Photograph courtesy of SpringerImages Database, Springer Publishing Company

2. Pseudomonas Folliculitis

Pseudomonas folliculitis

A. Type of gram-negative folliculitis
B. There is often a history of exposure to a hot tub or whirlpool within 12–48 hours
C. Edematous red pruritic follicular papules on the trunk
D. Most often caused by Pseudomonas aeruginosa
E. Resolves spontaneously

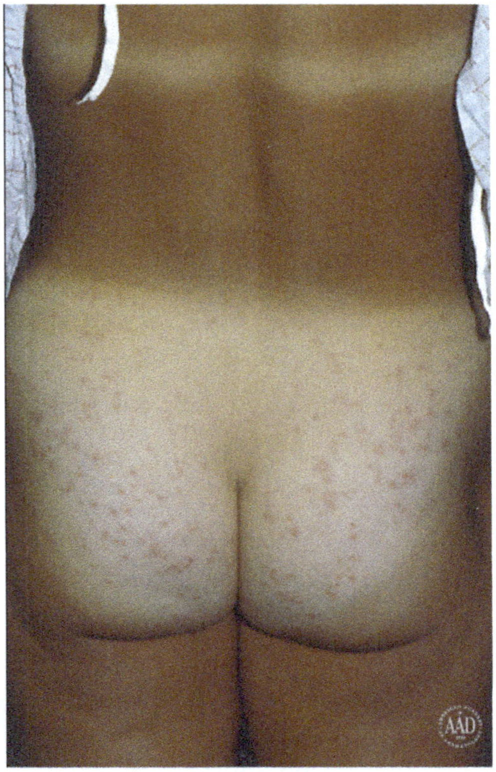

Pseudomonas folliculitis
Photograph courtesy of the American Academy of Dermatology

ii. Eosinophilic Pustular Folliculitis

Eosinophilic pustular folliculitis

A. Pruritic follicular edematous papules and pustules of the face, scalp, and upper trunk in the setting of HIV (CD4 usually < 300 cells/mm^3) or other immunosuppressed states
B. Improves with elevation of CD4 count with treatment

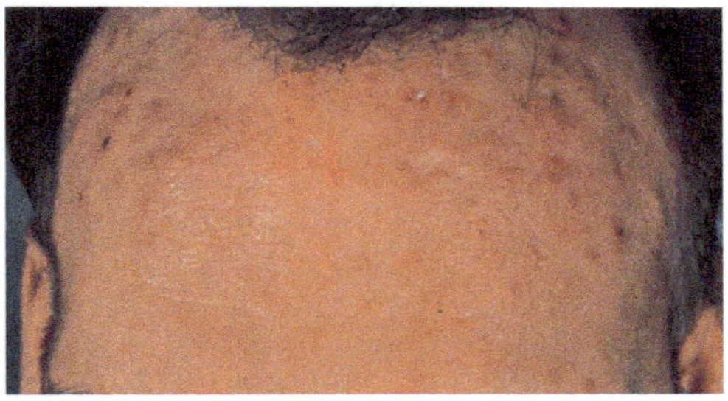

Eosinophilic pustular folliculitis
Photograph courtesy of SpringerImages Database, Springer Publishing Company

Eosinophilic pustular folliculitis

A. Pruritic follicular edematous papules and pustules of the upper trunk in the setting of HIV

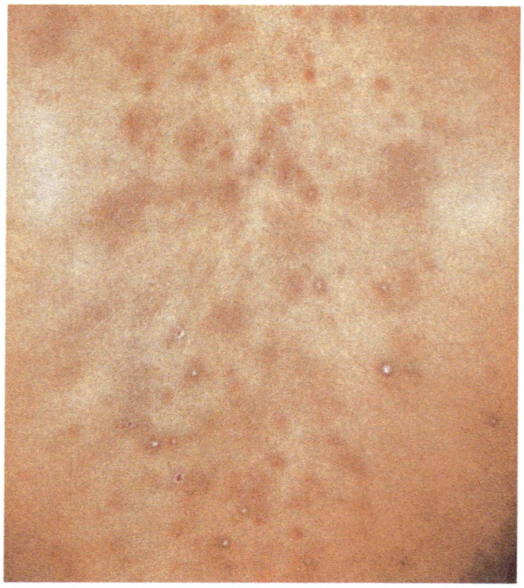

Eosinophilic pustular folliculitis
Photograph courtesy of SpringerImages Database, Springer Publishing Company

iii. Drug Induced Folliculitis

Drug induced folliculitis

A. May begin within 2 weeks of certain drugs (steroids, androgen hormones, chlorinated compounds, EGFR inhibitors, iodides, bromides, lithium, isoniazid, anticonvulsants)
B. Acute acneiform eruption of monomorphic red follicular papules and pustules on trunk, shoulders, upper arms (no comedones)

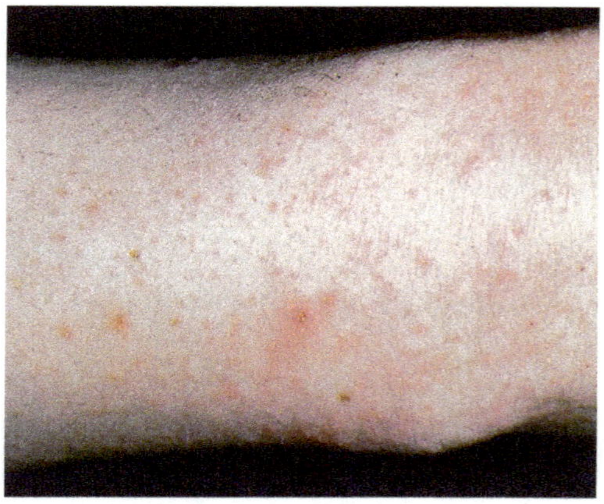

Drug induced folliculitis
Photograph courtesy of SpringerImages Database, Springer Publishing Company

Drug induced folliculitis

A. Acute acneiform eruption of monomorphic red follicular papules and pustules without comedones

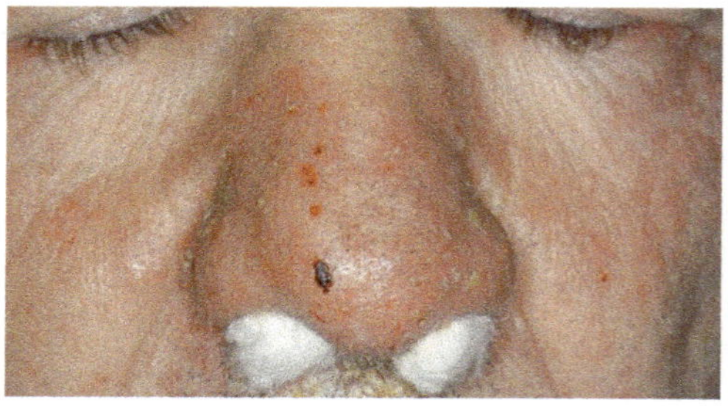

Drug induced folliculitis
Photograph courtesy of SpringerImages Database, Springer Publishing Company

e. Gonococcemia

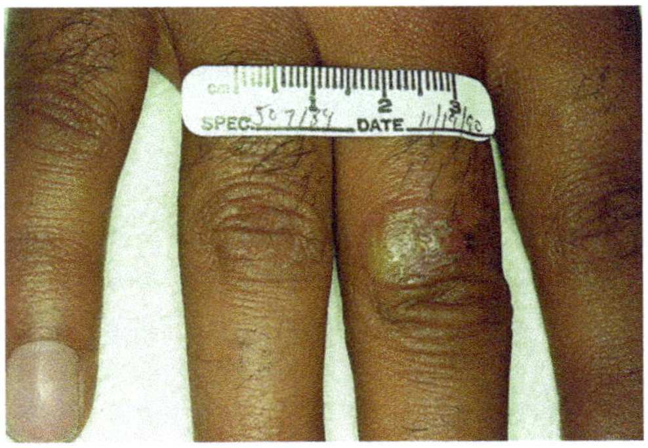

Gonococcemia
Photograph courtesy of SpringerImages Database, Springer Publishing Company

Gonococcemia

A. Fever, joint pain (large joints: knees, elbows, wrists, ankles)
B. Hemorrhagic vesiculopustules on the distal extremities most often over joints or palmoplantar surfaces
C. Lesions contain organisms and represent an embolic septic vasculitis

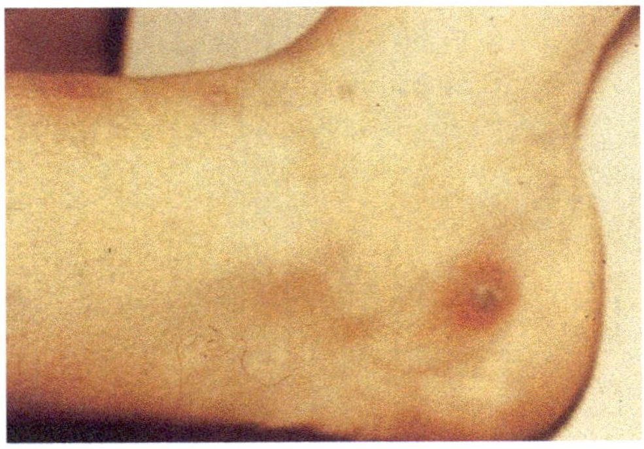

Gonococcemia
Photograph courtesy of SpringerImages Database, Springer Publishing Company

Gonococcemia

A. Hemorrhagic vesiculopustule on the heel

f. Meningococcemia

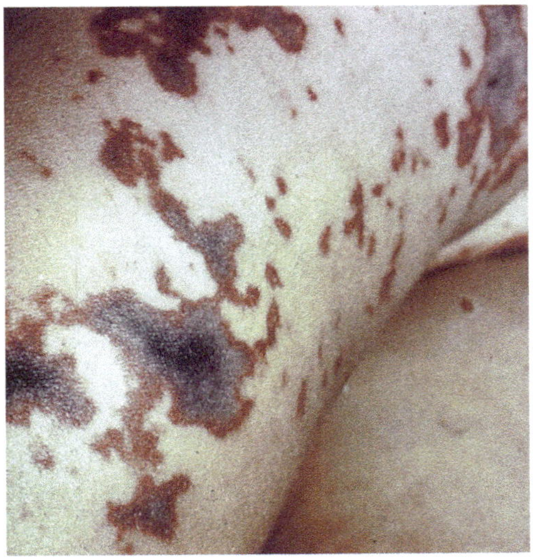

Meningococcemia
Photograph courtesy of SpringerImages Database, Springer Publishing Company

Meningococcemia

A. Endotoxin of Neisseria meningitides may cause shock, multiorgan failure, and purpura fulminans (rapidly progressing medical emergency)
B. Mainly occurs in infants, adolescents, and young adults
C. Reservoir is nasopharynx, leading to respiratory transmission
D. Acute form
   1. Angular geometric petechial and purpuric plaques and ischemic necrosis (gun metal gray interior is characteristic), most common on the trunk and lower extremities, bullous hemorrhagic lesions may also occur
   2. Fever, chills, myalgias, headache, hypotention
   3. Meningitis, encephalitis, pneumonia, arthritis, pericarditis, myocarditis, purpura fulminans
E. Chronic form
   1. Recurrent episodes of fever, arthralgia, and the development of red macules, papules, and tender nodules
   2. Resolve, then recur within 2–10 days

g. Impetigo

i. Non Bullous Impetigo

Non bullous impetigo

A. Staphylococcus aureus is the most common cause
B. Nasal carriers at great risk, more common in children than adults
C. Begins as a red macule, which evolves into a vesicle or pustule, then a superficial erythematous erosion with honey-colored yellow crust and extension of satellite lesions to the surrounding skin
D. The face (around the nose and mouth) is a common location
E. Usually resolves within 2 weeks without scarring without treatment

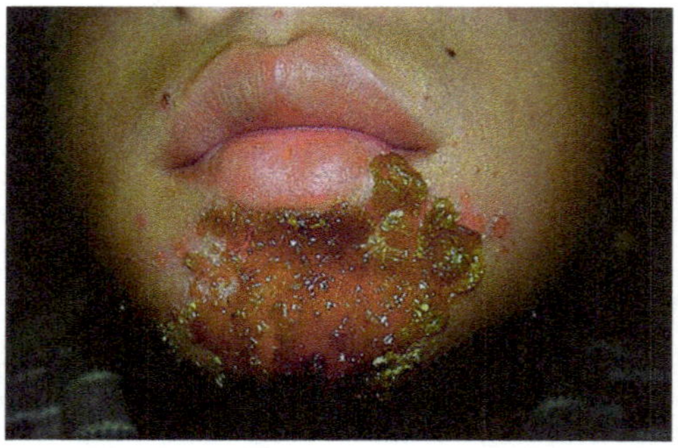

Non bullous impetigo
Photograph courtesy of SpringerImages Database, Springer Publishing Company

Non bullous impetigo

A. Superficial erythematous erosions with honey-colored yellow crust and extension of satellite lesions to the surrounding skin
B. Most common around the perinasal and perioral areas

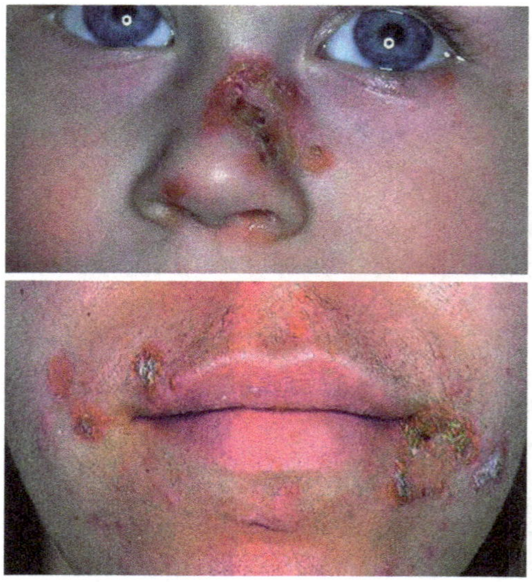

Non bullous impetigo
Photograph courtesy of SpringerImages Database, Springer Publishing Company

ii. Bullous Impetigo

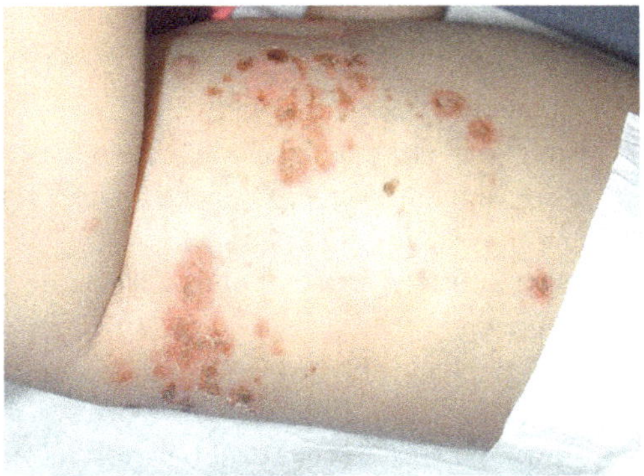

Bullous impetigo
Photograph courtesy of SpringerImages Database, Springer Publishing Company

Bullous impetigo

A. Small vesicles evolve into 1–2 cm superficial flaccid transparent bullae
B. Bullae rupture quickly leaving erosions with collarettes of scale forming rings of scale (bullae may not be seen because of early rupture)
C. Occurs on intertriginous areas (groin, buttocks, perineum, and axillae) most often but can occur anywhere (face, trunk, extremities)
D. Most common in infants, young children, and immunocompromised adults
E. Heal without treatment in 3–6 weeks without scarring
F. Exfoliative toxin may disseminate and cause staphylococcal scalded skin syndrome

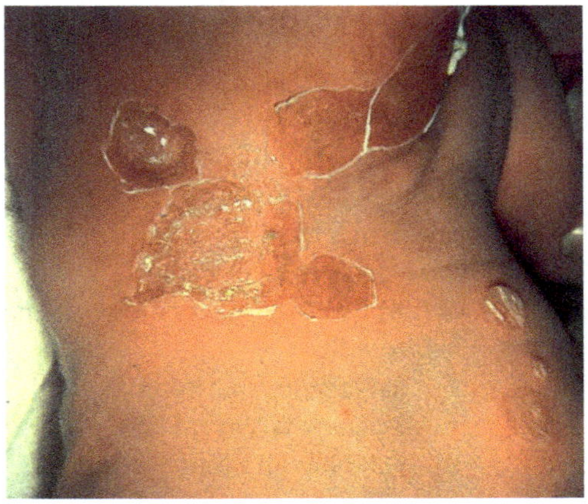

Bullous impetigo
Photograph courtesy of SpringerImages Database, Springer Publishing Company

Bullous impetigo

A. Flaccid bullae and erosions with collarettes of scale forming rings of scale

h. Leishmaniasis

Leishmaniasis

A. Protozoan infection spread by the bite of the sand fly
B. Clinical manifestations depend on host cell–mediated immune response and the species of Leishmania
C. Most common presentation is a papule at the site of inoculation that ulcerates
D. Four clinical subtypes
   1. Cutaneous
      a. A small papule develops at the inoculation site which enlarges over several weeks into a nodule or plaque that ulcerates with rolled border which may be mistaken for basal cell carcinoma (top figure)
      b. Lesions are most often solitary but may be multiple with satellites or sporotrichoid spread
      c. Most resolve spontaneously within several months with scarring
      d. Common on exposed sites: face (chiclero ulcer—lesion on the ear), neck, arms, legs
   2. Diffuse cutaneous
      a. Usually seen in patients with reduced cell-mediated immunity
      b. Multiple keloid-like lesions on the face and limbs (middle figure)
      c. Nasal infiltration may be present
   3. Mucocutaneous
      a. May develop after months to years
      b. Infiltration and ulceration of the nose, lips, or oropharynx (bottom figure)
      c. Lesions range from edema of the lips and nose to perforation of nasal and/or laryngeal cartilage and palate with extensive loss of nose and mouth tissue producing a "Tapir face" (espundia)
   4. Visceral (kala-azar)
      a. Parasite spreads to liver, bone marrow, and spleen producing fever, wasting, cough, adenopathy, and hepatosplenomegaly
      b. Post-kala-azar dermal leishmaniasis is a sequela of treated or untreated visceral leishmaniasis with skin-colored nodules and visceral symptoms

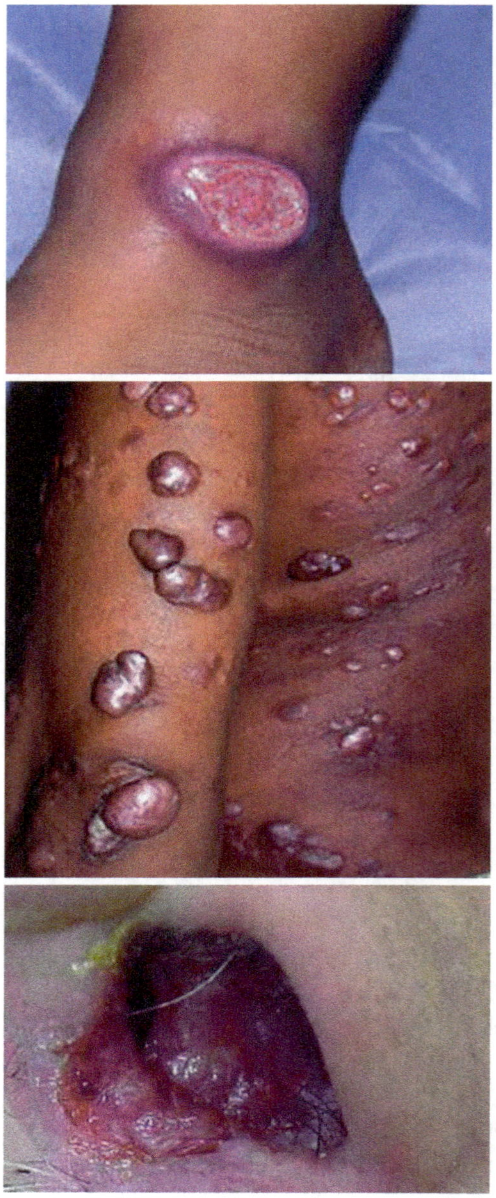

Leishmaniasis
Photograph courtesy of SpringerImages Database, Springer Publishing Company

i. Local Cutaneous Leishmaniasis

Local cutaneous leishmaniasis

A. A small papule develops at the inoculation site which enlarges over several weeks into a nodule or plaque that ulcerates with rolled border

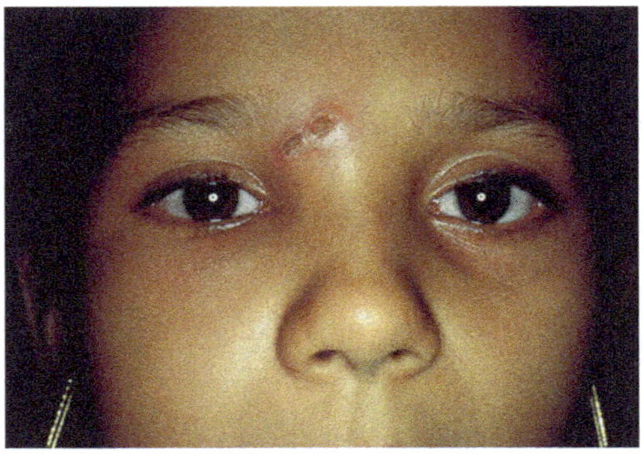

Local cutaneous leishmaniasis
Photograph courtesy of SpringerImages Database, Springer Publishing Company

Local cutaneous leishmaniasis

A. Multiple facial ulcerated plaques with rolled borders ("oriental sores")

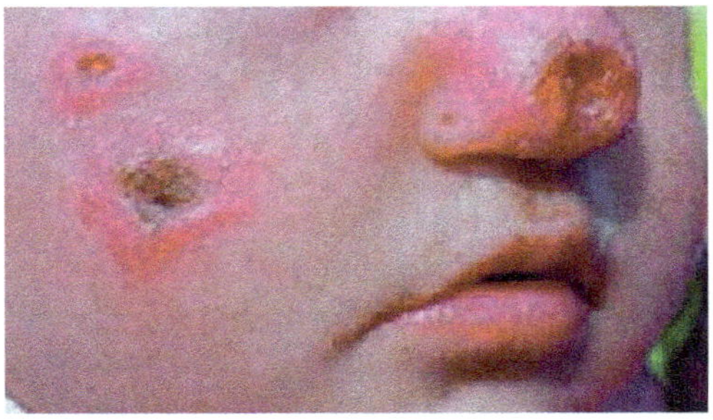

Local cutaneous leishmaniasis
Photograph courtesy of SpringerImages Database, Springer Publishing Company

ii. Mucocutaneous Leishmaniasis

Mucocutaneous leishmaniasis

A. Infiltration and ulceration of the nose, lips, and oropharynx

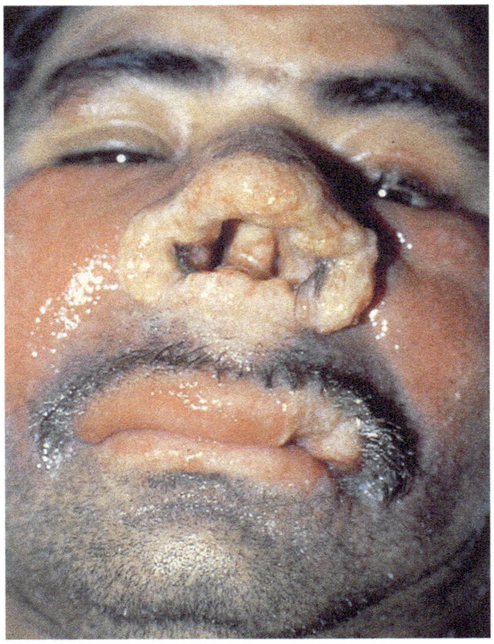

Mucocutaneous leishmaniasis
Photograph courtesy of SpringerImages Database, Springer Publishing Company

iii. Diffuse Cutaneous Leishmaniasis

Diffuse cutaneous leishmaniasis

A. Multiple keloid-like facial lesions and nasal infiltration

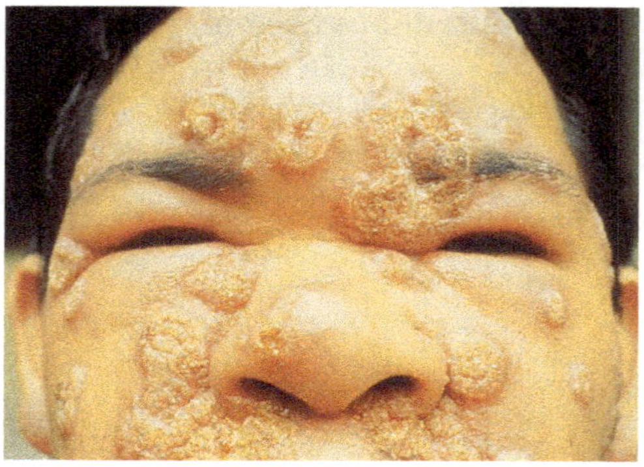

Diffuse cutaneous leishmaniasis
Photograph courtesy of SpringerImages Database, Springer Publishing Company

i. Leprosy

i. Tuberculoid Leprosy

Tuberculoid leprosy

A. Few organisms (strong cell-mediated immunity against the organism)
B. Few lesions, usually less than five
C. Hypopigmented or red dry scaly hairless plaques with sharply defined elevated grainy borders that slope down to an atrophic hypopigmented anesthetic center
D. Superficial nerves proximal to the lesion may be enlarged
E. Spontaneously resolve within 3 years

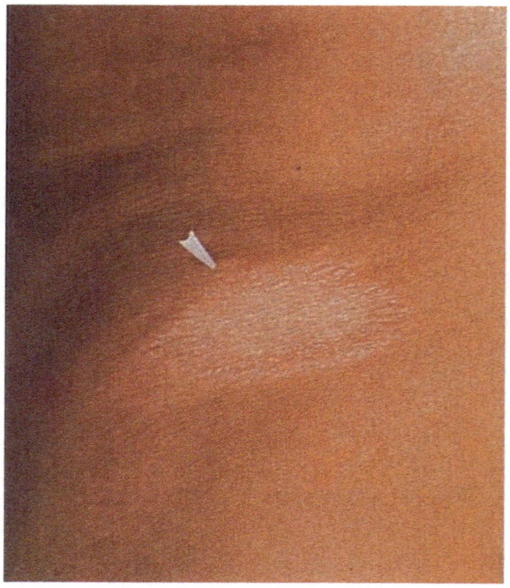

Tuberculoid leprosy
Photograph courtesy of SpringerImages Database, Springer Publishing Company

ii. Borderline Tuberculoid Leprosy

Borderline leprosy
A. Intermediate features between lepromatous and tuberculoid leprosy
B. Red, anesthetic, scaly, well-demarcated, infiltrated plaque with central clearing and alopecia
C. Small satellite lesions help to classify this lesion clinically as borderline tuberculoid rather than borderline lepromatous leprosy

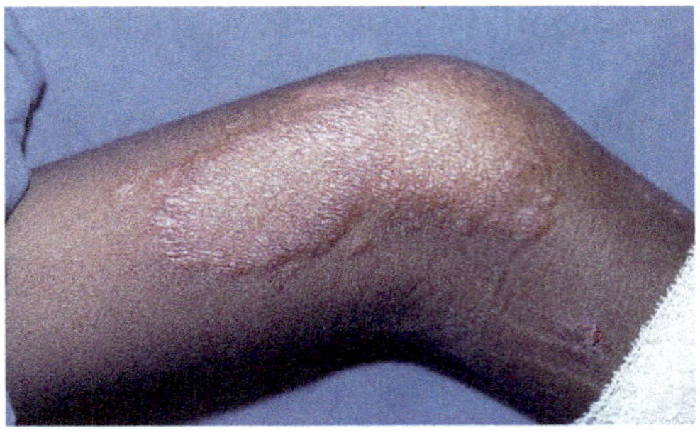

Borderline tuberculoid leprosy
Photograph courtesy of SpringerImages Database, Springer Publishing Company

Borderline tuberculoid leprosy
A. Well-demarcated, red, anesthetic plaque with a thick granular margin associated with satellite lesions

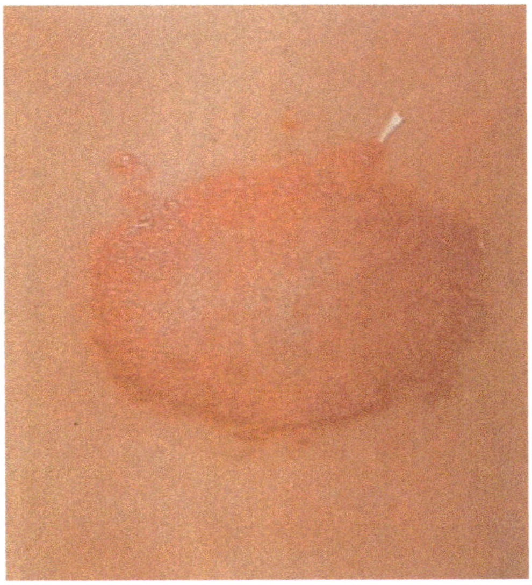

Borderline tuberculoid leprosy
Photograph courtesy of SpringerImages Database, Springer Publishing Company

Borderliine tuberculoid leprosy
A. Red brown, anesthetic plaque with satellite lesions

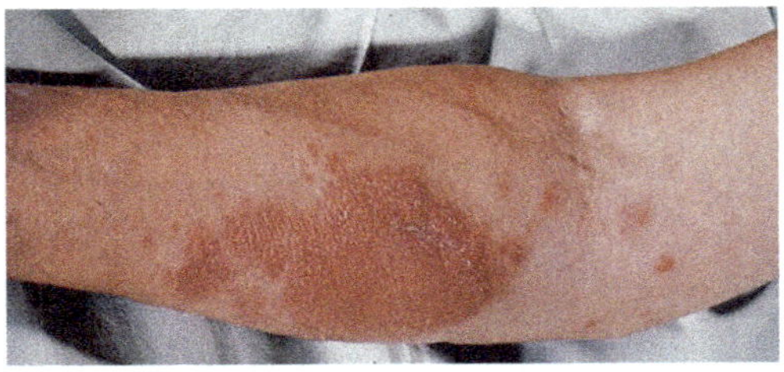

Borderline tuberculoid leprosy
Photograph courtesy of SpringerImages Database, Springer Publishing Company

iii. Borderline Lepromatous Leprosy

Borderline lepromatous leprosy

A. Diffuse, symmetric, widespread infiltration of the buttocks and lower extremities with brownish-red plaques

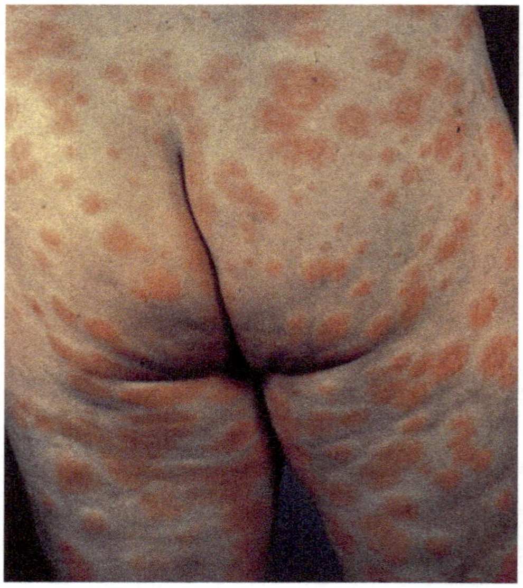

Borderline lepromatous leprosy
Photograph courtesy of SpringerImages Database, Springer Publishing Company

iv. Lepromatous Leprosy

Lepromatous leprosy

A. Multiple organisms in the dermis and nasal secretions (weak cell-mediated immunity against the organism)
B. Diffuse, symmetric, widespread infiltration of the skin with brownish-red papules, plaques, and nodules (top figure)
   1. The face is often involved resulting in leonine facies, loss of hair in involved skin (madarosis—loss of eyebrows), saddle nose, and bilateral earlobe infiltration (bottom figure)
   2. The buttocks and lower extremities are frequently involved
C. Enlarged peripheral nerves with anesthesia
D. Ocular problems (lagophthalmous, anesthesia of cornea and conjunctiva)

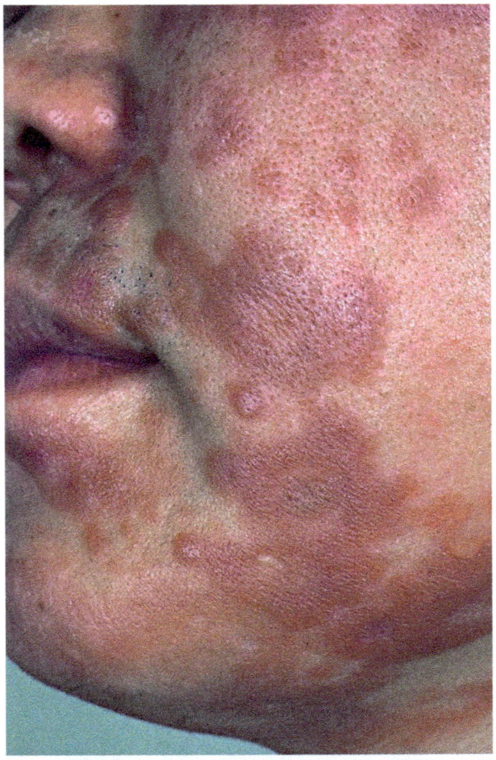

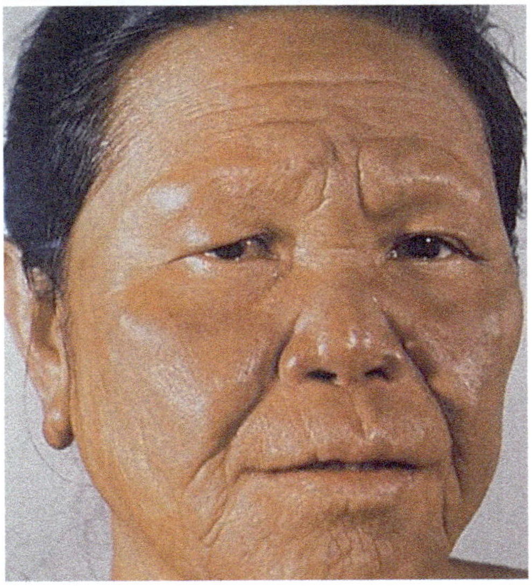

Lepromatous leprosy
Photograph courtesy of SpringerImages Database, Springer Publishing Company

v. Reversal Reactions

1. Type 1 Reversal Reaction

Reversal Reactions

A. May develop during treatment and are characterized by acute inflammation
B. Causes: treatment (antibiotics), pregnancy, other infections, mental stress
C. Type 1 reversal reaction: inflammation of existing plaques due to enhanced cell-mediated immunity, may affect any type of leprosy, especially borderline

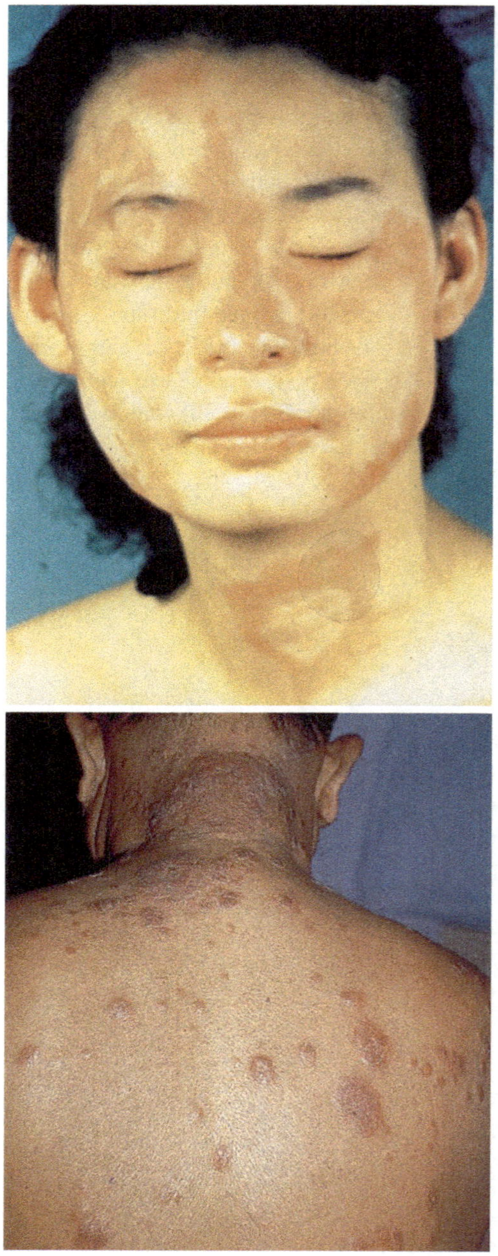

Type 1 reversal reactions
Photograph courtesy of SpringerImages Database, Springer Publishing Company

2. Type 2 Reversal Reactions

Type 2 Reversal Reactions

A. Mainly occurs in lepromatous leprosy or borderline leprosy undergoing treatment
B. Caused by the formation of immune complexes and small vessel immune complex mediated vasculitis in association with excessive humoral reaction
C. Erythema nodosum leprosum is most common with the development of multiple papulonodules
D. Lucio phenomenon—thrombosis and necrotizing small vessel vasculitis resulting in severe ulcerations

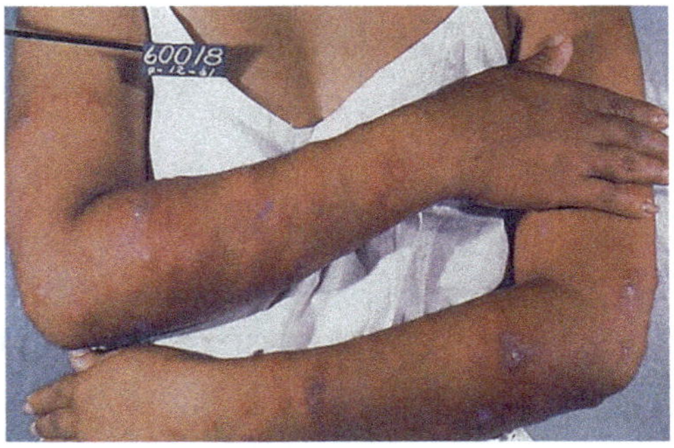

Type 2 reversal reactions
Photograph courtesy of SpringerImages Database, Springer Publishing Company

Type 2 Reversal Reactions

A. Lucio phenomenon—thrombosis and necrotizing small vessel vasculitis resulting in severe ulcerations

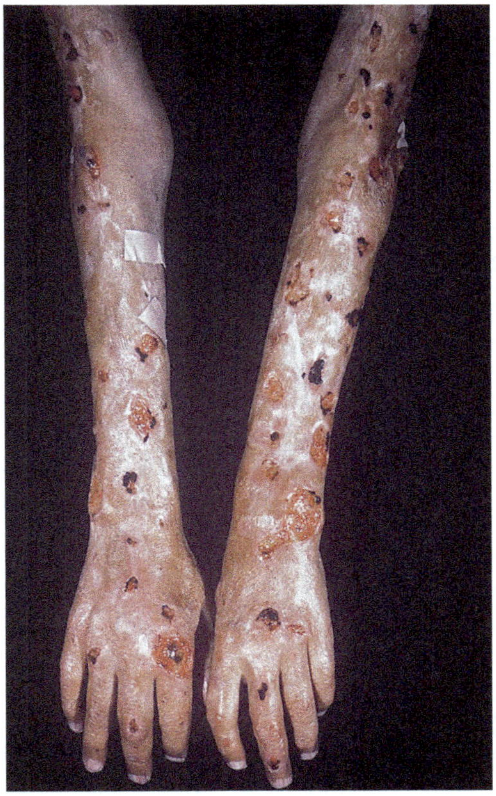

Type 2 reversal reactions
Photograph courtesy of SpringerImages Database, Springer Publishing Company

j. Mycobacterial Infections

i. Cutaneous Tuberculosis

1. Tuberculosis Verrucosa Cutis

Tuberculosis verrucosa cutis

A. Inoculation of mycobacterium tuberculosis at sites prone to trauma in previously infected person (patient has immunity against the organism)
B. Small asymptomatic indurated wart-like papule with surrounding inflammatory rim which enlarges in a serpiginous manner to form a red brown verrucous plaque

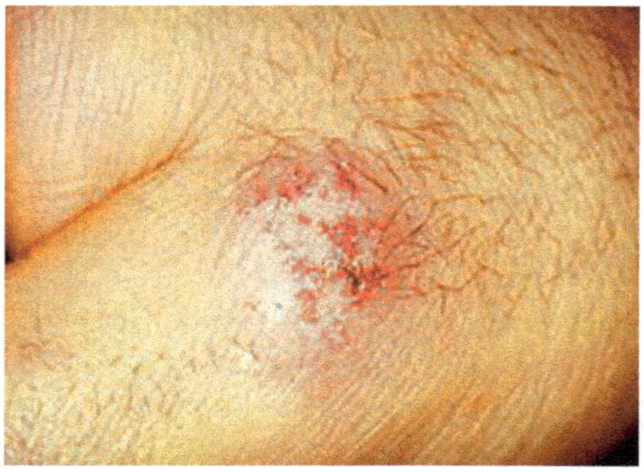

Tuberculosis verrucosa cutis
Photograph courtesy of SpringerImages Database, Springer Publishing Company

2. Scrofuloderma

Mycobacterium tuberculosis scrofuloderma

A. Results from extension of underlying disease
B. Original focus of tuberculosis may be from underlying nodes, bones, joints, epididymis
C. Firm deep-seated subcutaneous nodule that has accumulated inflammatory material and necrotic tissue (suppurative nodule); nodule becomes fluctuant, drains, ulcerates, and forms sinus tracts
D. Multiple ulcers can appear and heal with keloids and retracted scars

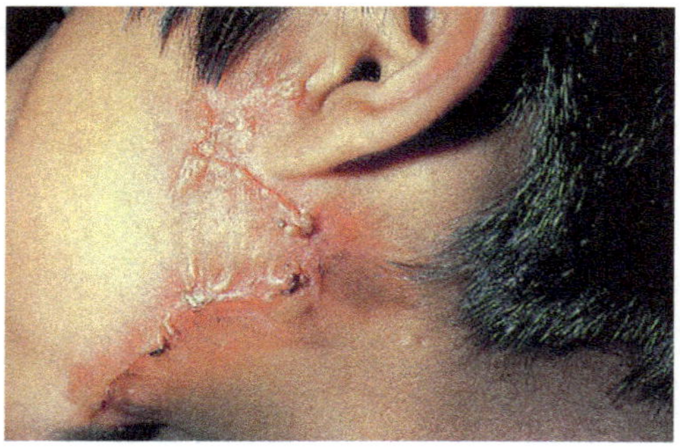

Scrofuloderma
Photograph courtesy of SpringerImages Database, Springer Publishing Company

3. Lupus Vulgaris

Lupus vulgaris

A. Occurs in a previously sensitized person
B. Can develop secondarily from tuberculosis verrucosa cutis, scrofuloderma, or other endogenous and exogenous sources
C. Red plaque that expands with central scarring and tissue destruction
D. Most commonly occurs on the head and neck (nose, cheeks, earlobe, oral mucosa)

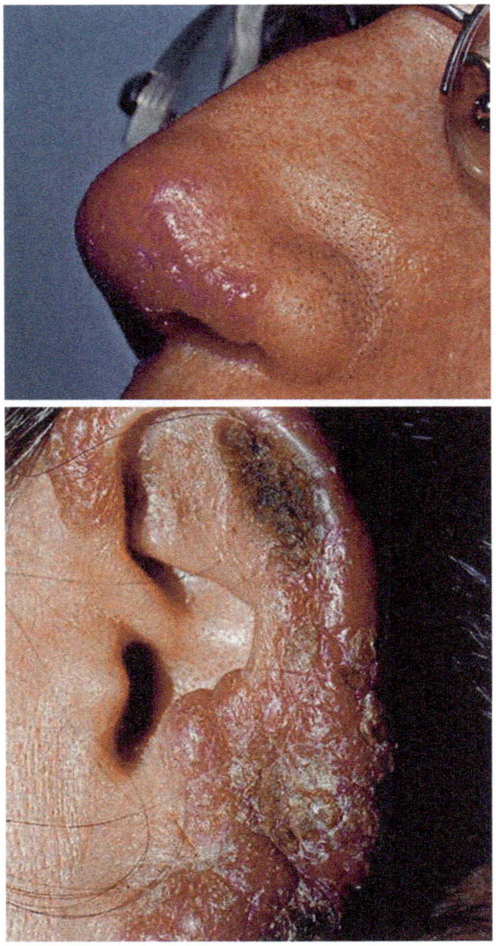

Lupus vulgaris
Photograph courtesy of SpringerImages Database, Springer Publishing Company

4. Erythema Nodosum Leprosum (Nodular Vasculitis)

Erythema induratum (nodular vasculitis)

A. Lobular panniculitis classically associated with tuberculosis, but similar lesions can be idiopathic or induced by infections or drugs
B. Most common in young to middle-age women
C. Symptoms begin after exposure to cold temperatures
D. Tender red to violaceous subcutaneous nodules or plaques on the posterior lower legs, nodules may ulcerate and heal with scarring

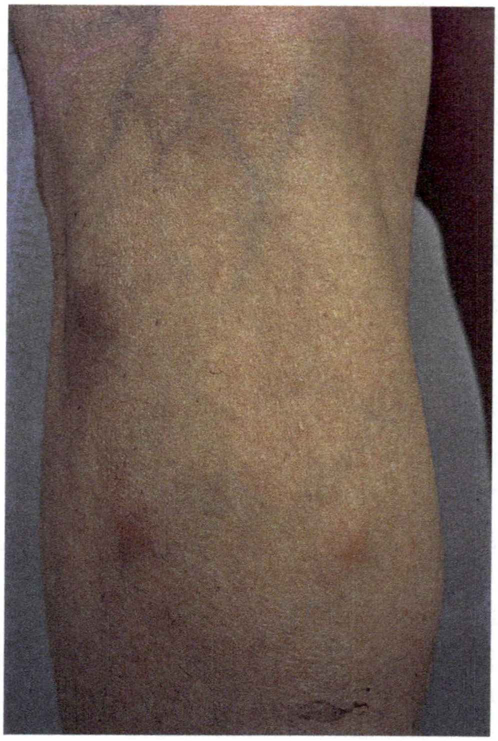

Erythema nodosum leprosum (nodular vasculitis)
Photograph courtesy of SpringerImages Database, Springer Publishing Company

ii. Non Tuberculous Mycobacterial Infections

1. Mycobacterium Ulcerans (Buruli Ulcer)

Mycobacterium ulcerans (Buruli Ulcer)

A. Seen in Africa and Australia
B. Subcutaneous nodule becomes fluctuant and ulcerates within 1–2 months
C. Ulcer is painless, without adenopathy or systemic illness, has a deep necrotic base with undermined edges, and may expand up to 15 cm and destroy bone
D. Most commonly occurs on the extremities (lower greater than upper)

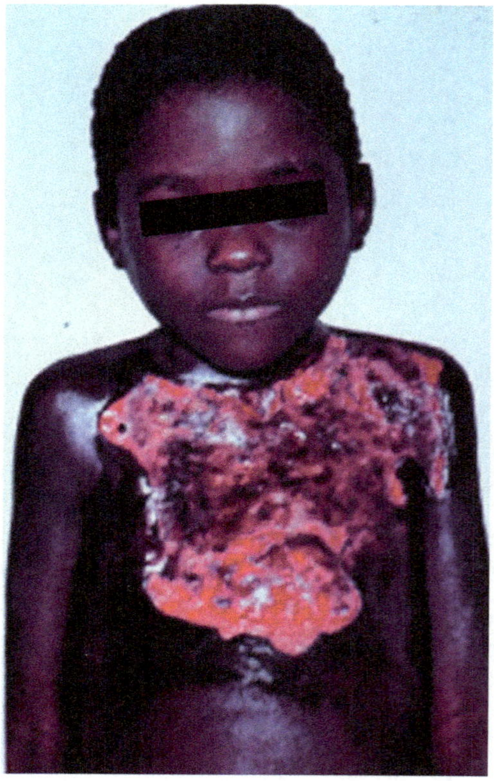

Mycobacterium ulcerans (buruli ulcer)
Photograph courtesy of SpringerImages Database, Springer Publishing Company

2. Mycobacterium Marinum

Mycobacterium marinum

A. Infection usually occurs after exposure to contaminated fresh or salt water on breaks in the skin (e.g., cleaning fish tanks with breaks in the skin, "fish tank granuloma")
B. Requires a portal of entry (traumatized skin)
C. Most common atypical mycobacterium infection
D. After an Incubation of 2–3 weeks, a blue red inflammatory nodule or pustule develops at the site of inoculation (hands, finger most common)
E. The nodule or pustule evolves into a crusted ulcer, suppurative abscess, or verrucous nodule
F. Multiple lesions may develop along the course of draining lymphatics on the distal limbs (sporotrichoid lymphocutaneous spread)
   1. M. marinum is the most common etiology of lymphocutaneous spread among nontuberculous mycobacterial infections

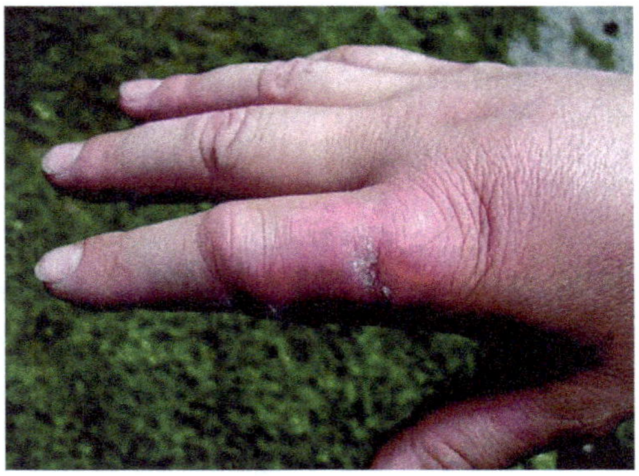

Mycobacterium marinum
Photograph courtesy of SpringerImages Database, Springer Publishing Company

k. Pitted Keratolysis

Pitted keratolysis

A. Predisposing factors: hyperhidrosis, prolonged occlusion
B. Most commonly caused by kytococcus sedentarius (Corynebacterium species)
C. Small 1–7 mm crater-like depressions (shallow round pits) in the stratum corneum on weight-bearing regions of the soles of the feet and rarely the palms, pits may coalesce to large craters or rings of craters
D. Hyperhidrosis and malodor are common
E. Most common in adolescent males

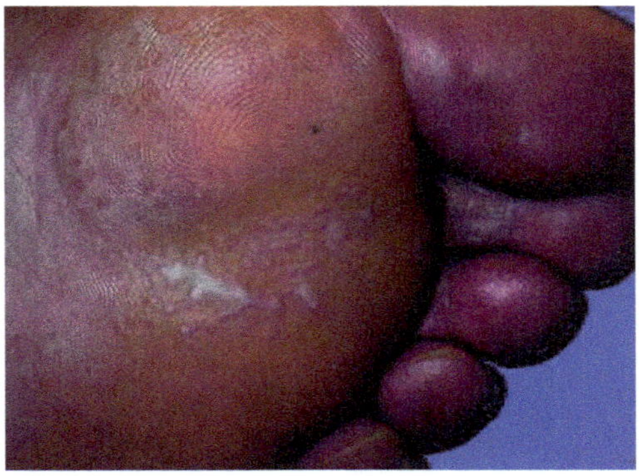

Pitted keratolysis
Photograph courtesy of SpringerImages Database, Springer Publishing Company

l. Rocky Mountain Spotted Fever

Rocky mountain spotted fever

A. The organism (Rickettsia rickettsia) resides in arthropod hosts (tick, flea, louse, mite)
B. The organism is transmitted by the arthropod (most commonly the tick, dermacentor variabalis) when it feeds; the organism then attaches to endothelial cells
C. Fever, headache, myalgias, nausea, vomiting, and abdominal pain occur in the first 3 days after the tick bite
D. Rash appears between days 3 and 6 initially as red macules on the wrists and ankles, followed by centripetal spread to the trunk
E. The macules develop into petechiae and purpuric papules on the palms and soles, dorsal hands or feet, wrists or ankles
F. Retiform purpura may develop

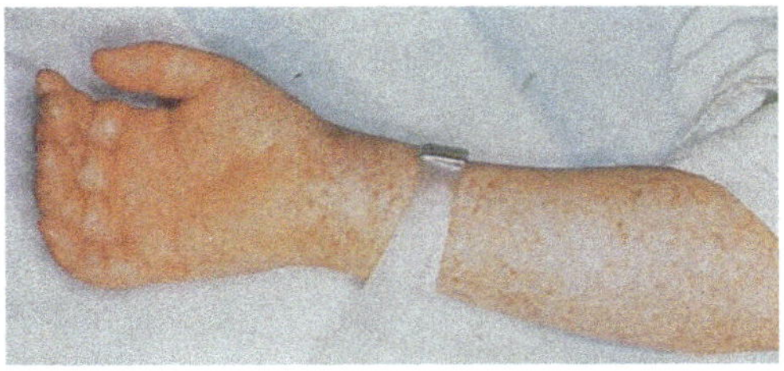

Rocky mountain spotted fever
Photograph courtesy of SpringerImages Database, Springer Publishing Company

Rocky mountain spotted fever

A. Petechiae and purpuric papules on dorsal hands and wrists with centripetal spread to the trunk (top figure)
B. Retiform purpura and necrosis on the trunk (bottom figure)

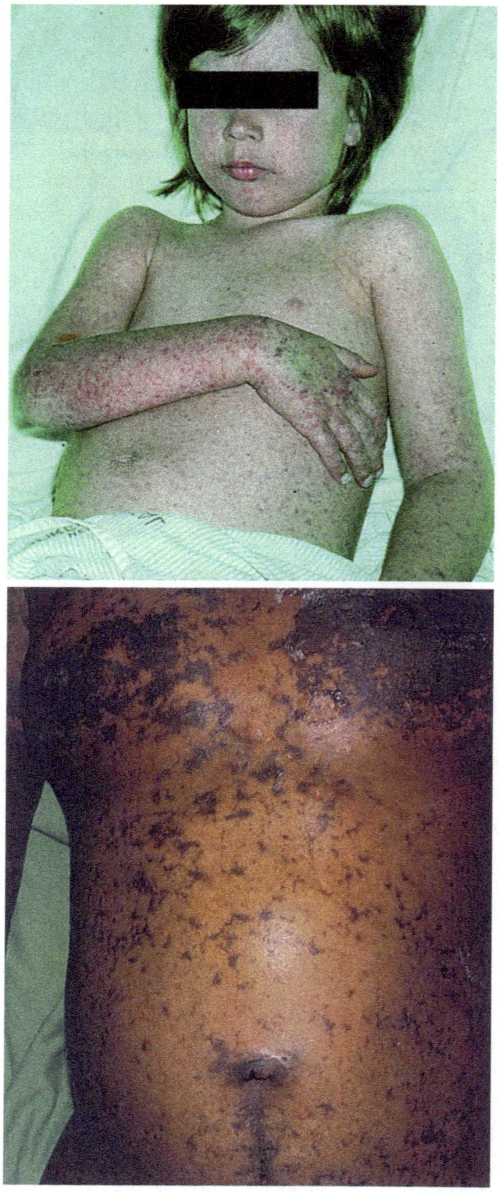

Rocky mountain spotted fever
Photograph courtesy of SpringerImages Database, Springer Publishing Company

m. Syphilis

i. Primary Syphilis

1. Chancre (Primary Syphilis)

Chancre (primary syphilis)

A. Chancre: single round oval indurated painless ulcer at site of inoculation
B. Regional adenopathy may be present
C. Occurs 3 weeks after exposure and spontaneously resolves in a few weeks

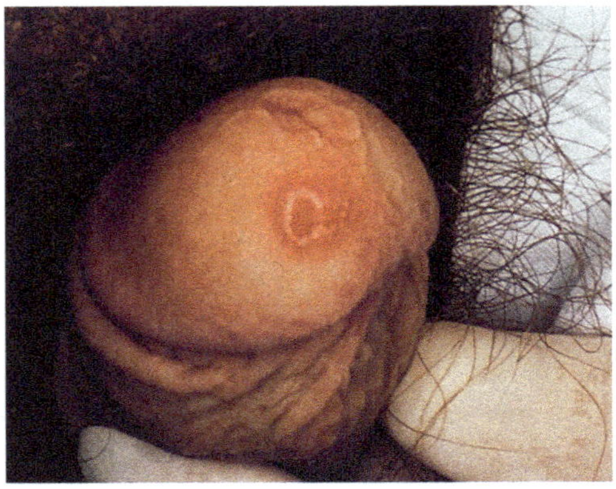

Chancre (primary syphilis)
Photograph courtesy of SpringerImages Database, Springer Publishing Company

Chancre (primary syphilis)

A. Chancre of the glans penis

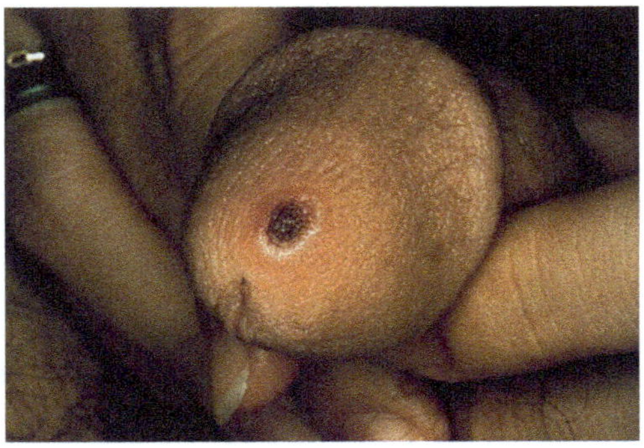

Chancre (primary syphilis)
Photograph courtesy of SpringerImages Database, Springer Publishing Company

ii. Secondary Syphilis

1. Generalized Papulosquamous Eruption (Secondary Syphilis)

Generalized Papulosquamous Eruption (Secondary Syphilis)

A. Occurs 3–6 weeks after chancre resolves, results from hematogenous and lymphatic dissemination of treponemes
B. Resolves in weeks to months without treatment, may relapse
C. Prodrome fever, malaise, sore throat, adenopathy, weight loss, headache, muscle ache
D. Generalized papulosquamous eruption of pink, violaceous, red brown papules ("copper pennies") resembling pityriasis rosea
   1. Most common manifestation of secondary syphilis
   2. The palms and soles are the most common sites, where lesions typically have a collarette of scale

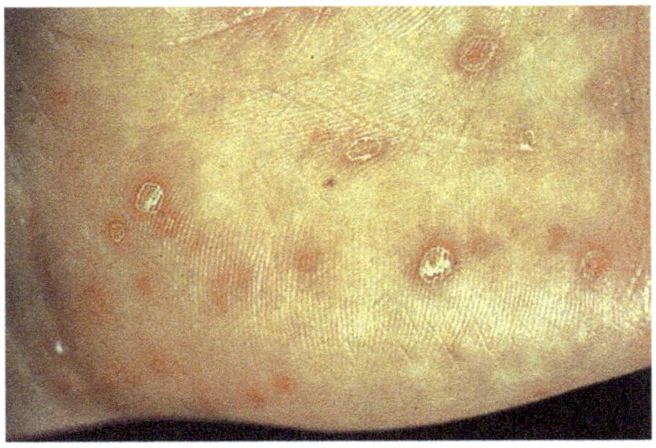

Generalized papulosquamous eruption (secondary syphilis)
Photograph courtesy of SpringerImages Database, Springer Publishing Company

Generalized Papulosquamous Eruption (Secondary Syphilis)

A. Papulosquamous eruption of red brown papules with collarettes of scale on the soles and ankles

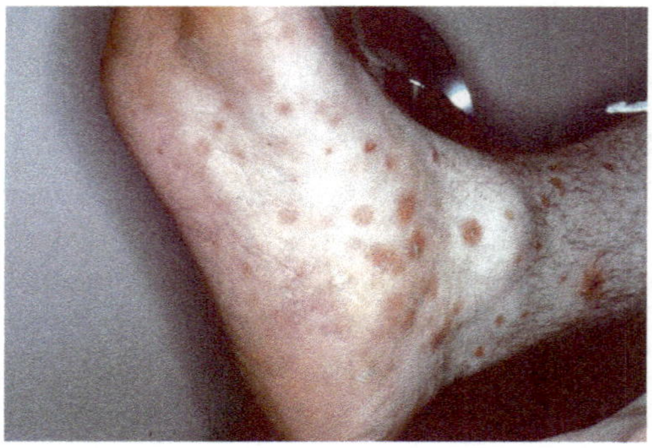

Generalized papulosquamous eruption (secondary syphilis)
Photograph courtesy of SpringerImages Database, Springer Publishing Company

Generalized Papulosquamous Eruption (Secondary Syphilis)

A. Generalized papulosquamous eruption of red brown macules and papules ("copper pennies") favoring lines of cleavage similar to pityriasis rosea

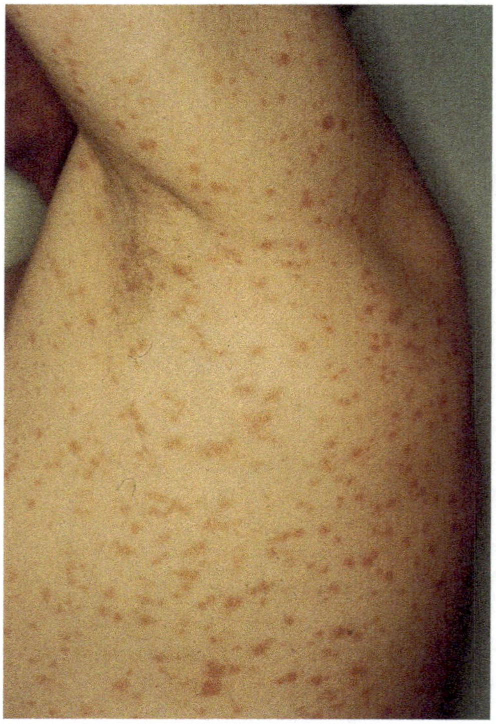

Generalized papulosquamous eruption (secondary syphilis)
Photograph courtesy of SpringerImages Database, Springer Publishing Company

2. Mucous Patches (Secondary Syphilis)

Mucous patches (secondary syphilis)

A. Mucous patches: large gray plaques or shallow erosions with a red areola
B. Highly contagious

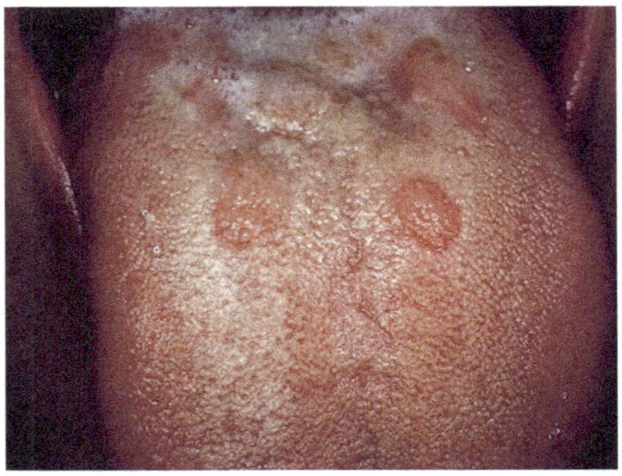

Mucous patches (secondary syphilis)
Photograph courtesy of SpringerImages Database, Springer Publishing Company

3. Split Papules of the Oral Commissure (Secondary Syphilis)

Split papules of oral commissure (secondary syphilis)

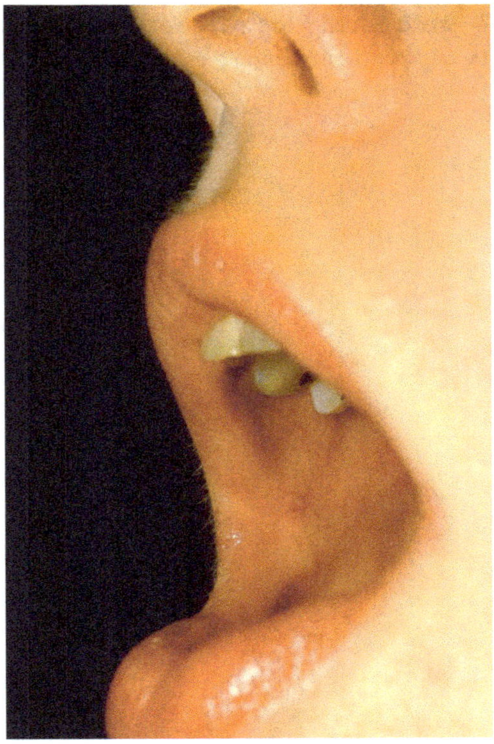

Split papules of the oral commissure (secondary syphilis)
Photograph courtesy of Mayo Clinic, Department of Dermatology, Rochester, MN

Split papules of oral commissure (secondary syphilis)

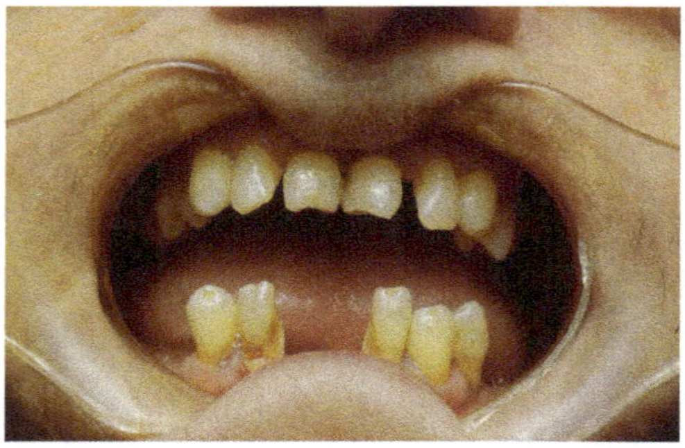

Split papules of the oral commissure (secondary syphilis)
Photograph courtesy of Mayo Clinic, Department of Dermatology, Rochester, MN

4. Moth Eaten Alopecia (Secondary Syphilis)

Patchy non-scarring moth eaten alopecia (secondary syphillis)

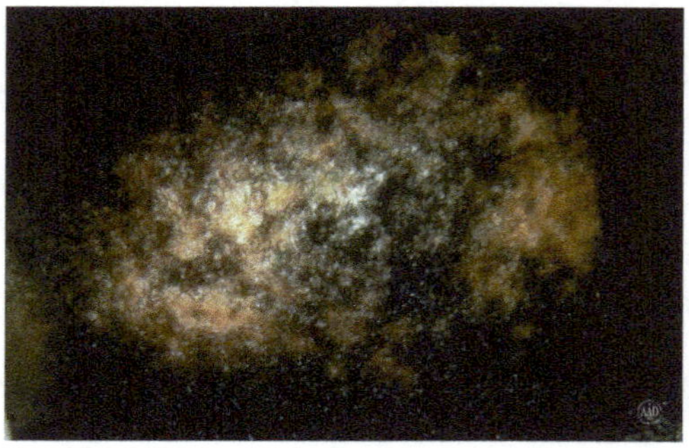

Moth eaten alopecia (secondary syphilis)
Photograph courtesy of the American Academy of Dermatology

5. Annular Secondary Syphilis

Annular secondary syphilis

A. Annular or figurate plaques with central hyperpigmentation most commonly seen on the anogenital areas, palms and soles, axilla, and particularly the face.
B. Commonly seen in patients of African descent

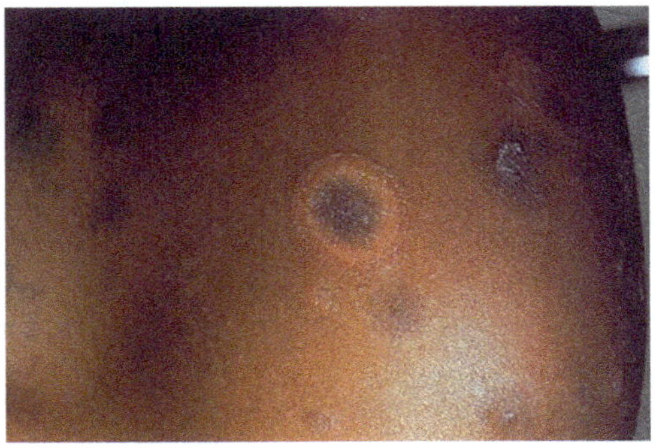

Annular secondary syphilis
Photograph courtesy of SpringerImages Database, Springer Publishing Company

6. Condyloma Lata (Secondary Syphilis)

Condyloma lata of secondary syphilis

A. Moist erythematous plaques in the anogenital area that resemble condyloma acuminata
B. Highly infectious

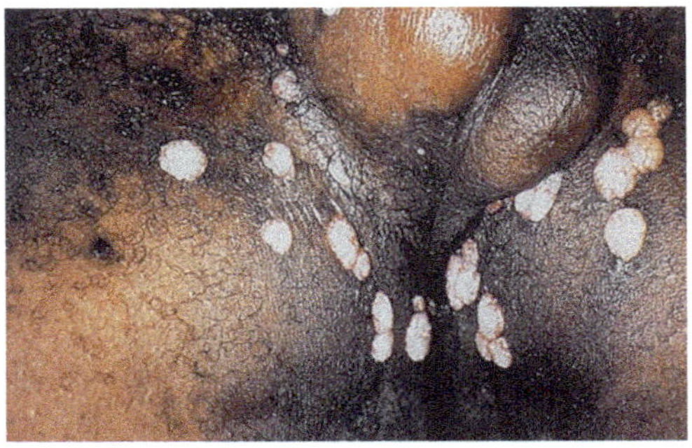

Condyloma lata (secondary syphilis)
Photograph courtesy of SpringerImages Database, Springer Publishing Company

iii. Tertiary Syphilis

1. Gummas (Tertiary Syphilis)

Gummas (Tertiary syphilis)

A. Months to years after initial infection
B. Caused by granulomatous inflammation of the skin, central nervous system, cardiovascular system
C. Gummas
   1. Most common feature of late syphilis
   2. Locally destructive lesions of the skin, bones (pain, swelling, limited range of motion), liver, oral cavity, upper respiratory tract, myocardium
   3. Nodules (top figure) or ulcerative plaques (bottom figure) sometimes with an arciform pattern (borders may be serpiginous or kidney shaped), most common on the lower legs but may occur anywhere
D. Central nervous system
   1. Neurosyphilis can occur in primary, secondary, or tertiary syphilis (most common)
   2. Infarctions cause hemiparesis, hemiplegia
   3. Parenchymal invasion may result in paresis, dementia
   4. Tabes dorsalis, diplopia, paresthesias, loss of vibratory and position sense
E. Heart and great vessels
   1. 15–30 years after infection
   2. Endarteritis

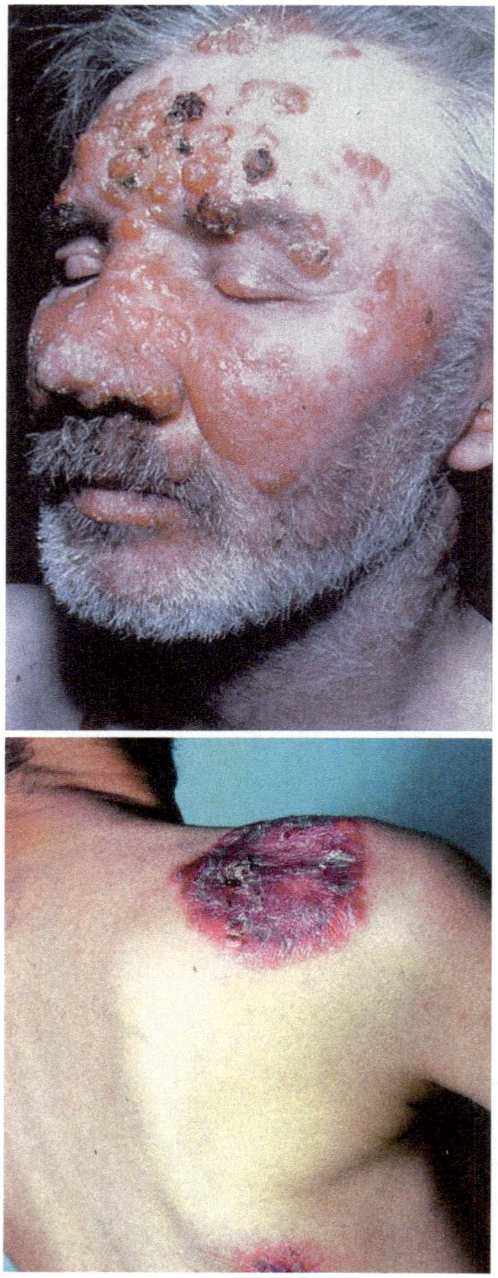

Gummas (tertiary syphilis)
Photograph courtesy of SpringerImages Database, Springer Publishing Company

Chapter X

Infestations and Bites

56 Cutaneous Larva Migrans

Cutaneous larva migrans

A. Caused by the dog and cat hookworm (ancylostoma braziliens)
B. Common in the southeastern USA or Caribbean
C. Acquired by walking or sitting on the ground (usually a beach) contaminated by animal feces
D. Most common on the distal lower extremities and buttocks
E. Larvae burrow through intact skin resulting serpiginous and pruritic edematous, vesicular, linear streaks representing the path of the organism in the epidermis
F. Symptoms start 1–6 days after exposure, organism moves 1–2 cm per day and dies in 2–8 weeks without treatment

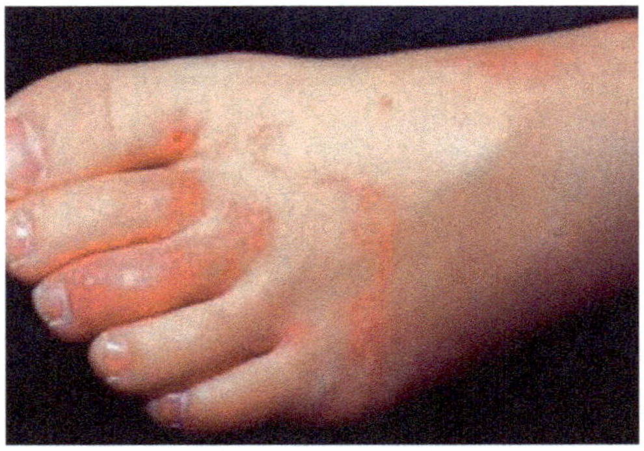

Cutaneous larva migrans
Photograph courtesy of SpringerImages Database, Springer Publishing Company

H.M. Gloster, Jr. et al., *Absolute Dermatology Review: Mastering Clinical Conditions on the Dermatology Recertification Exam*, DOI 10.1007/978-3-319-03218-4_56, © Springer International Publishing Switzerland 2016

57 Bed Bugs and Fleas

Bed bugs and fleas

A. Grouped or disseminated, erythematous, pruritic urticarial small papules which may be excoriated and may have a central hemorrhagic punctum
B. Typically grouped or distributed linearly: "breakfast, lunch and dinner" most indicative of flea bites or bed bug bites

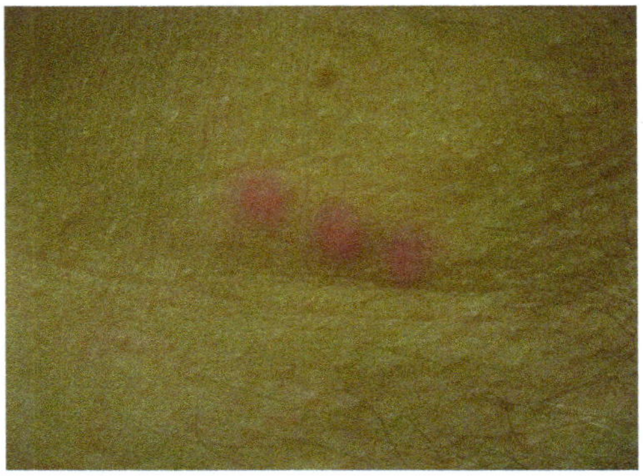

Bed bugs and fleas
Photograph courtesy of SpringerImages Database, Springer Publishing Company

Bed bugs and fleas

A. Grouped pruritic urticarial small papules with a central hemorrhagic punctum

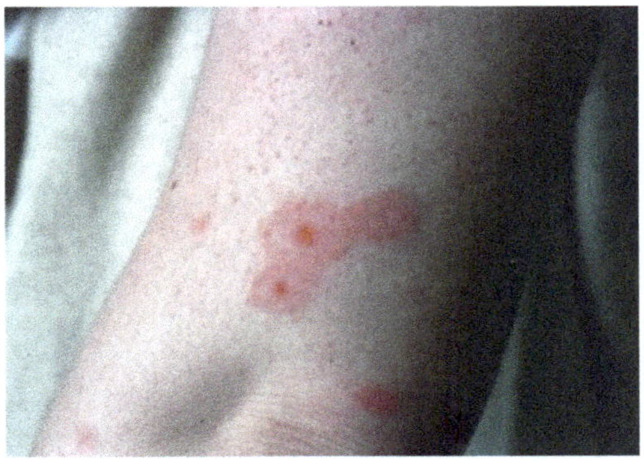

Bed bugs and fleas
Photograph courtesy of SpringerImages Database, Springer Publishing Company

H.M. Gloster, Jr. et al., *Absolute Dermatology Review: Mastering Clinical Conditions on the Dermatology Recertification Exam*, DOI 10.1007/978-3-319-03218-4_57,

58 Brown Recluse Spider Bite

Brown recluse spider bite.

A. The spider has a dark brown fiddle on its back, a small body, and long legs
B. Bite causes local necrotic reactions due to sphingomyelinase D
C. Initially, there is erythema, then central vesiculation or duskiness with a blanched halo, followed by hemorrhagic bullae with necrosis

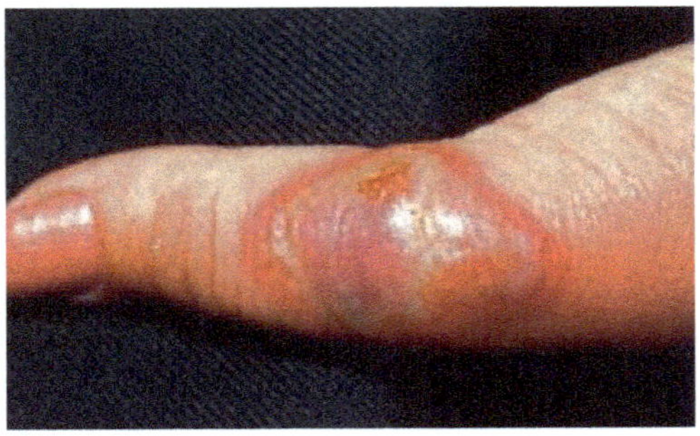

Brown recluse spider bite
Photograph courtesy of SpringerImages Database, Springer Publishing Company

H.M. Gloster, Jr. et al., *Absolute Dermatology Review: Mastering Clinical Conditions on the Dermatology Recertification Exam*,
DOI 10.1007/978-3-319-03218-4_58, © Springer International Publishing Switzerland 2016

59 Scabies

Scabies

A. Extremely pruritic, excoriated red–pink papules, papulovesicles, and small linear burrows
B. Commonly affects folds of the body:
    1. Interdigital finger web spaces
    2. Flexor wrists, axillae, ankles, buttocks, waist, periumbilical area
    3. Men: penis (pink papules on the glans are a classic sign) and scrotum
    4. Women: areola, nipples, inframammary, vulva
    5. Infants: acral vesiculopustules

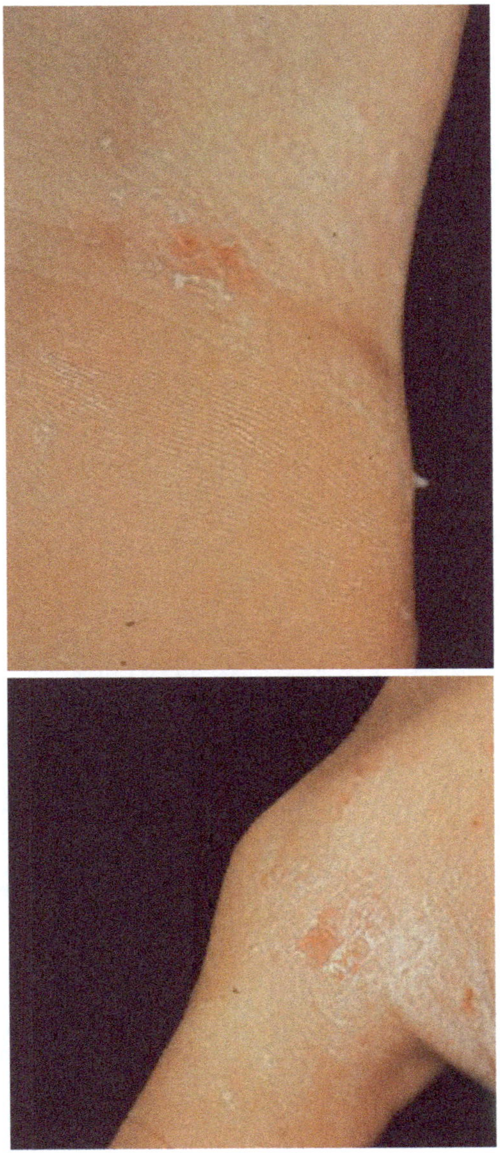

Scabies
Photograph courtesy of SpringerImages Database, Springer Publishing Company

H.M. Gloster, Jr. et al., *Absolute Dermatology Review: Mastering Clinical Conditions on the Dermatology Recertification Exam*,
DOI 10.1007/978-3-319-03218-4_59, © Springer International Publishing Switzerland 2016

Scabies

A. Pink papules on the glans penis and scrotum are a classic sign of scabies

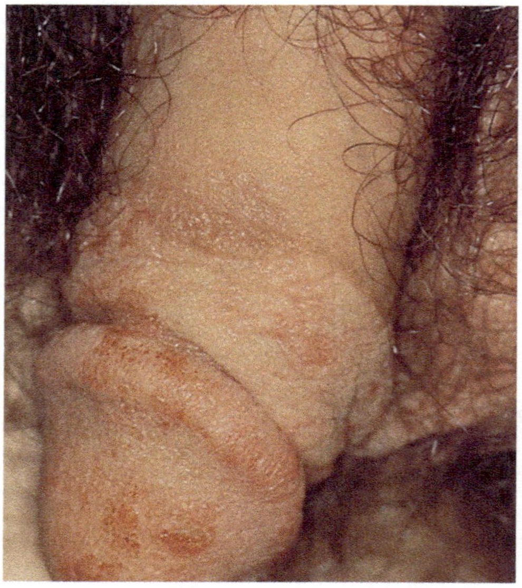

Scabies
Photograph courtesy of SpringerImages Database, Springer Publishing Company

60 Norwegian Crusted Scabies

Norwegian (crusted) scabies

A. Seen most often in the immunocompromised or those unable to scratch
B. Minimal pruritus, large number of mites, contagious
C. Acral (including subungual) hyperkeratosis

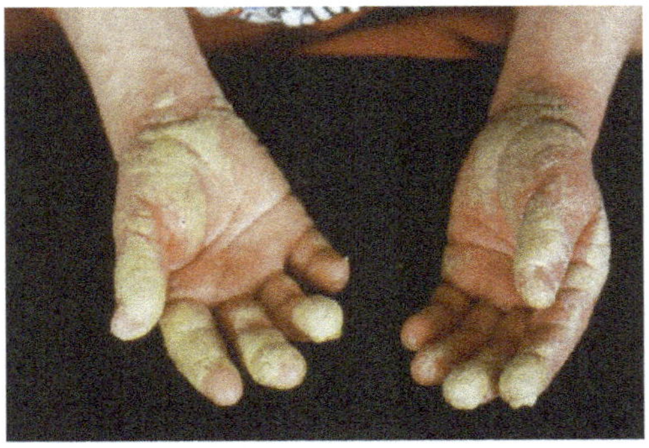

Norwegian crusted scabies
Photograph courtesy of SpringerImages Database, Springer Publishing Company

H.M. Gloster, Jr. et al., *Absolute Dermatology Review: Mastering Clinical Conditions on the Dermatology Recertification Exam*, DOI 10.1007/978-3-319-03218-4_60, © Springer International Publishing Switzerland 2016

61 Lice

a. Pubic Lice

Pubic lice

A. Diagnosed by finding nits attached to hair shafts (appear as small dots of firm material along the hair shaft) or adult lice clinging to base of pubic hairs
B. Pruritus, erythema, excoriations
C. Macula caerulea—slate gray to blue macules on trunk and thighs in those with chronic lice

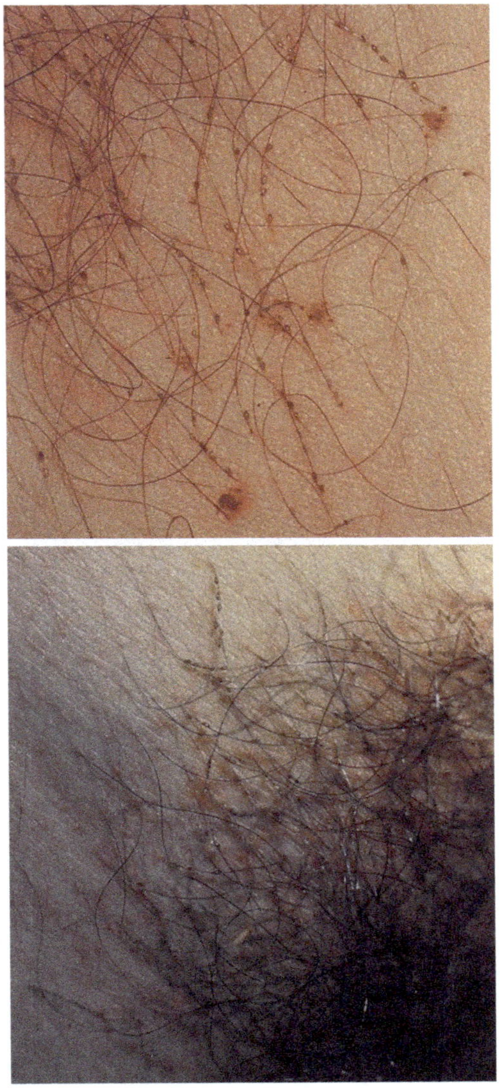

Pubic lice
Photograph courtesy of SpringerImages Database, Springer Publishing Company

H.M. Gloster, Jr. et al., *Absolute Dermatology Review: Mastering Clinical Conditions on the Dermatology Recertification Exam*, DOI 10.1007/978-3-319-03218-4_61, © Springer International Publishing Switzerland 2016

b. Head Lice

Head lice

A. Diagnosed by finding eggs (nits) attached to scalp hairs (Top figure) or adult lice (Bottom figure)
B. Pruritus, excoriations, erythema, pyoderma, scale

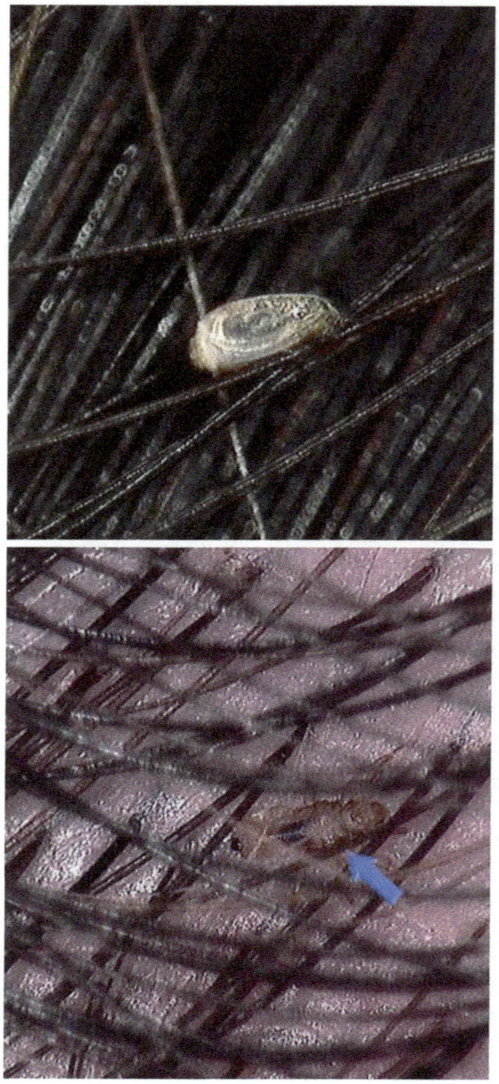

Head lice
Photograph courtesy of SpringerImages Database, Springer Publishing Company

62 Tunga Penetrans (Tungiasis)

Tunga penetrans (tungiasis)

A. Caused by the burrowing female sand flea (tunga penetrans)
B. Endemic in Caribbean islands
C. Papulonecrotic lesions on the feet, usually near great toenail, less commonly soles and toe webs
D. Female burrows into the dermis, then the flea's belly enlarges up to 1 cm to create a nodule with central punctum through which eggs are ejected, then the female dies and is sloughed off, often leading to secondary infection

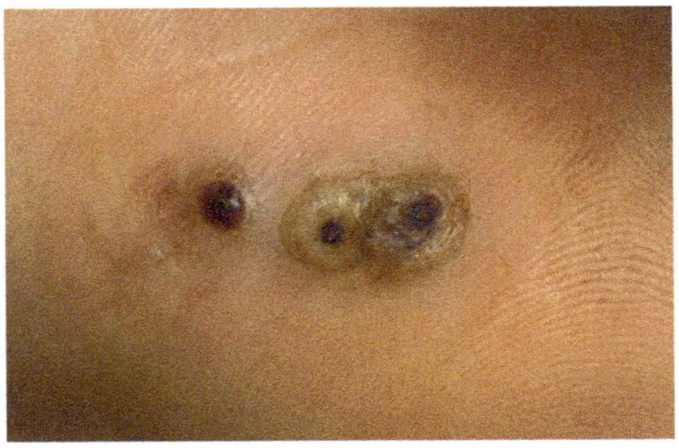

Tunga penetrans (tungiasis)
Photograph courtesy of SpringerImages Database, Springer Publishing Company

H.M. Gloster, Jr. et al., *Absolute Dermatology Review: Mastering Clinical Conditions on the Dermatology Recertification Exam*,
DOI 10.1007/978-3-319-03218-4_62, © Springer International Publishing Switzerland 2016

Chapter XI

Hair, Nails, and Mucous Membranes

Alopecias 63

a. Non Scarring Alopecias

i. Telogen Effluvium

Telogen effluvium

A. Nonscarrring alopecia in which a stressful event such as pregnancy, childbirth, medication changes, severe weight loss, surgery, major illness, or extreme psychological distress triggers a shift of an abnormal percentage of hairs from anagen into telogen
B. Diffuse thinning of hair on entire scalp
C. Hair pluck (trichogram—hair pull) showing greater than 20 % (normal 5–10 %) telogen hairs (club-shaped bulb with no attached root sheath)
D. Hairs may be easily extracted by gentle pulling

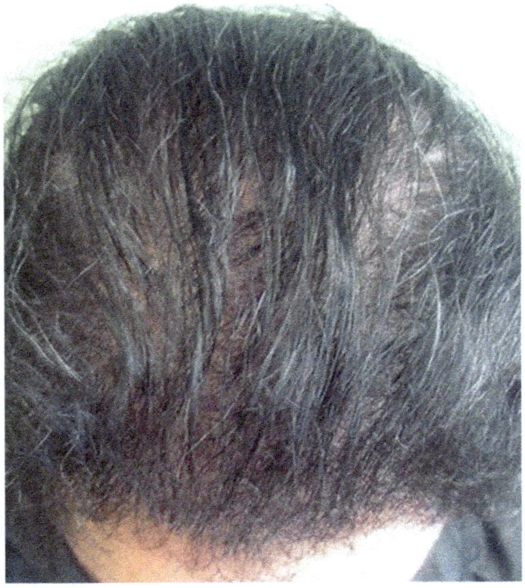

Telogen effluvium
Photograph courtesy of SpringerImages Database, Springer Publishing Company

H.M. Gloster, Jr. et al., *Absolute Dermatology Review: Mastering Clinical Conditions on the Dermatology Recertification Exam*, DOI 10.1007/978-3-319-03218-4_63, © Springer International Publishing Switzerland 2016

ii. Anagen Effluvium

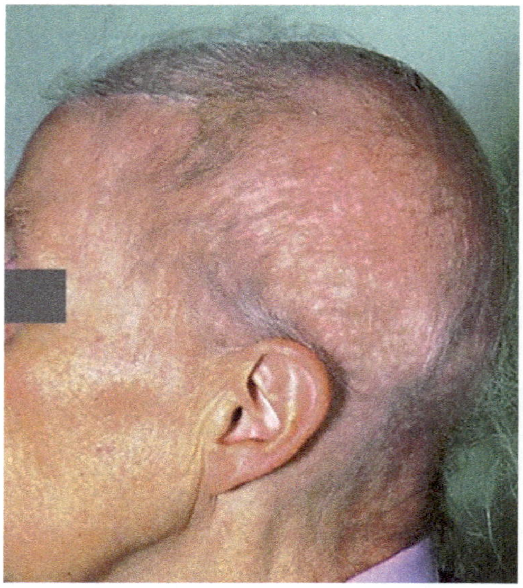

Anagen effluvium
Photograph courtesy of SpringerImages Database, Springer Publishing Company

Anagen effluvium

A. Diffuse nonscarring alopecia primarily of the scalp but also eyebrows and pubic hairs
B. Caused by chemotherapy drugs, which lead to an abrupt stop in mitotic activity
C. Occurs 2–3 weeks after drug is initiated, reversible when drug stopped, straight hair may grow back curly

iii. Androgenetic Alopecia

1. Female Pattern Androgenetic Alopecia

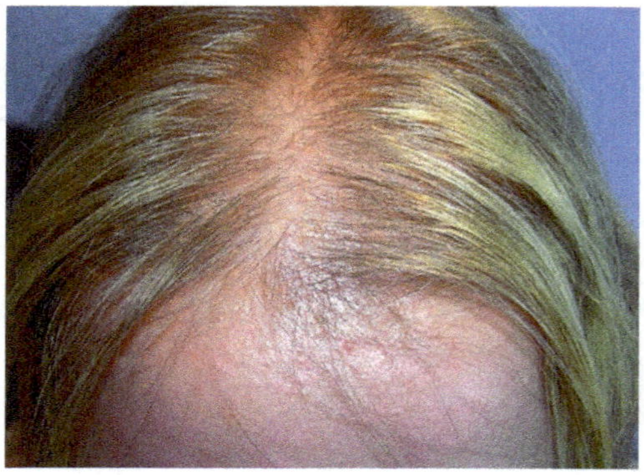

Female pattern androgenetic alopecia
Photograph courtesy of SpringerImages Database, Springer Publishing Company

Female pattern androgenetic alopecia (female pattern hair loss)

A. Non scarring alopecia
B. Thinning of crown with preservation of frontal hairline
C. Hair loss at crown is heaviest near the frontal hairline, but the hairline is preserved
D. Examination of the midline part reveals decreased hair density producing a "Christmas tree pattern"
E. A part at the crown is much thinner than one at the occiput
F. Often starts with widening of part and progresses to balding and thinning along both sides of part line

2. Male Pattern Androgenetic Alopecia

Male pattern androgenetic alopecia (male pattern hair loss).

A. Nonscarring alopecia with thinning at the vertex and frontotemporal region and recession of the frontal hairline

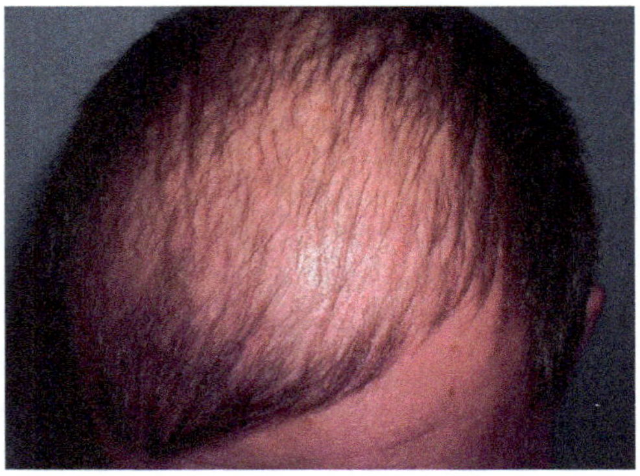

Male pattern androgenetic alopecia
Photograph courtesy of SpringerImages Database, Springer Publishing Company

iv. Trichotillomania

Trichotillomania:

A. Nonscarring alopecia
B. Self-induced plucking or twisting and breaking of hair often associated with psychological stress or personality disorder
C. Onset childhood or early adolescents, more common in young girls
D. Incomplete or distorted follicular anatomy with patches of alopecia with bizarre shapes, irregular borders, and broken hairs of varying lengths
E. Frontal scalp, eyebrows, and eyelashes most commonly involved or may be confined to one side of the scalp

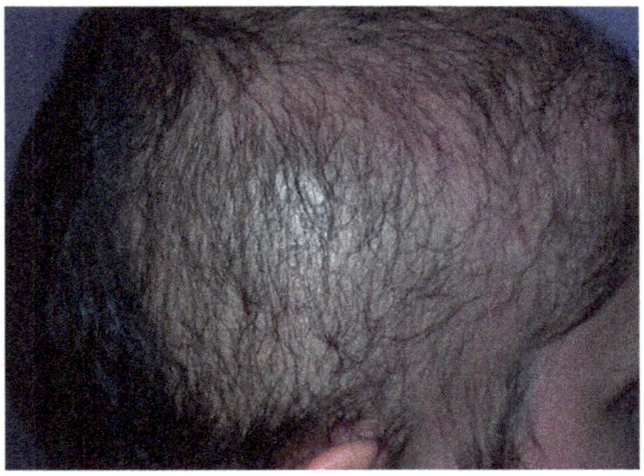

Trichotillomania
Photograph courtesy of SpringerImages Database, Springer Publishing Company

Trichotillomania

A. Incomplete or distorted follicular anatomy with patches of alopecia with bizarre shapes, irregular borders, and broken hairs of varying lengths

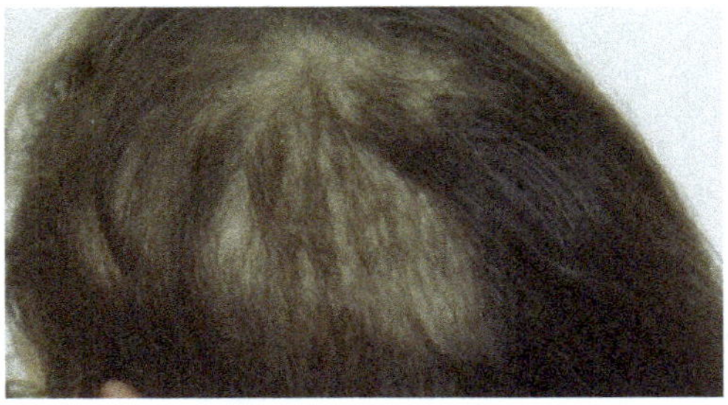

Trichotillomania
Photograph courtesy of SpringerImages Database, Springer Publishing Company

v. Alopecia Areata

Alopecia areata:

A. Nonscarring alopecia
B. Most commonly presenting as circular smooth patches of hair loss with short "exclamation point" hairs (distal end broader than proximal end) at margins
C. Gray hair often spared
D. Can lead to total scalp hair loss (totalis), complete body and scalp hair loss (universalis), or band like along temple and occipital scalp (ophiasis)
E. Nails also involved
   1. Pits most common
   2. Trachonychia—sandpaper-like roughness due to excessive longitudinal ridging
   3. Brittle nails, onycholysis, koilonychias

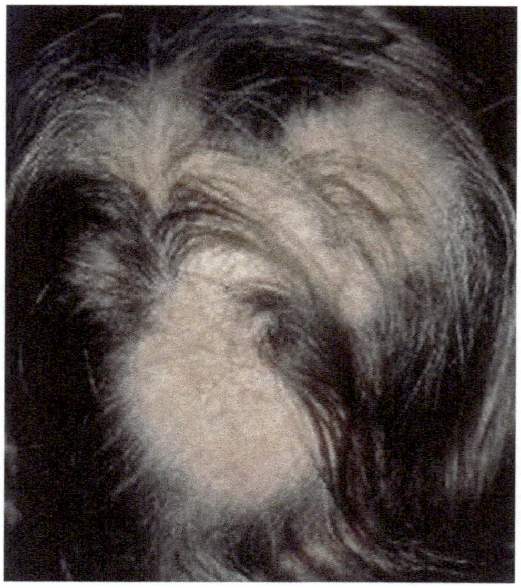

Alopecia areata
Photograph courtesy of SpringerImages Database, Springer Publishing Company

Alopecia areata (ophiasis pattern)

A. Bandlike smooth patches of hair loss along the temple and occipital scalp

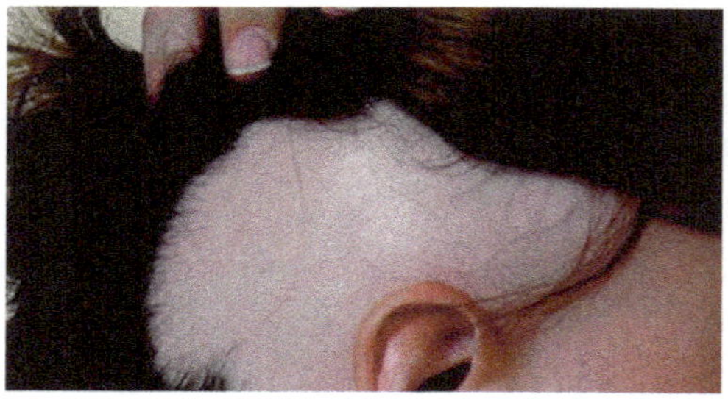

Alopecia areata
Photograph courtesy of SpringerImages Database, Springer Publishing Company

Alopecia areata (totalis pattern)

A. Total scalp hair loss

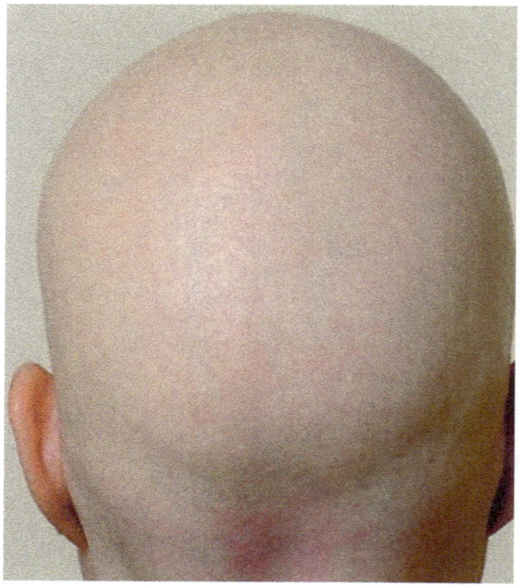

Alopecia areata
Photograph courtesy of SpringerImages Database, Springer Publishing Company

b. Scarring Alopecias

i. Central Centrifugal Cicatricial Alopecia

Central centrifugal cicatricial alopecia

A. Slowly progressive scarring alopecia centered on crown or vertex
B. Expands symmetrically and centrifugally with most disease activity (inflammation) at periphery surrounding the hairless zone
C. Most often in blacks; eventual burnout after years, 3:1 female to male

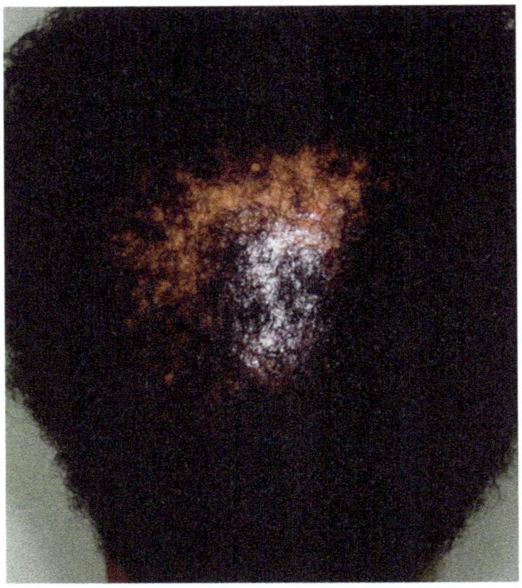

Central centrifugal cicatricial alopecia
Photograph courtesy of SpringerImages Database, Springer Publishing Company

ii. Lichen Planopilaris

1. Early-Stage Lichen Planopilaris

Early-Stage Lichen Planopilaris

A. Inflammatory scarring alopecia
B. Pruritic and tender
C. Scattered foci of hair loss on the scalp with multiple keratotic plugs (follicular hyperkeratosis, scale) surrounded by a violaceous rim (perifollicular erythema)

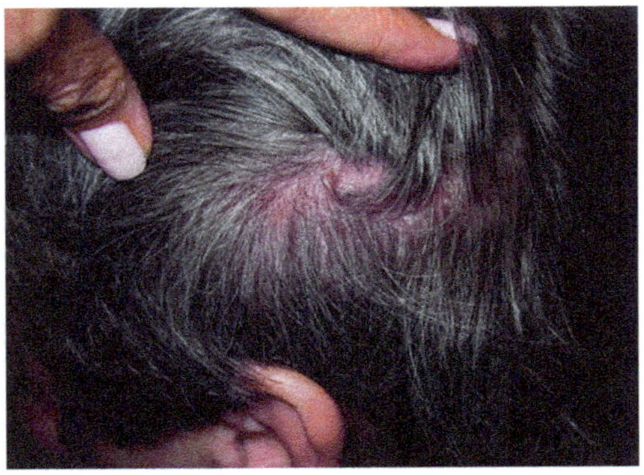

Early-stage lichen planopilaris
Photograph courtesy of SpringerImages Database, Springer Publishing Company

2. Late-Stage Lichen Planopilaris

Late-Stage Lichen planopilaris

A. Later stages show scarring alopecia with loss of follicular openings
B. Minimal perifollicular erythema is present most often at the margins

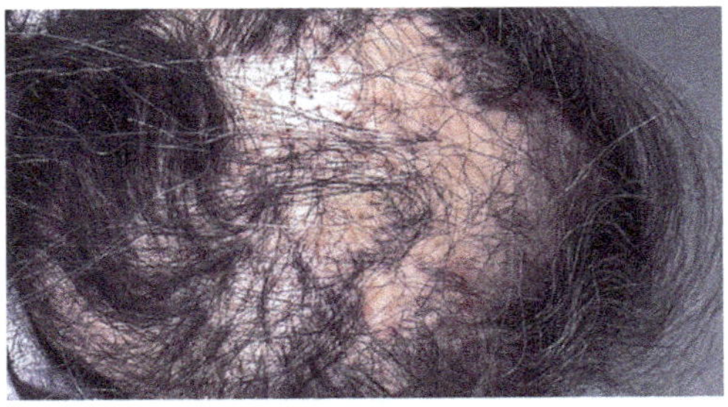

Late-stage lichen planopilaris
Photograph courtesy of SpringerImages Database, Springer Publishing Company

iii. Discoid Lupus Erythematosus

Discoid lupus erythematosus.

A. Scarring alopecia
B. Pruritic and tender
C. Erythema, atrophy, dilated plugged pores, alopecia

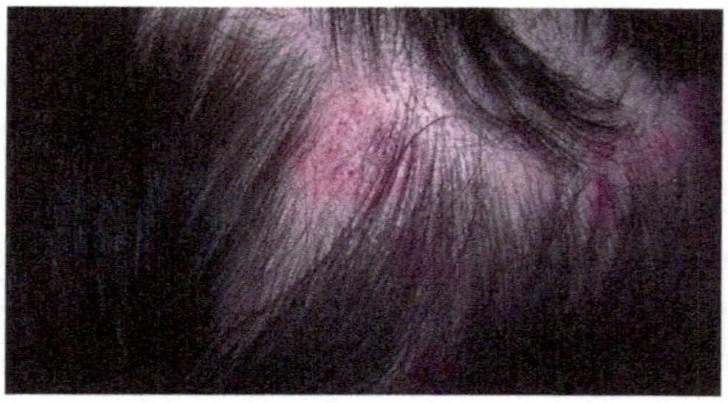

Discoid lupus erythematosus
Photograph courtesy of SpringerImages Database, Springer Publishing Company

Discoid Lupus Erythematosus

A. Scarring alopecia with atrophy, follicular plugs, hyperpigmentation, and hypopigmentation

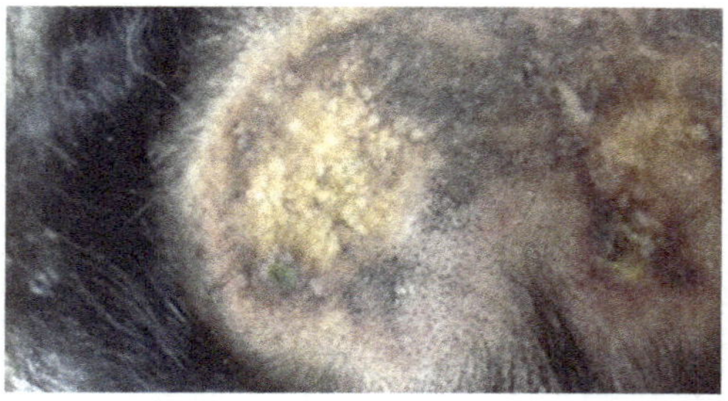

Discoid lupus erythematosus
Photograph courtesy of Hugh Gloster, MD

Discoid Lupus Erythematosus

A. Central hypopigmentation and peripheral hyperpigmentation is common in blacks

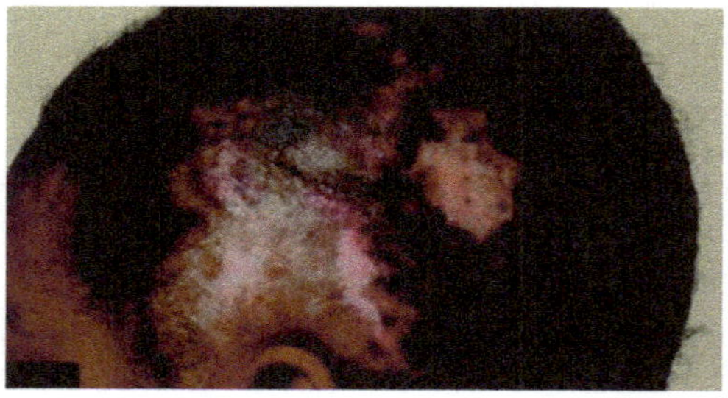

Discoid lupus erythematosus
Photograph courtesy of SpringerImages Database, Springer Publishing Company

iv. Dissecting Cellulitis

Dissecting cellulitis.

A. More common in young black men
B. Begins with the formation of multiple pustules, abscesses, or firm nodules on the posterior vertex or occiput
C. Lesions evolve into interconnecting boggy fluctuant oval and linear ridges that eventually discharge purulent foul-smelling material
D. Advanced disease is characterized by scarring alopecia
E. May be part of the follicular occlusion triad (dissecting cellulitis, hidradenitis suppurative, acne conglobata), but isolated scalp disease often seen

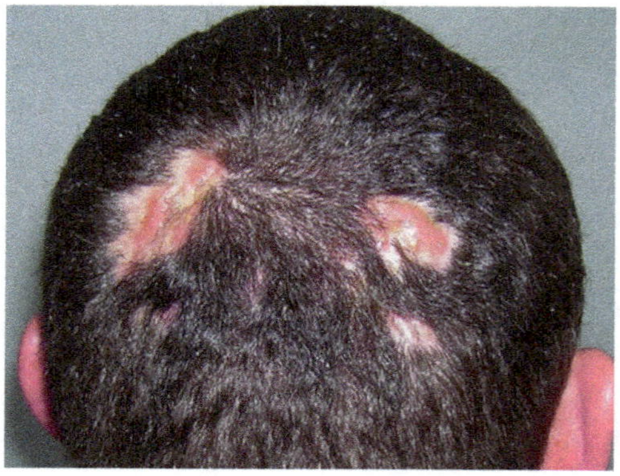

Dissecting cellulitis
Photograph courtesy of SpringerImages Database, Springer Publishing Company

Dissecting Cellulitis

A. Interconnecting boggy fluctuant oval and linear ridges that discharge purulent foul-smelling material

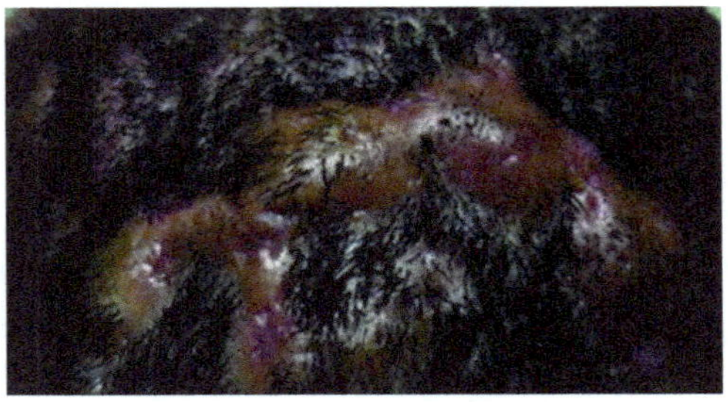

Dissecting cellulitis
Photograph courtesy of SpringerImages Database, Springer Publishing Company

v. Folliculitis Decalvans

Folliculitis Decalvans

A. Highly inflammatory form of scarring alopecia with absent follicular ostia that mainly involves vertex and occipital scalp
B. Perifollicular papules and pustules, erosions, erythema, and hemorrhagic crusts
C. Tufted follicles (multiple hairs emerging from one dilated follicle)
D. Variably sized irregular patches of scarring alopecia

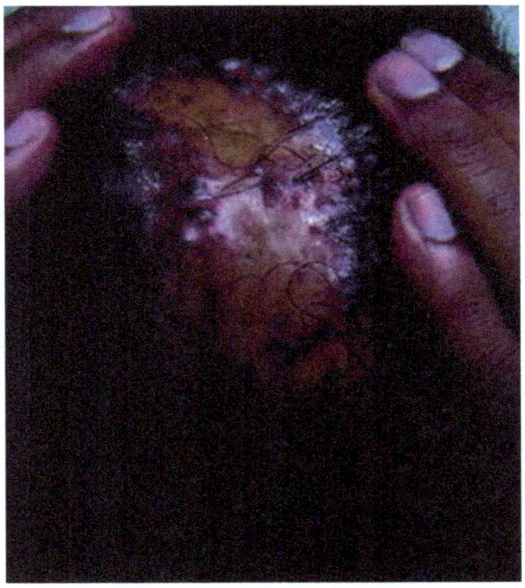

Folliculitis decalvans
Photograph courtesy of SpringerImages Database, Springer Publishing Company

Folliculitis Decalvans

A. Absent follicular ostia, tufted follicles, perifollicular papules, and erythema

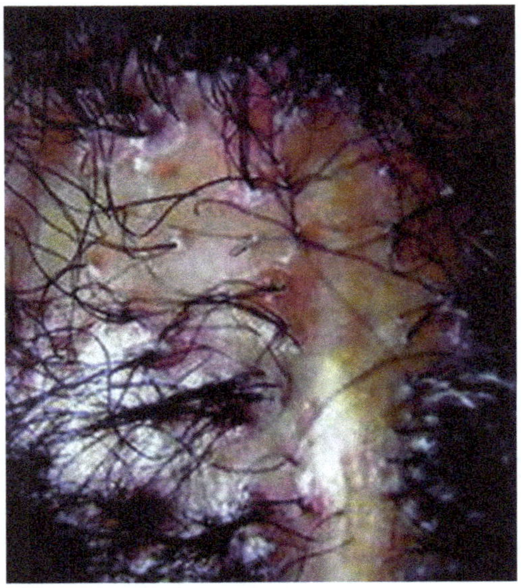

Folliculitis decalvans
Photograph courtesy of SpringerImages Database, Springer Publishing Company

vi. Acne Keloidalis Nuchae

1. Early-Stage Acne Keloidalis Nuchae

Early-Stage Acne Keloidalis Nuchae

A. Early lesions are characterized by persistent follicular and perifollicular papules and plaques on the posterior neck and occipital scalp

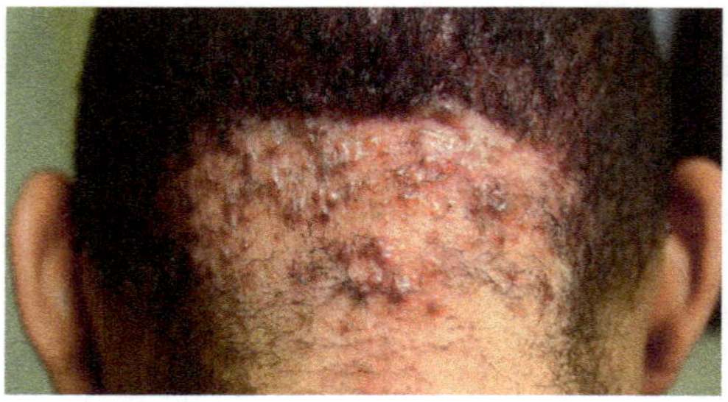

Early-stage acne keloidalis nuchae
Photograph courtesy of SpringerImages Database, Springer Publishing Company

2. Late-Stage Acne Keloidalis Nuchae

Late-Stage Acne Keloidalis Nuchae:

A. Keloid-like papules coalesce into plaques associated with scarring alopecia, tufted hairs, broken hair shafts, abscesses, and draining sinus tracts

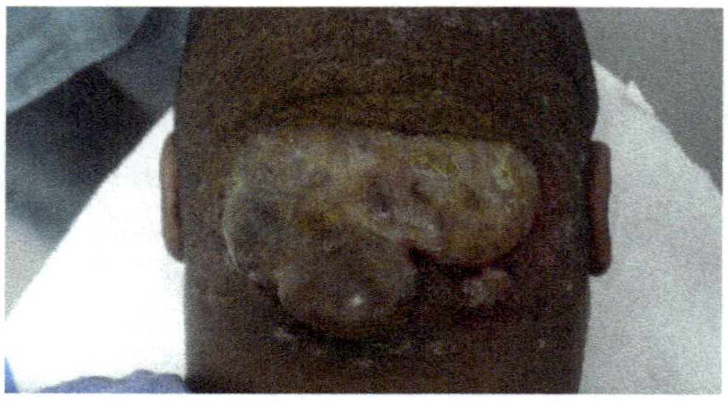

Late-stage acne keloidalis nuchae
Photograph courtesy of Hugh Gloster, MD

vii. Frontal Fibrosing Alopecia

Frontal fibrosing alopecia

A. Most common in postmenopausal women
B. Clinical variant of lichen planopilaris
C. Perifollicular erythema, follicular hyperkeratosis, and scarring affecting the frontotemporal hairline leading to progressive recession of the frontotemporal hairline in a band-like fashion
D. Frequent nonscarring alopecia of the eyebrows is present

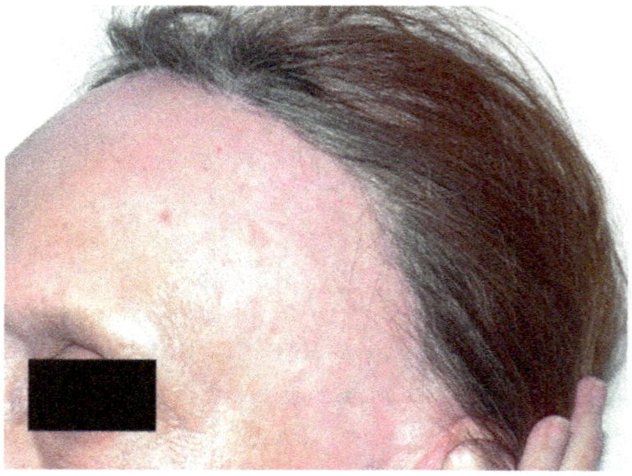

Frontal fibrosing alopecia
Photograph courtesy of SpringerImages Database, Springer Publishing Company

viii. Traction Alopecia

Traction alopecia

A. Most common presentation: black women, age 30–40 years, several years history of bitemporal hair loss
B. Pattern of progressive scarring alopecia determined by type of traction
C. Pulling the hair back will lead to alopecia at periphery of scalp in the frontotemporal area
D. Initially, hair loss is temporary and can regrow, but alopecia may be permanent if excess traction continues for years

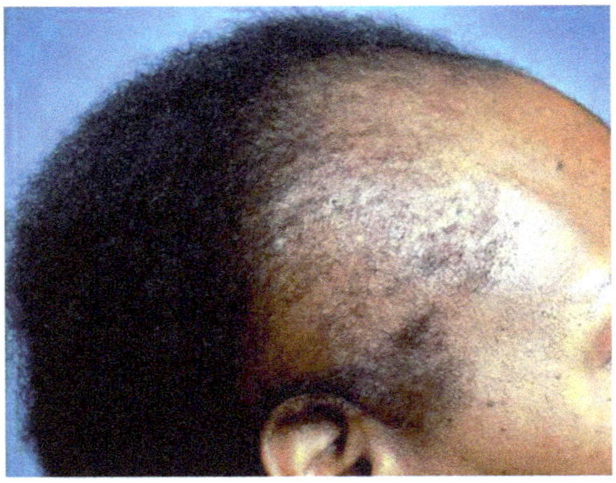

Traction alopecia
Photograph courtesy of SpringerImages Database, Springer Publishing Company

Traction alopecia

A. Bitemporal scarring alopecia as a result of pulling the hair back for years

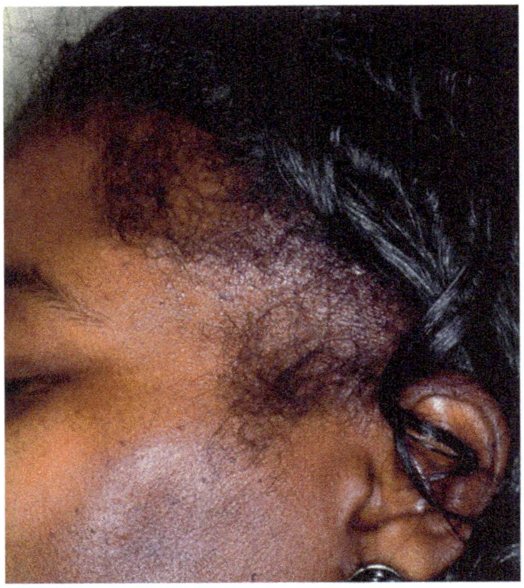

Traction alopecia
Photograph courtesy of SpringerImages Database, Springer Publishing Company

Nail Disease

64

a. Trachyonychia

Trachonychia

A. Also known as 20 nail dystrophy and sandpaper nails
B. Nail roughness due to excessive longitudinal ridging, often associated with thinning—the nails appear to have been sandpapered in a longitudinal direction
C. Several nails usually affected (not always all 20)
D. More common in children
E. Associated conditions include alopecia areata (most common), lichen planus, psoriasis, eczema

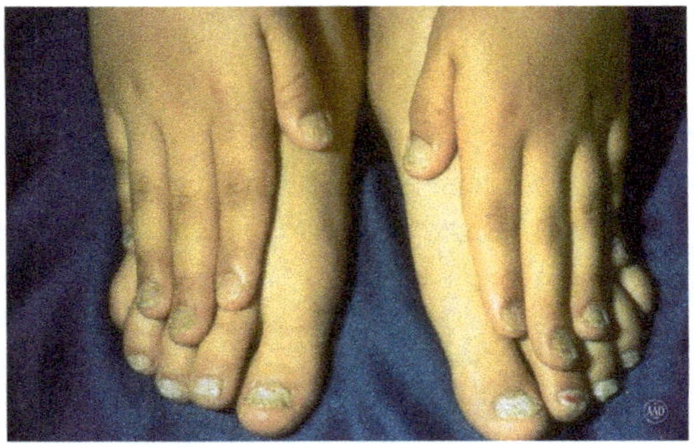

Trachyonychia
Photograph courtesy of the American Academy of Dermatology

b. Beau's Lines

Beau's lines

A. One or more transverse depressions of the nail plate due to temporary interruption of the mitotic activity of the proximal nail matrix
B. Depression grows distally with the nail plate
C. Multiple lines indicate repeated damage
D. Most commonly caused by mechanical trauma (manicures, picking) or dermatologic disease of the proximal nail fold (eczema, chronic paronychia)
E. Involvement of all nails at the same level may indicate a systemic disease (severe or febrile illness, erythroderma, drugs)

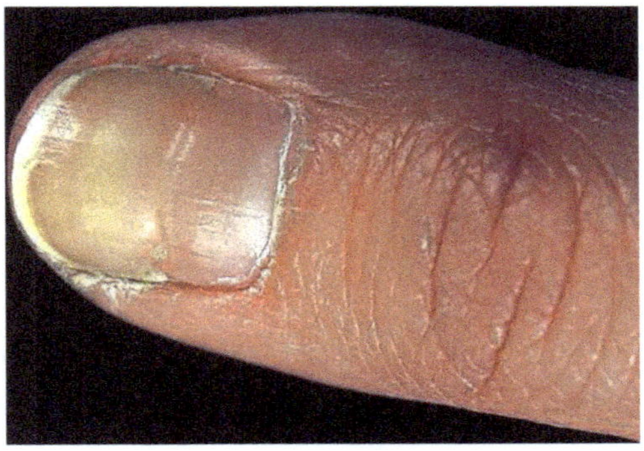

Beau's Lines
Photograph courtesy of SpringerImages Database, Springer Publishing Company

H.M. Gloster, Jr. et al., *Absolute Dermatology Review: Mastering Clinical Conditions on the Dermatology Recertification Exam*,
DOI 10.1007/978-3-319-03218-4_64,

c. Half and Half Nails (Lindsay's Nails)

Half and half nails (Lindsay's nails)
  A. Type of apparent leukonychia
  B. Leukonychia of proximal half of nail
  C. May be seen in patients with chronic renal failure

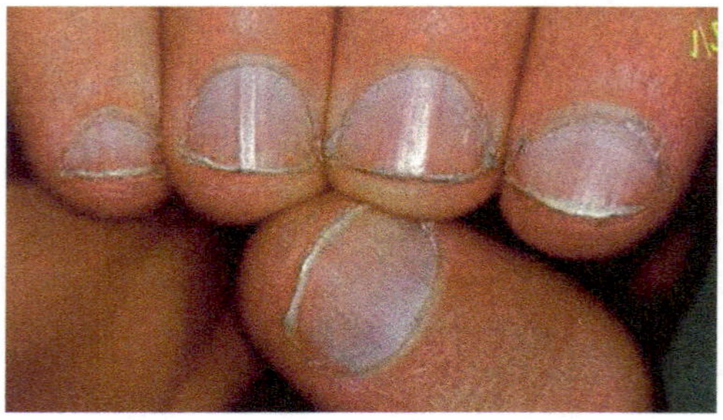

Half and half nails (Lindsay's nails)
Photograph courtesy of SpringerImages Database, Springer Publishing Company

d. Yellow Nail Syndrome

Yellow nail syndrome
  A. Thick, hard, yellow/yellow–green discoloration, excessive curvature (transversely and longitudinally), and absent cuticles of the nails
  B. Associated with lymphedema and respiratory disease

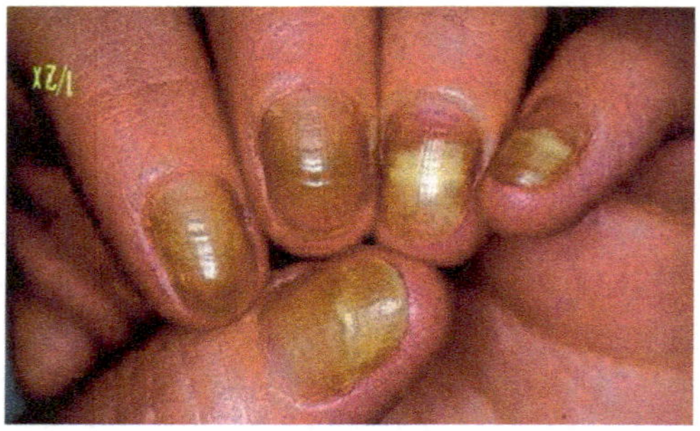

Yellow nail syndrome
Photograph courtesy of SpringerImages Database, Springer Publishing Company

e. Onychorrhexis

Onychorrhexis
  A. Longitudinal ridging and fissuring
  B. May be seen in lichen planus

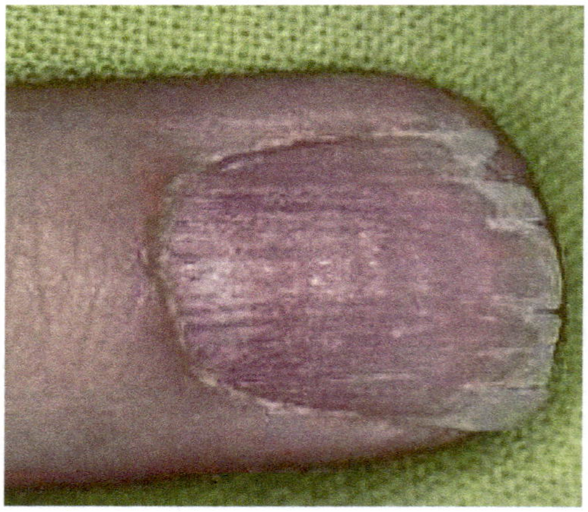

Onychorrhexis
Photograph courtesy of SpringerImages Database, Springer Publishing Company

f. Punctate Leukonychia

Leukonychia punctata

A. Variant of true leukonychia
B. Small white spots of nail plate that grow with the nail
C. Caused by trauma
D. Most common in children

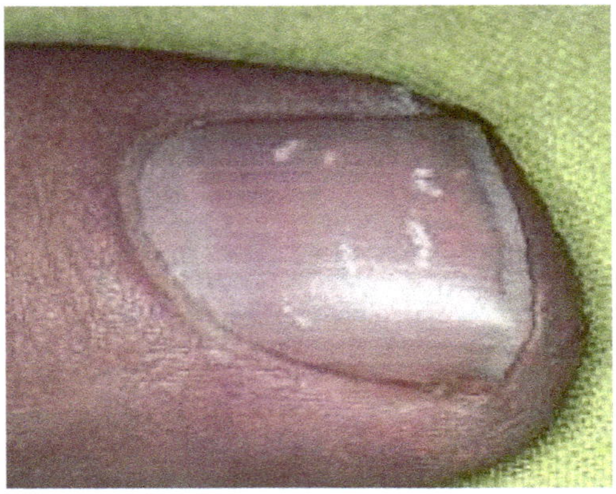

Punctate leukonychia
Photograph courtesy of SpringerImages Database, Springer Publishing Company

g. Striate Leukonychia

Leukonychia striata

A. Variant of true leukonychia
B. One or more transverse white parallel lines on the nail plate
C. Most often caused by trauma (e.g., fingernails of women as a result of manicures, toenails as a result of trauma from shoes)
D. Mees' lines (white transverse bands seen in arsenic or thallium poisoning) are a type of striate leukonychia
E. Must be distinguished from apparent leukonychia (nail bed discoloration) and pseudoleukonychia (nail plate invasion by fungi)

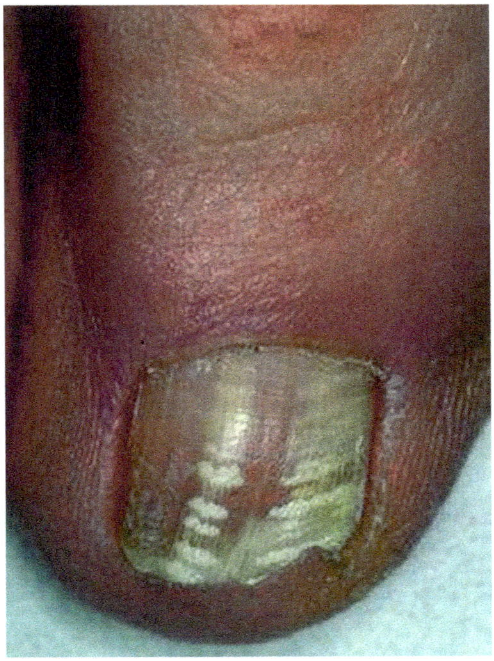

Striate leukonychia
Photograph courtesy of SpringerImages Database, Springer Publishing Company

h. Onychomadesis

Onychomadesis

A. Proximal nail detachment, usually traumatic
B. Onychomadesis in multiple digits may indicate a systemic cause
C. Caused by a complete arrest of nail matrix activity

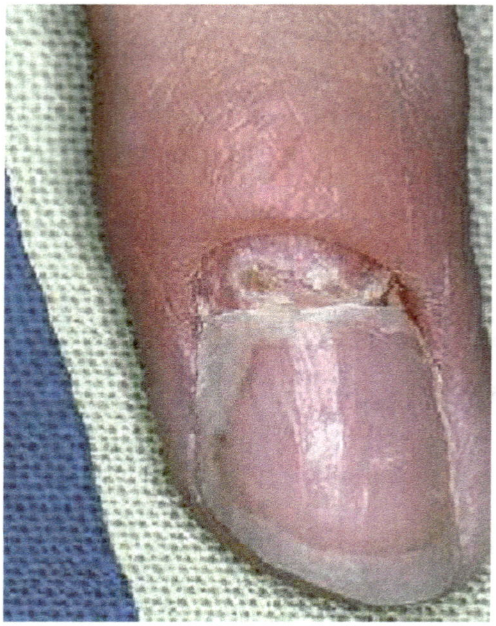

Onychomadesis
Photograph courtesy of SpringerImages Database, Springer Publishing Company

i. Koilonychia

Koilonychia

A. Spoon nails (upward eversion of lateral edges)
B. Physiological in children, in adults may be occupational or associated with iron deficiency anemia

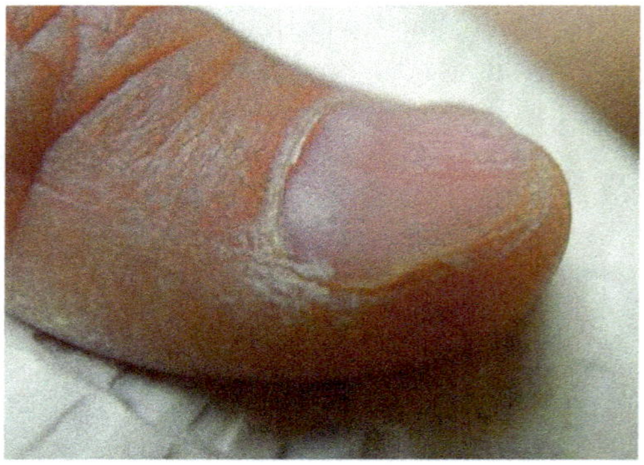

Koilonychia
Photograph courtesy of SpringerImages Database, Springer Publishing Company

j. Terry's Nails

Terry's nails (also see Chap. 7, section 48c(iv))

A. Type of apparent leukonychia (white discoloration of nail bed that fades with pressure)
B. Leukonychia of whole nail obscuring the lunula and sparing the distal 1–2 mm band of color in the nail bed
C. Seen in normal people and those with cirrhosis of the liver

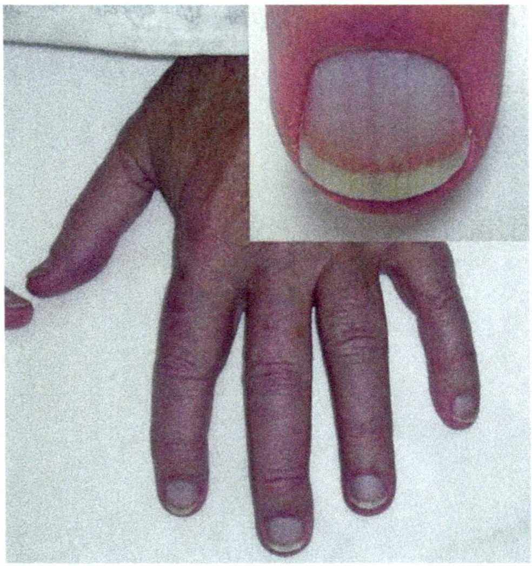

Terry's nails
Photograph courtesy of SpringerImages Database, Springer Publishing Company

k. Clubbing

Clubbing

A. Bulbous digits with enlarged and excessively curved nail plates
B. Lovibond's sign: greater than 180 degree angle between the proximal nail fold and the nail plate
C. Associations:
   1. Pulmonary disease: bronchiectasis and neoplasms
   2. Hypertrophic osteoarthropathy
   3. Bilateral clubbing: neoplasms, pulmonary and cardiac disease

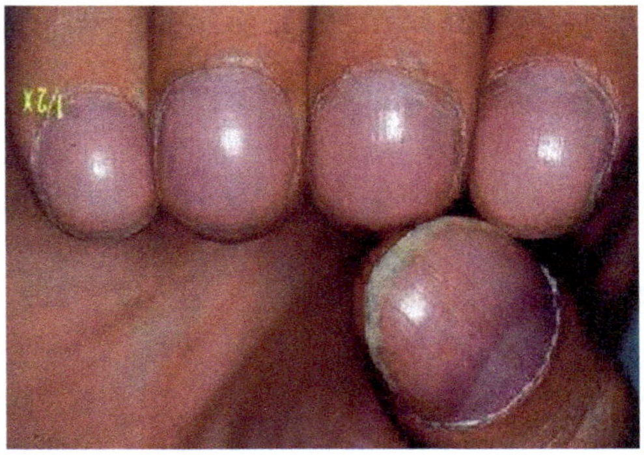

Clubbing
Photograph courtesy of SpringerImages Database, Springer Publishing Company

I. Psoriatic Nail Disease

Psoriatic nail disease

A. Nail pits and onycholysis (distal nail plate detachment from the nail bed)

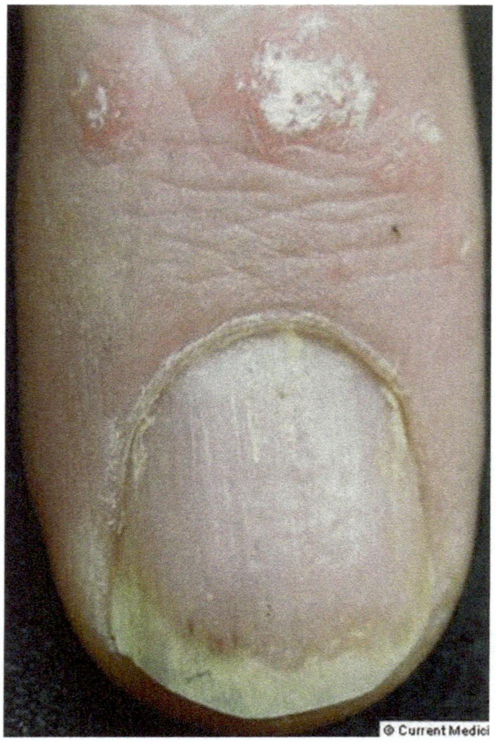

Psoriatic nail disease
Photograph courtesy of SpringerImages Database, Springer Publishing Company

Psoriatic nail disease

A. Nail pits, onycholysis, yellow discoloration of the nail plate, and subungual debris

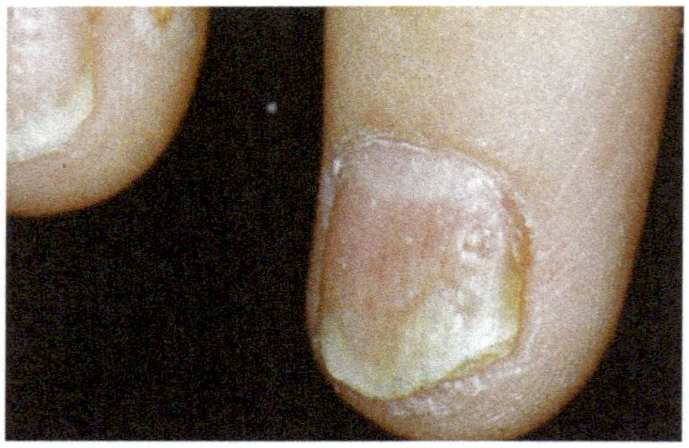

Psoriatic nail disease
Photograph courtesy of SpringerImages Database, Springer Publishing Company

Psoriatic nail disease

A. Nail pits, salmon patches, and distal onycholysis

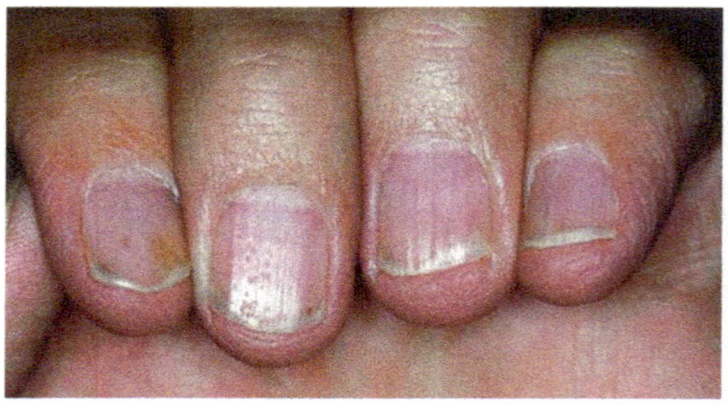

Psoriatic nail disease

65 Mucous Membrane Disease

a. Geographic Tongue (Benign Migratory Glossitis)

Geographic tongue (benign migratory glossitis)

A. Benign disorder of unknown etiology, may be more common in psoriatics or atopics
B. Well-delineated erythematous patches partially surrounded by yellow–white thin serpiginous borders
C. Lateral and dorsal tongue
D. May migrate, usually asymptomatic but may burn slightly
E. Differs from candidiasis, characterized by white patches on oral mucosa (cheese-like curds) that are easily wiped off to reveal an erythematous base

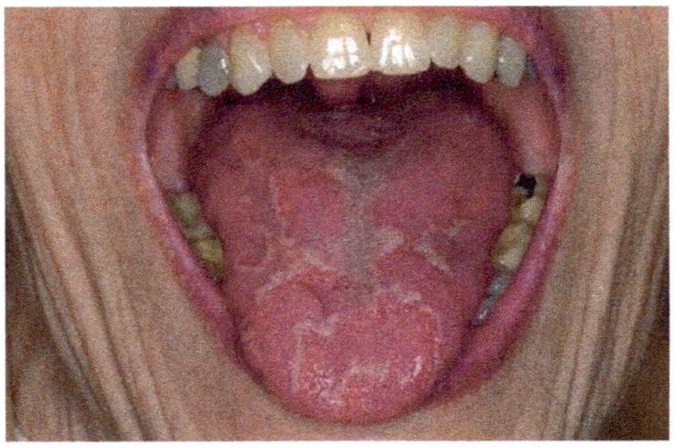

Geographic tongue (benign migratory glossitis)
Photograph courtesy of SpringerImages Database, Springer Publishing Company

b. Oral Hairy Leukoplakia

Oral hairy leukoplakia

A. Ebstein-Barr virus (human herpes virus 4) associated mucosal condition that usually represents an early sign of HIV infection
B. Most common in patients with HIV infection, also seen in other immunosuppressed states
C. Asymptomatic, vertically oriented, white shaggy, hairy, feathery ridges forming white corrugated plaques on the lateral sides of the tongue
D. Plaques are adherent and not easily removed by mechanical force (unlike candiasis, which can be removed with a tongue blade leaving an erythematous base)
E. No malignant potential
F. Lesions can come and go

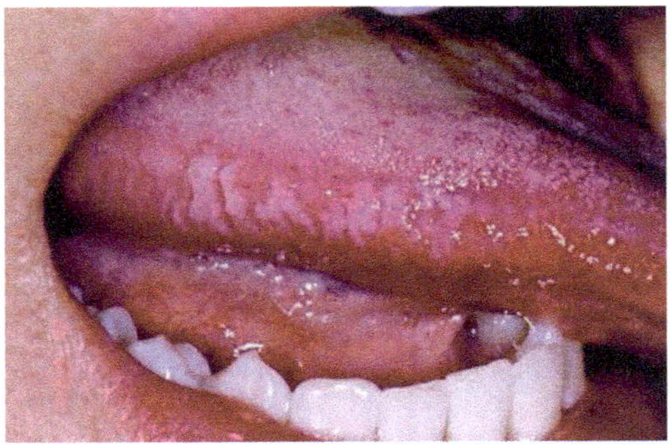

Oral hairy leukoplakia
Photograph courtesy of SpringerImages Database, Springer Publishing Company

H.M. Gloster, Jr. et al., *Absolute Dermatology Review: Mastering Clinical Conditions on the Dermatology Recertification Exam*,
DOI 10.1007/978-3-319-03218-4_65, © Springer International Publishing Switzerland 2016

Oral hairy leukoplakia

A. Vertically oriented, white shaggy, hairy, feathery ridges forming white corrugated plaques on the lateral sides of the tongue

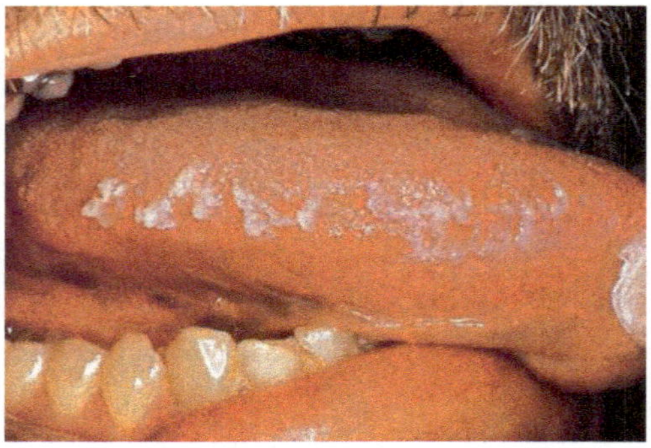

Oral hairy leukoplakia
Photograph courtesy of SpringerImages Database, Springer Publishing Company

c. Aphthous Stomatitis

i. Minor Aphthous Stomatitis

Minor aphthous stomatitis

A. Painful, shallow, less than 5 mm, round creamy white ulcers with sharp borders and a red halo located on the oral mucosa
B. May be recurrent
C. Heal without scar in 1–2 weeks
D. Most common cause of oral ulcers (20 % of population), peak onset second decade

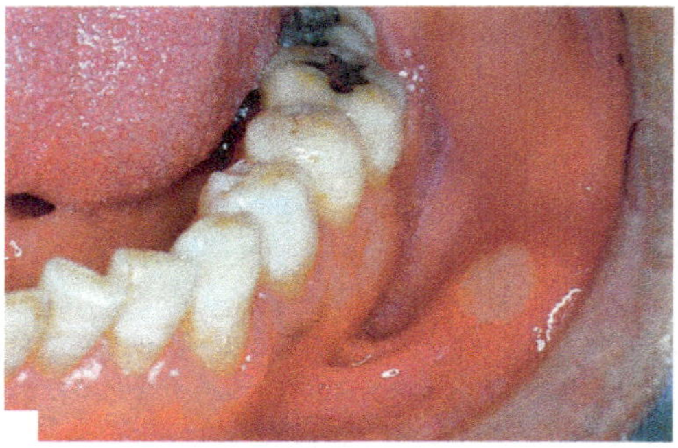

Minor aphthous stomatitis
Photograph courtesy of SpringerImages Database, Springer Publishing Company

ii. Major Aphthous Stomatitis

Major aphthous stomatitis

A. Larger (greater than 1cm) ulcers, deeper, persist up to 6 weeks, may heal with scarring
B. Associated with pain, fever, malaise

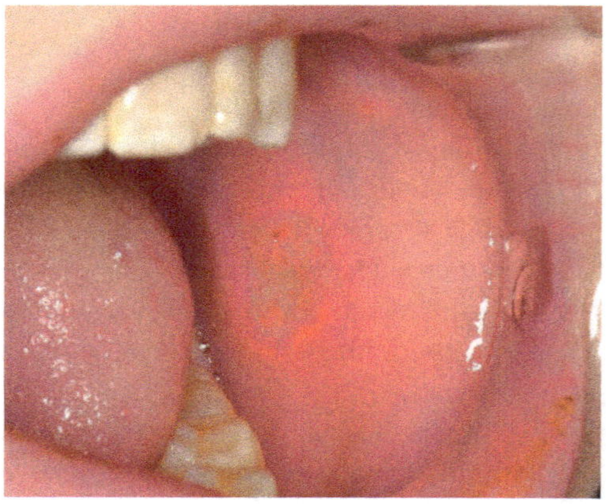

Major aphthous stomatitis
Photograph courtesy of SpringerImages Database, Springer Publishing Company

Chapter XII

Benign Neoplasms

Accessory Tragus

66

Accesory Tragus

A. Dome-shaped skin-colored papules or nodules that primarily arise in the preauricular area
B. May also occur on the mandibular cheek (jawline) or neck along anterior border of the sternocleidomastoid muscle

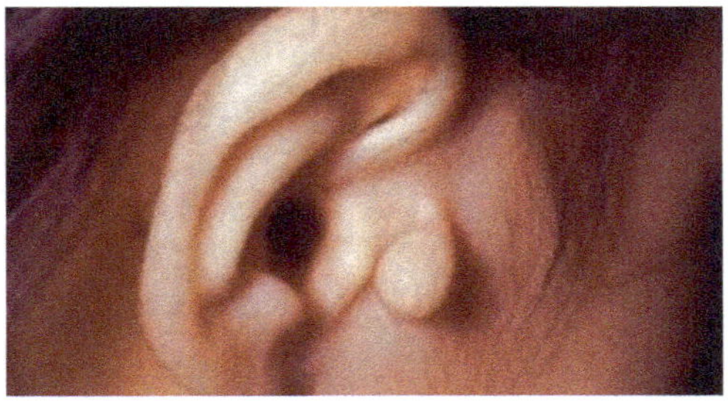

Accessory tragus
Photograph courtesy of SpringerImages Database, Springer Publishing Company

H.M. Gloster, Jr. et al., *Absolute Dermatology Review: Mastering Clinical Conditions on the Dermatology Recertification Exam*,
DOI 10.1007/978-3-319-03218-4_66,

67 Accessory (Supernumerary) Digit

Accessory (supernumerary) digit

A. Congenital
B. Rudimentary digit most commonly on the lateral ulnar hand near fifth digit
C. Nerve bundles histologically

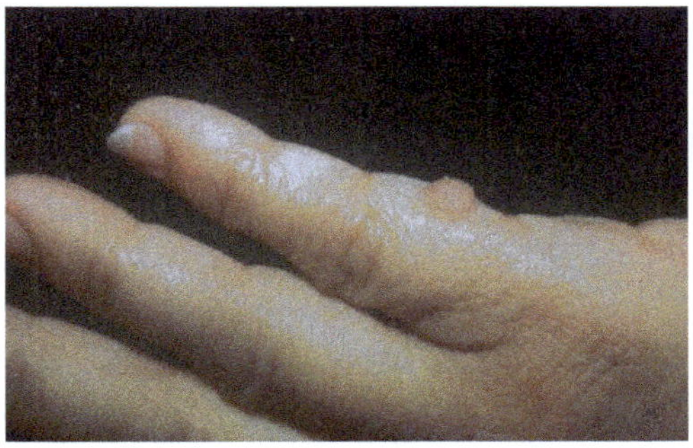

Accessory (supernumerary) digit
Courtesy of the American Academy of Dermatology

H.M. Gloster, Jr. et al., *Absolute Dermatology Review: Mastering Clinical Conditions on the Dermatology Recertification Exam*,
DOI 10.1007/978-3-319-03218-4_67,

68 Acquired Digital Fibrokeratoma

Acquired digital fibrokeratoma

A. Solitary, skin-colored to pink, keratotic, exophytic papulonodule with a collarette of elevated skin at the base
B. The finger is the most common site, but also occurs on toes
C. Trauma may be a predisposing factor
D. Usually occurs in middle-age adults
E. Differential diagnosis includes accessory (supernumerary digit, periungual fibroma, verruca vulgaris

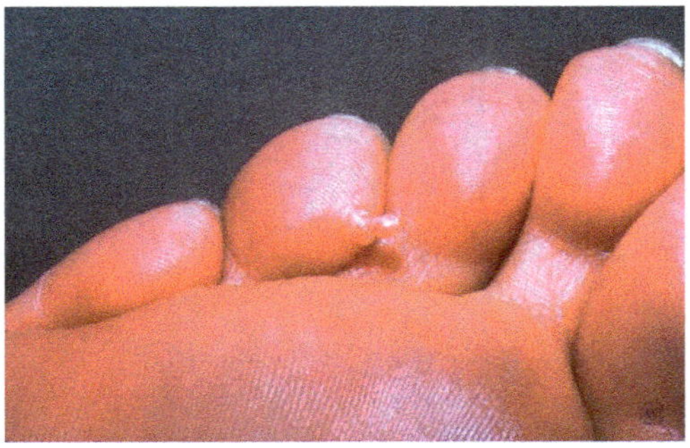

Acquired digital fibrokeratoma
Courtesy of the American Academy of Dermatology

H.M. Gloster, Jr. et al., *Absolute Dermatology Review: Mastering Clinical Conditions on the Dermatology Recertification Exam*,
DOI 10.1007/978-3-319-03218-4_68, © Springer International Publishing Switzerland 2016

69 Adnexal Tumors

a. Trichoepithelioma

Solitary trichoepithelioma

A. Skin-colored papule or nodule on the face, especially the nose
B. More common than multiple trichoepitheliomas
C. Not inherited

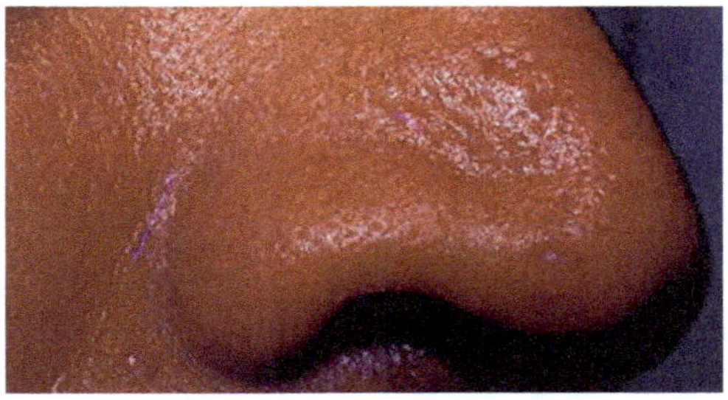

Trichoepithelioma
Photograph courtesy of SpringerImages Database, Springer Publishing Company

H.M. Gloster, Jr. et al., *Absolute Dermatology Review: Mastering Clinical Conditions on the Dermatology Recertification Exam*, DOI 10.1007/978-3-319-03218-4_69, © Springer International Publishing Switzerland 2016

b. Multiple Trichoepitheliomas

Multiple Trichoepitheliomas (epithelioma adenoides cysticum: Brooke-Spiegler Syndrome)

A. Numerous round skin-colored firm papules or nodules, 2–8 mm in diameter, on the central face (melolabial fold, nose, forehead, upper lip)
B. Autosomal dominant traiit
C. May appear along with cylindromas

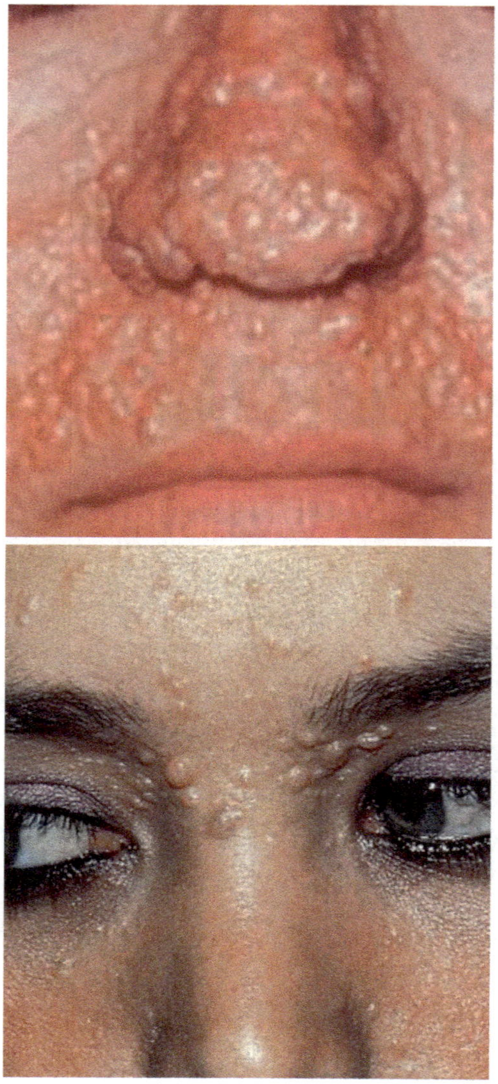

Multiple trichoepitheliomas
Photograph courtesy of SpringerImages Database, Springer Publishing Company

c. Cylindroma

Cylindroma

A. Solitary
   1. Smooth, firm rubbery pink, red, or blue dome-shaped few mm–to–few cm nodules that commonly occur on the scalp
   2. Solitary lesions appear sporadically
B. Multiple cylindromas
   1. Numerous rounded masses on the scalp beginning in second or third decade, may resemble a "bunch of grapes"
   2. May surround the scalp to form "turban tumors"
   3. Multiple lesions should prompt consideration for the Brooke-Spiegler syndrome or multiple cylindromatosis
   4. Autosomal dominant

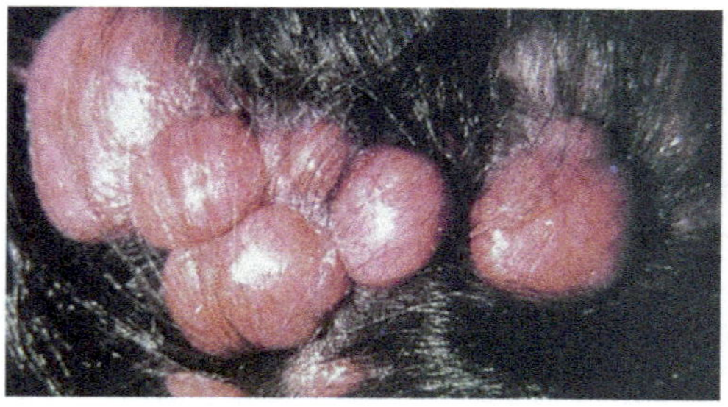

Cylindroma
Photograph courtesy of SpringerImages Database, Springer Publishing Company

Cylindromas

A. Numerous rounded masses on the scalp resembling a "bunch of grapes"

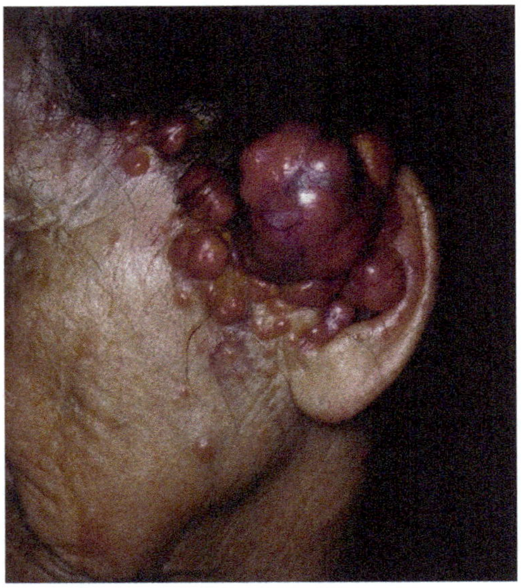

Cylindroma
Photograph courtesy of SpringerImages Database, Springer Publishing Company

d. Syringoma

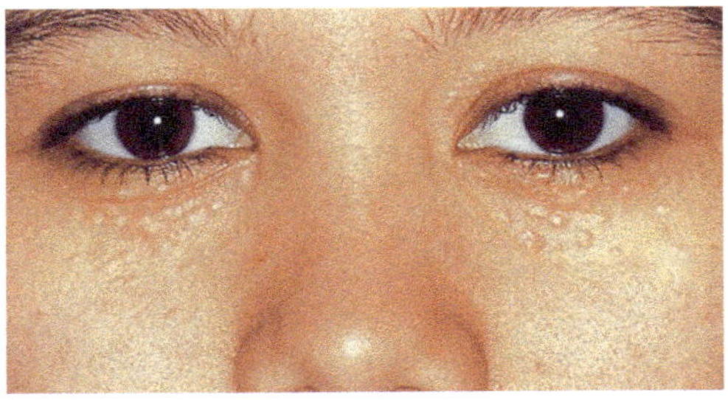

Syringoma
Photograph courtesy of SpringerImages Database, Springer Publishing Company

Syringoma

A. Small (1–3 mm), symmetrical, firm skin-colored to yellow papules
B. Usually occur in periorbital location (especially eyelids) and upper cheeks
C. May be eruptive, especially on trunk (usually ventral surfaces such as the neck and upper chest, penis)
    1. Eruptive variant more common in blacks and Asians
D. More common in women, Asians

e. Nevus Sebaceous

Nevus Sebaceous

A. Usually involves the scalp or face
B. Birth: slightly raised and subtle plaque or plaques
C. Childhood: the plaque thickens slightly and becomes a salmon-colored, yellow/orange waxy hairless plaque (top figure)
D. Adolescents: the plaque thickens with a pebbly or verrucous surface and increases in size with puberty (bottom figure)
E. When the face and neck are involved, the lesions are usually small yellow–white papules that coalesce into linear plaques
F. Adnexal neoplasms may develop within nevus sebaceous in 10–20 % by fourth to seventh decade
   1. Incidence of basal cell carcinoma is less than 1 % (BCC is the most common malignancy)
   2. Trichoblastoma is the most common neoplasm overall (syringocystadenoma papilliferum is the second most common)

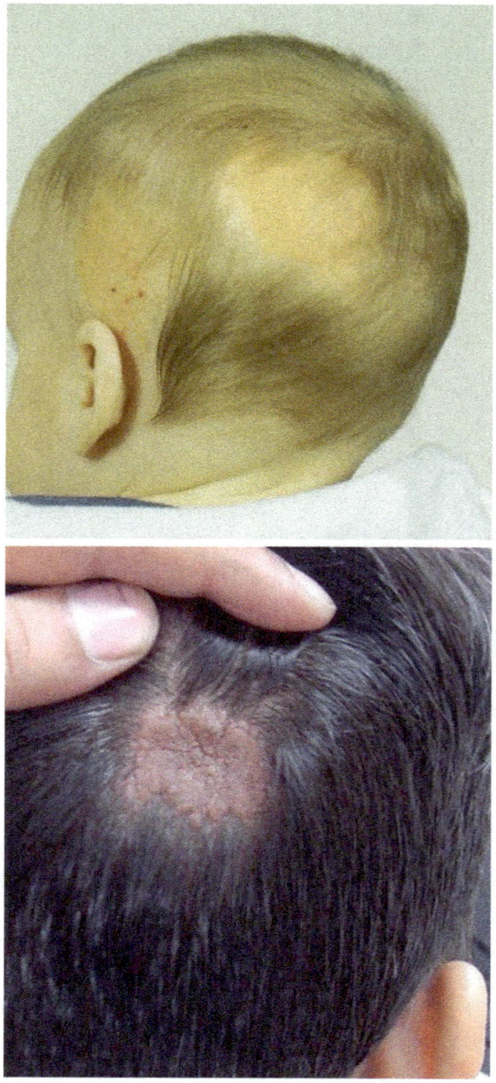

Nevus sebaceous
Photograph courtesy of SpringerImages Database, Springer Publishing Company

Nevus sebaceous

A. When the face and neck are involved, the lesions are usually small yellow–white papules that coalesce into linear plaques

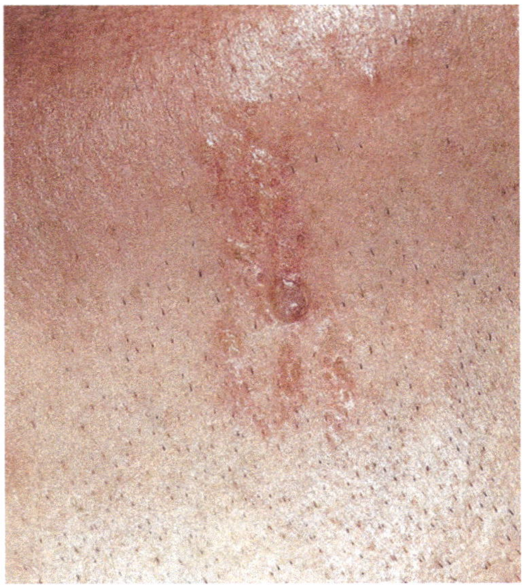

Nevus sebaceous
Photograph courtesy of SpringerImages Database, Springer Publishing Company

f. Trichofolliculoma

Trichofolliculoma

A. Solitary skin-colored dome-shaped nodule with central pore and diagnostic wool-like tuft of white hair emerging from the pore
B. Usually occur on the face

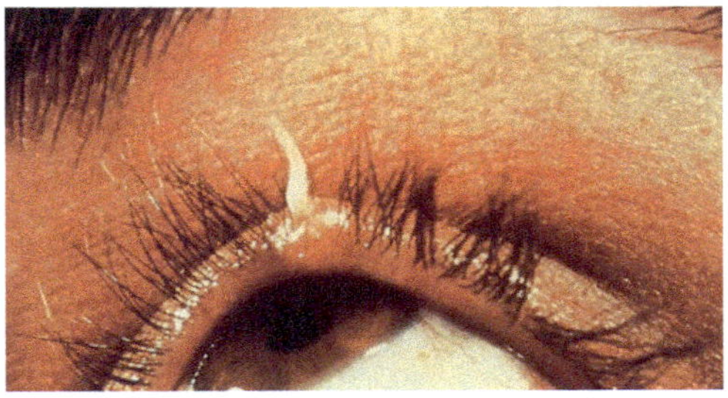

Trichofolliculoma
Photograph courtesy of SpringerImages Database, Springer Publishing Company

g. Poroma

Poroma

A. Sessile, soft, red nodule most commonly on sole or side of foot (less often palm) that easily bleeds
B. Grows and protrudes from cup-shaped shallow depression

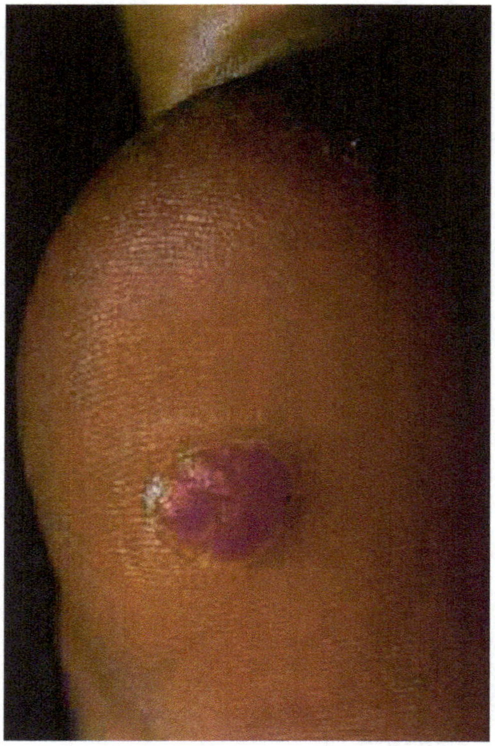

Poroma
Photograph courtesy of SpringerImages Database, Springer Publishing Company

70 Becker's Nevus

Becker's nevus

A. Unilateral hyperpigmented and hypertrichotic (hair usually develops after pigment) patch or slightly elevated plaque with irregular borders
B. Tan to brown patch slowly expands several centimeters and develops a pebbly surface, acne lesions, and hypertrichosis at puberty
C. Hairs become coarser and darker with time, pigment fades with time
D. Usually occurs on the shoulder, upper chest, scapula (shoulder girdle)
E. Typically occurs in younger men (onset in adolescence or the second or third decade)

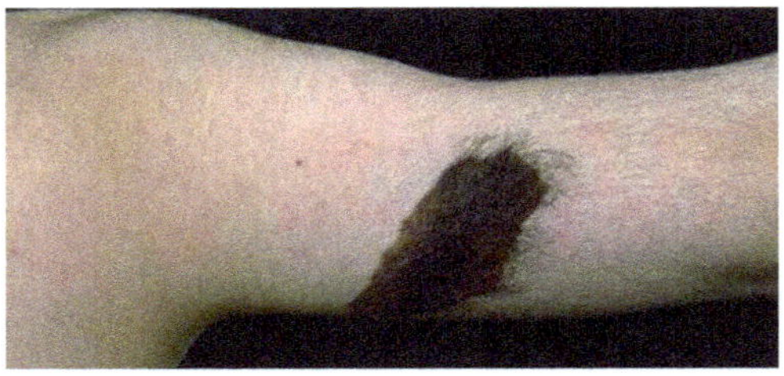

Becker's nevus
Photograph courtesy of SpringerImages Database, Springer Publishing Company

H.M. Gloster, Jr. et al., *Absolute Dermatology Review: Mastering Clinical Conditions on the Dermatology Recertification Exam*, DOI 10.1007/978-3-319-03218-4_70, © Springer International Publishing Switzerland 2016

Cysts 71

a. Epidermoid Cyst

Epidermoid cyst

A. Most common type of cyst
B. Skin-colored to yellow dermal nodules that may have a punctum, which represents the follicle from which the cyst derived

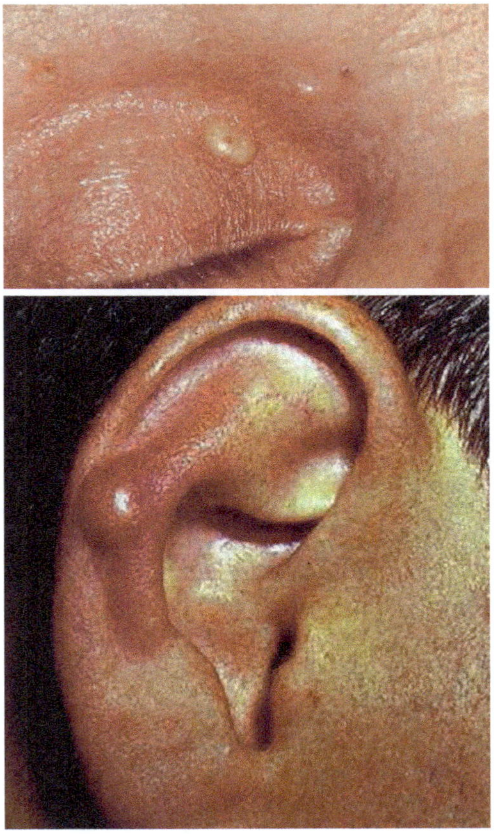

Epidermoid cyst
Photograph courtesy of SpringerImages Database, Springer Publishing Company

H.M. Gloster, Jr. et al., *Absolute Dermatology Review: Mastering Clinical Conditions on the Dermatology Recertification Exam*, DOI 10.1007/978-3-319-03218-4_71, © Springer International Publishing Switzerland 2016

b. Milia

Milia

A. Tiny superficial epidermoid cysts
B. Multiple firm tiny (1–3 mm) white papules that may have an umbliticated surface

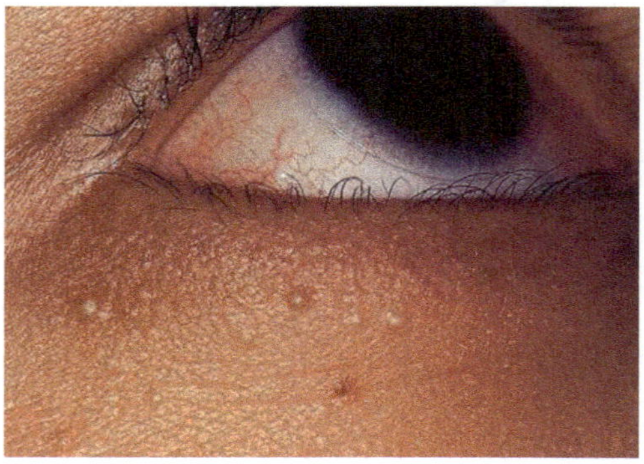

Milia
Photograph courtesy of SpringerImages Database, Springer Publishing Company

c. Steatocystoma Multiplex

Steatocystoma multiplex

A. Multiple to few 1 mm to 1 cm yellow to flesh-colored dermal cysts that drain oily fluid if punctured
B. Most common on the chest, axillae, and groin
C. Onset may correspond to puberty
D. May be inherited as an autosomal dominant condition
E. May occur in association with eruptive vellus hair cysts and pachonychia congenita type II

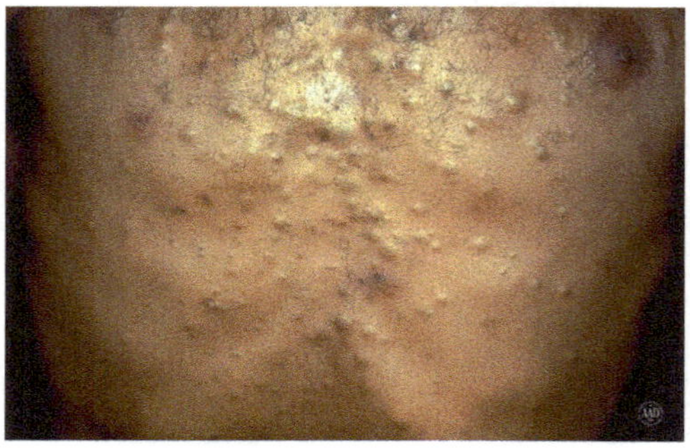

Steatocystoma Multiplex
Photograph courtesy of the American Academy of Dermatology

d. Eruptive Vellus Hair Cysts

Eruptive vellus hair cyst

A. Occlusion of vellus hair follicle with cystic dilation
B. Numerous small skin-colored to brown dome-shaped papules
C. Most common on the chest wall, abdomen, extremities
D. May be autosomal dominantly inherited
E. May be seen in conjunction with steatocystoma multiplex and pachonychia congenita type II

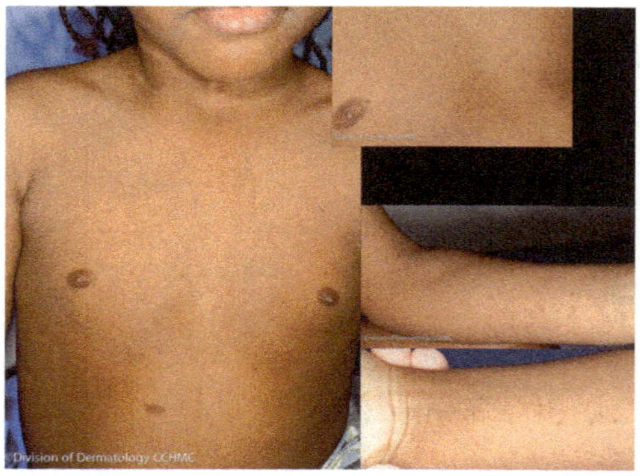

Eruptive vellus hair cysts
Photograph courtesy of Kara Shah, M.D, PhD, CCHMC (Cincinnati, OH), Department of Dermatology

72 Dermatofibroma

Dermatofibroma

A. The legs are the most common site
B. Firm, minimally elevated (or depressed) to dome-shaped papule, usually less than 1 cm
C. Commonly hyperpigmented in dark skin or tan–pink with rim of hyperpigmentation in light skin
D. May exhibit the "dimple sign" when pinched: a dimple-like depression in the overlying skin due to the downward movement of the tumor while being fixed to overlying skin
E. May arise at sites of trauma or arthropod bites and may be pruritic or painful

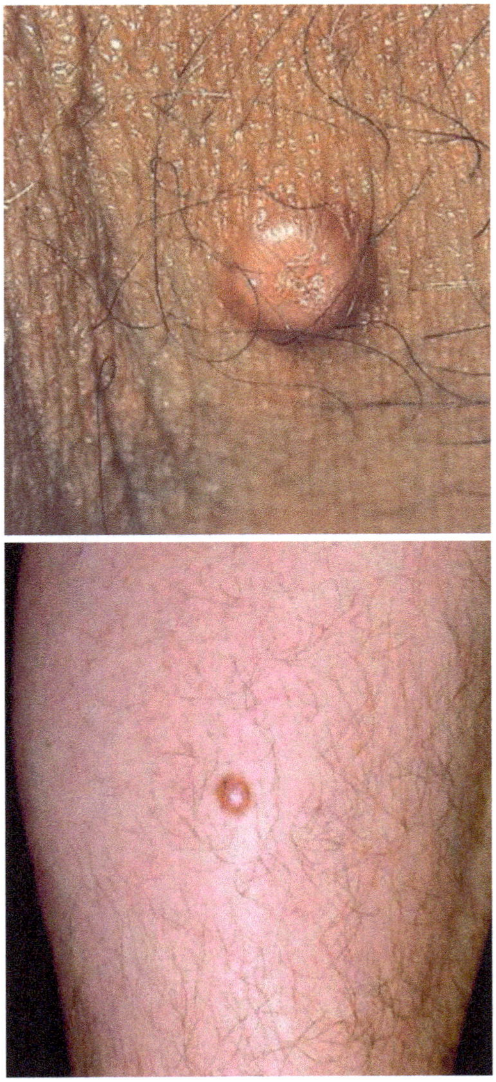

Dermatofibroma
Photograph courtesy of SpringerImages Database, Springer Publishing Company

H.M. Gloster, Jr. et al., *Absolute Dermatology Review: Mastering Clinical Conditions on the Dermatology Recertification Exam*, DOI 10.1007/978-3-319-03218-4_72, © Springer International Publishing Switzerland 2016

a. Dermatofibroma (Dermoscopy)

Dermatofibroma (dermoscopy)

A. Central white scar-like patch
B. Peripheral delicate pigment network due to hyperpigmented rete ridges

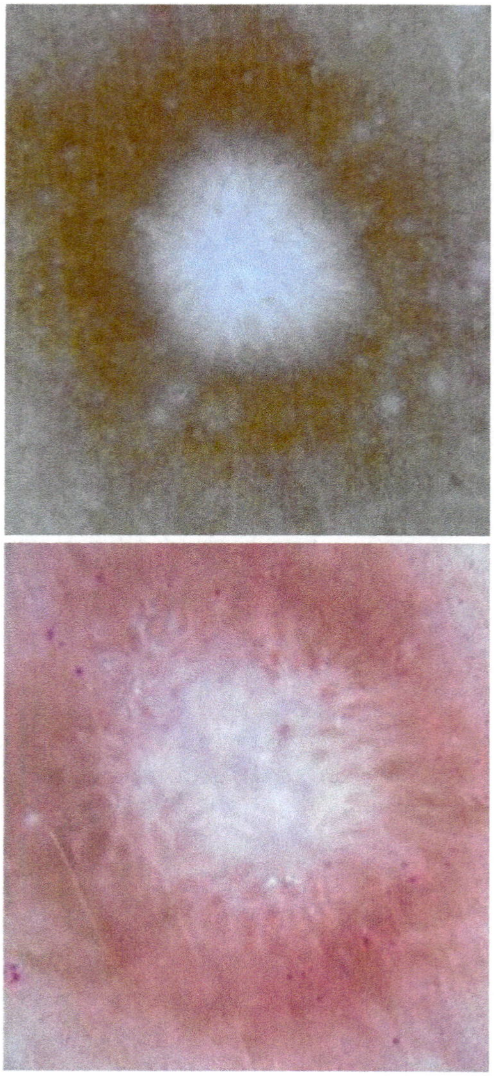

Dermatofibroma (dermoscopy)
Photograph courtesy of SpringerImages Database, Springer Publishing Company

Melanocytic Nevi

73

a. Halo Nevus

Halo Nevus

A. White halo around a brown papule, which is a nevus
B. Erythema often precedes the halo
C. Most common on the upper back in teenagers with a lot of nevi (mean age 15 years)
D. 20 % also have vitiligo
E. May occur with infliximab therapy, common in Turner Syndrome
F. Usually the nevus regresses over months to years and leaves a white macule which repigments over years
G. In adults over 40, new onset of multiple halo nevi may be a sign of an ocular or cutaneous melanoma elsewhere. In patients who also have melanoma, the halo may be asymmetric and irregular

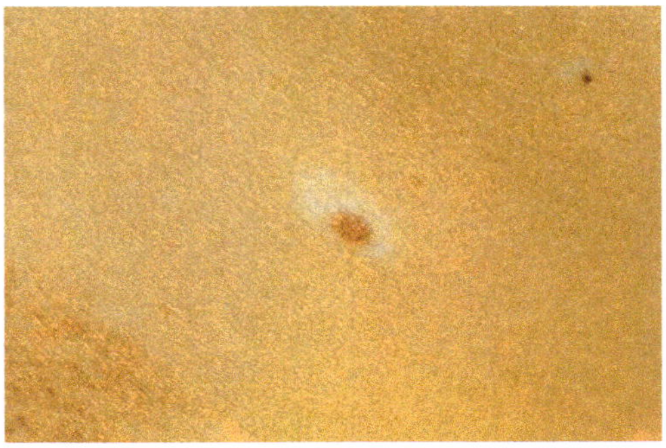

Halo nevus
Photograph courtesy of SpringerImages Database, Springer Publishing Company

i. Halo Nevus (Dermoscopy)

Halo Nevus (dermoscopy)

A. Symmetric white structureless area surrounding a nevus with a globular pattern

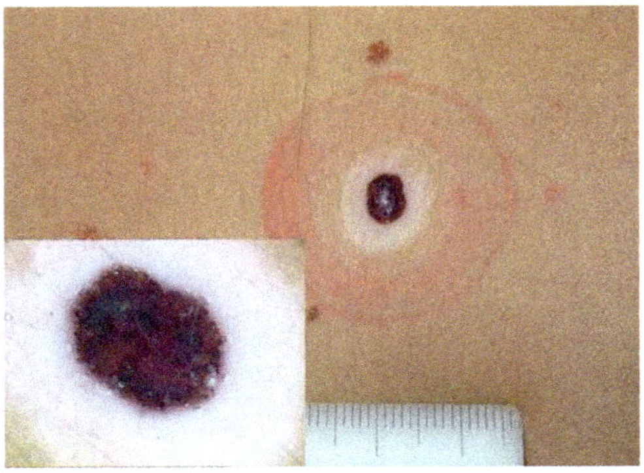

Halo nevus (dermoscopy)
Photograph courtesy of SpringerImages Database, Springer Publishing Company

H.M. Gloster, Jr. et al., *Absolute Dermatology Review: Mastering Clinical Conditions on the Dermatology Recertification Exam*,
DOI 10.1007/978-3-319-03218-4_73,

b. Congentinal Nevus

Congenital nevus

A. Present at birth
B. Grow in proportion to the growth of the patient
C. Usually round or oval, fairly symmetric, well demarcated, slightly raised and tan at birth, some have pebbly surface
D. With age, become more elevated, darken, become more verrucous, and may be covered with course hairs
E. When small (less than 1.5 cm), melanoma risk is no greater than with acquired nevi

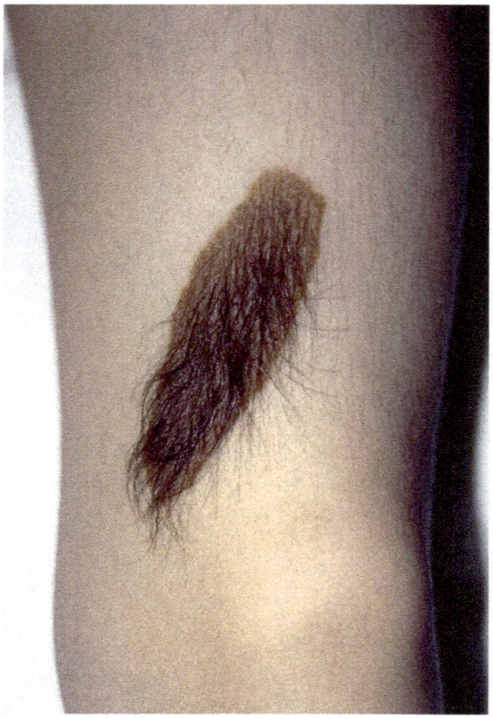

Congentinal nevus
Photograph courtesy of SpringerImages Database, Springer Publishing Company

i. Large Congenital Nevus

Large Congenital nevus (greater than 20 cm)

A. Slightly higher risk of developing melanoma than ordinary nevi
B. 70 % of melanomas that develop in large or giant congenital melanocytic nevi develop by the age of 10
C. Increased risk of neurocutaneous melanosis and noncutaneous melanoma

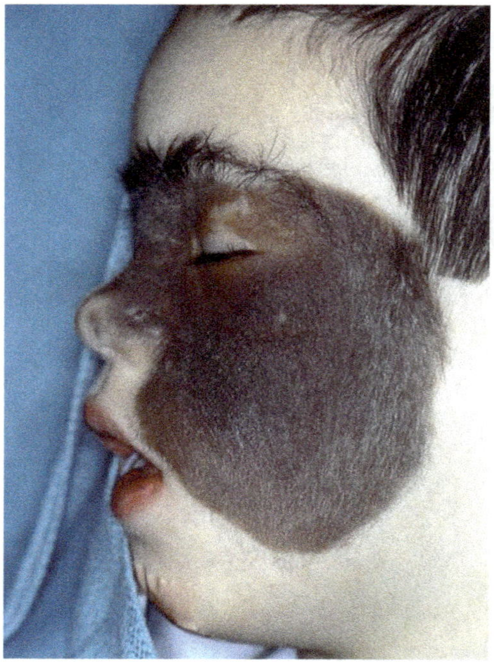

Large congenital nevus
Photograph courtesy of SpringerImages Database, Springer Publishing Company

ii. Congenital Nevus (Dermoscopy)

Congenital nevus (dermoscopy)

A. Globules, diffuse background pigmentation (structureless), milia-like cysts, hypertrichosis, perifollicular pigmentation, hyphae-like structures
B. Most common patterns: reticular, globular, reticular-globular, diffuse brown pigmentation, and multicomponent

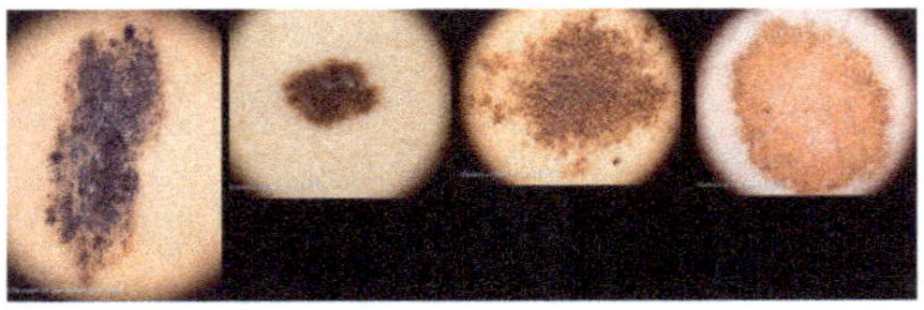

Congenital nevus (dermoscopy)
Photograph courtesy of Kara Shah, M.D, PhD, CCHMC (Cincinnati, OH), Department of Dermatology

c. Junctional Nevi

Junctional nevus

A. Symmetric, medium to dark brown flat macule with regular borders (usually dark brown center with lighter brown rim)
B. Melanocytic nests at the junction of the epidermis and dermis

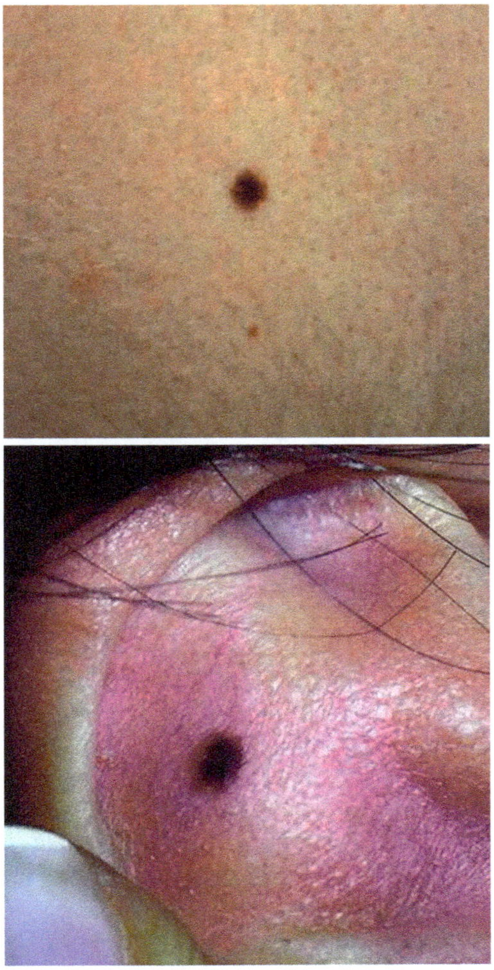

Junctional nevi
Photograph courtesy of SpringerImages Database, Springer Publishing Company

i. Junctional Nevi (Dermoscopy)

Junctional nevus (dermoscopy)

A. Uniform pigment network, homogenous in color, fading out toward the periphery

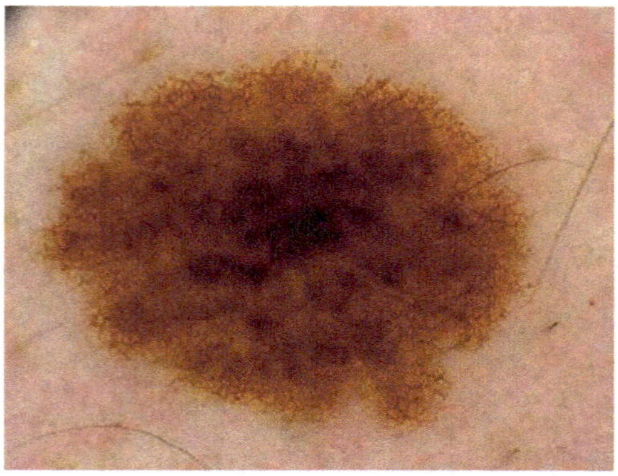

Junctional nevi (dermoscopy)
Photograph courtesy of SpringerImages Database, Springer Publishing Company

d. Compound Nevus

Compound nevus

A. Light brown to medium brown papule with combined features of junctional and intradermal nevi (usually lighter than junctional nevi)
B. Intraepidermal melanocyte and subepidermal nevus cell proliferations

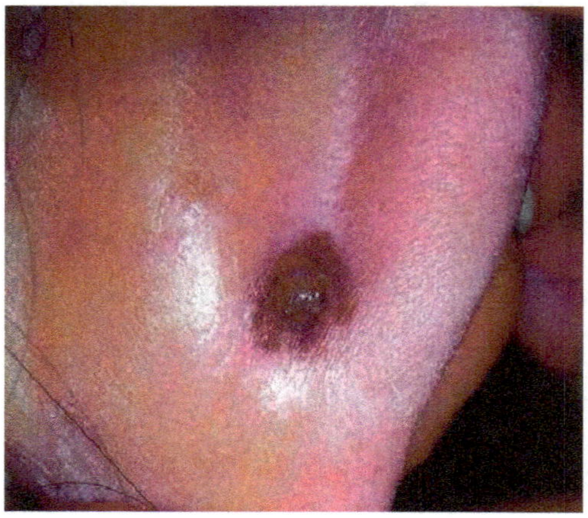

Compound nevus
Photograph courtesy of SpringerImages Database, Springer Publishing Company

i. Compound Nevus (Dermoscopy)

Compound nevus (dermoscopy)

A. Globular architecture with multiple round to ovoid globules sometimes forming a cobblestone pattern

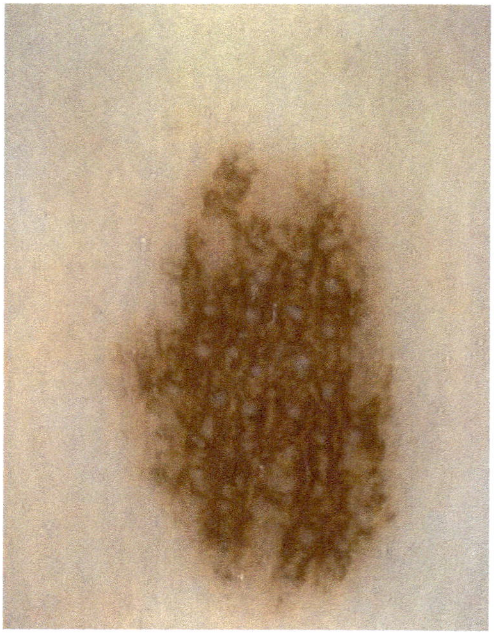

Compound nevus (dermoscopy)
Courtesy of the American Academy of Dermatology

e. Intradermal Nevus

Intradermal nevus

A. Skin-colored or light brown papule with nests of nevus cells in the upper dermis
B. Lesions may be dome shaped, sessile, pedunculated, or polypoid

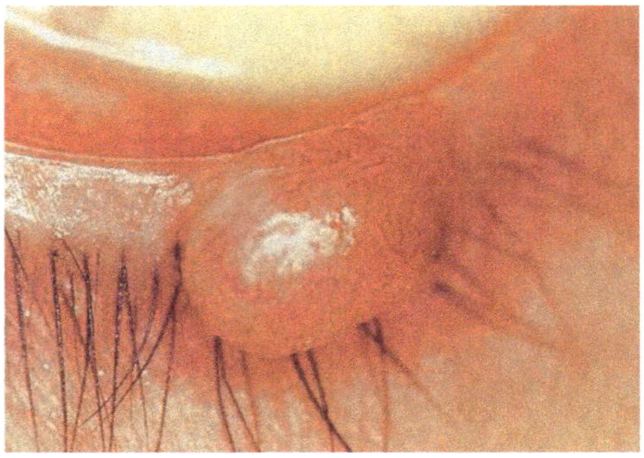

Intradermal nevus
Photograph courtesy of SpringerImages Database, Springer Publishing Company

Intradermal nevus

A. Skin-colored or light brown papule

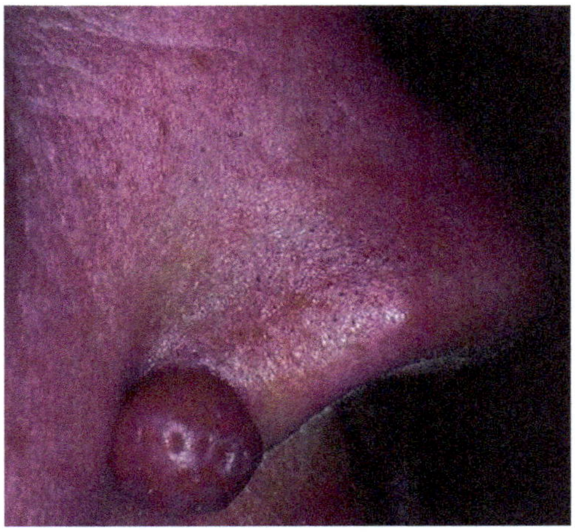

Intradermal nevus
Photograph courtesy of SpringerImages Database, Springer Publishing Company

f. Nevus Spilus

Nevus spilus

A. Tan patch (1–4 cm) with superimposed speckles
B. Dark speckles can be a variety of different pigmented lesions (lentigos, junctional or compound nevi, spitz nevi, blue nevi, and occasionally atypical nevi and congenital nevi)

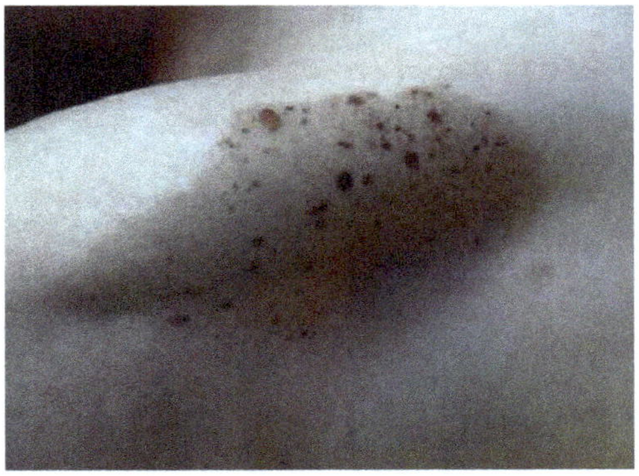

Nevus spilus
Photograph courtesy of SpringerImages Database, Springer Publishing Company

g. Spitz Nevus

Spitz nevus

A. Reddish pink or pigmented dome-shaped well-circumscribed papule or nodule (average size of 8 mm) usually in children or young adults
B. Most commonly occurs on the head and neck
C. Histologic features can be confused with melanoma

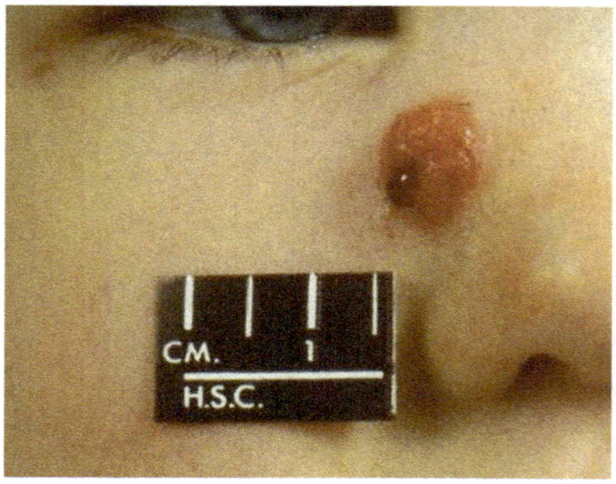

Spitz nevus
Photograph courtesy of SpringerImages Database, Springer Publishing Company

i. Spitz Nevus (Dermoscopy)

Spitz nevus (dermoscopy)

A. Dotted vessels and typical negative pigment network (reticular depigmentation) at the periphery

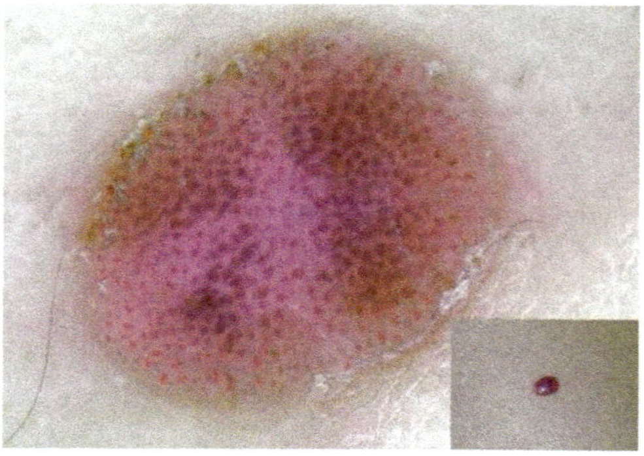

Spitz nevus (dermoscopy)
Photograph courtesy of SpringerImages Database, Springer Publishing Company

h. Blue Nevus

i. Common Blue Nevus

Common blue nevus

A. Well-circumscribed, solitary, dome-shaped blue, blue gray, or blue black papule or nodule, usually less than 1 cm
B. 50 % dorsal hands and feet
C. Onset childhood or adolescents

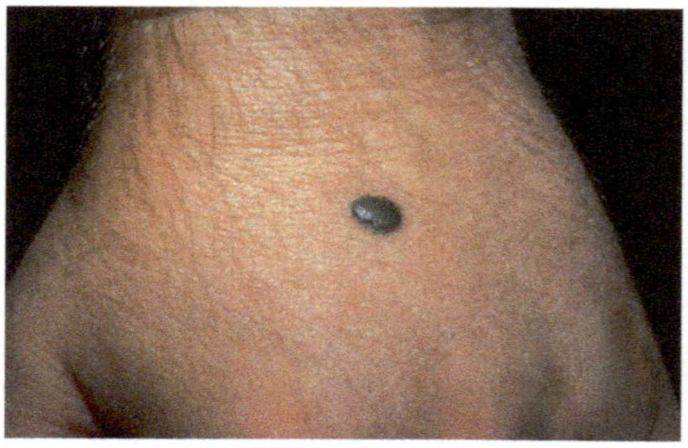

Common blue nevus
Photograph courtesy of the American Academy of Dermatology

ii. Cellular Blue Nevus

Cellular blue nevus
A. Blue to blue gray or black nodules or plaques, usually greater than 1 cm
B. Buttocks, sacrococcygeal area, scalp
C. Middle-aged women

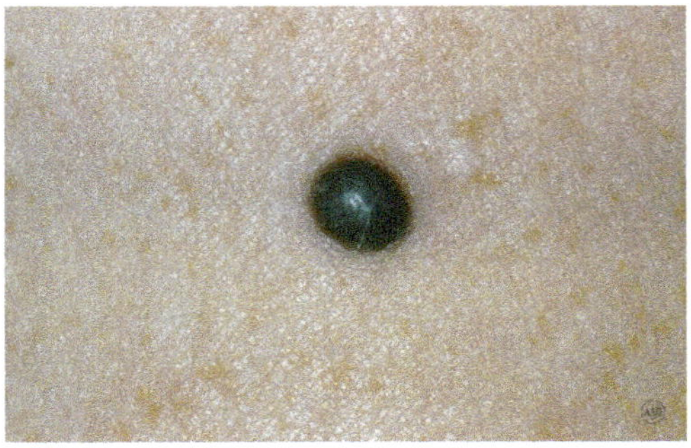

Cellular blue nevus
Photographs courtesy of the American Academy of Dermatology

iii. Blue Nevus (Dermoscopy)

Blue nevus (dermoscopy)
A. Homogenous pattern: homogenous blue gray to blue black pigmentation

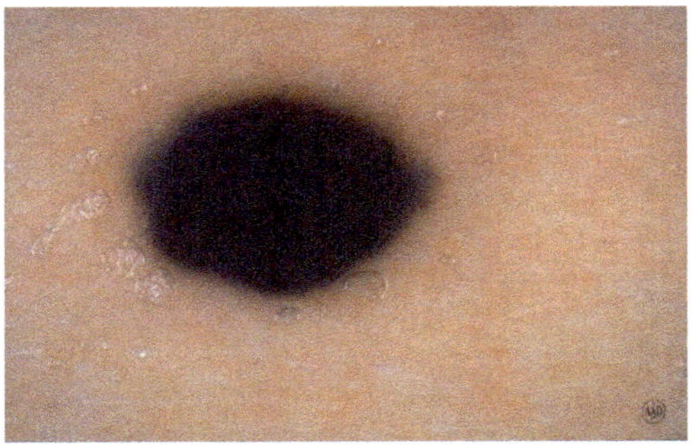

Blue nevus (dermoscopy)
Courtesy of the American Academy of Dermatology

i. Nevus of Ito (Nevus Fuscoceruleus Acromiodeltoides)

Nevus of Ito (nevus fuscoceruleus acromiodeltoides)
A. Dermal hypermelanosis (increased melanocytes)
B. Usually present at birth but may develop in later life
C. More common in Asians and other dark-skin races
D. Unilateral, flat, blue black, or slate gray pigmentation on the supraclavicular, scapular, or deltoid regions (distributed along the lateral supraclavicular and lateral brachial nerves)

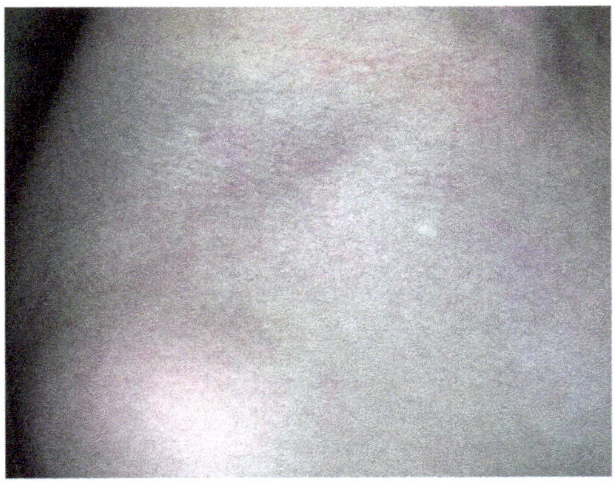

Nevus of ito (nevus fuscoceruleus acromiodeltoides)
Photograph courtesy of SpringerImages Database, Springer Publishing Company

Nevus of Ito (nevus fuscoceruleus acromiodeltoides)

A. Speckled pigmentation on the neck which is supplied by the lateral supraclavicular nerve

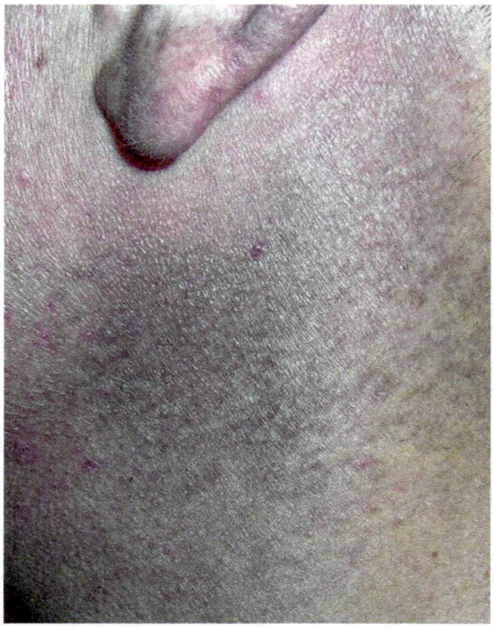

Nevus of ito (nevus fuscoceruleus acromiodeltoides) Photograph courtesy of SpringerImages Database, Springer Publishing Company

j. Nevus of Ota (Nevus Fuscoceruleus Ophthalmomaxillaris)

Nevus of Ota (nevus fuscoceruleus ophthalmomaxillaris)

A. Dermal hypermelanosis (increased melanocytes)
B. Blue brown, gray to black unilateral facial patch (rarely bilateral) composed of a confluence of individual macules one to several millimeters in diameter (figure a)
C. Favors the first two branches of cranial nerve 5 on the face (VI and V2)
D. Ipsilateral sclera involved (figure b)
E. More common in Asians and blacks, more common than Nevus of Ito
F. Most present at birth, sometimes appears around puberty, may extend with time and persists for life

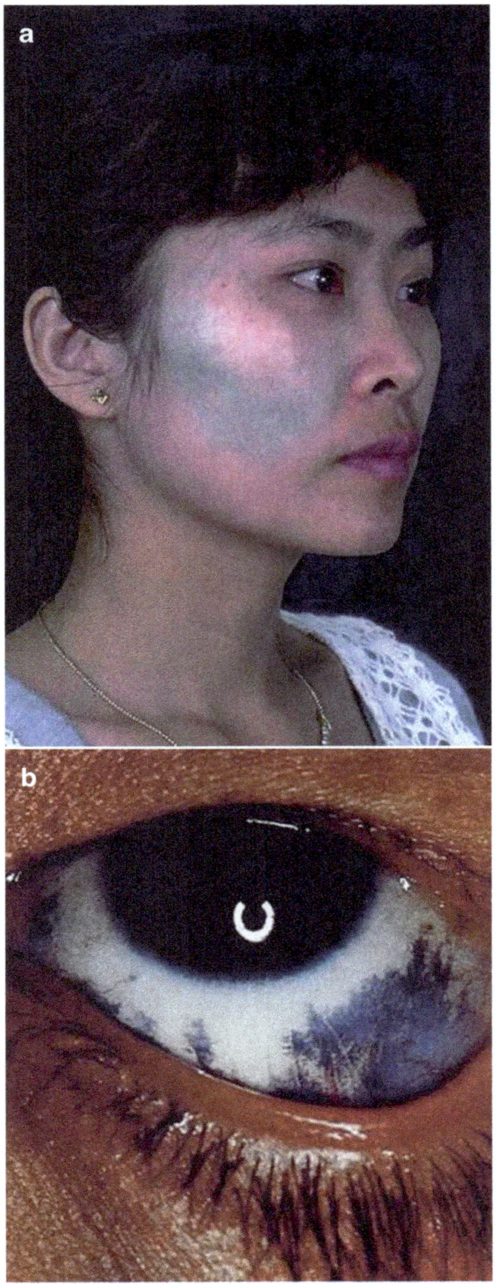

Nevus of ota (nevus fuscoceruleus ophthalmomaxillaris) Photograph courtesy of SpringerImages Database, Springer Publishing Company

k. Nevus Comedonicus

Nevus comedonicus

A. Groups of dilated follicular openings with dark keratin plugs resembling comedones
B. May express keratinaceous material from plugs

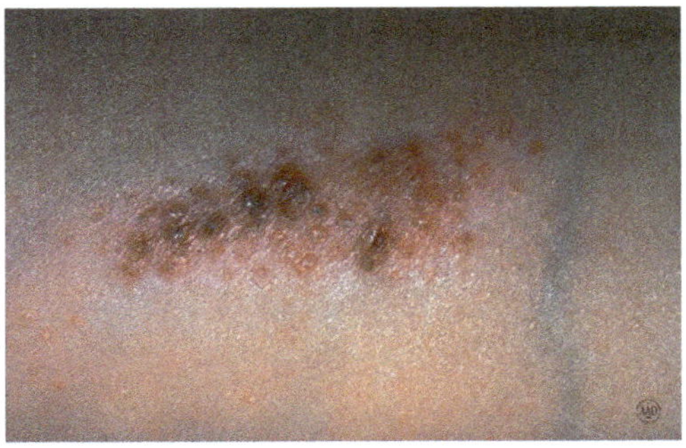

Nevus comedonicus
Courtesy of the American Academy of Dermatology

74 Mucocele

Mucocele

A. Caused by rupture or blockage of a minor salivary gland duct with resultant spillage of mucus into submucosal tissue
B. Sudden onset of a painless, soft, dome-shaped, bluish translucent papule or nodule, usually solitary, few mm to over 1 cm
C. Superficial lesions appear vesicular, deep lesions have a bluish tinge, very deep lesions have no color
D. Most common on the lower labial mucosa or floor of the mouth but may also occur wherever there are minor salivary glands (ventral tongue, buccal mucosa, posterior hard palate)
E. Typically undergo multiple cycles of swelling, rupturing, and refilling (chronic and recurrent)

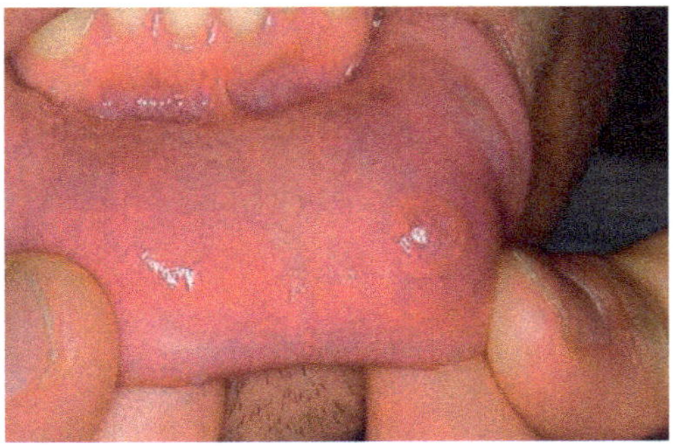

Mucocele
Photograph courtesy of SpringerImages Database, Springer Publishing Company

Mucocele

A. Mucocele of the anterior ventral tongue. The lesion appears white due to ulceration from chronic trauma

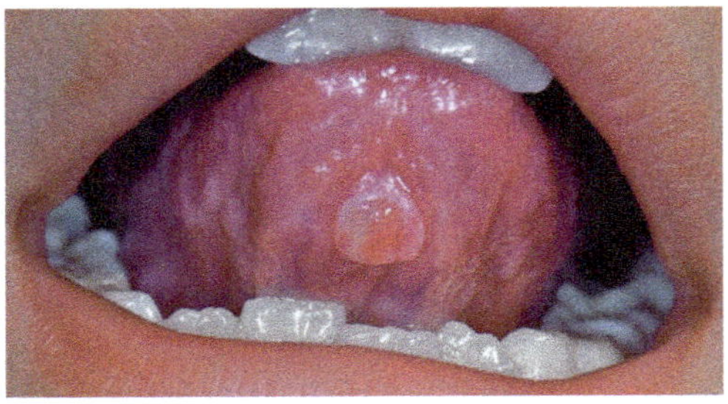

Mucocele
Photograph courtesy of SpringerImages Database, Springer Publishing Company

H.M. Gloster, Jr. et al., *Absolute Dermatology Review: Mastering Clinical Conditions on the Dermatology Recertification Exam*,
DOI 10.1007/978-3-319-03218-4_74, © Springer International Publishing Switzerland 2016

75 Pyogenic Granuloma

Pyogenic granuloma

A. Rapidly growing, solitary, friable, dome-shaped red papule or nodule of granulation tissue that frequently ulcerates and bleeds
B. A collarette of hyperplastic epithelium is usually present
C. Most common sites are the gingiva, lip, and finger
D. May develop after minor trauma
E. Most common in children and young adults
F. Often occurs on the gingiva of pregnant women

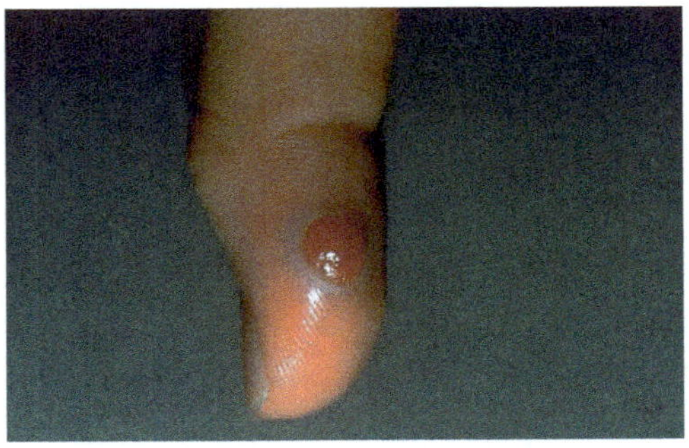

Pyogenic granuloma
Courtesy of the American Academy of Dermatology

Pyogenic granuloma

A. Rapidly growing, solitary, friable, dome-shaped red papule of granulation tissue on the gingiva

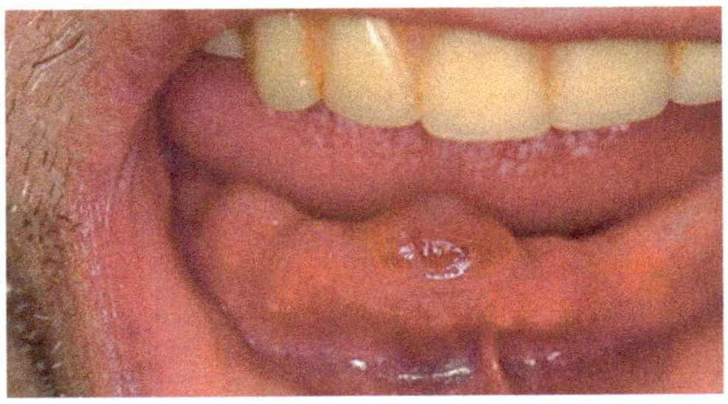

Pygognenic granuloma
Photograph courtesy of SpringerImages Database, Springer Publishing Company

H.M. Gloster, Jr. et al., *Absolute Dermatology Review: Mastering Clinical Conditions on the Dermatology Recertification Exam*, DOI 10.1007/978-3-319-03218-4_75, © Springer International Publishing Switzerland 2016

76 Seborrheic Keratosis

Seborrheic keratoses

A. Tan, brown, or black well-demarcated macules, papules, or plaques
B. May be solitary but usually are multiple, 1–5 cm in diameter
C. Common, benign, begin fourth decade
D. May occur anywhere except palms, soles, lips, mucous membranes
E. Distinguishing features from other pigmented lesions:
    1. Keratotic plugging with follicular prominence (horn pseudocysts)
    2. Velvety papillomatous surface
    3. Verrucous stuck on appearance

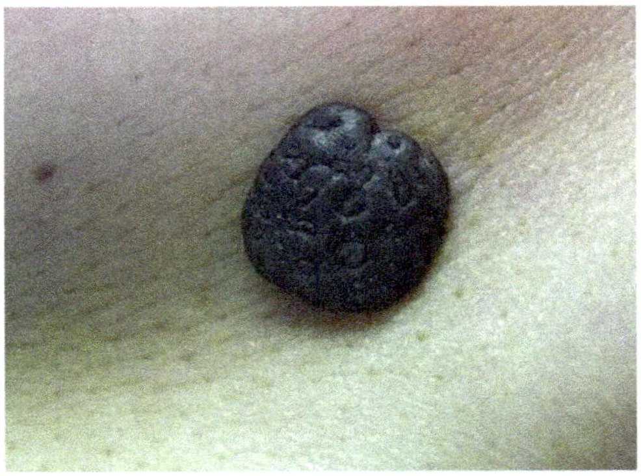

Seborrheic keratosis
Photograph courtesy of SpringerImages Database, Springer Publishing Company

Seborrheic keratoses

A. Brown plaques with a cobblestone surface and "stuck-on" appearance

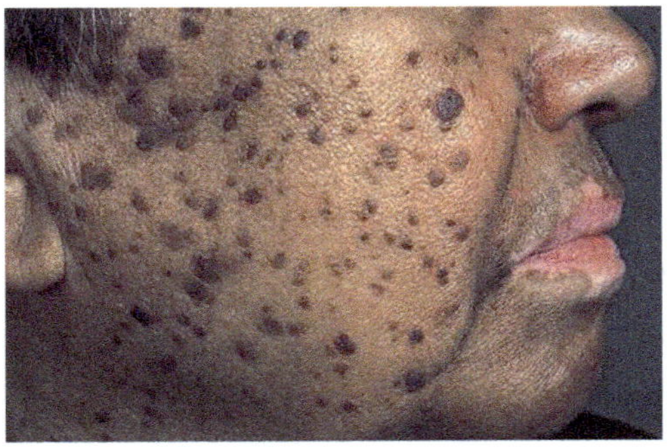

Seborrheic keratosis
Photograph courtesy of SpringerImages Database, Springer Publishing Company

H.M. Gloster, Jr. et al., *Absolute Dermatology Review: Mastering Clinical Conditions on the Dermatology Recertification Exam*, DOI 10.1007/978-3-319-03218-4_76, © Springer International Publishing Switzerland 2016

Seborrheic keratoses

A. Multiple brown plaques with papillomatous surfaces and a verrucous stuck-on appearance

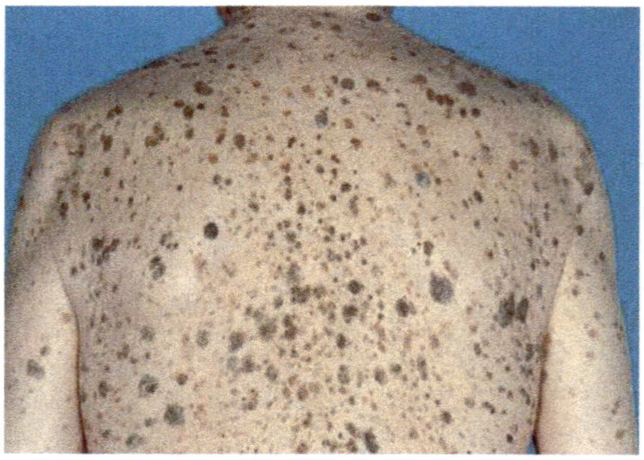

Seborrheic keratosis
Photograph courtesy of SpringerImages Database, Springer Publishing Company

a. Seborrheic Keratosis (Dermoscopy)

Seborrheic keratosis (dermoscopy)

A. Comedo-like openings (white arrows in figure b) – black targetoid globules
B. Milia-like cysts (black arrow in figure b)– white shining globules
C. Appears stuck on with sharp circumscription

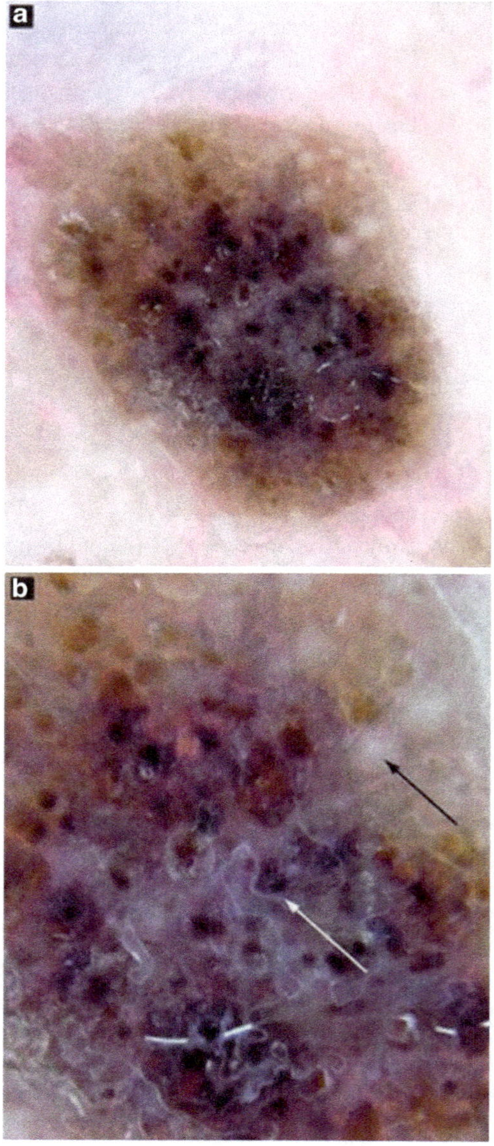

Seborrheic keratosis (dermoscopy)
Photograph courtesy of SpringerImages Database, Springer Publishing Company

77 Skin Tags

Skin tag (achrocordon)

A. Common lesions, favor the neck, axilla, and groin
B. Soft skin-colored to slightly hyperpigmented pedunculated papules
C. Single or multiple, 1–2 mm in diameter, may itch or become painful secondary to irritation

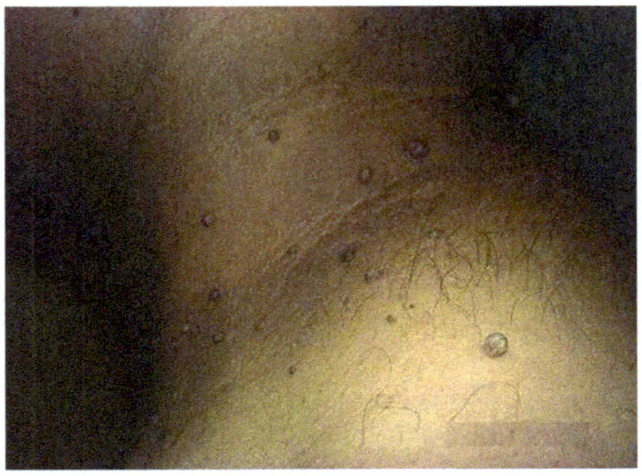

Skin tags
Photograph courtesy of SpringerImages Database, Springer Publishing Company

H.M. Gloster, Jr. et al., *Absolute Dermatology Review: Mastering Clinical Conditions on the Dermatology Recertification Exam*, DOI 10.1007/978-3-319-03218-4_77, © Springer International Publishing Switzerland 2016

78 Supernumerary Nipples

Supernumerary nipples

A. Focal remnants of embryologic mammary tissue

B. Small soft pink or brown papule with or without a surrounding areola located along the milk lines (mammary ridges) that extend from anterior axillary fold to the upper medial thigh bilaterally (including the vulva)

C. Most common on the inframammary chest, usually single and unilateral but may be multiple

D. Usually sporadic (1–6 % in the general population) but 10 % familial

E. May develop any disorders that occur in normally positioned breasts (e.g., variation with hormonal cycle, fibrocystic changes, fibroadenomas, cancer)

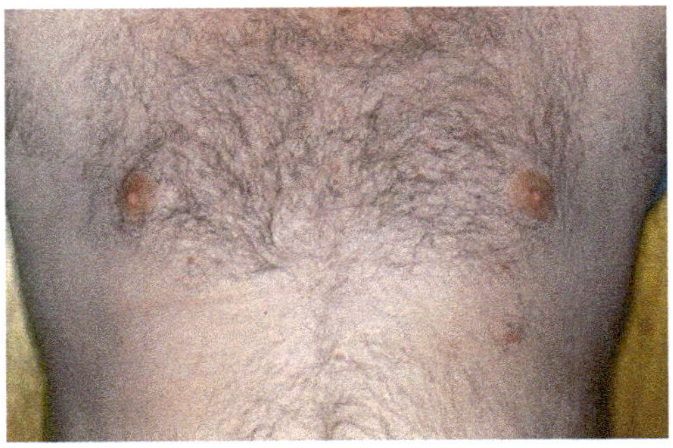

Supernumerary nipples
Photograph courtesy of SpringerImages Database, Springer Publishing Company

H.M. Gloster, Jr. et al., *Absolute Dermatology Review: Mastering Clinical Conditions on the Dermatology Recertification Exam*, DOI 10.1007/978-3-319-03218-4_78, © Springer International Publishing Switzerland 2016

Supernumerary nipple

A. Brown papule without a surrounding areola located along the "milk line" (mammary ridges) on the supramammary chest

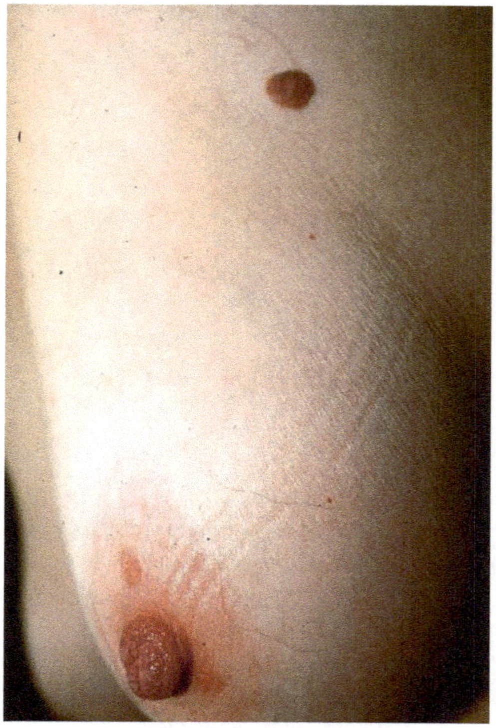

Supernumerary nipples
Photograph courtesy of SpringerImages Database, Springer Publishing Company

79 Confluent and Reticulated Papillomatosis

Confluent and reticulated papillomatosis (CARP)

A. Onset puberty, more common in women over men and blacks over whites
B. Multiple, brown, verrucous, papillomatous papules confluent centrally and reticulated peripherally
C. Most common on the central chest but also may occur on the upper abdomen and central back

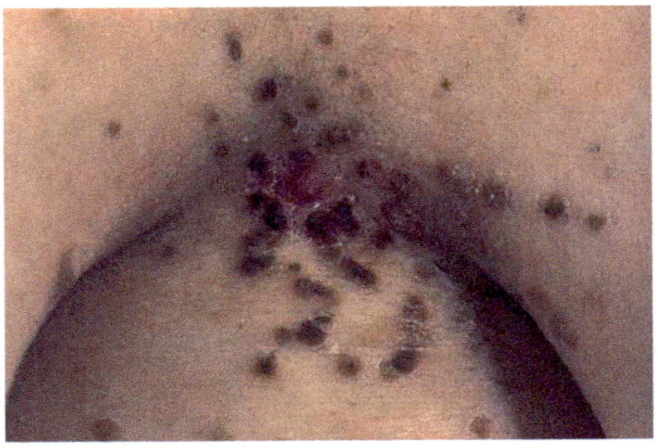

Confluent and reticulated papillomatosis
Photograph courtesy of SpringerImages Database, Springer Publishing Company

H.M. Gloster, Jr. et al., *Absolute Dermatology Review: Mastering Clinical Conditions on the Dermatology Recertification Exam*, DOI 10.1007/978-3-319-03218-4_79,

80 Epidermal Nevus

Epidermal nevus

A. Onset usually early childhood (80 % within first year), expands until the start of grade school
B. Hyperpigmented to flesh-colored, papillomatous, verrucous papules and plaques in a linear or swirled array
C. Most commonly on neck, trunk, and extremities

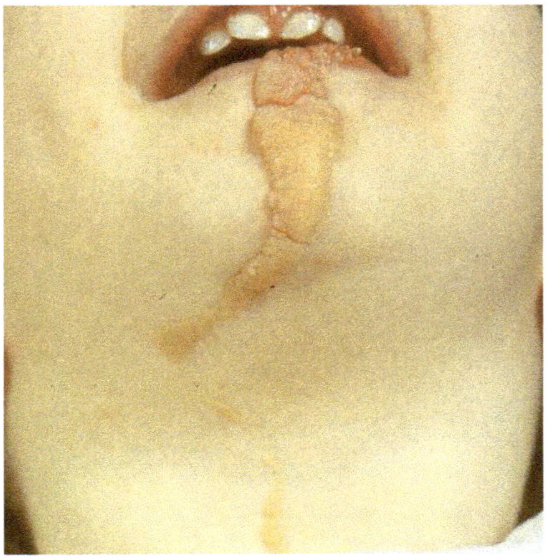

Epidermal nevus
Photograph courtesy of SpringerImages Database, Springer Publishing Company

H.M. Gloster, Jr. et al., *Absolute Dermatology Review: Mastering Clinical Conditions on the Dermatology Recertification Exam*, DOI 10.1007/978-3-319-03218-4_80, © Springer International Publishing Switzerland 2016

81 Inflammatory Linear Epidermal Nevus

Inflammatory linear verrucous epidermal nevus (ILVEN)

A. Linear psoriasiform scaly pruritic red papules coalesce to form a unilateral linear plaque usually on one extremity
B. Most appear before the age of five, more common in girls (4:1 male-to-female ratio)
C. Persists for years

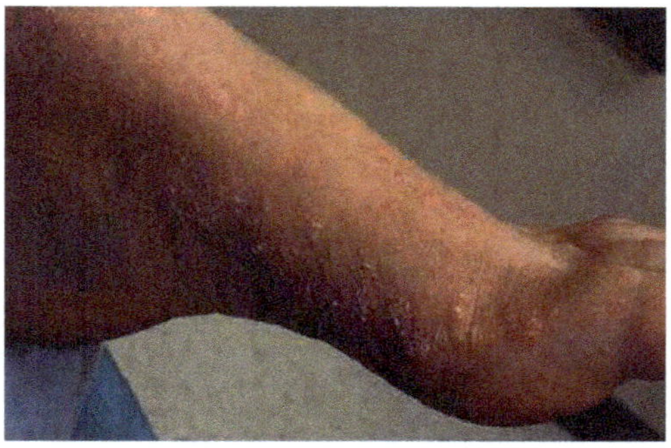

Inflammatory linear epidermal nevus
Photograph courtesy of SpringerImages Database, Springer Publishing Company

Inflammatory linear verrucous epidermal nevus (ILVEN)

A. Linear psoriasiform scaly pruritic red papules coalesce to form a unilateral linear plaque usually on one extremity

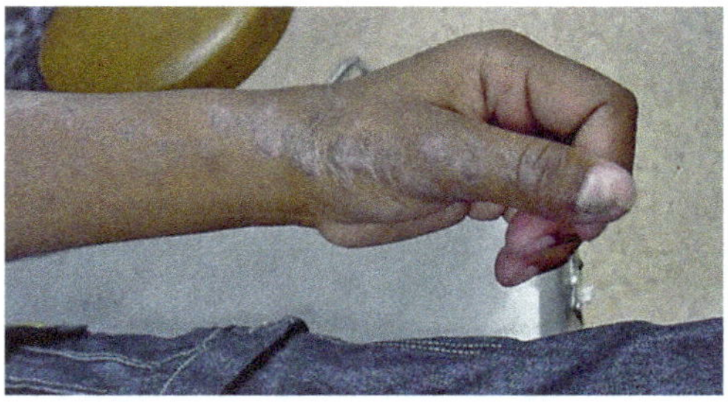

Inflammatory linear epidermal nevus
Photograph courtesy of SpringerImages Database, Springer Publishing Company

H.M. Gloster, Jr. et al., *Absolute Dermatology Review: Mastering Clinical Conditions on the Dermatology Recertification Exam*,
DOI 10.1007/978-3-319-03218-4_81, © Springer International Publishing Switzerland 2016

Chapter XIII

Malignant and Premalignant Neoplasms

82 Actinic Keratosis

Actinic keratosis:

A. Discrete, erythematous, rough scaly keratotic papules and plaques
B. Most often occur in the elderly on sun-damaged skin

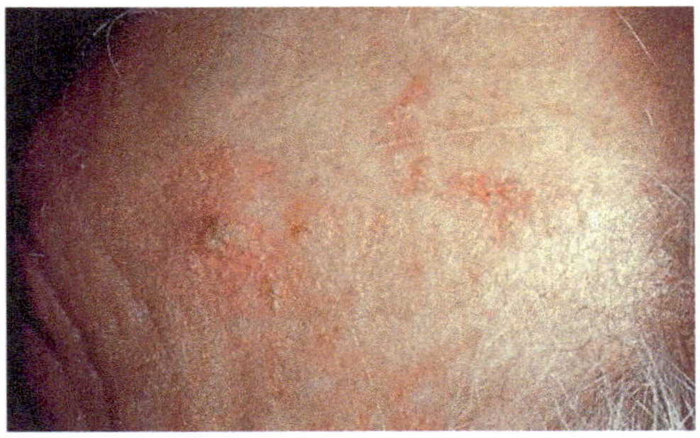

Actinic keratosis
Photograph courtesy of SpringerImages Database, Springer Publishing Company

a. Hypertrophic Actinic Keratosis

Hypertrophic Actinic Keratosis

A. Hyperkeratotic papule most often occur in the elderly on sun-damaged skin

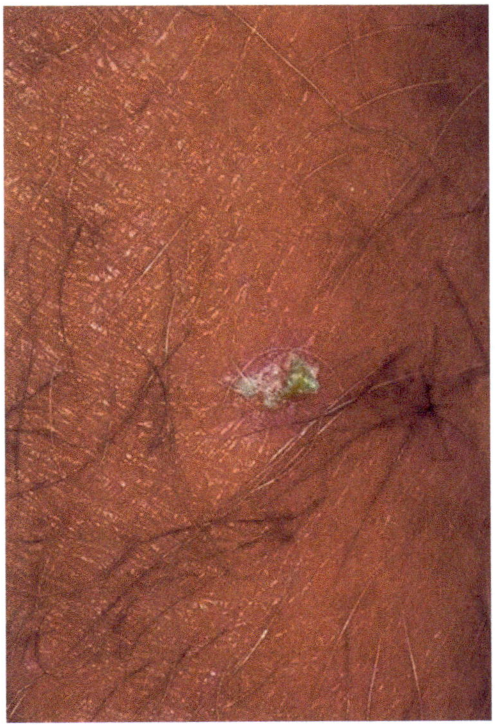

Hypertrophic actinic keratosis
Photograph courtesy of SpringerImages Database, Springer Publishing Company

H.M. Gloster, Jr. et al., *Absolute Dermatology Review: Mastering Clinical Conditions on the Dermatology Recertification Exam*,
DOI 10.1007/978-3-319-03218-4_82, © Springer International Publishing Switzerland 2016

b. Pigmented Actinic Keratosis

Pigmented Actinic Keratosis

A. Hyperpigmented, rough, keratotic plaques that most often occur in the elderly on sun-damaged skin

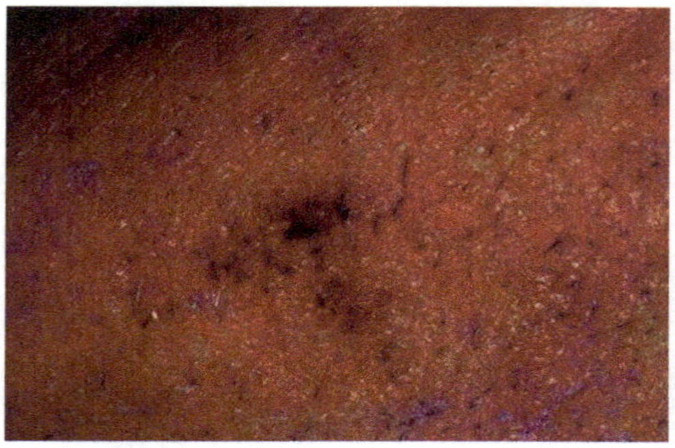

Pigmented actinic keratosis
Photograph courtesy of SpringerImages Database, Springer Publishing Company

83 Actinic Cheilitis

Actinic cheilitis

A. Erythematous scaly red papules and plaques on the lower vermillion lip
B. Erythema and scale may be diffuse with leukoplakia, crusting, atrophic changes, and loss of vermillion border definition

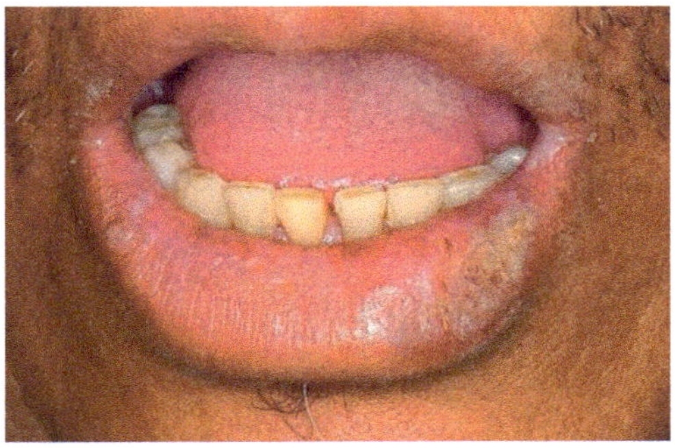

Actinic cheilitis
Photograph courtesy of SpringerImages Database, Springer Publishing Company

H.M. Gloster, Jr. et al., *Absolute Dermatology Review: Mastering Clinical Conditions on the Dermatology Recertification Exam*, DOI 10.1007/978-3-319-03218-4_83, © Springer International Publishing Switzerland 2016

84 Angiosarcoma

Angiosarcoma

A. Rare malignant tumor of vascular origin most commonly seen on the scalp and face of the elderly (2:1 male predominance)
B. Typically begins as a bruise-like patch with a peripheral red ring that spreads centrifugally
C. Eventually characterized by the development of violaceous elevated satellite nodules and plaques that bleed and ulcerate
D. May be associated with facial swelling and edema
E. Head tilt: classic maneuver to indicate angiosarcoma in which the lesion becomes very indurated and violaceous after putting head in a dependent position for 2 minutes

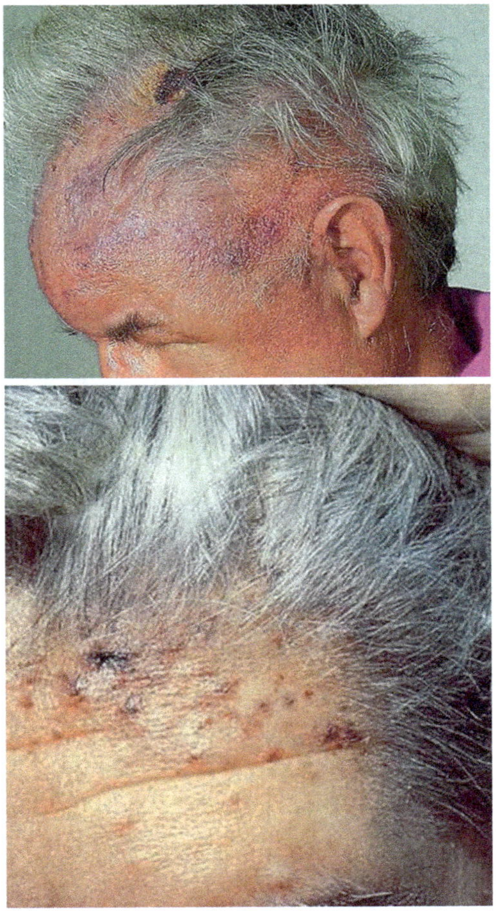

Angiosarcoma
Photograph courtesy of SpringerImages Database, Springer Publishing Company

H.M. Gloster, Jr. et al., *Absolute Dermatology Review: Mastering Clinical Conditions on the Dermatology Recertification Exam*, DOI 10.1007/978-3-319-03218-4_84, © Springer International Publishing Switzerland 2016

a. Angiosarcoma-Stewart Treves Syndrome

Angioscarcoma – Stewart Treves Syndrome

A. Angiosarcoma may also arise in areas of chronic lymphedema
B. Most cases (over 90 %) associated with lymphedema arise after mastectomy and lymph node dissection (Stewart-Treves syndrome), characterized by brawny nonpitting edema with violaceous nodules on the inner arm 4–27 years after onset of lymphedema

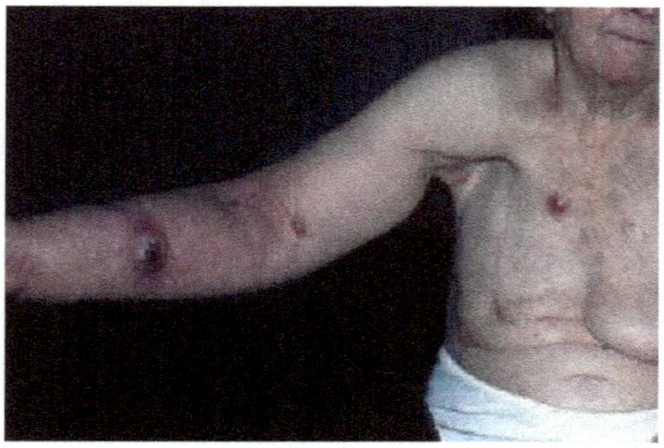

Angiosarcoma Stewart-Treves syndrome
Photograph courtesy of SpringerImages Database, Springer Publishing Company

Angioscarcoma – Stewart Treves Syndrome

A. Angiosarcoma may also appear on sites previously irradiated for breast cancer (average of 6 years after radiation therapy) as infiltrative plaques or nodules on the abdominal or chest wall

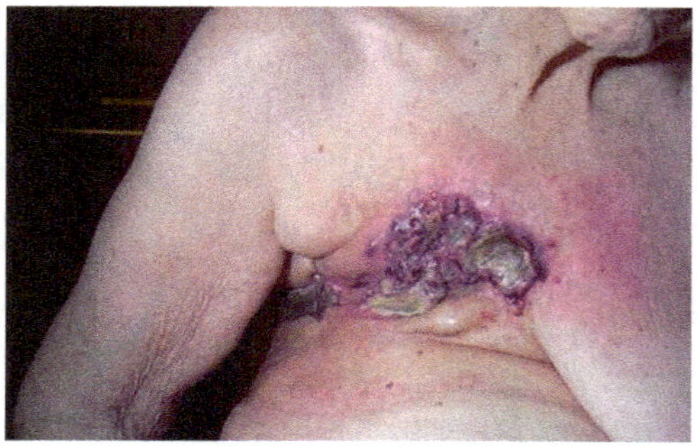

Angiosarcoma Stewart-Treves syndrome
Photograph courtesy of SpringerImages Database, Springer Publishing Company

85 Cutaneous Metastases

Cutaneous metastases

A. Most common tumors to metastastize to the skin in men are melanoma, lung, and colon cancer. In women, breast and melanoma are most prevalent
B. Usually presents as a firm, painless red nodule (figure: cutaneous metastasis of colorectal cancer on the scrotum), but multiple lesions may occur
C. May also present as patches, papules, infiltrated or indurated plaques, ulcers, and tumor nodules
D. Occur in 5 % of patients with internal cancers
E. Often in the vicinity of the primary tumor

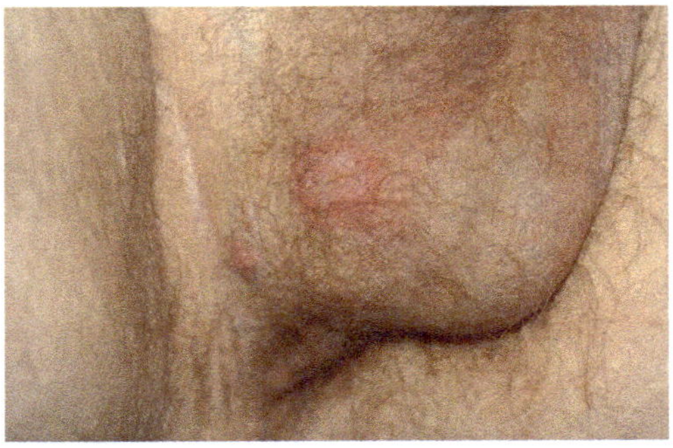

Cutaneous metastases
Photograph courtesy of SpringerImages Database, Springer Publishing Company

Cutaneous metastases

A. Multiple cutaneous metastatic nodules on the back from esophageal adenocarcinoma

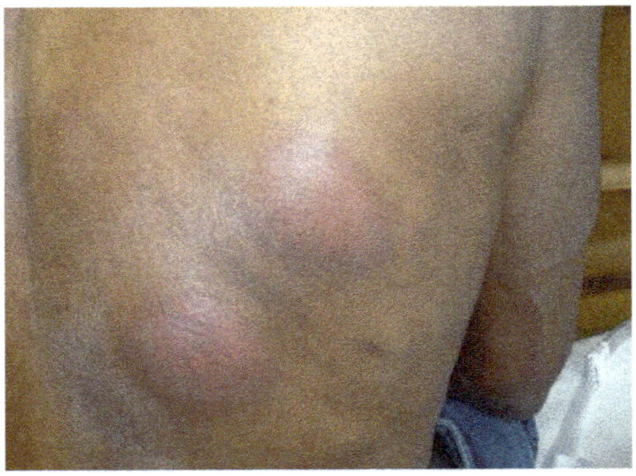

Cutaneous metastases
Photograph courtesy of SpringerImages Database, Springer Publishing Company

H.M. Gloster, Jr. et al., *Absolute Dermatology Review: Mastering Clinical Conditions on the Dermatology Recertification Exam*,
DOI 10.1007/978-3-319-03218-4_85,

a. Cutaneous Metastases to the Scalp

Cutaneous metastasis to the scalp

A. A vascular nodule is the most common presentation
B. Most common primary tumors are squamous cell carcinoma of the oral cavity, lung or renal cancer (men), and breast cancer (women)

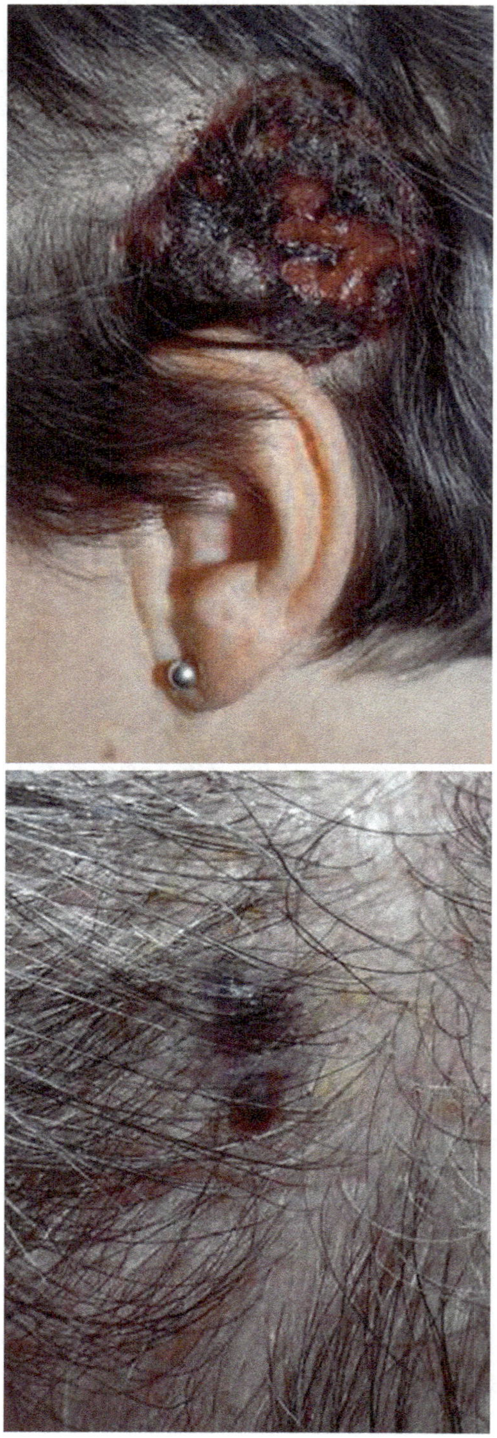

Cutaneous metastases to the scalp from cancer of the colon
Photograph courtesy of SpringerImages Database, Springer Publishing Company

b. Cutaneous Metastases to the Abdomen

i. Sister Mary Joseph Nodule

Cutaneous metastases to the abdomen

A. May develop from intra-abdominal tumors (e.g., colon cancer) and cancers arising in the pelvis
B. Sister Mary Joseph nodule: periumbilical plaque with scale and crust that represents a cutaneous metastasis of gastrointestinal malignancies (gastric, colon, ovarian, pancreatic)

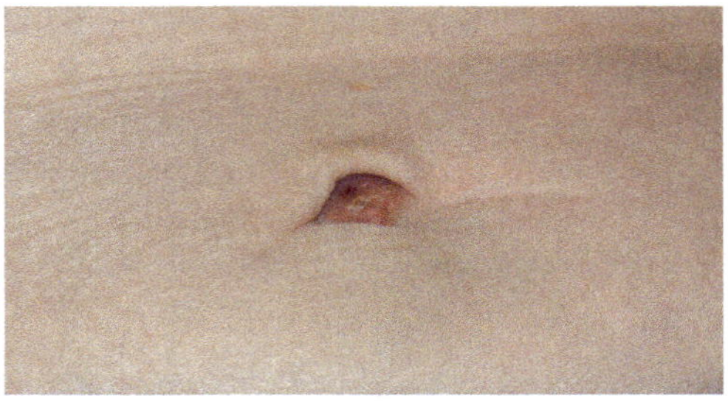

Sister Mary Joseph nodule
Courtesy of Mayo Clinic Department of Dermatology (Rochester, Mn)

c. Cutaneous Metastases of Breast Cancer

i. Cancer en Cuirasse

Cutaneous metastases of breast cancer

A. Cancer en cuirasse: indurated, fibrotic, morphea-like plaques with a peau d'orange appearance

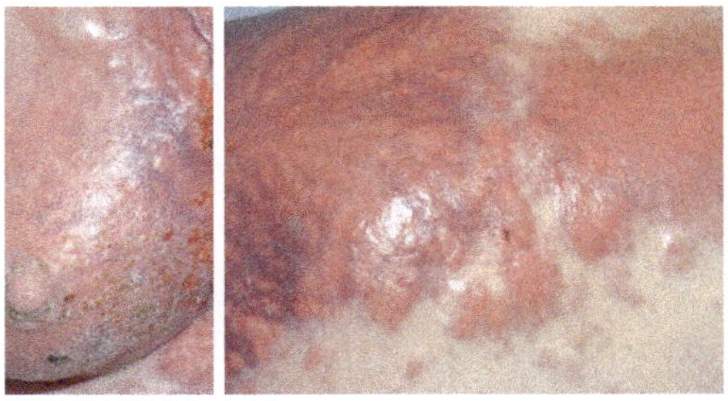

Cutaneous metastases of breast cancer (cancer en Cuirasse)
Photograph courtesy of SpringerImages Database, Springer Publishing Company

ii. Paget's Disease

Cutaneous metastases of breast cancer

A. Paget's disease: unilateral, eczematous, psoriasiform scaly plaque around the areola and nipple due to extension of an underlying ductal adenocarcinoma of the breast

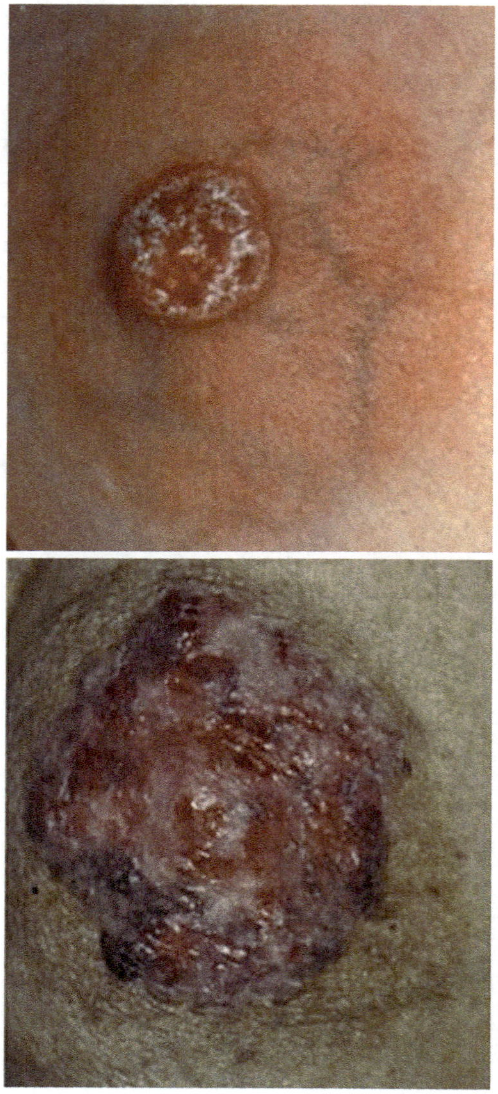

Cutaneous metastases of breast cancer (Paget's disease)
Photograph courtesy of SpringerImages Database, Springer Publishing Company

iii. Inflammatory Carcinoma (Carcinoma Erysipeloides)

Cutaneous metastases of breast cancer

A. Inflammatory carcinoma (carcinoma erysipeloides): red, edematous patch with spreading border, skin dimpling and induration ressembling erysipelas or cellulitis (tumor cells in dilated lymphatics)

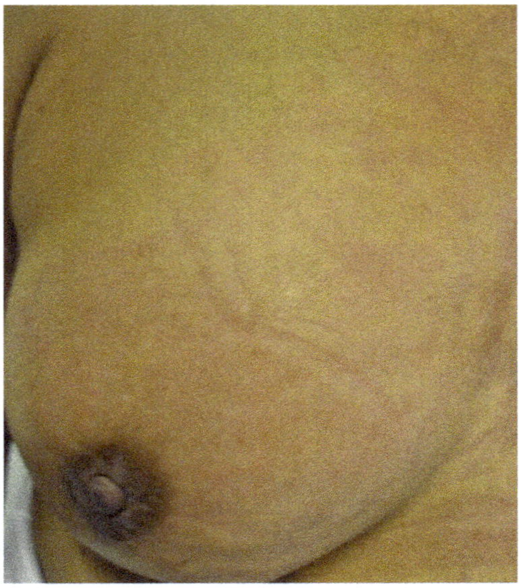

Cutaneous metastases of breast cancer (inflammatory carcinoma – carcinoma erysipeloides)
Photograph courtesy of SpringerImages Database, Springer Publishing Company

Cutaneous metastases of breast cancer

A. Inflammatory carcinoma (carcinoma erysipeloides): red, edematous, warm, tender patch with spreading border and skin dimpling (peau d'orange) and induration
B. Affected breast may be enlarged

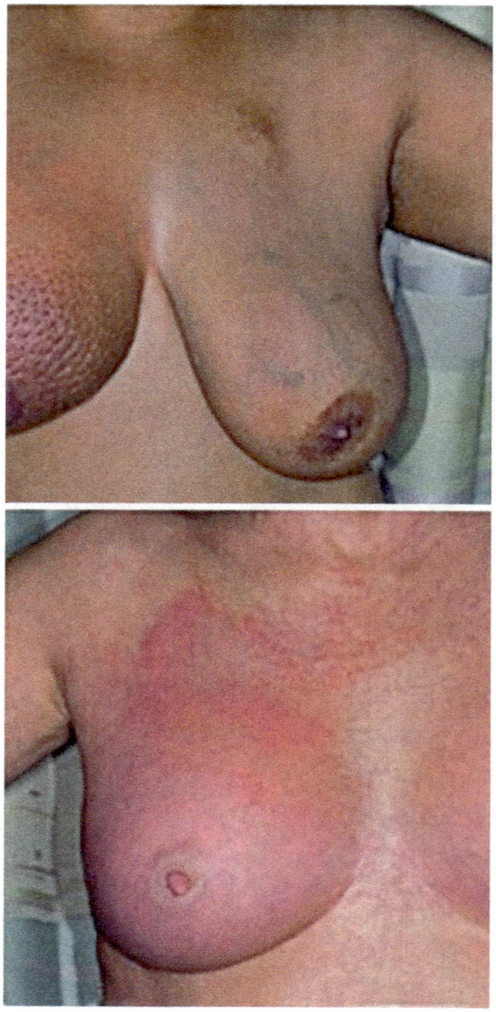

Cutaneous metastases of breast cancer (inflammatory carcinoma – carcinoma erysipeloides)
Photograph courtesy of SpringerImages Database, Springer Publishing Company

Dermatofibrosarcoma Protuberans 86

Dermatofibrosarcoma protuberans

A. Occurs most commonly on the trunk, followed by the proximal extremities, then head and neck
B. Slow-growing (over many years), asymptomatic skin-colored indurated plaque
C. Slowly enlarges and develops violaceous to red-brown nodules within the plaques

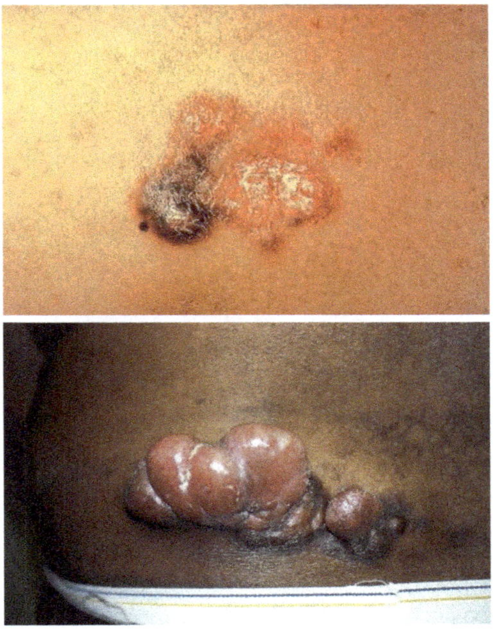

Dermatofibrosarcoma protuberans
Photographs courtesy of SpringerImages Database, Springer Publishing Company

H.M. Gloster, Jr. et al., *Absolute Dermatology Review: Mastering Clinical Conditions on the Dermatology Recertification Exam*, DOI 10.1007/978-3-319-03218-4_86, © Springer International Publishing Switzerland 2016

87 Kaposi's Sarcoma

Kaposi's sarcoma

A. Human herpesvirus-8 induced neoplasm
B. Clinically characterized by reddish-purple or violaceous patches, papules, and plaques that progress in a multifocal fashion, frequently follow the skin lines, and may ulcerate and result in edema
C. There are four types of Kaposi's sarcoma: classic, African-endemic, iatrogenic immunosuppression, and AIDS related

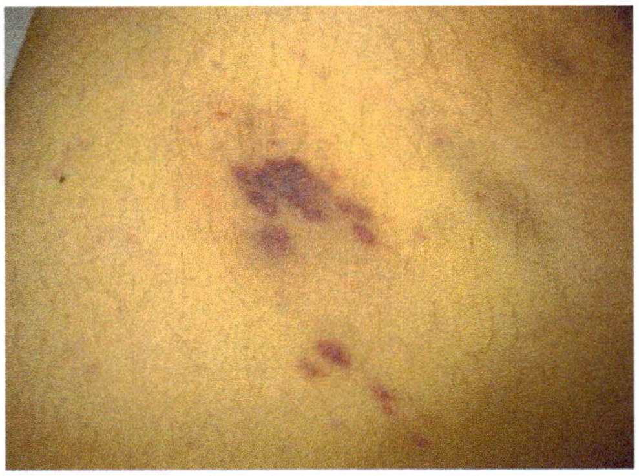

Kaposi's sarcoma
Photograph courtesy of SpringerImages Database, Springer Publishing Company

a. Classic Kaposi's Sarcoma

Classic Kaposi's sarcoma

A. Slow-growing pink, red, violaceous macules on distal lower extremities that may coalesce to large plaques or develop into nodules or polypoid tumors
B. Most common in Ashkenazi Jews or individuals of Mediterranean or Eastern European descent
C. Iatrogenic immunosuppression-type Kaposi's sarcoma has a similar clinical presentation to classic Kaposi's sarcoma but may regress when immunosuppression is removed

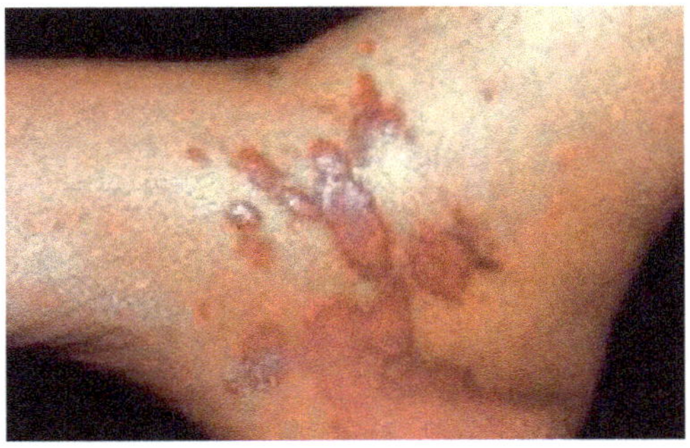

Classic Kaposi's sarcoma
Photograph courtesy of SpringerImages Database, Springer Publishing Company

H.M. Gloster, Jr. et al., *Absolute Dermatology Review: Mastering Clinical Conditions on the Dermatology Recertification Exam*, DOI 10.1007/978-3-319-03218-4_87, © Springer International Publishing Switzerland 2016

b. African Endemic Kaposi's Sarcoma

African endemic Kaposi's sarcoma

A. Mainly males, 9 % of cancers in equatorial Africa
B. Nodular, florid, infiltrative, and lymphadenopathic variants exist

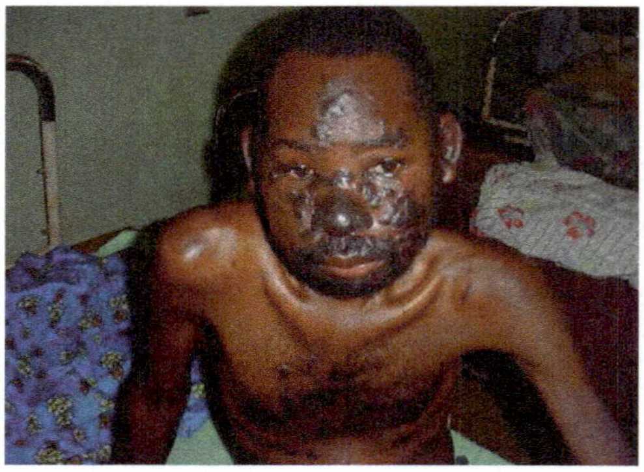

African endemic Kaposi's sarcoma
Photograph courtesy of SpringerImages Database, Springer Publishing Company

c. AIDS Related Kaposi's Sarcoma

AIDS related Kaposi's Sarcoma

A. Seen in 40 % of men who became HIV infected (CD4 < 200) by homosexual contact
B. Cutaneous lesions begin as red or purple patches that become elevated and evolve into nodules and plaques
C. Mucosa, trunk, and midface are common sites
D. Tumors may involve the viscera (gastrointestinal, lungs, nodes) or oral cavity

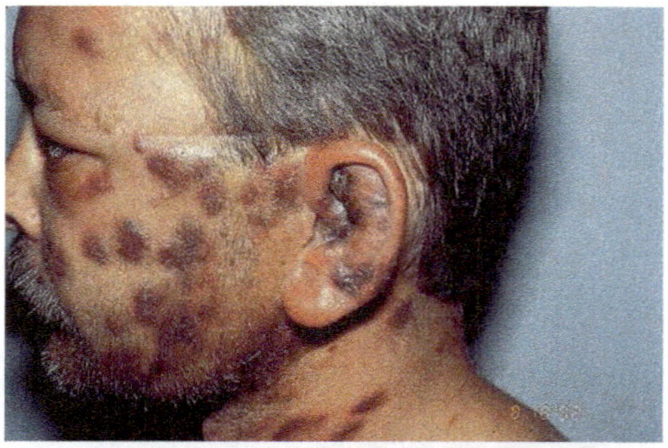

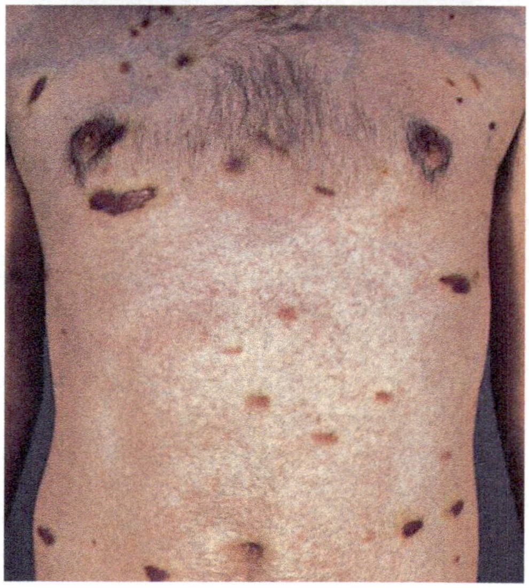

AIDS related Kaposi's sarcoma
Photograph courtesy of SpringerImages Database, Springer Publishing Company

88 Keratoacanthoma

Keratoacanthoma

A. Typically begins as a rapidly enlarging dome-shaped pink or skin-colored nodule which evolves within a few weeks into a nodule with a rolled, shouldered border and central crater filled with keratotic plug
B. May be locally destructive
C. May resolve over months to leave an atrophic scar
D. Most occur on sun-exposed skin of head, neck, or extremities of those over the age of 50
E. Solitary variant is most common

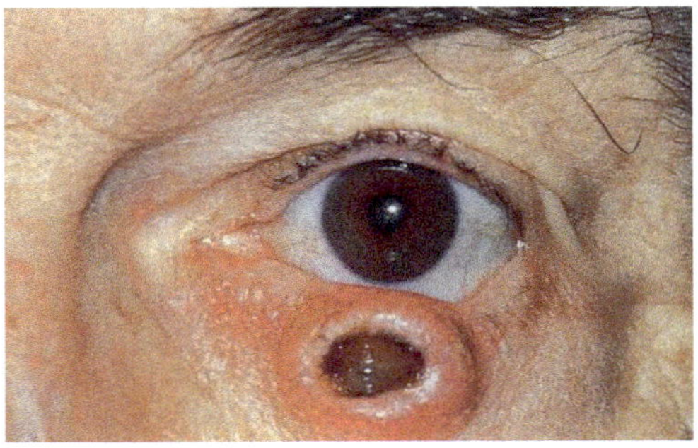

Keratoacanthoma
Photograph courtesy of SpringerImages Database, Springer Publishing Company

Keratoacanthoma

A. May be difficult to distinguish form squamous cell carcinoma of the keratoacanthoma type

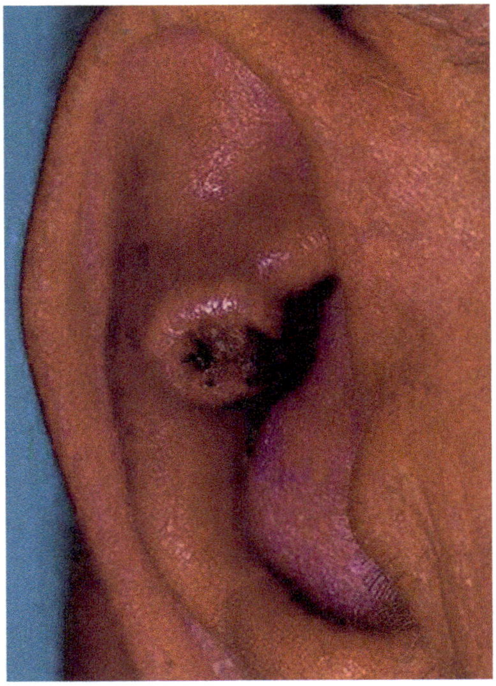

Keratoacanthoma
Photograph courtesy of SpringerImages Database, Springer Publishing Company

H.M. Gloster, Jr. et al., *Absolute Dermatology Review: Mastering Clinical Conditions on the Dermatology Recertification Exam*, DOI 10.1007/978-3-319-03218-4_88, © Springer International Publishing Switzerland 2016

Keratoacanthoma

A. Sharply circumscribed rapidly growing crateriform nodule with keratotic core

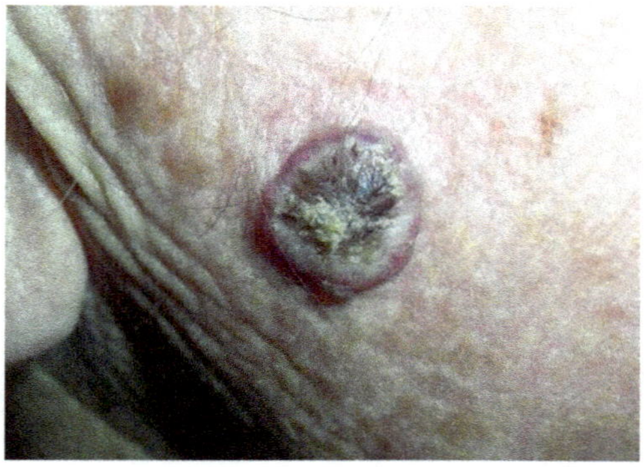

Keratoacanthoma
Photograph courtesy of SpringerImages Database, Springer Publishing Company

89 Malignant Melanoma

a. Superficial Spreading Melanoma

Superficial spreading melanoma

A. Most common type in fair skin (60–70 % of melanomas)
B. Most commonly develops between the ages of 40 and 60 years on the trunk of men and legs of women
C. May arise de novo or within a preexisting nevus
D. Asymmetric brown to black macule with irregular borders and variegated color (may have shades of light or dark brown, black, red, pink, blue, white)

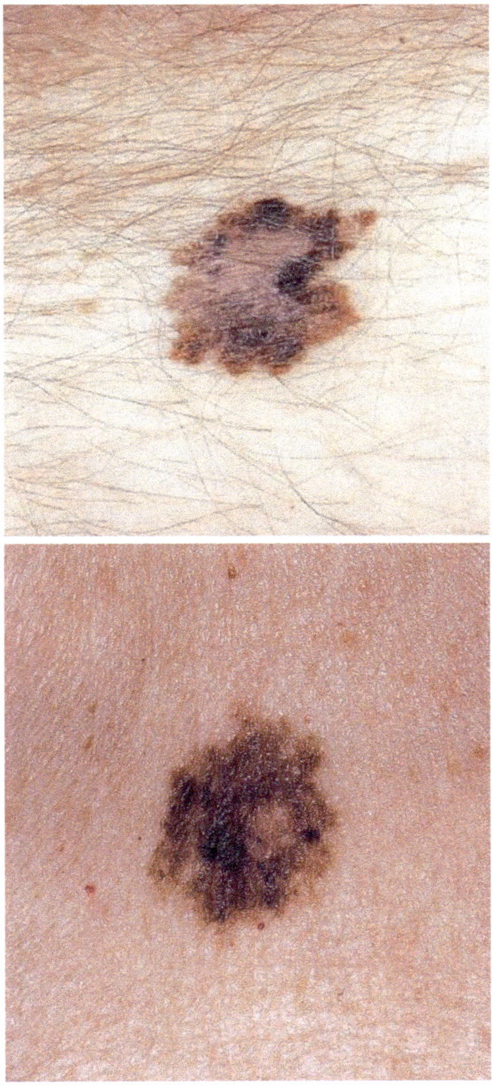

Superficial spreading melanoma
Photograph courtesy of SpringerImages Database, Springer Publishing Company

H.M. Gloster, Jr. et al., *Absolute Dermatology Review: Mastering Clinical Conditions on the Dermatology Recertification Exam*,
DOI 10.1007/978-3-319-03218-4_89, © Springer International Publishing Switzerland 2016

Superficial spreading melanoma with typical notched borders

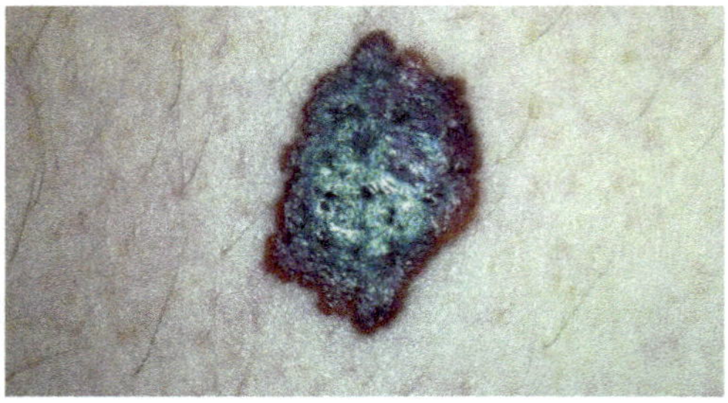

Superficial spreading melanoma
Photograph courtesy of SpringerImages Database, Springer Publishing Company

b. Nodular Melanoma

Nodular melanoma

A. Second most common type of melanoma in fair skin (10–30 %)
B. Most commonly occurs after the age of 60 on the trunk, head, and neck
C. Arises de novo
D. Blue to black nodule (sometimes red or pink), may ulcerate or bleed, may grow rapidly
E. Usually diagnosed at a thicker, more advanced stage with poor prognosis

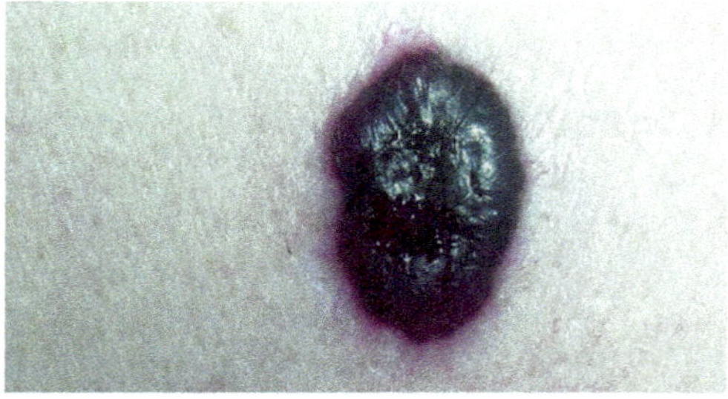

Nodular melanoma
Photograph courtesy of SpringerImages Database, Springer Publishing Company

Nodular melanoma

A. Blue to black nodule which may grow rapidly

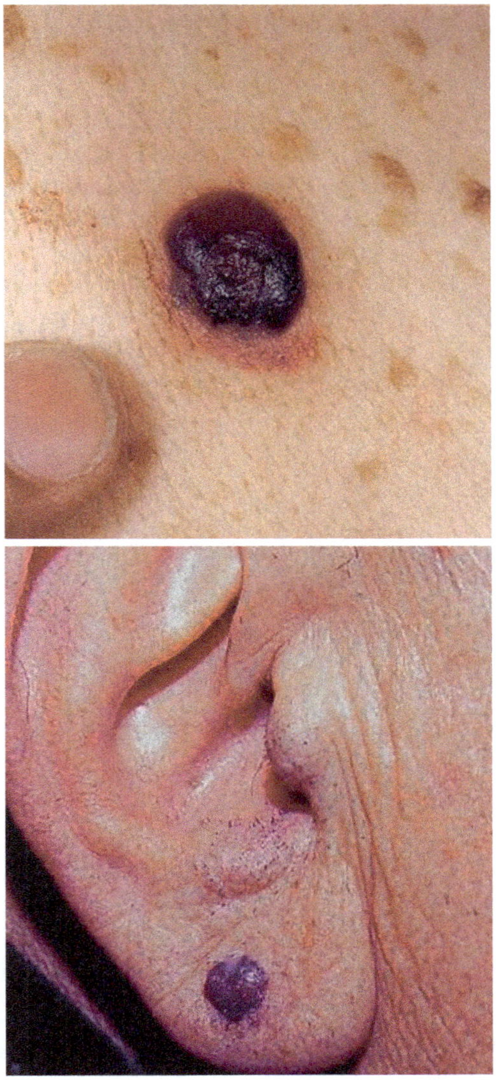

Nodular melanoma
Photograph courtesy of SpringerImages Database, Springer Publishing Company

c. Lentigo Maligna Melanoma

Lentigo maligna melanoma

A. Third most common type of melanoma in fair skin (10 %)
B. Most commonly arises in the seventh decade on the sun-exposed facial skin (especially the nose and cheek)
C. Asymmetric tan to brown or black macule with varied color and irregular borders
D. Slow-growing radial growth phase for years as lentigo maligna (in situ), clinical signs of invasion and progression to lentigo maligna melanoma are nodule formation and flecks of dark brown or black pigmentation

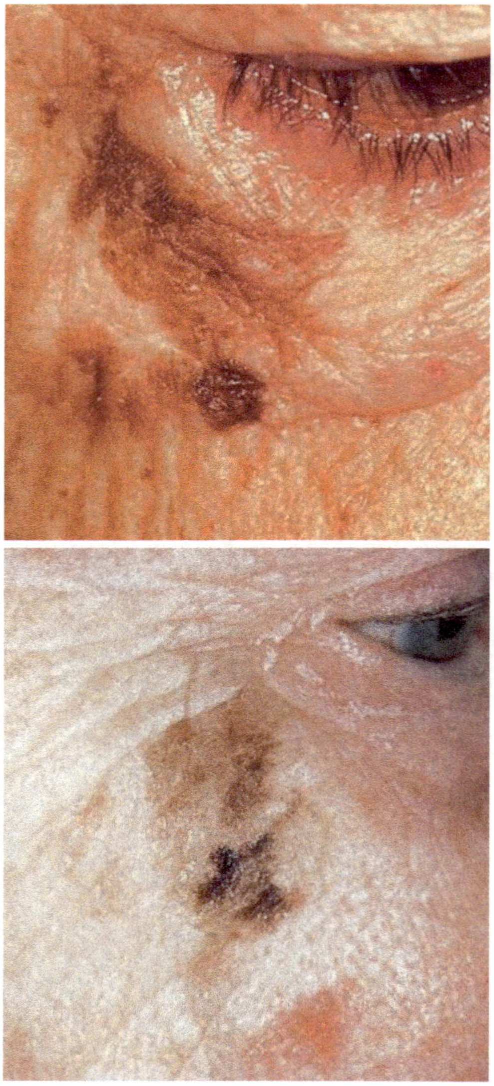

Lentigo maligna melanoma
Photograph courtesy of SpringerImages Database, Springer Publishing Company

d. Acral Lentiginous Melanoma

Acral lentiginous melanoma

A. Uncommon (5 % of melanomas)
B. Most common type in darker races (e.g., Blacks and Asians)
C. Usually presents in the seventh decade
D. Asymmetric brown to black macule with varied colors and irregular borders on the palms, soles, or nail apparatus
E. Usually diagnosed at advanced stage with poor prognosis

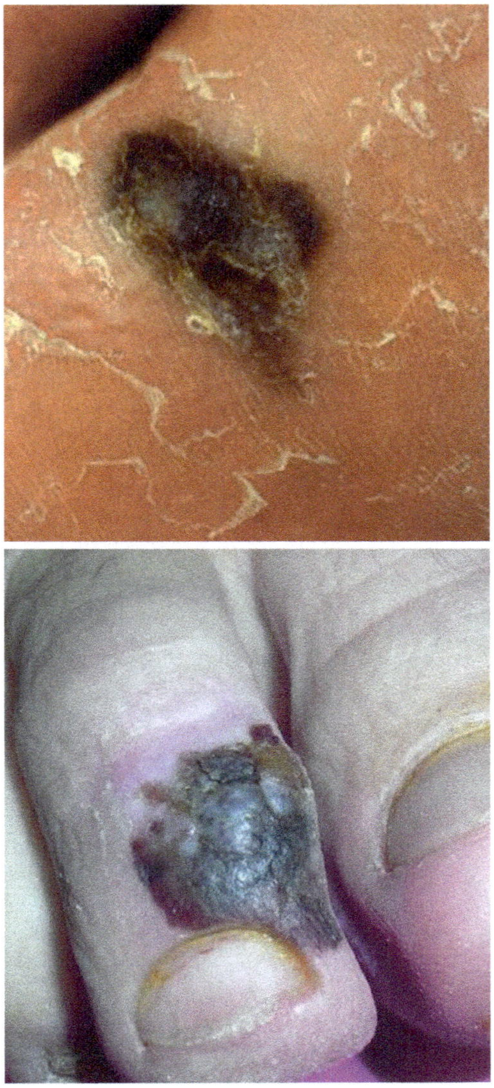

Acral lentiginous melanoma
Photograph courtesy of SpringerImages Database, Springer Publishing Company

i. Acral Lentiginous Melanoma of the Nail Apparatus

Acral lentiginous melanoma of the nail apparatus

A. Irregular hyperpigmented lines on the nail plate with varied color and width of the band
B. Dark bands may have a triangular shape (broad end against nail fold)
   1. Band width is usually greater than 3 mm
C. Hutchinson's sign: pigment extending onto the hyponichium or beyond the lateral or proximal nail fold

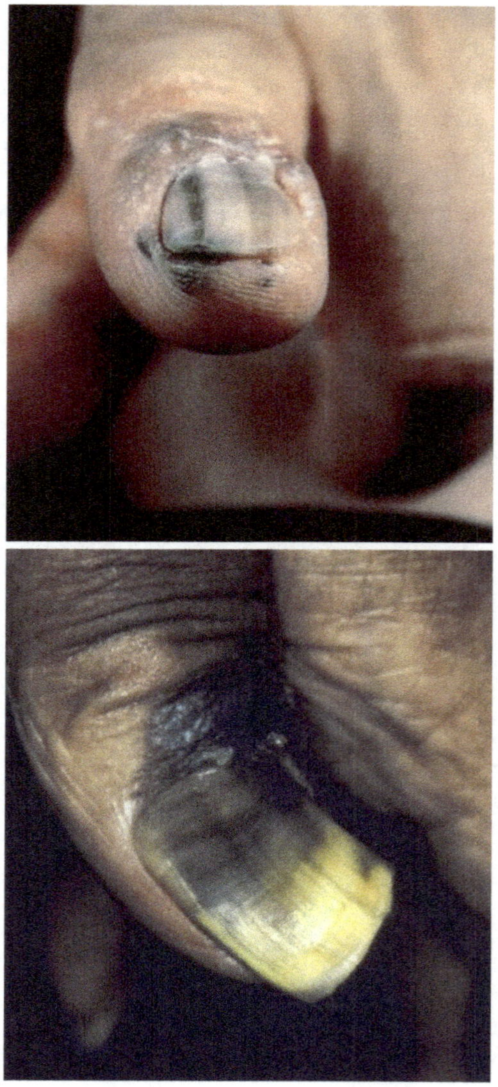

Acral lentiginous melanoma of the nail apparatus
Photographs courtesy of SpringerImages Database, Springer Publishing Company and Hugh Gloster, MD

e. Dermoscopy in Melanoma

Dermoscopy in melanoma

A. Asymmetry of color and structure
B. Multiple colors
C. Atypical network
D. Streaks at the periphery (radial streaming or pseudopods)
E. Irregular dots or globules
F. Irregular blood vessels
G. Blue-white veil
F. Regression structures
G. Blotches

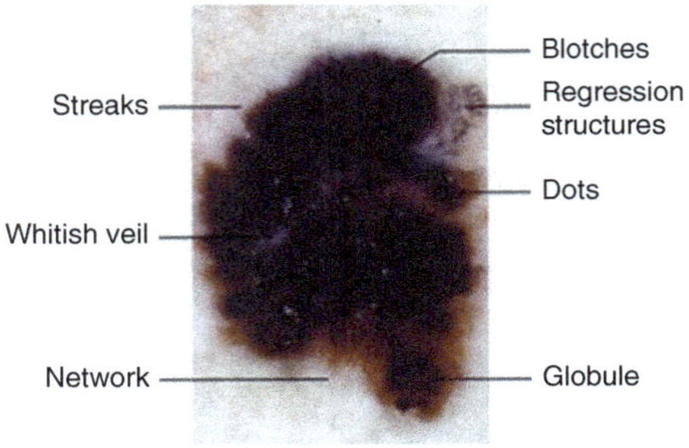

Dermoscopy in melanoma
Photographs courtesy of SpringerImages Database, Springer Publishing Company

Dermoscopy, superficial spreading melanonoma

A. Atypical pigment network (varying shades, chaotic)
B. Blue white veil in center
C. Streaks and pseudopods at the periphery
D. Irregularly distributed dots and globules

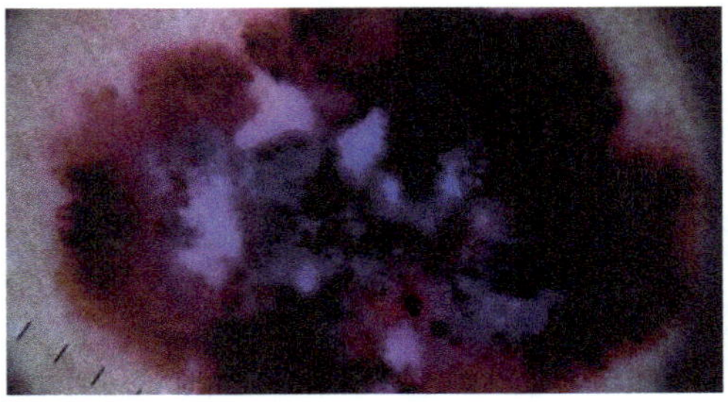

Dermoscopy in melanoma
Photographs courtesy of SpringerImages Database, Springer Publishing Company

Basal Cell Carcinoma

90

a. Superficial Basal Cell Carcinoma

Superficial basal cell carcinoma

A. Well-circumscribed thin plaque with a thin rolled border
B. Commonly seen on the trunk and extremities
C. May closely resemble eczema, psoriasis, or tinea; may be differentiated from these entities by the rolled border

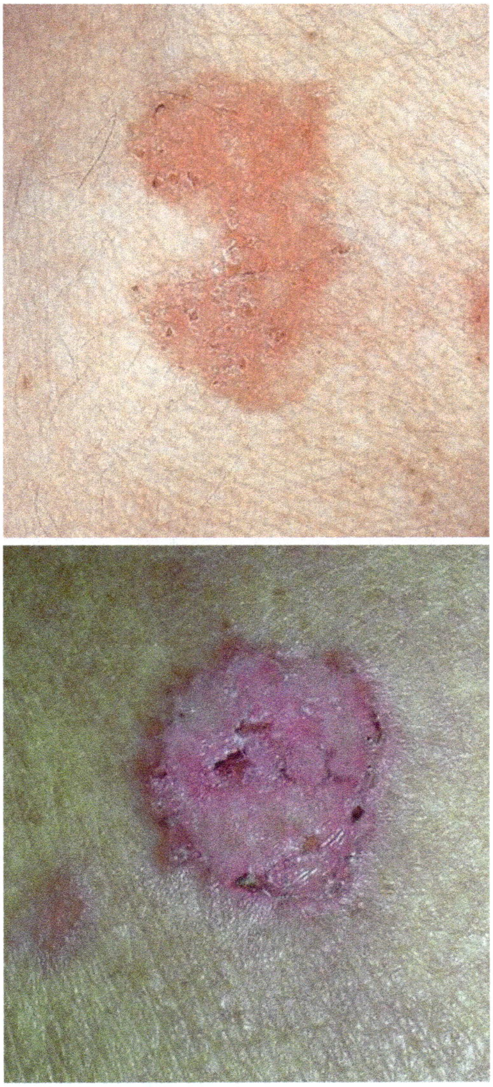

Superficial basal cell carcinoma
Photographs courtesy of SpringerImages Database, Springer Publishing Company

H.M. Gloster, Jr. et al., *Absolute Dermatology Review: Mastering Clinical Conditions on the Dermatology Recertification Exam*, DOI 10.1007/978-3-319-03218-4_90, © Springer International Publishing Switzerland 2016

b. Nodular Basal Cell Carcinoma

Nodular basal cell carcinoma

A. Papule or nodule with elevated pearly rolled borders and telangiectasias which may ulcerate
B. Usually occurs on sun-exposed skin, especially the head and neck

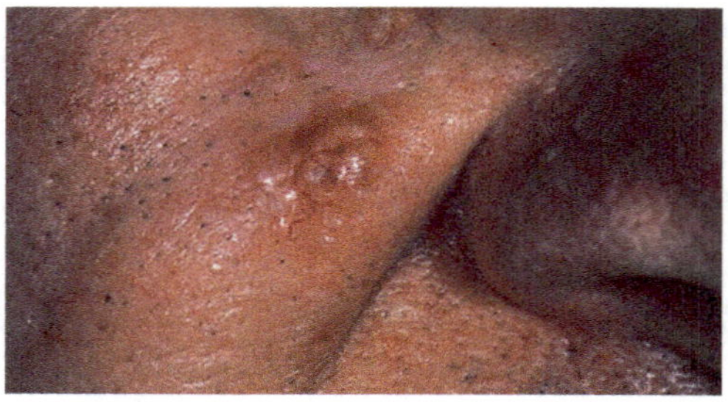

Nodular basal cell carcinoma
Photographs courtesy of SpringerImages Database, Springer Publishing Company

Nodular basal cell carcinoma

A. Pearly, telangiectatic papule with a rolled border

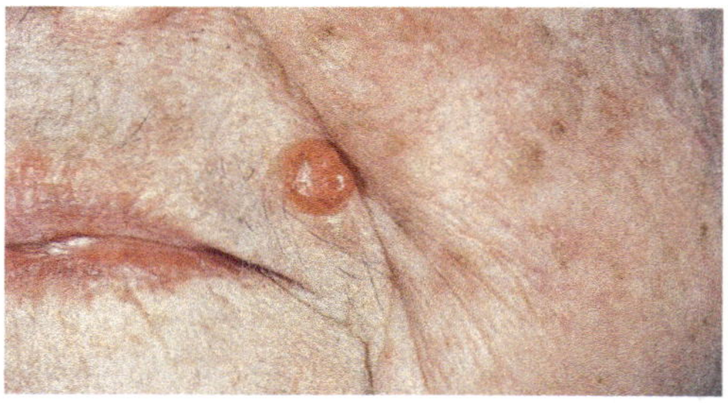

Nodular basal cell carcinoma
Photographs courtesy of SpringerImages Database, Springer Publishing Company

i. Dermoscopy of Nodular Basal Cell Carcinoma

Dermoscopy of nodular basal cell carcinoma

A. Arborizing tree-like telangiectasias with foci of microulceration

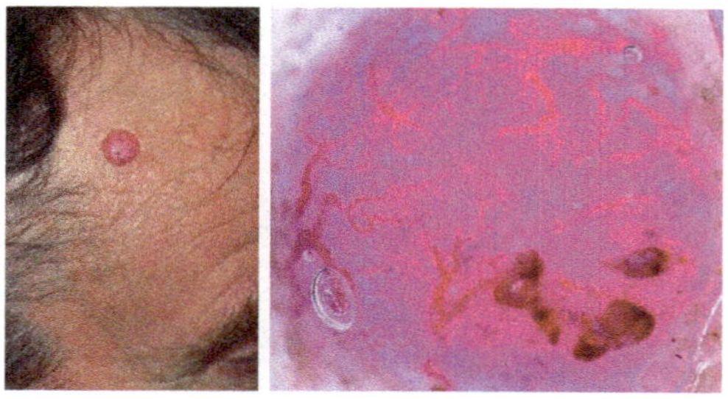

Dermoscopy of nodular basal cell carcinoma
Photograph courtesy of SpringerImages Database, Springer Publishing Company

c. Morpheaform Basal Cell Carcinoma

Morpheaform basal cell carcinoma

A. Indurated plaque resembling a scar, a plaque of morphea, or lichen sclerosus et atrophicus
B. The typical telangiectatic, pearly features of nodular basal cell carcinoma are not present
C. May be subtle in appearance and have subclinical extensions that may not be apparent on physical examination

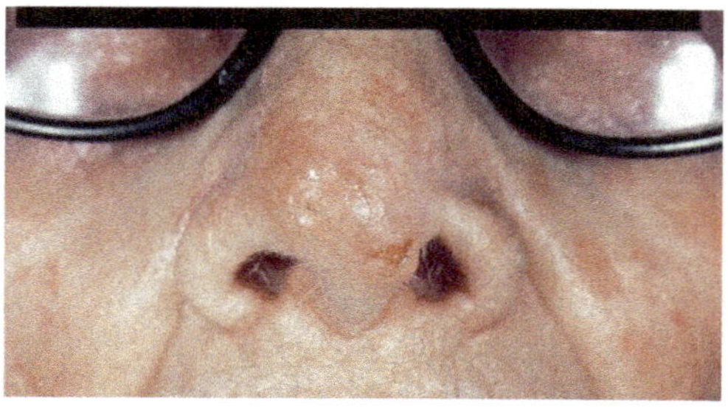

Morpheaform basal cell carcinoma
Photograph courtesy of SpringerImages Database, Springer Publishing Company

Morpheaform basal cell carcinoma

A. Flat, pale, waxy, poorly demarcated indurated plaque on the lower eyelid

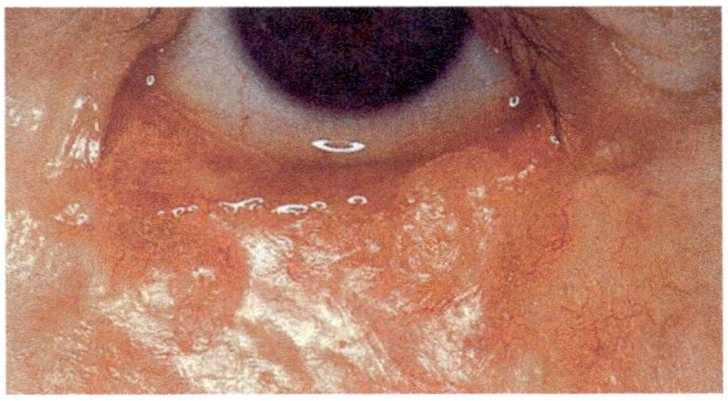

Morpheaform basal cell carcinoma
Photograph courtesy of SpringerImages Database, Springer Publishing Company

d. Pigmented Basal Cell Carcinoma

Pigmented basal cell carcinoma

A. More common in people of color
B. Pearly plaques with rolled borders and telangiectases that vary in color from blue to brown to black

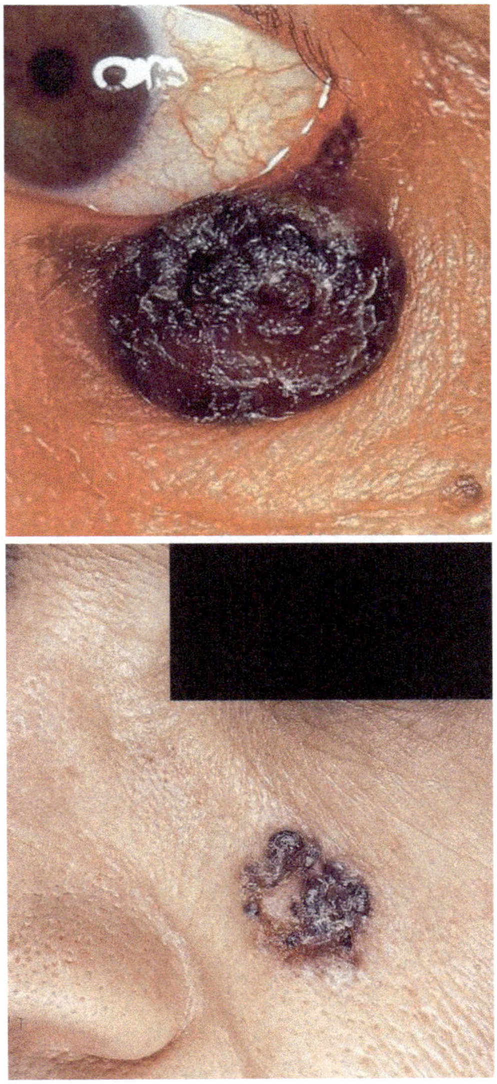

Pigmented basal cell carcinoma
Photograph courtesy of SpringerImages Database, Springer Publishing Company

i. Dermoscopy of Pigmented Basal Cell Carcinoma

Dermoscopy of pigmented basal cell carcinoma

A. Arborizing telangiectasias
B. Blue gray ovoid nests and globules
C. Spokewheel areas

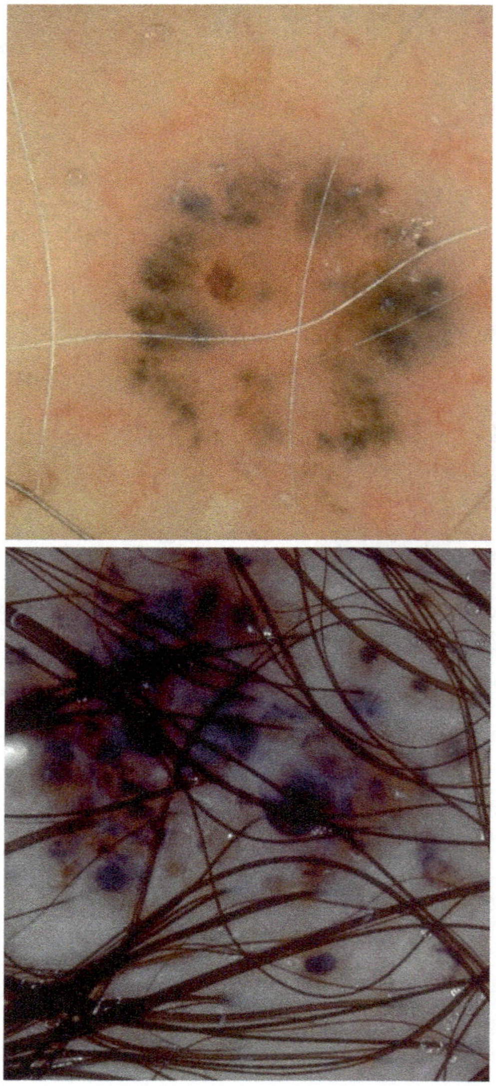

Dermoscopy of pigmented basal cell carcinoma
Photograph courtesy of SpringerImages Database, Springer Publishing Company

Squamous Cell Carcinoma 91

a. Squamous Cell Carcinoma In Situ (Bowen's Disease)

Squamous cell carcinoma in situ (Bowen's disease)
  A. Red scaly superficial patch or plaque on sun-exposed area

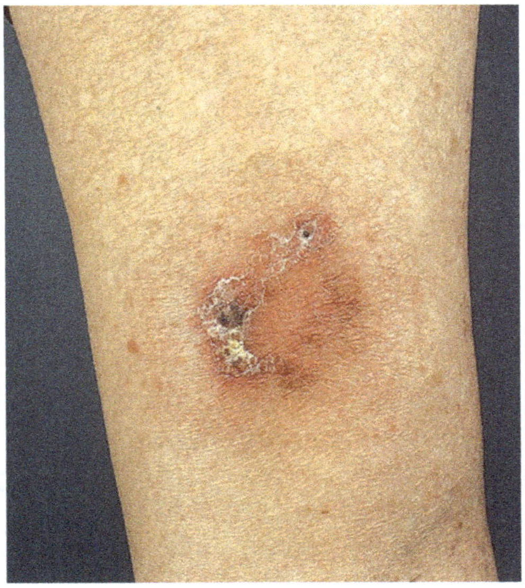

Squamous cell carcinoma in situ
Photograph courtesy of SpringerImages Database, Springer Publishing Company

b. Invasive Squamous Cell Carcinoma

Invasive squamous cell carcinoma
  A. May be a papulonodule, a plaque, papillomatous or exophytic with variable scale, or hyperkeratotic, crusted, eroded, or ulcerated
  B. Primarily occurs on sun-exposed skin

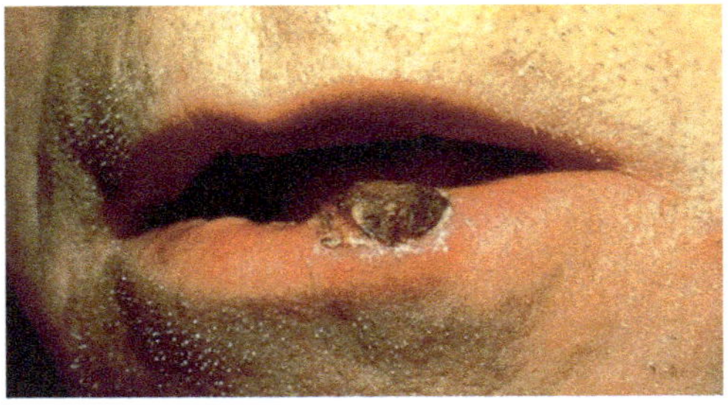

Invasive squamous cell carcinoma
Photograph courtesy of SpringerImages Database, Springer Publishing Company

H.M. Gloster, Jr. et al., *Absolute Dermatology Review: Mastering Clinical Conditions on the Dermatology Recertification Exam*, DOI 10.1007/978-3-319-03218-4_91, © Springer International Publishing Switzerland 2016

Invasive squamous cell carcinoma
A. Ulcerated plaque on the right temple

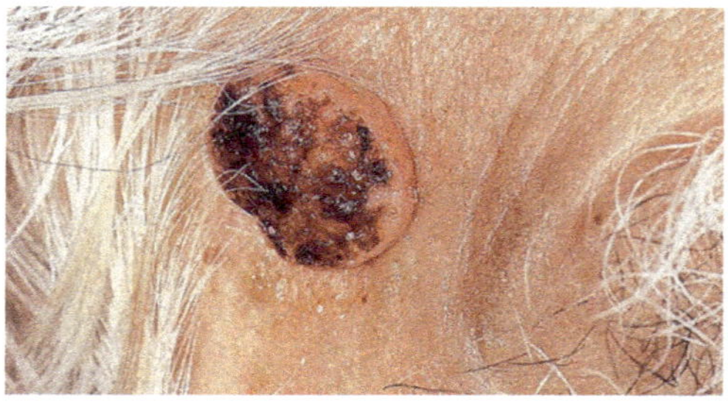

Invasive squamous cell carcinoma
Photograph courtesy of SpringerImages Database, Springer Publishing Company

Invasive squamous cell carcinoma
A. Ulcerated nodule on the right lower eyelid

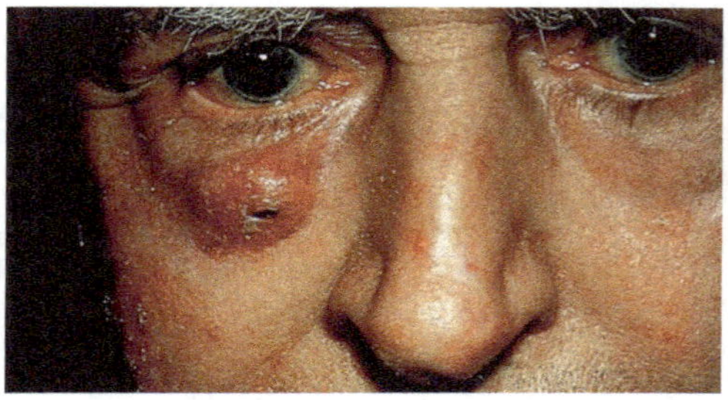

Invasive squamous cell carcinoma
Photograph courtesy of SpringerImages Database, Springer Publishing Company

c. Erythroplasia of Queyrat

Erythroplasia of Querat
A. Well-demarcated velvety eroded red plaque on the glans penis or vulva
B. SCC in situ of the glans penis

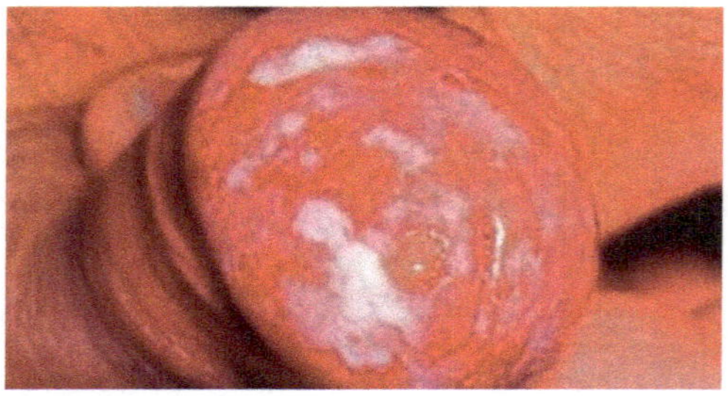

Erythroplasia of queyrat
Photograph courtesy of SpringerImages Database, Springer Publishing Company

Erythroplasia of Querat
A. Well-demarcated velvety eroded red plaque on the glans penis

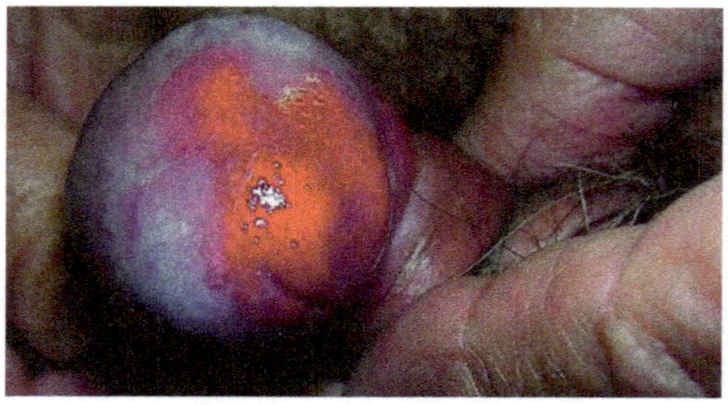

Erythroplasia of queyrat
Photograph courtesy of SpringerImages Database, Springer Publishing Company

d. Verrucous Carcinoma

Verrucous carcinoma
  A. Large exophytic tumors with a verrucous surface
  B. Associated with human papilloma virus
  C. Gradual penetration (bulldozing) into underlying tissues
  D. Three types
    1. Epithelioma cuniculatum
    2. Giant condyloma acuminatum of the genitalia (Bushke-Lowenstein)
    3. Oral florid papillomatosis

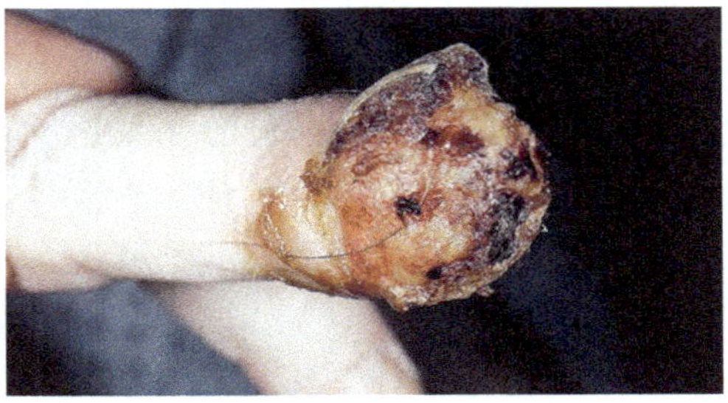

Verrucous carcinoma
Photograph courtesy of SpringerImages Database, Springer Publishing Company

i. Epithelioma Cuniculatum

Epithelioma cuniculatum
  A. Rabbit burrow appearance
  B. Often presents on the plantar foot as a boggy exophytic plaque
  C. May be misdiagnosed as verruca vulgaris

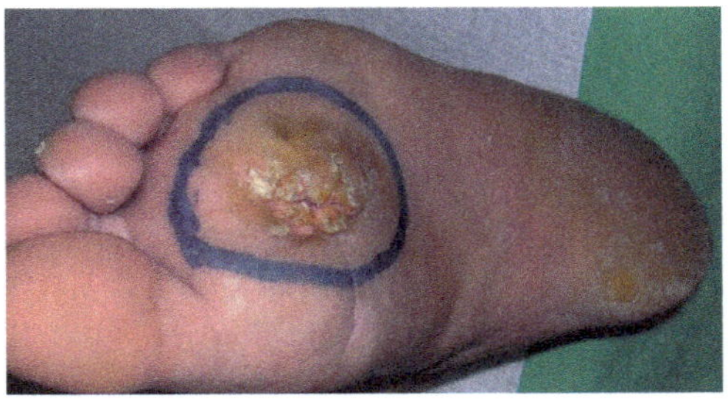

Epithelioma cuniculatum
Photograph courtesy of SpringerImages Database, Springer Publishing Company

Epithelioma cuniculatum
  A. Boggy exophytic plaque on the plantar foot

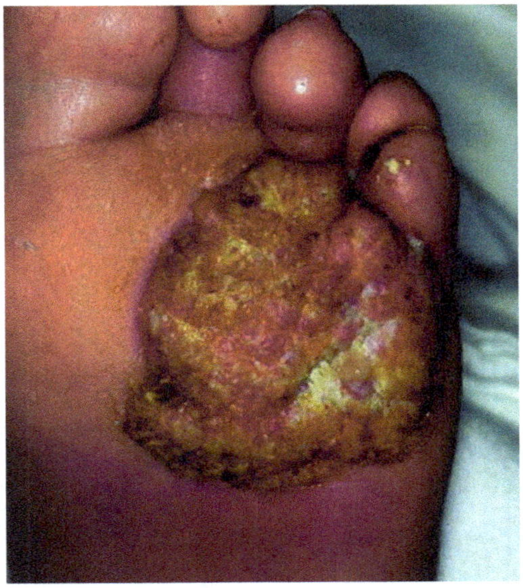

Epithelioma cuniculatum
Photograph courtesy of SpringerImages Database, Springer Publishing Company

ii. Giant Condyloma of the Genitalia (Buschke-Lowenstein Tumor)

Giant condyloma of the genitalia (Buschke-Lowenstein Tumor)
  A. Verrucous carcinoma of the anorectal or external genital area

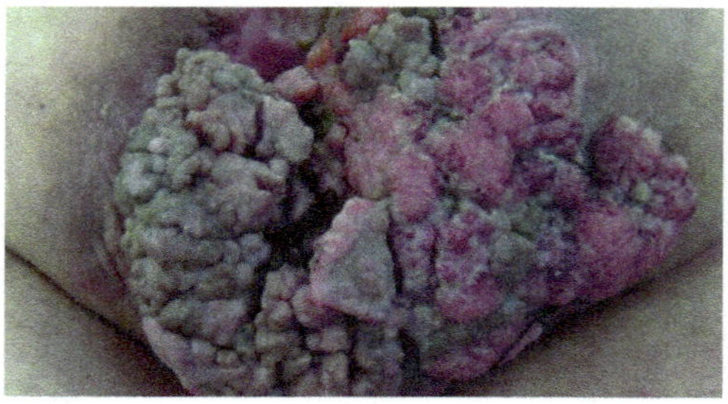

Giant condyloma of the genitalia (Buschke-Lowenstein tumor)
Photograph courtesy of SpringerImages Database, Springer Publishing Company

iii. Oral Florid Papillomatosis

Oral florid papillomatosis
  A. White verrucous lesions on the oral cavity or nasal sinuses that may be exophytic (cauliflower-like) and extensive
  B. May progress to verrucous carcinoma

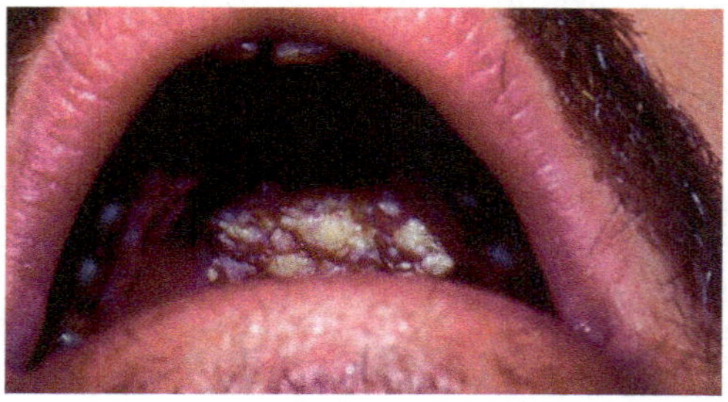

Oral florid papillomatosis
Photograph courtesy of SpringerImages Database, Springer Publishing Company

92 Extramammary Paget's Disease

Extramammary Paget's disease (EMP)

A. Slowly expanding sharply demarcated pink or red plaque most commonly on the vulva in women and perianal area in men
B. Scattered areas of white scale within the pink or red plaque give a "strawberries and cream" appearance
C. Most commonly occurs in elderly caucasians
D. Primary EMP
   1. Most common type (over 75 % of patients)
   2. Arises as a primary intraepithelial adenocarcinoma
E. Secondary EMP
   1. 10–20 % of patients
   2. Cutaneous extension of underlying adnexal adenocarcionma or an underlying visceral malignancy (colorectal or bladder most commonly but also prostate, cervical, ovarian, endometrial)

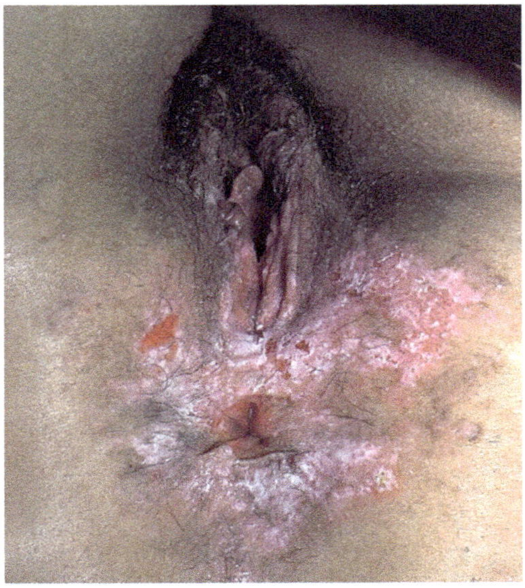

Extramammary paget's disease
Photograph courtesy of SpringerImages Database, Springer Publishing Company

H.M. Gloster, Jr. et al., *Absolute Dermatology Review: Mastering Clinical Conditions on the Dermatology Recertification Exam*,
DOI 10.1007/978-3-319-03218-4_92,

Cutaneous Lymphomas

93

a. T Cell Lymphomas

i. Mycosis Fungoides

1. Patch Stage Mycosis Fungoides

Patch stage Mycosis Fungoides (MF)

A. Most common type of cutaneous T cell lymphoma
B. Protracted course over years
C. Clinical features
   1. Erythematous finely scaling patches with variable degrees of atrophy
   2. Poikilodermatous variant: mottled hyperpigmentation or hypopigmentation, atrophy, telangiectasia
   3. Generalized hypopigmented lesions can be seen in dark skin or juvenile MF
   4. Most commonly seen on the buttocks and covered sites of the trunk in a "bathing trunk" distribution

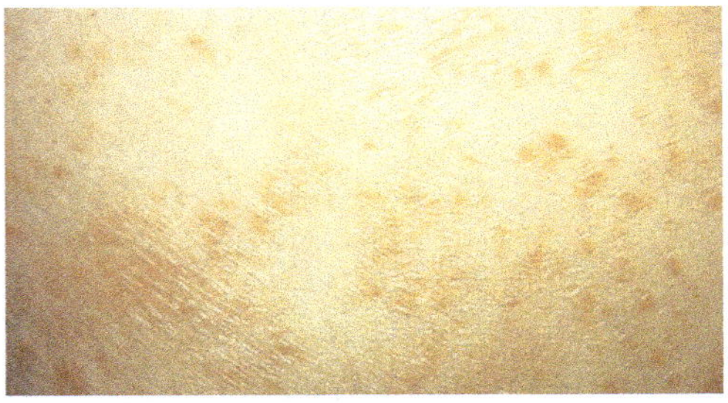

Patch stage mycosis fungoides
Photograph courtesy of SpringerImages Database, Springer Publishing Company

a. Patch Stage Mycosis Fungoides (Hypopigmented Variant)

Patch stage mycosis fungoides (hypopigmented variant)

A. More common in dark-skinned individuals
B. Ill-defined, pruritic, hypopigmented macules and patches
C. May be preceded by chronic eczema or dermatitis
D. May resemble vitiligo, pityriasis alba, tinea versicolor, tinea corporis, sarcoid, postinflammatory hypopigmentation

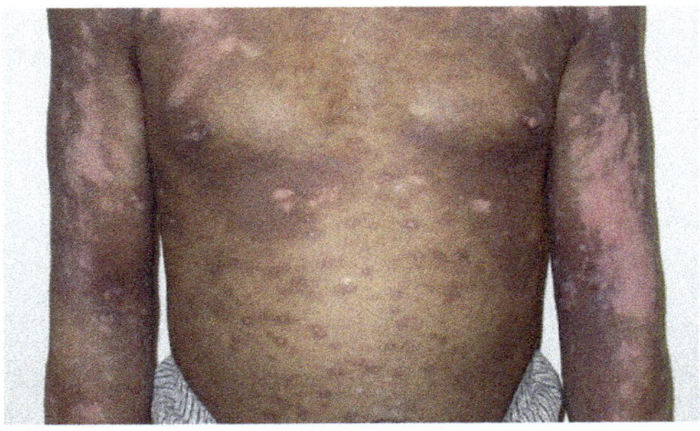

Patch stage mycosis fungoides (hypopigmented variant)
Photograph courtesy of Hugh Gloster, MD

H.M. Gloster, Jr. et al., *Absolute Dermatology Review: Mastering Clinical Conditions on the Dermatology Recertification Exam*, DOI 10.1007/978-3-319-03218-4_93, © Springer International Publishing Switzerland 2016

Patch stage mycosis fungoides (hypopigmented variant)

A. Generalized hypopigmented lesions can be seen in dark-skin individuals

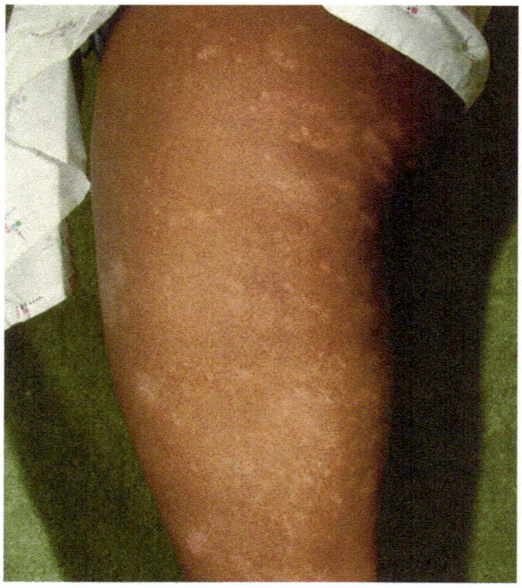

Patch stage mycosis fungoides (hypopigmented variant)
Photograph courtesy of SpringerImages Database, Springer Publishing Company

2. Plaque Stage Mycosis Fungoides

Mycosis fungoides, plaque stage

A. Infiltrated red-brown scaling plaques which may enlarge to several centimeters and have an annular, polycyclic, or horseshoe pattern
B. Raised borders with central clearing may occur, resembling tinea cruris or annular erythema

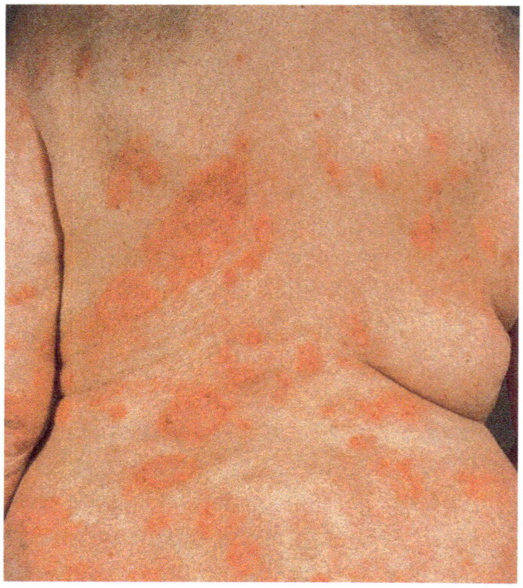

Mycosis fungoides, plaque stage
Photograph courtesy of SpringerImages Database, Springer Publishing Company

3. Pagetoid Reticulosis

Pagetoid reticulosis

A. Localized plaque-stage mycosis fungoides
B. Solitary psoriasiform or hyperkeratotic patch or plaque on an extremity which is slowly progressive

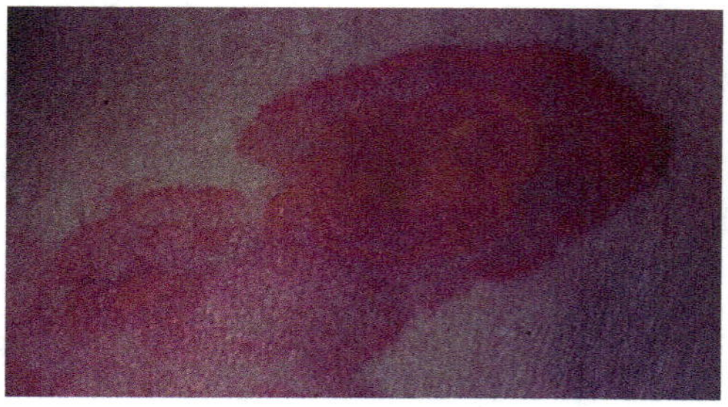

Pagetoid reticulosis
Photograph courtesy of SpringerImages Database, Springer Publishing Company

4. Tumor Stage Mycosis Fungoides

Mycosis fungoides, tumor stage

A. Combination of patches, plaques, and tumors with ulceration

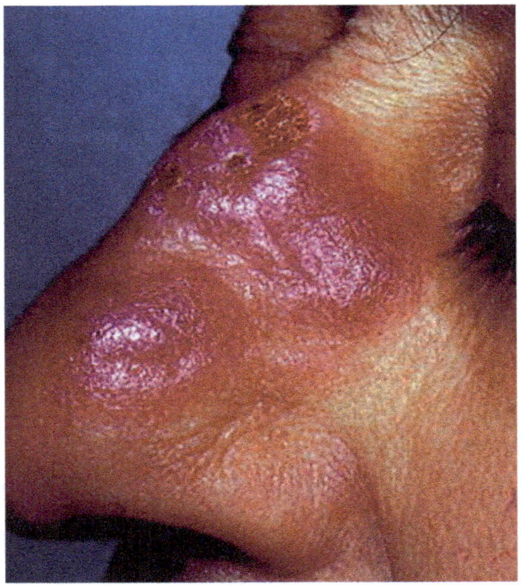

Tumor stage mycosis fungoides
Photograph courtesy of SpringerImages Database, Springer Publishing Company

Mycosis fungoides, tumor stage

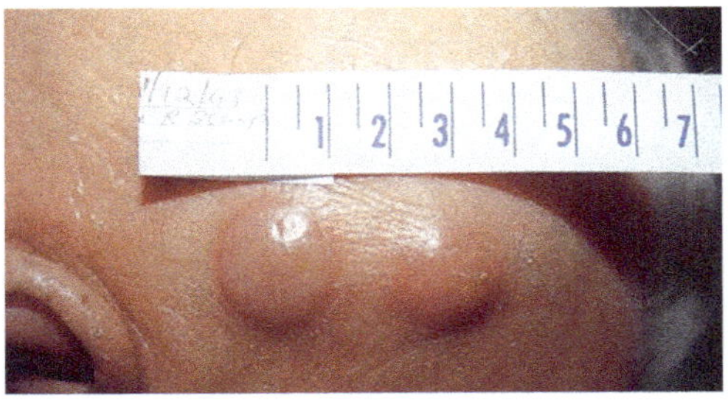

Tumor stage mycosis fungoides
Photograph courtesy of SpringerImages Database, Springer Publishing Company

ii. Folliculotropic Cutaneous T-Cell Lymphoma

Folliculotropic cutaneous T-cell lymphoma

A. Folliculotropic infiltrates sparing epidermis
B. Pruritic, grouped follicular papules, acneiform lesions, and indurated plaques
C. Most commonly occur on the head and neck
D. Infiltrated plaques in eyebrow area with alopecia are common
E. Most cases show mucinous degeneration of hair follicles (follicular mucinosis)

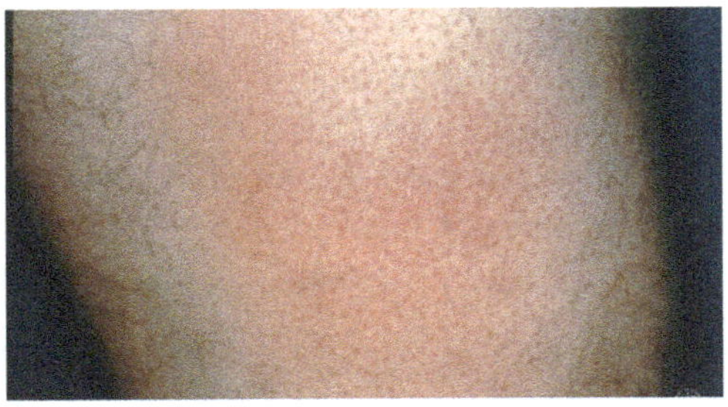

Folliculotropic cutaneous T-cell lymphoma
Photograph courtesy of the American Academy of Dermatology

Folliculotropic cutaneous T-cell lymphoma

A. Pruritic, grouped follicular papules and indurated plaques
B. Most commonly occur on the head and neck

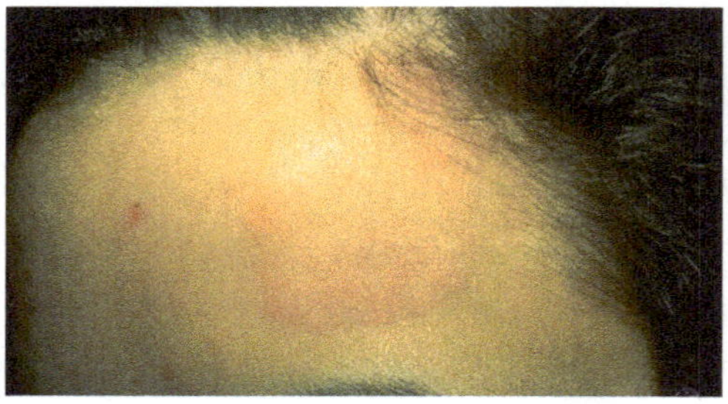

Folliculotropic cutaneous T-cell lymphoma
Photograph courtesy of the American Academy of Dermatology

Folliculotropic cutaneous T-cell lymphoma

A. Infiltrated plaques on the scalp with alopecia are common

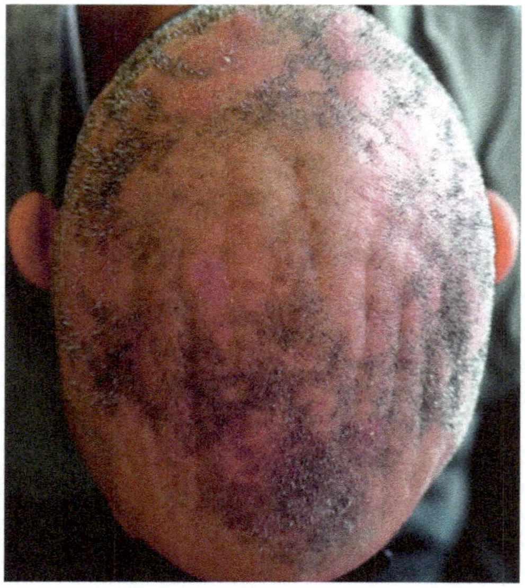

Folliculotropic cutaneous T-cell lymphoma
Photograph courtesy of SpringerImages Database, Springer Publishing Company

iii. Granulomatous Slack Skin

Granulomatous slack skin

A. Variant of cutaneous T cell lymphoma
B. Circumscribed areas of pendulous lax skin with a predilection for the axilla or groin
C. One third of cases are associated with Hodgkins Lymphoma

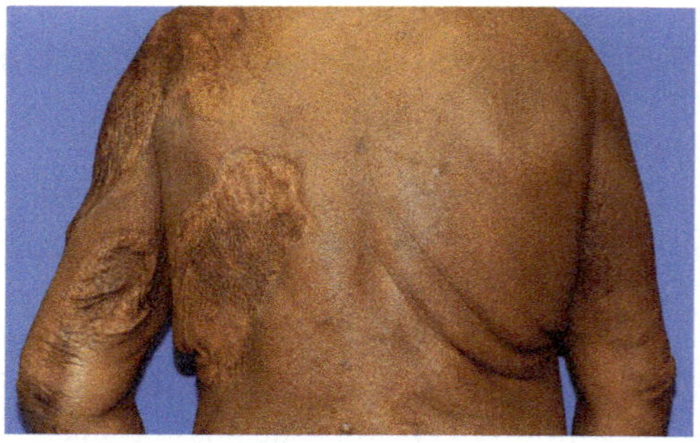

Granulomatous slack skin
Courtesy of Mayo Clinic, Department of Dermatology, Rochester, MN

Granulomatous slack skin

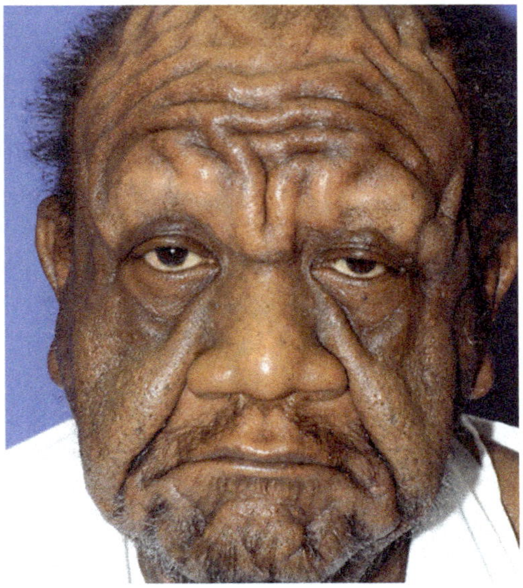

Granulomatous slack skin
Courtesy of Mayo Clinic, Department of Dermatology, Rochester, MN

Granulomatous slack skin

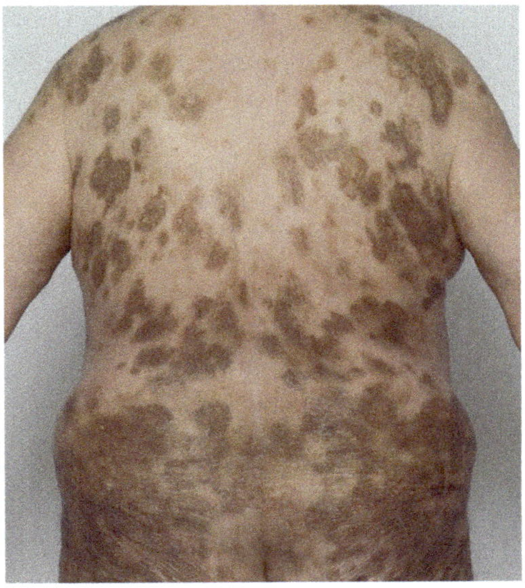

Granulomatous slack skin
Courtesy of Mayo Clinic, Department of Dermatology, Rochester, MN

iv. Sezary Syndrome

Sezary syndrome

A. Neoplastic T cells (sezary cells) in the skin, lymph nodes, and peripheral blood
B. Generalized adenopathy and erythroderma, which may be associated with intense pruritus, exfoliation, edema, lichenification, alopecia, nail dystrophy, and palmoplantar hyerkeratosis
C. Poor prognosis with 25 % 5 year survival

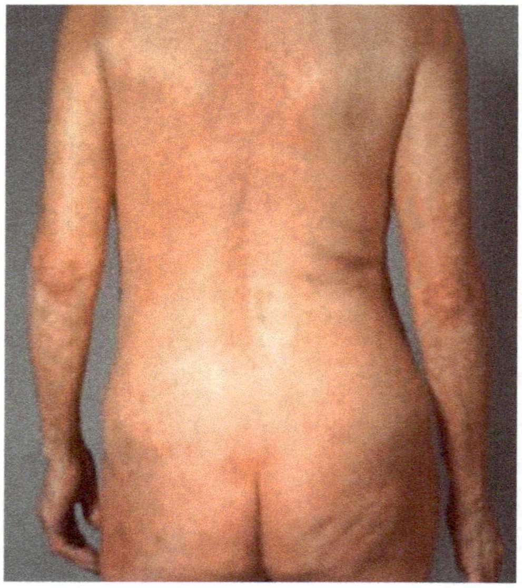

Sezary syndrome
Photograph courtesy of SpringerImages Database, Springer Publishing Company

v. Primary Cutaneous CD 30+ Anaplastic Large Cell Lymphoma

Primary cutaneous CD 30+ anaplastic large cell lymphoma

A. Solitary or localized nodules or tumors with ulceration
B. Lesions may partially or completely regress

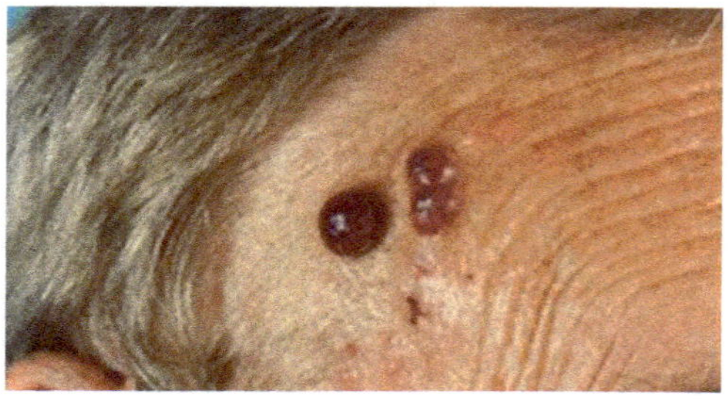

Primary cutaneous CD 30+ anaplastic large cell lymphoma
Photograph courtesy of SpringerImages Database, Springer Publishing Company

vi. Lymphomatoid Papulosis

Lymphomatoid papulosis

A. Asymptomatic, chronic, recurrent self-healing red brown papules and nodules (1 to 100) that develop central hemorrhage, necrosis, and crusting
B. Lesions disappear within 3–8 weeks, resulting in skin lesions in different stages of evolution and regression (hallmark: papulonecrotic lesions at different stages of evolution)
C. Most commonly on the trunk and extremities
D. Lesions disappear to leave hyperpigmented or hypopigmented macules, atrophic varioliform scars, or do not ulcerate at all and resolve with no marks
E. Disease lasts months to years
F. In 20 % may be preceded by, associated with, or followed by another type of cutaneous or systemic lymphoma
G. Good prognosis

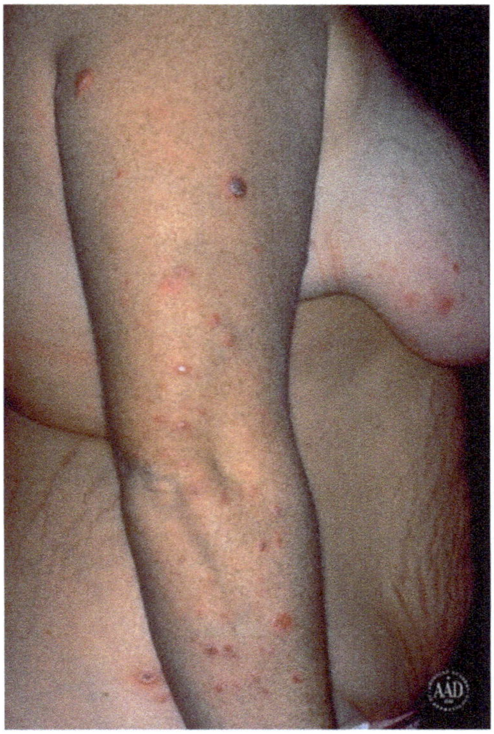

Lymphomatoid papulosis
Courtesy of the American Academy of Dermatology

Lymphomatoid papulosis

A. Papulonecrotic lesion with central hemorrhage and necrosis

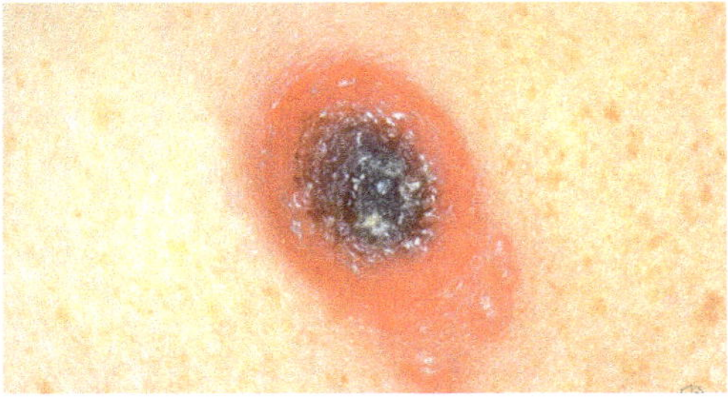

Lymphomatoid papulosis
Courtesy of the American Academy of Dermatology

Lymphomatoid papulosis

A. Papulonecrotic lesions at different stages of evolution

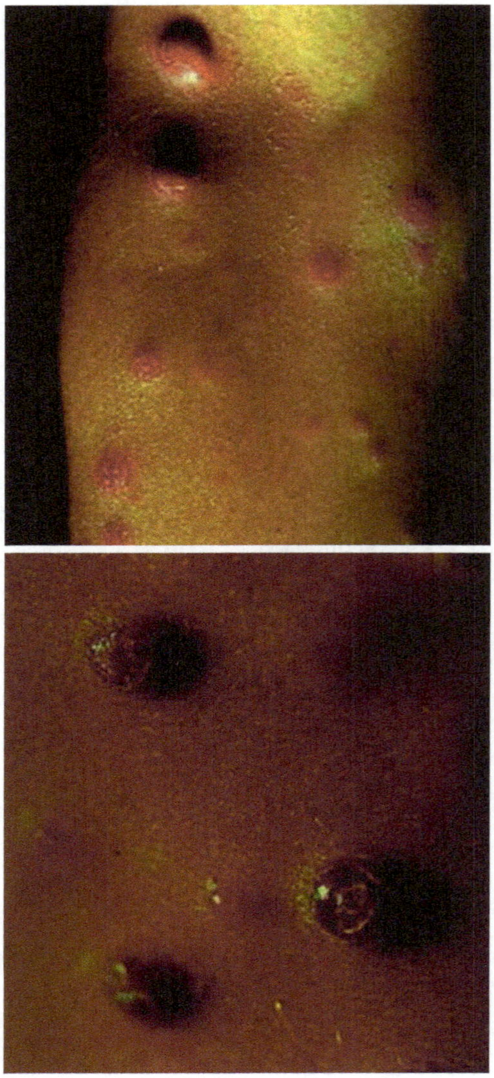

Lymphomatoid papulosis
Photograph courtesy of SpringerImages Database, Springer Publishing Company

vii. Subacute Panniculitis-Like T Cell Lymphoma

Subcutaneous panniculitis-like T-cell lymphoma

A. Lymphoma involving subcutaneous tissue
B. Solitary or multiple subcutaneous nodules or deeply seated plaques 1–20 cm in diameter on the trunk or extremities that resolve with lipoatrophy
C. Indolent course, may be preceded for years by seemingly benign panniculitis
D. 20 % have associated autoimmune disease (usually systemic lupus erythematosus) and may show overlapping clinical and histopathologic features of lupus panniculitis
E. 15 % have associated hemophagocytic syndrome, which carries a poor prognosis

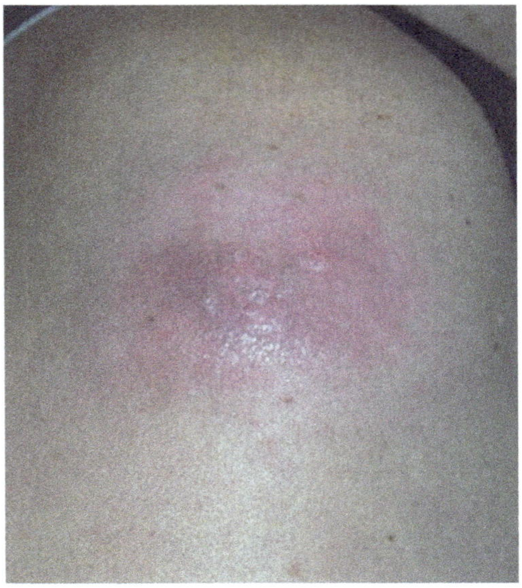

Subcutaneous panniculitis-like T-cell lymphoma
Photograph courtesy of SpringerImages Database, Springer Publishing Company

b. B Cell Lymphomas

i. Follicular Center Lymphoma

Follicular center lymphoma

A. B cell lymphoma
B. Indolent clinical behavior (slowly increases in size) and favorable prognosis (95 % 5 year survival)
C. Asymptomatic, single red plaque or tumor
D. Most commonly occurs on the head and neck, especially the scalp and forehead
E. May also occur on the back (Crosti's lymphoma) as red or purple plaques or tumors often surrounded by patches of erythema

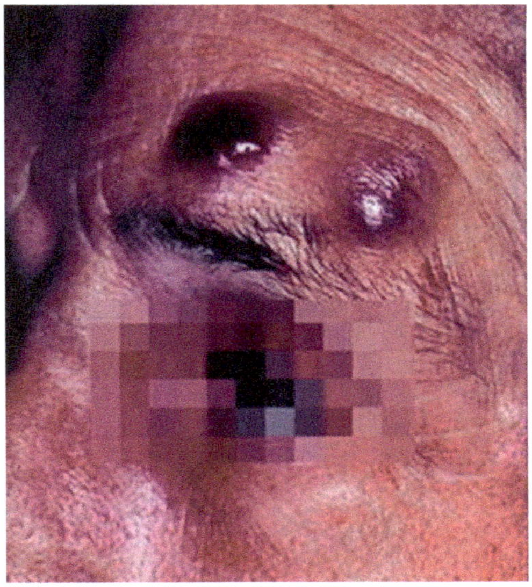

Follicular center lymphoma
Photograph courtesy of SpringerImages Database, Springer Publishing Company

ii. Marginal Zone Lymphoma

Marginal zone lymphoma

A. B cell lymphoma
B. Indolent growth, good prognosis, 98 % 5 year survival
C. Asymptomatic, red to purple papules, plaques, and nodules that do not ulcerate
D. Most commonly occurs on the extremities (upper extremities more common than lower extremities) or trunk

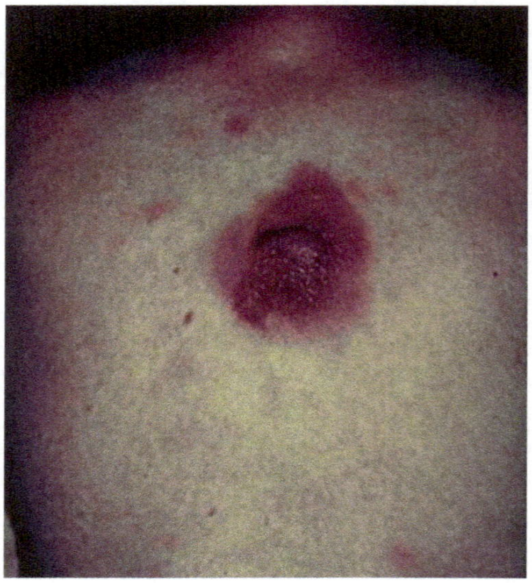

Marginal zone lymphoma
Photograph courtesy of SpringerImages Database, Springer Publishing Company

iii. Diffuse Large B Cell Lymphoma

Diffuse large b-cell lymphoma

A. Solitary or clustered red to red-brown nodules on the distal aspect of one or both legs
B. Less favorable prognosis

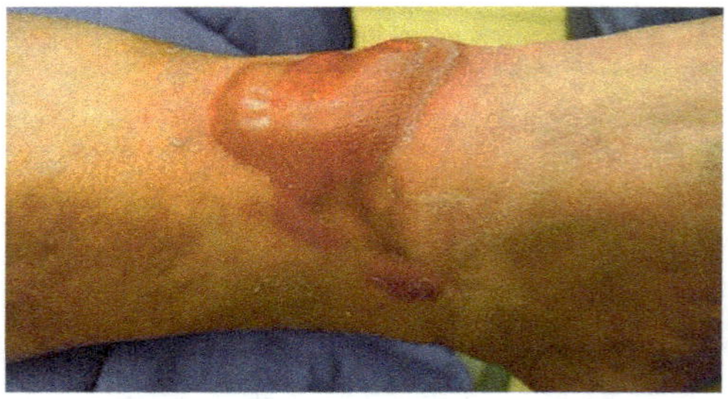

Diffuse large b-cell lymphoma
Photograph courtesy of SpringerImages Database, Springer Publishing Company

Chapter XIV

Disorders Due to Physical Agents

94 Chondrodermatitis Nodularis Helicis

Chondrodermatitis nodularis helicis

A. Unilateral, small (less than 1 cm), tender, red, dome-shaped papulonodules with central crust or keratin-filled crater on the ear
B. Most commonly occurs on the helix (figure a) in men and the antihelix (figure b) in women
C. Most patients are over the age of 50
D. Caused by mechanical trauma to the margin of the helix, exacerbated by thinning of the epidermis and dermis by time, photodamage, or cold

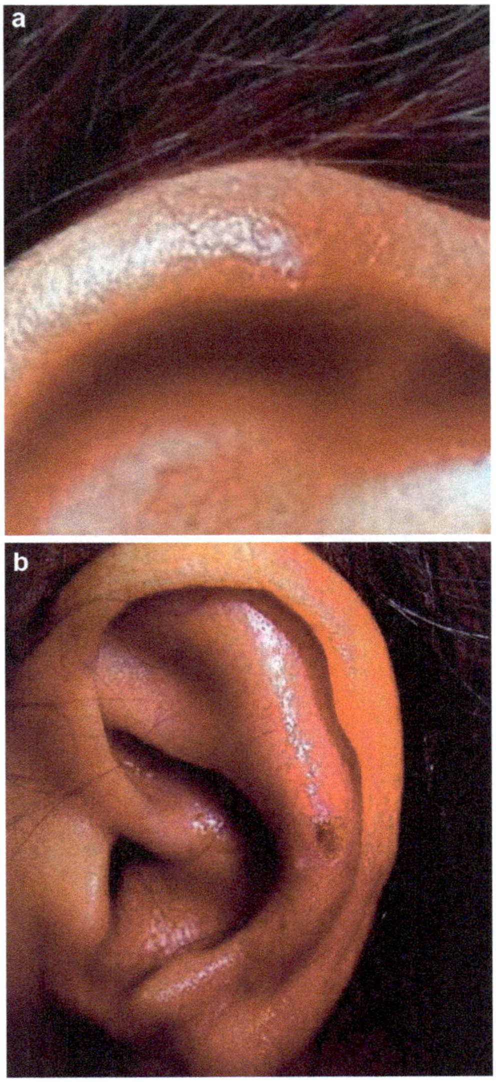

Chondrodermatitis nodularis helicis
Photograph courtesy of SpringerImages Database, Springer Publishing Company

H.M. Gloster, Jr. et al., *Absolute Dermatology Review: Mastering Clinical Conditions on the Dermatology Recertification Exam*,
DOI 10.1007/978-3-319-03218-4_94, © Springer International Publishing Switzerland 2016

95 Factitial Disease

Factitial disease (dermatitis artifacta)

A. Psychocutaneous disease in which patients inflict cutaneous lesions on themselves
B. Usually an unconscious process in which patients deny creating the lesions themselves
C. Most have borderline personality disorder
D. Often induced by foreign objects (carving with sharp instruments, applying chemicals, injecting substances)
E. Located on areas easily reached by the hands
F. More common in women (8:1 male-to-female ratio), onset is usually in adolescence or young adulthood
G. Present with erosions, ulcers (figure a), or unusual bizarre shapes without primary skin lesions, especially with linear or angulated edges arranged regularly that suggest external induction (figure b)

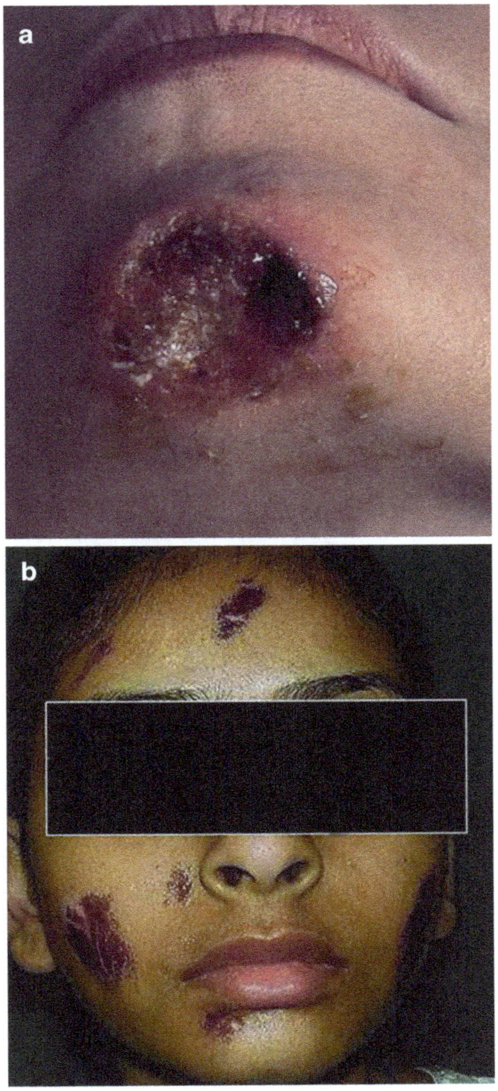

Factitial Disease
Photograph courtesy of SpringerImages Database, Springer Publishing Company

H.M. Gloster, Jr. et al., *Absolute Dermatology Review: Mastering Clinical Conditions on the Dermatology Recertification Exam*, DOI 10.1007/978-3-319-03218-4_95, © Springer International Publishing Switzerland 2016

96 Prurigo Nodularis

Prurigo nodularis

A. Produced by chronic repetitive scratching or picking
B. Underlying disorder associated with pruritus is usually present (e.g., atopic, xerosis, systemic disorder, psychological condition)
C. More common in adults, especially middle-age women
D. Symmetrical, intensely pruritic, firm, dome-shaped, skin-colored, red brown, or hyperpigmented papulonodules with varying degrees of scale crust, erosion, and ulceration
E. Favors the extensor extremities (especially anterior thighs and legs), upper back, buttocks, lumbosacral area (areas easy to reach)

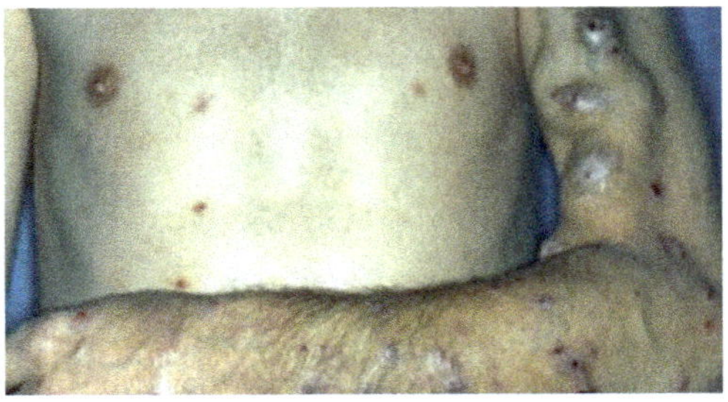

Prurigo nodularis
Photograph courtesy of SpringerImages Database, Springer Publishing Company

Prurigo nodularis

A. Typically spares difficult-to-reach areas such as the upper back ("butterfly sign")

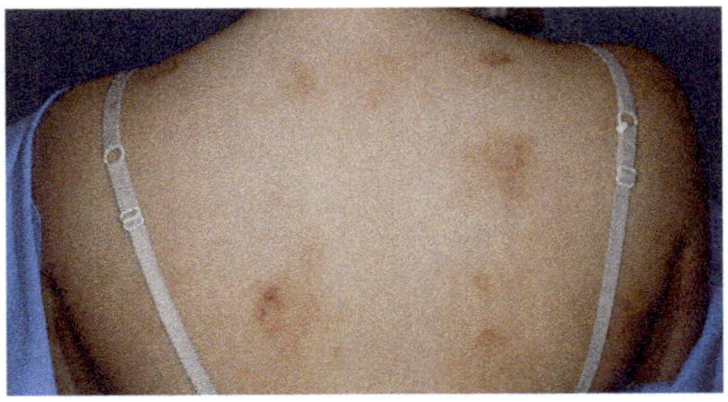

Prurigo nodularis
Photograph courtesy of Kara Shaw, MD

H.M. Gloster, Jr. et al., *Absolute Dermatology Review: Mastering Clinical Conditions on the Dermatology Recertification Exam*,
DOI 10.1007/978-3-319-03218-4_96, © Springer International Publishing Switzerland 2016

97 Trauma Induced Skin Disease

a. Talon Noir

Talon noir (black heel and palm)

A. Black or violet black macules on the palms and soles due to post-traumatic hemorrhage within the thickened stratum corneum
B. Usually unilateral, painless, and favors the edge of thick plantar or palmar skin
C. Occurs most often on the posterior edge of the plantar surface of one or both heels or the thenar eminence of the palm
D. Resolves with time or paring
E. Most often occurs in adolescents and young adults who participate in sports, especially basketball and tennis
G. Sudden stopping or landing on the floor or ground causes shearing forces that rupture papillary dermal capillaries and blood leaks in the epidermis and then the stratum corneum, where it remains for weeks to months
H. Paring the statum corneum will remove the hemoglobin deposits

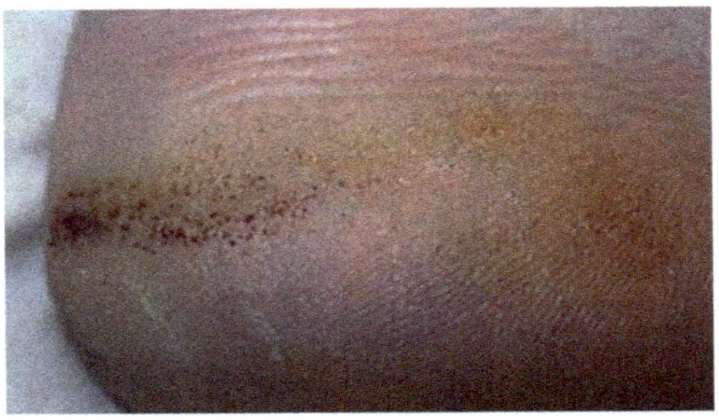

Talon noir
Photograph courtesy of SpringerImages Database, Springer Publishing Company

b. Erythema Ab Igne

i. Erythema Ab Igne (Early)

Erythema ab igne

A. Caused by chronic exposure to heat below the threshold of a thermal burn (e.g., hot water bottles, heating pads, radiators)
B. Common on the lumbosacral region (heat applied to relieve pain) and shins (in regions without central heat in homes)
C. Early: localized areas of reticulated blanchable erythema
D. There is a risk of squamous cell carcinoma (most common) or merkel cell carcinoma arising in affected areas

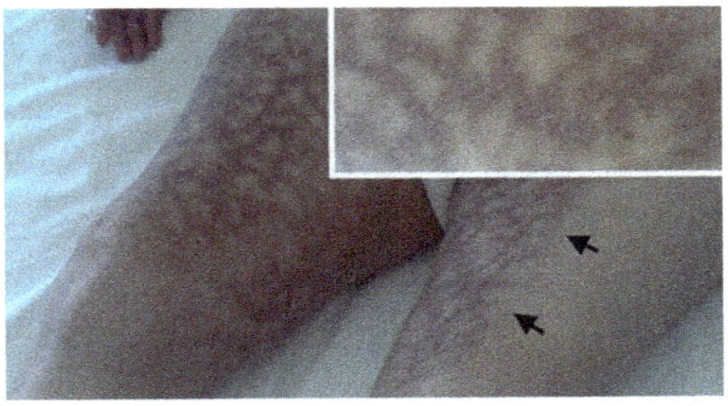

Erythema ab igne (early)
Photograph courtesy of SpringerImages Database, Springer Publishing Company

H.M. Gloster, Jr. et al., *Absolute Dermatology Review: Mastering Clinical Conditions on the Dermatology Recertification Exam*, DOI 10.1007/978-3-319-03218-4_97, © Springer International Publishing Switzerland 2016

ii. Erythema Ab Igne (Late)

Erythema ab igne

A. Late: hyperpigmented macules in a reticulated pattern, eventually overlying keratotic plaques and bullae may develop

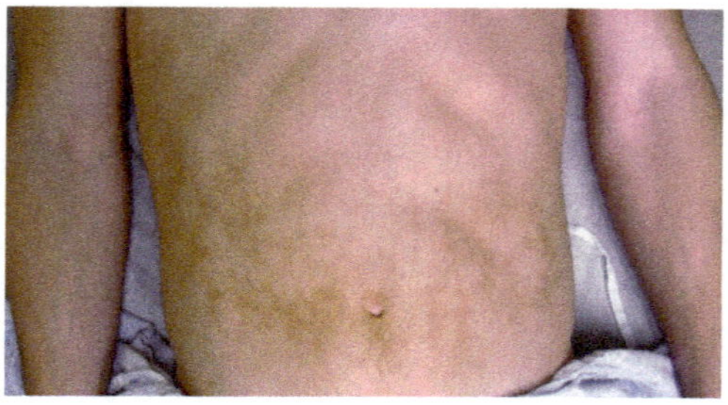

Erythema ab igne (late)
Photograph courtesy of SpringerImages Database, Springer Publishing Company

c. Corns

i. Hard Corns

Hard corns

A. Common on the dorsolateral fifth toe and dorsum of the interphalangeal joints of the lesser toes
B. Firm small dome-shaped papules or nodules with central translucent cores and an interruption in dermatoglyphics

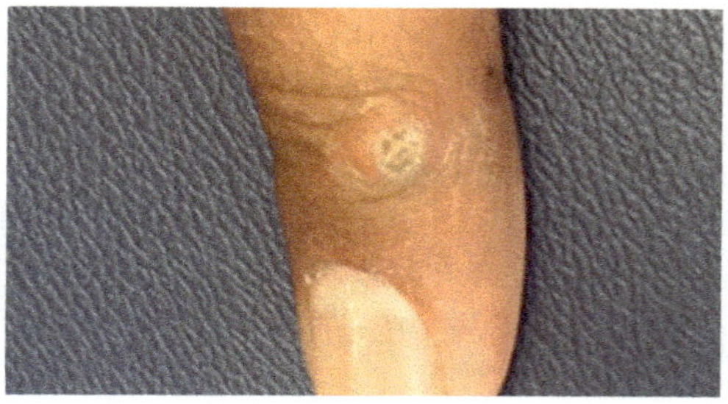

Hard corns
Photograph courtesy of Hugh Gloster, MD

ii. Soft Corns

Soft corns

A. Common in the web spaces and is often white and macerated
B. Caused by the absorption of moisture due to perspiration
C. May be painful
D. Opposing toes may exhibit kissing lesions

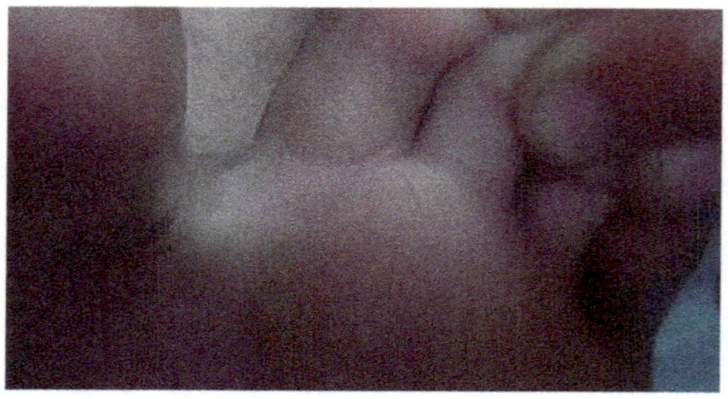

Soft corns
Photograph courtesy of SpringerImages Database, Springer Publishing Company

d. Calluses

Callus

A. Keratotic lesions resulting from repeated trauma (e.g., ill-fitting footwear, bony protuberances, specific activities)
B. Broad-based hyperkeratotiic plaques with increased skin markings

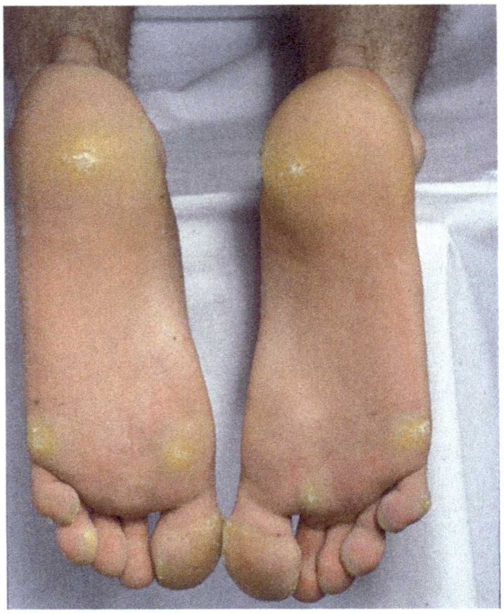

Calluses
Photograph courtesy of the Mayo Clinic Department of Dermatology, Rochester MN

e. Subungual Hematoma

Subungual hematoma

A. Red or red brown discrete area of discoloration under the nail
B. No Hutchinson's sign (extension of pigment on to the nail fold that may be seen in nail unit melanoma)
C. Develops because of trauma (patient may or may not recall the traumatic incident)
D. Dermoscopy: homogenous area, small and large globules, streaking
E. Becomes smaller over time and resolves once the nail grows out (fingernail: 6–8 months, toenail: 8–12 months)

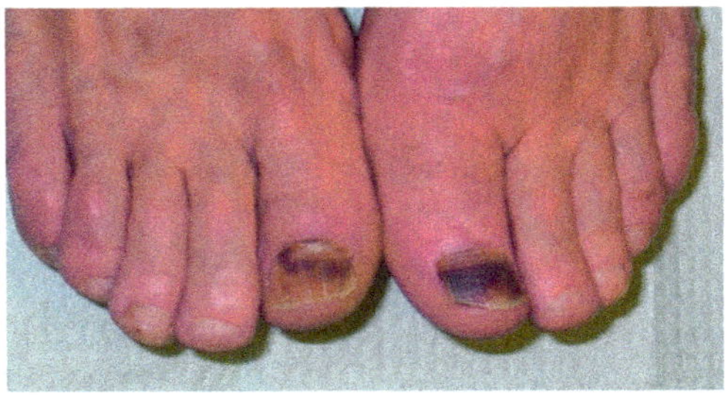

Subungual hematoma
Photograph courtesy of SpringerImages Database, Springer Publishing Company

f. Surgery Induced Ecchymoses

Surgery induced ecchymoses

A. The trauma of surgery results in the scattering of blood within tissue planes
B. Associated with edema and distortion of the anatomy but rarely compromises wound healing
C. Periorbital, perioral, and genital areas are susceptible; gravity plays a role
D. Increased risk in patients on blood thinners

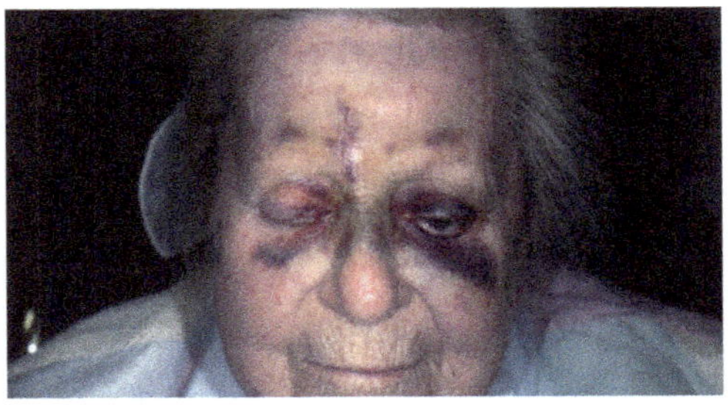

Surgery induced ecchymoses
Photograph courtesy of Hugh Gloster, MD

Surgery induced ecchymoses on the thigh

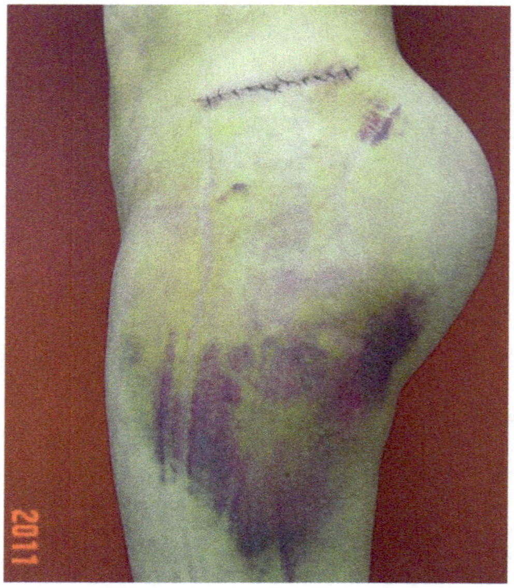

Surgery induced ecchymoses
Photograph courtesy of SpringerImages Database, Springer Publishing Company

g. Piezogenic Papules

Piezogenic pedal papules

A. Multiple tender skin-colored to yellow outpouchings on the medial and lateral aspects of the heels when standing
B. Usually bilateral
C. Secondary to herniation of subcutaneous fat through small tears in plantar fascia
D. Common in distance runners

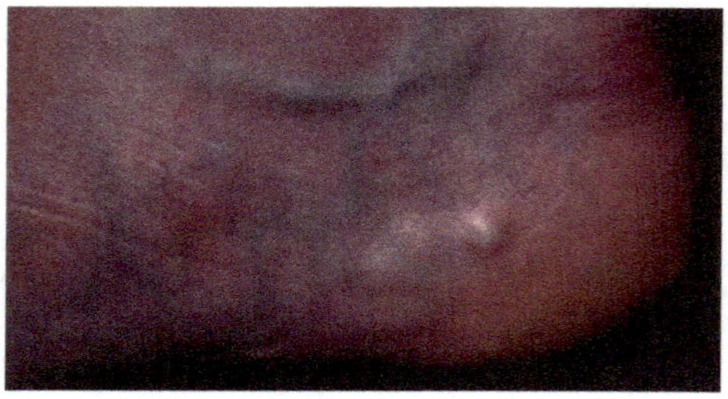

Piezogenic papules
Photograph courtesy of SpringerImages Database, Springer Publishing Company

h. Traumatic Tattoo

Traumatic tattoo

A. Blue-black macules in the area of trauma from explosive substances

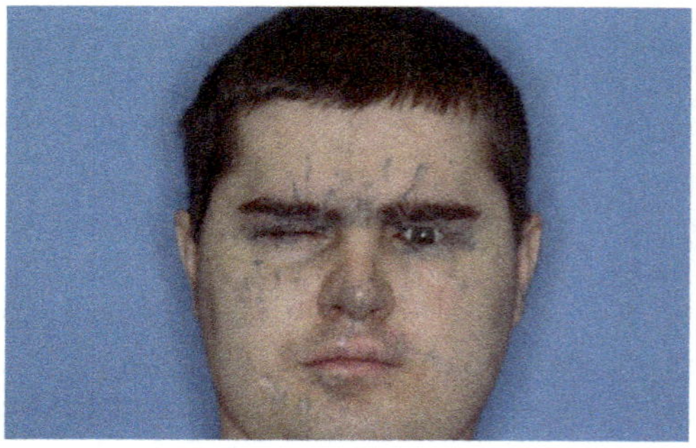

Traumatic tattoo
Photograph courtesy of SpringerImages Database, Springer Publishing Company

98 Photodermatoses

a. Phototoxicity

Phototoxicity

A. Can occur in any person who receives enough phototoxic drug together with sufficient exposure to ultraviolet light
B. Occurs as a result of a direct interaction of ultraviolet radiation with the drug (or a metabolite) in the skin, which leads to formation of reactive oxygen species and nonimmunologic cell damage
C. Most common drugs are tetracycline, nonsteroidal anti-inflammatory drugs, fluoroquinolones, amiodarone, psoralens, and phenothiazines
D. Clinically, resembles an exaggerated sunburn with erythema and bullae in sun-exposed areas followed by hyperpigmentation (figure a)
E. Photoonycholysis—nail plate separates from nail bed of several digits (figure b)

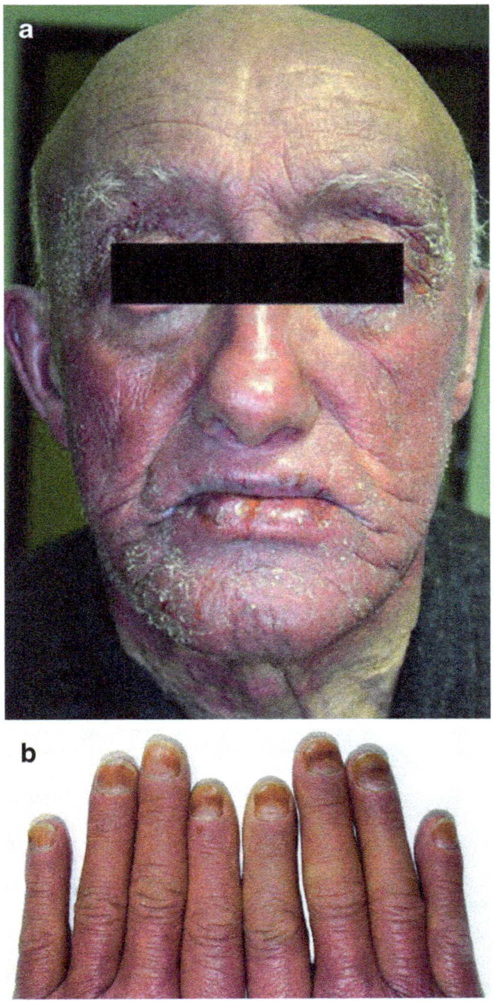

Phototoxicity
Photograph courtesy of SpringerImages Database, Springer Publishing Company

H.M. Gloster, Jr. et al., *Absolute Dermatology Review: Mastering Clinical Conditions on the Dermatology Recertification Exam*, DOI 10.1007/978-3-319-03218-4_98, © Springer International Publishing Switzerland 2016

Phototoxicity

A. Acute phototoxicity from amiodarone, mimicking sunburn and sparing the deep wrinkles

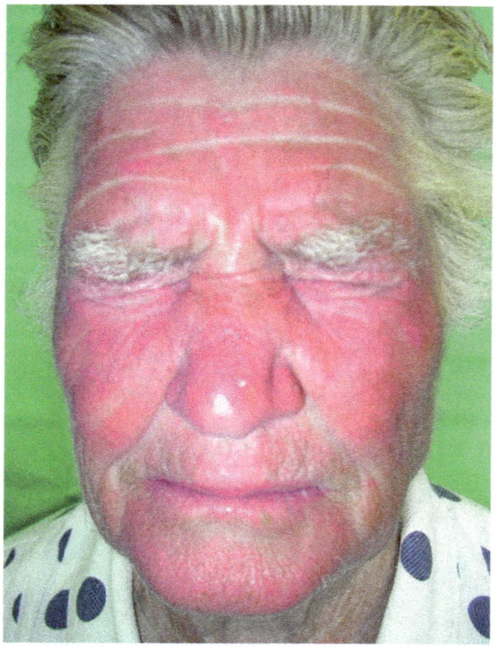

Phototoxicity
Photograph courtesy of SpringerImages Database, Springer Publishing Company

Phototoxicity (phytophotodermatitis)

A. Tissue damage results form a nonimmunologic interaction of ultraviolet light with furocoumarins (8- and 5-methoxypsoralen) in plants such as celery, limes and other citrus fruits, fig, mustard, scurf pea, buttercup
B. Photodistributed linear, geometric, bizarre patterned red patches, plaques, and bullae
C. After 1–2 weeks, linear, geometric, bizarre patterned hyperpigmented patches form which are slow to resolve

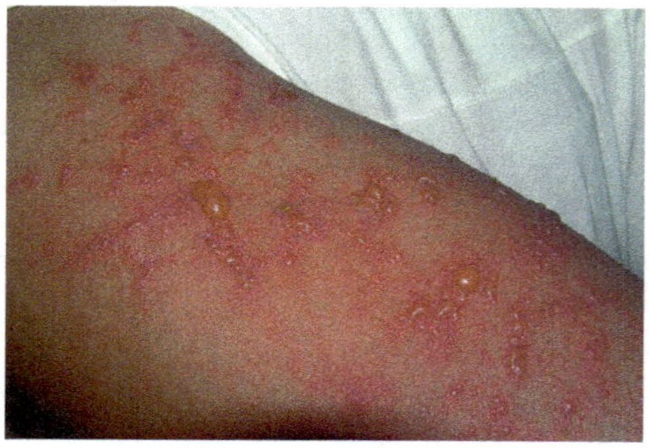

Phototoxicity
Photograph courtesy of SpringerImages Database, Springer Publishing Company

b. Photoallergy

Photoallergic reactions

A. Occur as a result of cell-mediated hypersensitivity to an allergen activated or produced by the effect of ultraviolet radiation on a drug (or its metabolite)
B. Ultraviolet radiation is required to convert the drug to an immunologically active compound
C. Most common drugs—thiazide diuretics, sulfonamide antibiotics, sulfonylureas, phenothiazines
D. Lesions occur on sun-exposed sites, are pruritic, may resemble dermatitis or lichen planus, and over time may lichenify
E. Chronic actinic dermatitis: chronic exposure to a photoallergic drug leads to extreme photosensitivity that persists months or years even after the drug is eliminated

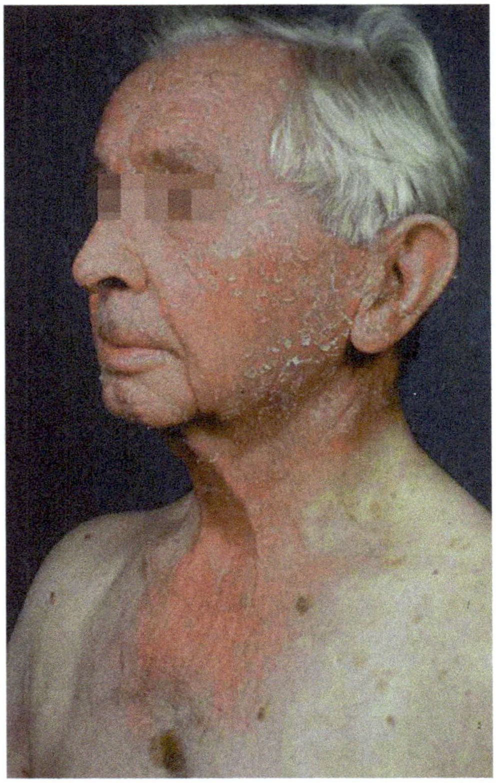

Photoallergy
Photograph courtesy of SpringerImages Database, Springer Publishing Company

Photoallergic reaction

A. Lichenoid lesions and pigmentation in the photoexposed areas

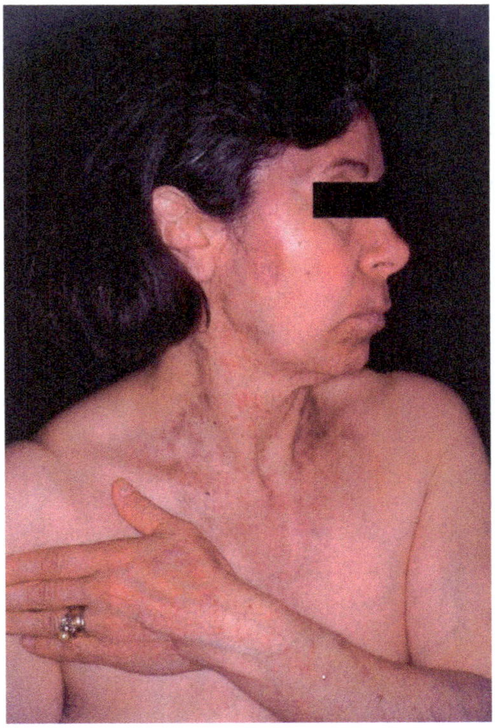

Photoallergy
Photograph courtesy of SpringerImages Database, Springer Publishing Company

c. Actinic Damage

i. Actinic Purpura

Actinic purpura

A. Ecchymoses from minor trauma due to poor dermal support of blood vessels in elderly patients with thin, actinically damaged skin

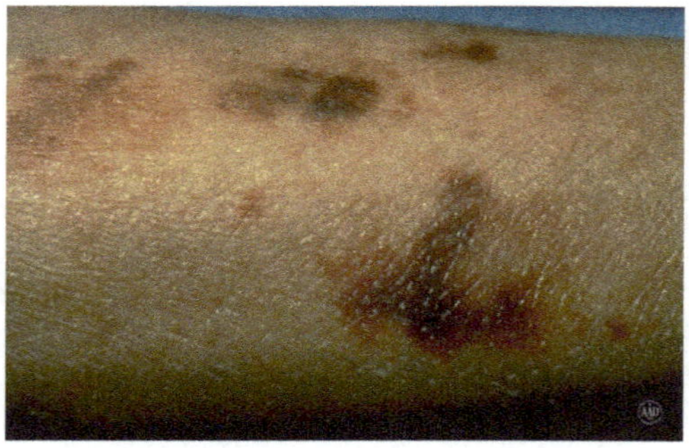

Actinic purpura
Courtesy of the American Academy of Dermatology

ii. Poikiloderma of Civatte

Poikiloderma of civatte

A. Atrophy, mild hyperpigmentation, and reticulated red–red brown mottled patches with telangiectasias (poikiloderma)
B. Arises on the lateral and inferior aspects of neck, usually sparing perifollicular skin and the central submental region

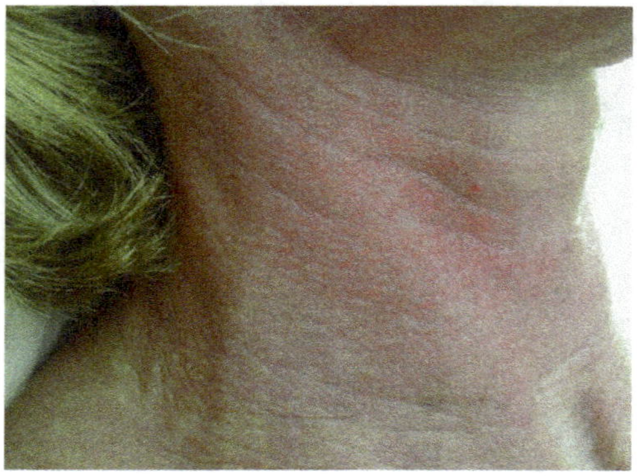

Poikiloderma of civatte
Photograph courtesy of SpringerImages Database, Springer Publishing Company

d. Polymorphous Light Eruption

Polymorphous light eruption (PMLE)

A. Most common photodermatosis
B. Usually occurs during spring or early summer, second or third decade of life
C. Pruritic erythematous grouped edematous papules, vesicles, or plaques within minutes to hours of sun exposure
D. Vesicles, bullae, papulovesicles, and confluent red swelling may occur, especially on the face
E. Most common on the face, ears, neck, outer arms, and dorsal hands, but there may be widespread involvement of sun-exposed areas
F. Helices of the ears (especially in boys) may be involved, often with vesicles (juvenile spring eruption)
G. In dark skin, most common morphology is grouped pinhead-sized papulovesicles on sun-exposed areas
H. Usually lasts for a few days

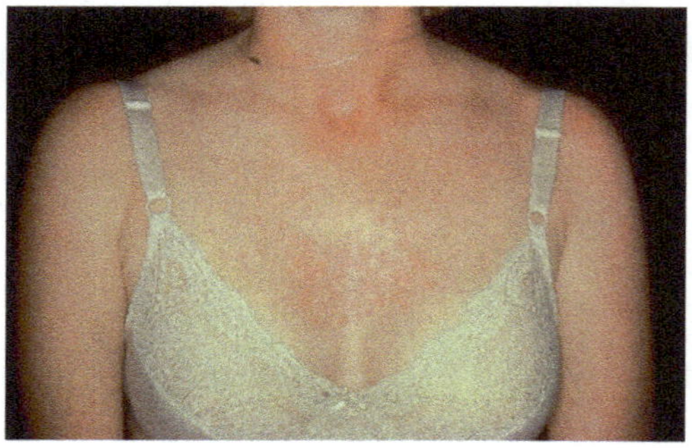

Polymorphous light eruption
Photograph courtesy of SpringerImages Database, Springer Publishing Company

Polymorphous light eruption (PMLE)

A. Pruritic erythematous grouped edematous papules, vesicles, or plaques within minutes to hours of sun exposure

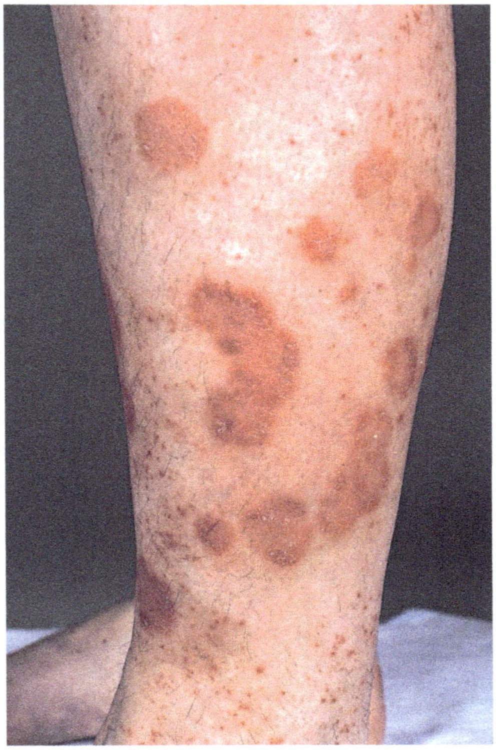

Polymorphous light eruption
Photograph courtesy of SpringerImages Database, Springer Publishing Company

e. Chronic Actinic Dermatitis

Chronic actinic dermatitis

A. Photodistributed eczematous dermatitis with sparing in the photo-protected area behind the ear and under the chin which may become generalized
B. Seen most often in older patients with regular sun exposure in warm climates
C. Chronic exposure to a photoallergic drug leads to extreme photosensitivity that persists months or years even after the drug is eliminated
D. Patch test sensitivity may exist to plant antigens, fragrances, topical meds

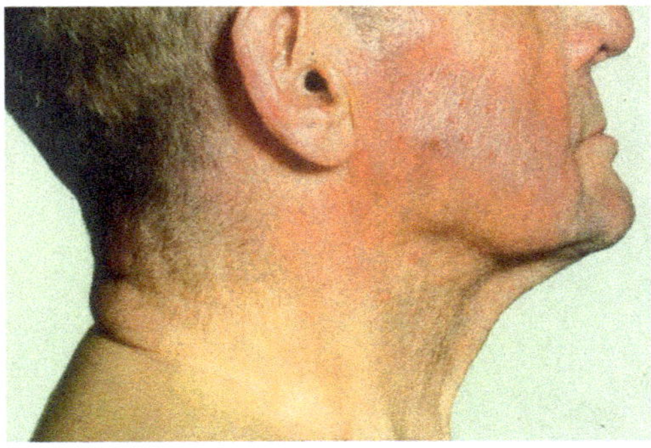

Chronic actinic dermatitis
Photograph courtesy of SpringerImages Database, Springer Publishing Company

Radiation Dermatitis 99

a. Acute Radiation Dermatitis

Acute radiation dermatitis

A. Erythema, edema, vesiculation, and desquamation may lead to hemorrhagic crusting and erosions, all within the area that received radiation therapy, which results in a well-demarcated patch or plaque with linear borders

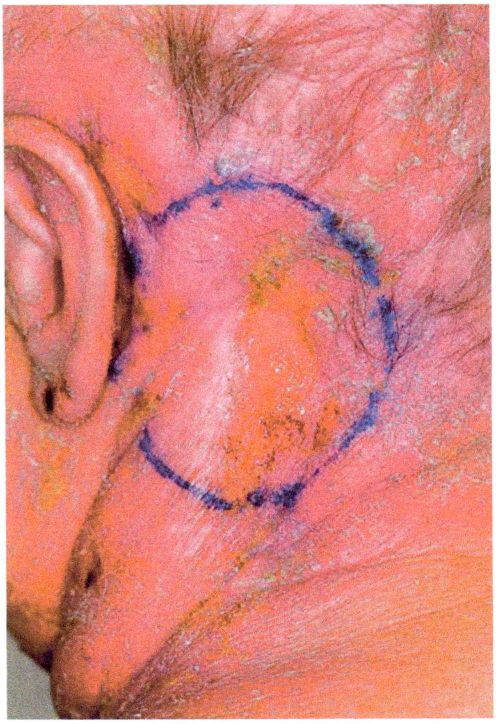

Acute radiation dermatitis
Photograph courtesy of SpringerImages Database, Springer Publishing Company

H.M. Gloster, Jr. et al., *Absolute Dermatology Review: Mastering Clinical Conditions on the Dermatology Recertification Exam*, DOI 10.1007/978-3-319-03218-4_99, © Springer International Publishing Switzerland 2016

b. Chronic Radiation Dermatitis

Chronic radiation dermatitis

A. Poikilodermatous changes (hyper- or hypopigmentation, telangiectasia, atrophy), scarring, alopecia, and ulceration within the area that received treatment
B. May present as a well-demarcated atrophic indurated white to yellow patch or plaque with telangiectasias and linear borders
C. Appears months to years after treatment

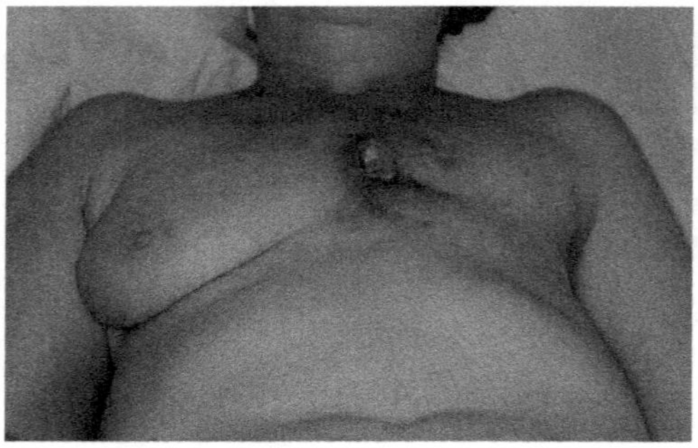

Chronic radiation dermatitis
Photograph courtesy of SpringerImages Database, Springer Publishing Company

Chapter XV

Drug Reactions, Erythemas, and Urticarias

Drug Reactions

100

a. Acute Generalized Exanthematous Pustulosis

Acute generalized exanthematous pustulosis (AGEP)

A. Acute, febrile drug reaction (90 % drug induced) characterized by numerous countless small nonfollicular sterile pustules arising within large areas of edematous erythema (figures a and b)
B. Begins on face and intertriginous areas (axilla and groin), then spreads over a few hours

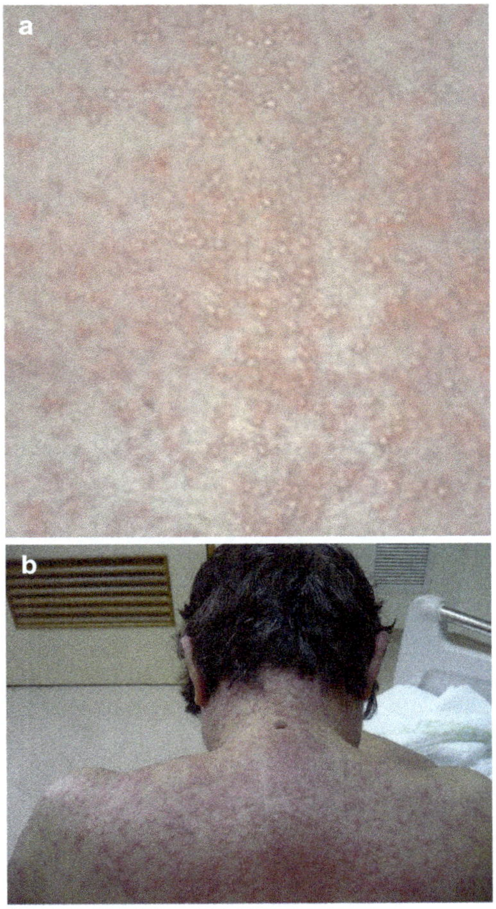

Acute generalized exanthematous pustulosis
Photograph courtesy of SpringerImages Database, Springer Publishing Company

H.M. Gloster, Jr. et al., *Absolute Dermatology Review: Mastering Clinical Conditions on the Dermatology Recertification Exam*, DOI 10.1007/978-3-319-03218-4_100,

b. Drug Induced Hyperpigmentation

Drug induced hyperpigmentation

A. Amiodarone: blue-grey hyperpigmentation on sun-exposed areas (figures a and b)

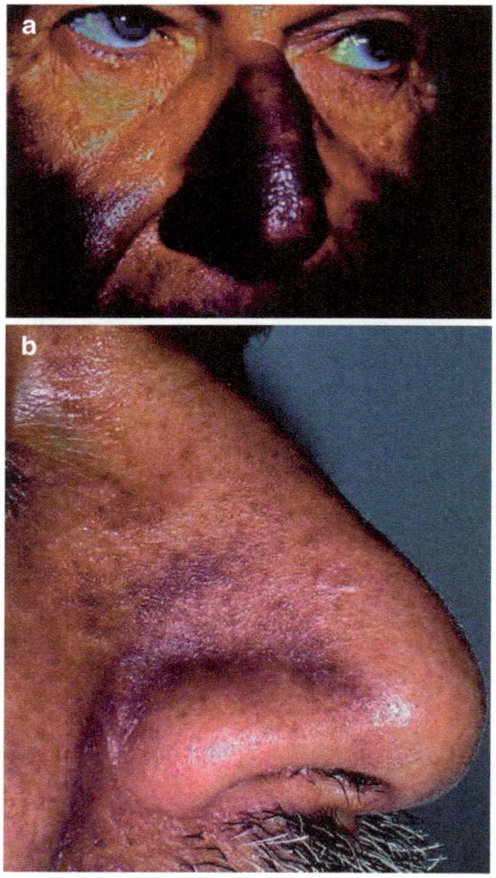

Drug induced hyperpigmentation
Photograph courtesy of SpringerImages Database, Springer Publishing Company

Drug induced hyperpigmentation

A. Minocycline
   1. Type 1: blue black discoloration in sites of inflammation and scars (e.g., acne), not dose related
   2. Type II: blue gray macules or patches within normal skin, usually the shins (figure a)
      a. May be misdiagnosed as ecchymoses
      b. More frequent with higher cumulative dose
   3. Type III: diffuse muddy brown pigmentation on sun-exposed areas (figure b)
      a. More frequent with higher cumulative doses
   4. Nails: blue black discoloration of the full nail plate of multiple nails

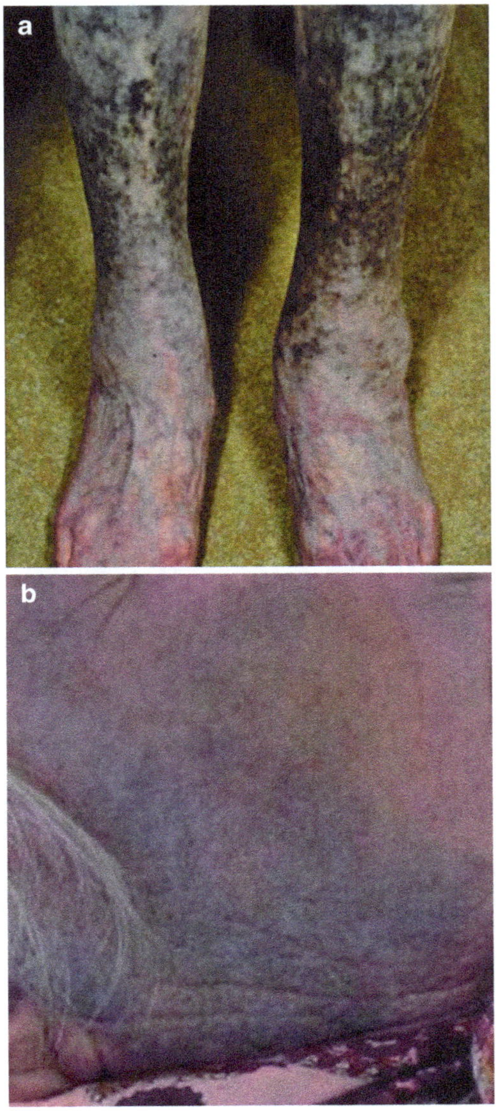

Drug induced hyperpigmentation
Photograph courtesy of SpringerImages Database, Springer Publishing Company

Drug induced hyperpigmentation

A. Type II minocycline-induced hyperpigmentation with blue gray patches on the shins

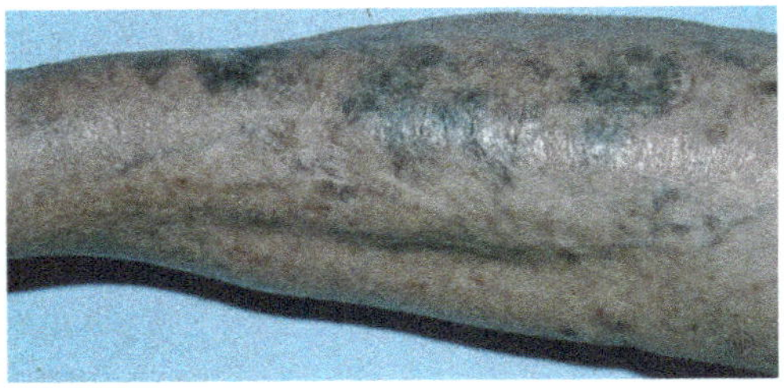

Drug induced hyperpigmentation
Photograph courtesy of the American Academy of Dermatology

c. Drug Reaction with Eosinophilia and Systemic Symptoms (DRESS)

Drug reaction with eosinophilia and systemic symptoms (DRESS)

A. Drug-induced hypersensitivity syndrome (anticonvulsants and sulfonamides most common)
B. Usually occurs 2–6 weeks after drug (later than most drug reactions)
C. Symptoms
   1. Fever
   2. Cutaneous eruption
      a. Morbilliform eruption, then edematous papules with follicular accentuation (figure a)
         – May also see vesicles/bullae (produced by dermal edema), pustules, erythroderma, exfoliative dermatitis
         – Most commonly on the face, upper trunk, and extremities
      b. Facial edema is the hallmark (figure b)
   3. Eosinophilia
   4. Adenopathy
   5. Sequelae
      a. Herpes virus reactivation
      b. Autoimmune diseases—more likely in young patients
         – Type 1 diabetes
         – Thyroiditis
         – Lupus
      c. End organ failure—more likely in elderly patients
         – Hepatitis: the liver is the most common and severe site of visceral involvement and is responsible for most deaths
         – Myocarditis
         – Pneumonitis
         – Nephritis

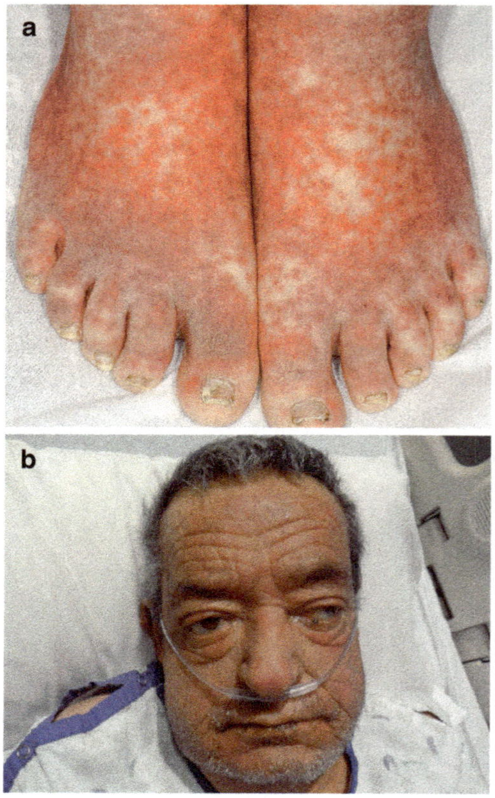

Drug reaction with eosinophilia and systemic symptoms
Photograph Courtesy of Adam Ingraffea, MD

d. Fixed Drug Eruption

Fixed drug eruption

A. First develops 1–2 weeks after exposure, then within 24 hours with subsequent exposures
B. May recur at the same sites
C. One or a few round sharply demarcated erythematous edematous plaques with a dusky violaceous hue (figure a)
   1. A central erosion or blister may develop
   2. Progressively fade over several days leaving dark brown postinflammatory hyperpigmentation
D. Favors periorificial and acral areas (lips, face, hands, feet, and genitals) but may be generalized (figure b)

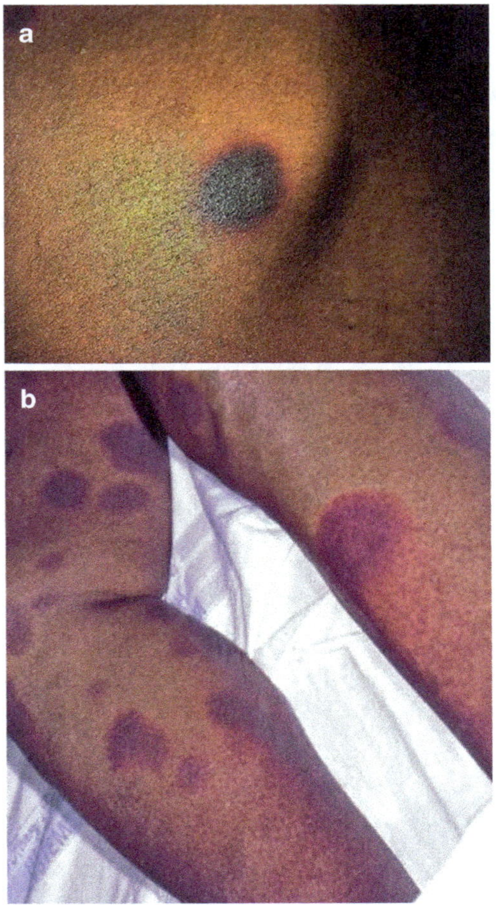

Fixed drug eruption
Photograph courtesy of SpringerImages Database, Springer Publishing Company

e. Erythema Multiforme

Erythema multiforme

A. Two types of target lesions
   1. Typical, with three different zones (bullseye or target-like appearance)
      a. Oval or circular pink urticarial plaques with a central dusky zone (may evolve into bullae or crust) surrounded by two concentric rings of erythema: one pale pink ring which is then surrounded by a pink red outermost ring (figures a and b)
      b. 1–4 cm in diameter
   2. Atypical papular, which has two zones with an ill-defined border
B. No mucosal involvement
C. Lesions favor the extremities and face (acrofacial)
   1. Symmetrically distributed acral lesions on palms (figure a), soles, dorsal hands and feet, extensor arms and legs
   2. Widespread target lesions in 10 %

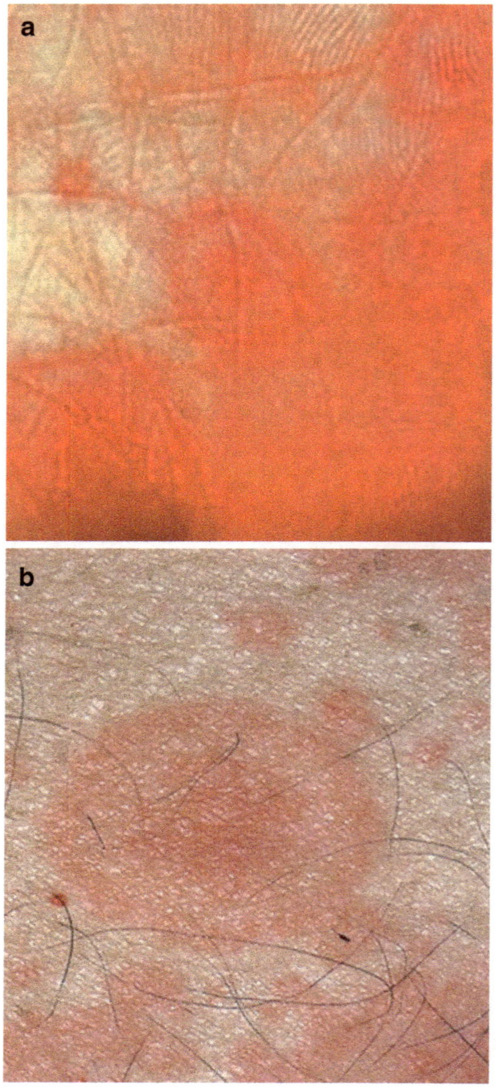

Erythema multiforme
Photograph courtesy of SpringerImages Database, Springer Publishing Company

Erythema multiforme

A. Targetoid plaques with central crusting on the leg

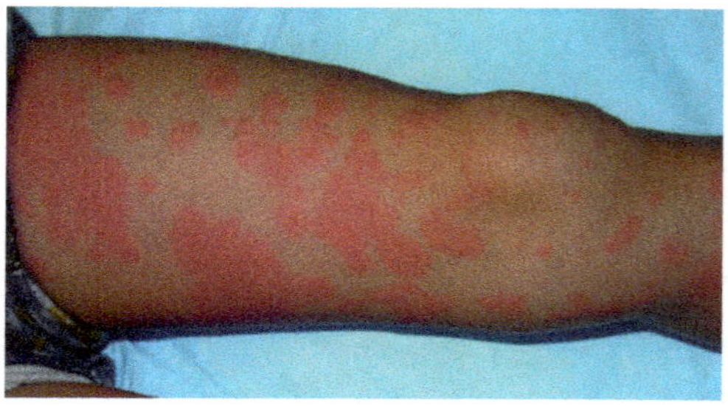

Erythema multiforme
Photograph courtesy of SpringerImages Database, Springer Publishing Company

f. Stevens Johnson Syndrome and Toxic Epidermal Necrolysis

Stevens-Johnson syndrome (SJS) and Toxic Epidermal Necrolysis (TEN)

A. Both are drug reactions of differing severity characterized by mucocutaneous tenderness, erythema, and extensive exfoliation with separation of skin at dermoepidermal junction
B. SJS may progress to TEN
C. Clinical features
   1. Tender erythema and erosions of mucosal areas—seen in 90 %
      a. Buccal area and lips (figure a)
      b. Ocular (conjunctival disease is very common)
      c. Genital mucosa
   2. Involvement of the epithelium of the respiratory and gastrointestinal tract (esophagitis, diarrhea) is also seen
   3. Skin lesions
      a. Atypical target lesions: coalescent dusky red or purpuric macules (figures a and b)
      b. At onset, the macules may have a dusky center, which then takes on a gray hue and may progress to multiple sites of epidermal detachment forming flaccid blisters (figure b)
      c. Lesions first appear on trunk, then spread to neck, face, proximal upper extremities
      d. Skin looks like wet cigarette paper when pulled away with trauma leaving large areas of raw bleeding dermis resembling scalded skin (figure b)
      e. Nikolsky sign—tangential pressure within an erythematous area induces a cleavage in the dermoepidermal junction
      f. Body surface area of epidermal attachment determines SJS, TEN, or overlap: SJS less than 10 %, SJS/TEN overlap 10–30 %, TEN greater than 30 %

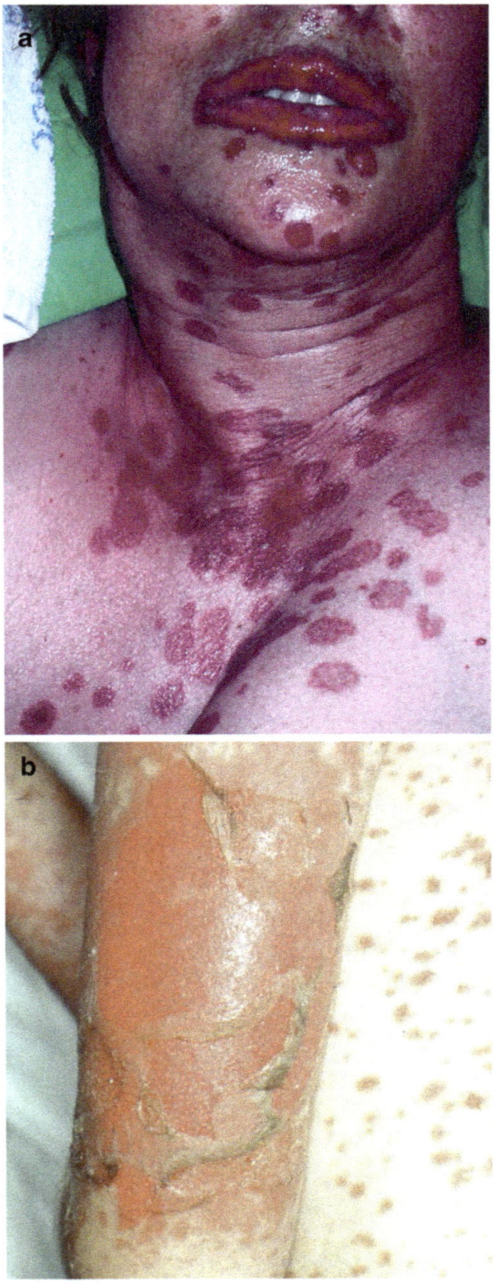

Stevens Johnson syndrome and toxic epidermal necrolysis
Photograph courtesy of SpringerImages Database, Springer Publishing Company

SJS/TEN overlap syndrome

A. Disseminated erosions and some bullae on the back of a patient with SJS/TEN overlap syndrome

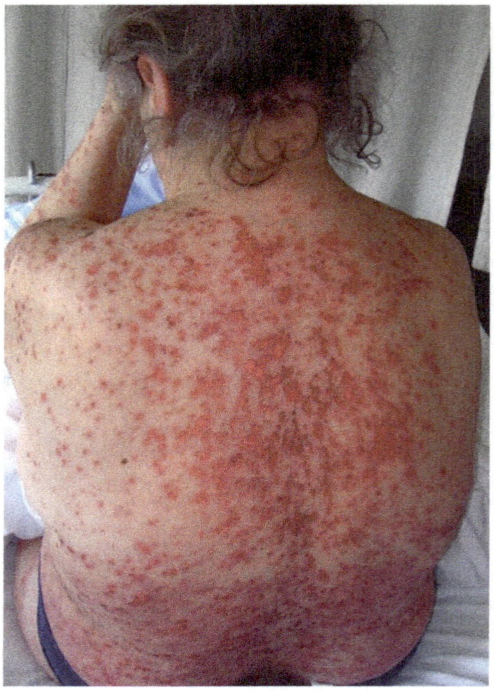

Stevens Johnson syndrome and toxic epidermal necrolysis overlap syndrome
Photograph courtesy of SpringerImages Database, Springer Publishing Company

Toxic epidermal necrolysis

A. Widespread epithelial loss greater than 30 % of the total body surface area in a TEN patient

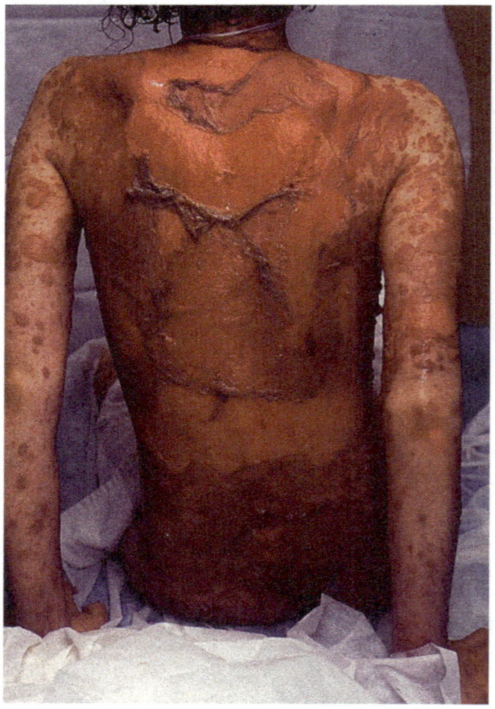

Toxic epidermal necrolysis
Photograph courtesy of SpringerImages Database, Springer Publishing Company

g. Steroid Induced Atrophy

i. Steroid Induced Epidermal Atrophy

Steroid-induced epidermal atrophy: fine wrinkling or shiny appearance of the skin

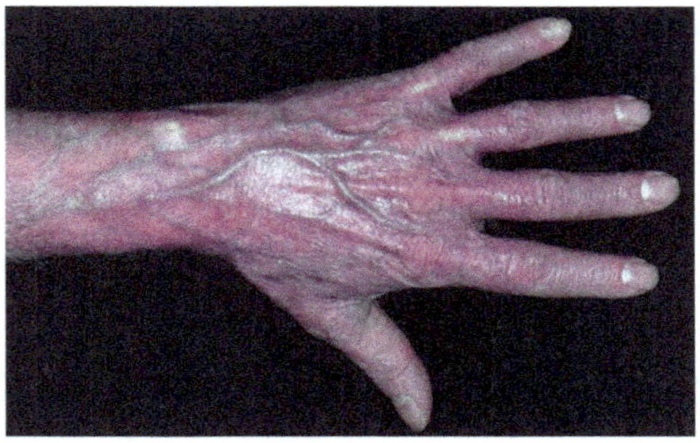

Steroid induced atrophy
Photograph courtesy of SpringerImages Database, Springer Publishing Company

ii. Steroid Induced Dermal Atrophy

Steroid induced dermal atrophy

A. Fragility
B. Visible vessels
C. Striae (figure a)
   1. Multiple symmetric well-defined linear atrophic depressions of the skin
   2. Initially appear as red to violaceous elevated lines (striae rubra), over time the color fades and lesions become atrophic and wrinkled (striae alba) and are permanent

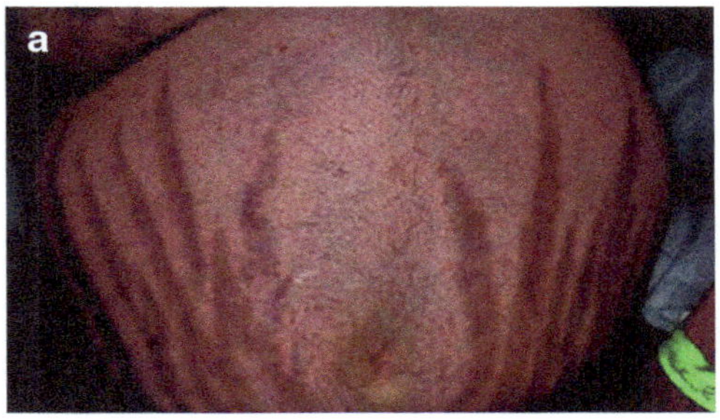

Steroid induced striae
Photograph courtesy of SpringerImages Database, Springer Publishing Company

iii. Steroid Induced Fat Atrophy

Steroid induced fat atrophy

A. Loss of fat causes a depression

B. Usually caused by steroid injections

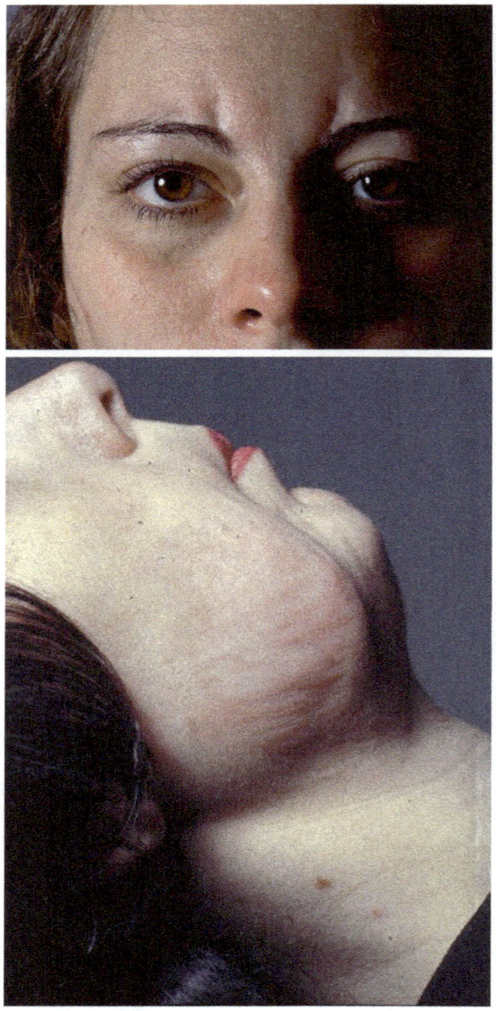

Steroid induced fat atrophy
Photograph courtesy of the Mayo Clinic Department of Dermatology, Rochester MN

h. Morbilliform Drug Eruption

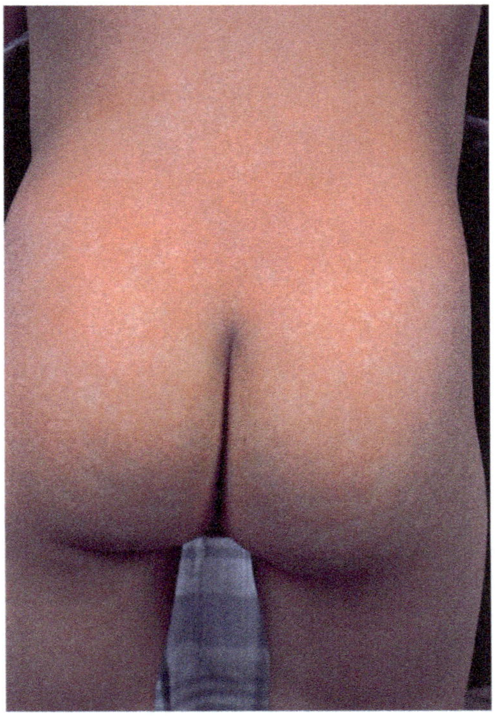

Morbilliform drug eruption
Photograph courtesy of SpringerImages Database, Springer Publishing Company

Morbilliform (exanthematous) drug eruptions

A. Most common drug reaction
B. Usually begins 7–14 days after medication is given, goes away in 1–2 weeks
C. Pruritic blanchable erythematous macules and papules that begin on the trunk and spread to the extremities in a symmetric fashion and progressively become confluent
D. Mucous membranes and palmoplantar surfaces are spared
E. Viral exanthems have a similar clinical presentation

Erythemas 101

a. Figurate Erythemas

i. Erythema Annulare Centrifigum

Erythema annulare centrifugum

A. May be a hypersensitivity reaction to many different antigens such as infections (especially dermatophytes), drugs, neoplasms, molds (e.g., blue cheese), food (e.g., tomatoes), and endocrinopathies
B. Firm pink papules which slowly expand centrifugally to form annular polycyclic plaques with scale trailing the leading edge and central clearing (figures a and b)
   1. A lesion may expand quickly more than 6 cm in 1–2 weeks
C. Superficial form
   1. Lesions are minimally elevated with scale at the inner margin (trailing scale)
   2. Pruritic, usually on hips and thighs
D. Deep form
   1. Advancing edges are elevated (infiltrated), and there is no trailing scale
   2. Nonpruritic

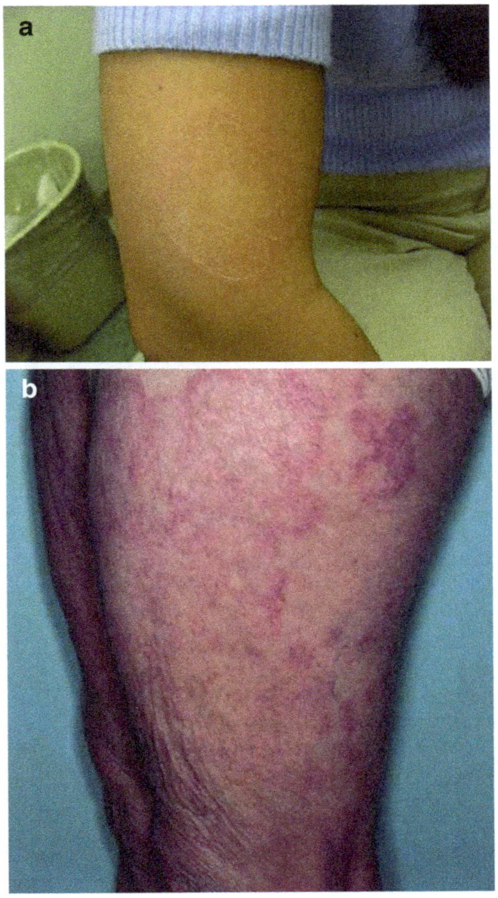

Figurate erythemas: erythema annulare centrifigum Photograph courtesy of SpringerImages Database, Springer Publishing Company

H.M. Gloster, Jr. et al., *Absolute Dermatology Review: Mastering Clinical Conditions on the Dermatology Recertification Exam*, DOI 10.1007/978-3-319-03218-4_101, © Springer International Publishing Switzerland 2016

ii. Erythema Gyratum Repens

Erythema gyratum repens

A. Migratory figurate wavy bands of erythema with trailing scale at the edge forming concentric rings with a wood grain appearance (rings within rings)
B. Rapid peripheral spread (up to 1 cm per day)
C. Paraneoplastic syndrome, usually lung cancer but also cancer of the breast, esophagus, and stomach
D. Resolves when cancer is treated

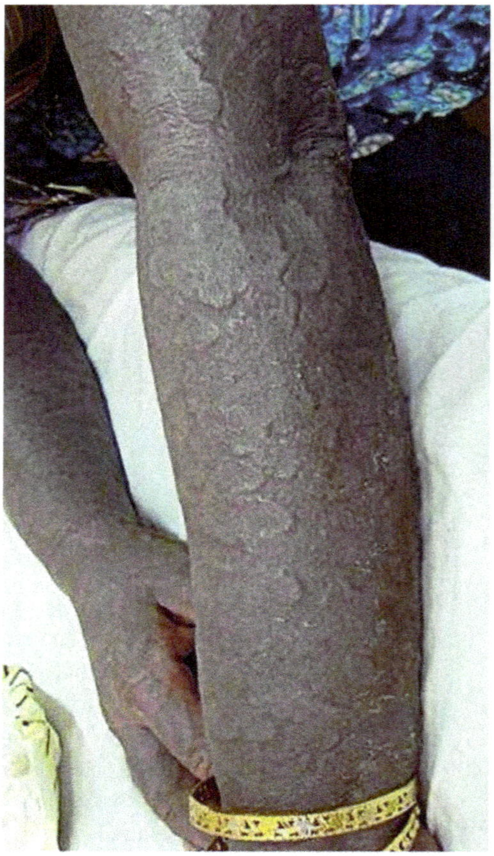

Figurate erythemas: erythema gyratum repens
Photograph courtesy of SpringerImages Database, Springer Publishing Company

iii. Erythema Chronicum Migrans

Erythema chronicum migrans

A. Develops at the site of a borrelia-infected tick bite, seen in 60–90 % of patients with Lyme disease
B. Annular nonscaling erythematous expanding superficial plaque with central clearing that is the initial cutaneous sign of Lyme disease (figures a and b)
C. Appears 1–2 weeks after the bite and resolves within 1 month
D. Light-colored center may give a bull's eye or target appearance with a red center at the tick bite site, around which is a lighter color, then a peripheral red rim
E. Target may expand up to 5 cm
F. Multiple lesions may be present in 25 % of patients due to spirochetemia or lymphatic spread

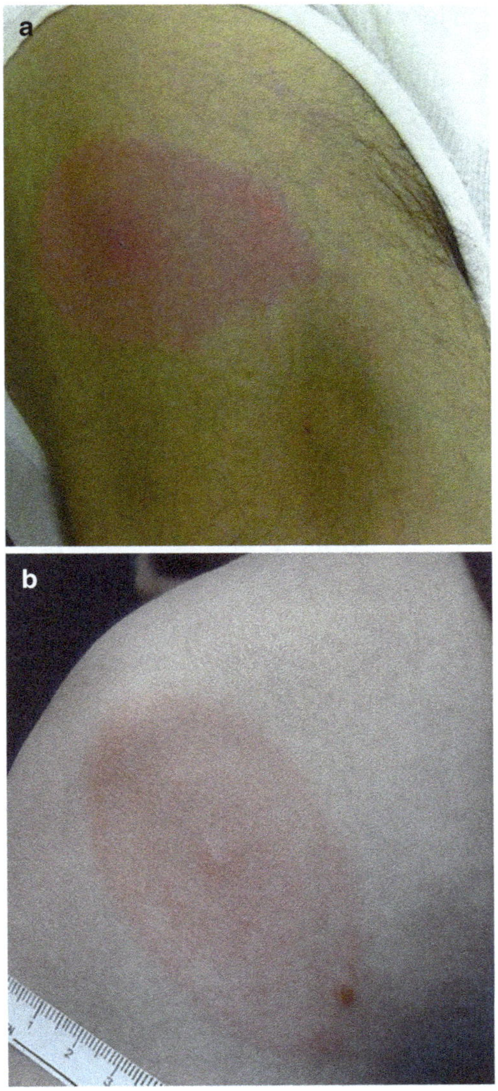

Figurate erythemas: erythema chronicum migrans
Photograph courtesy of SpringerImages Database, Springer Publishing Company

b. Necrolytic Acral Erythema

Necrolytic acral erythema

A. Associated with hepatitis C viral infection
B. Primarily involves acral sites (hands and feet, dorsum more common)
C. Flaccid blisters and erosions evolve into painful or pruritic red-brown thick hyperkeratotic plaques with thick brown scale
D. Waxes and wanes

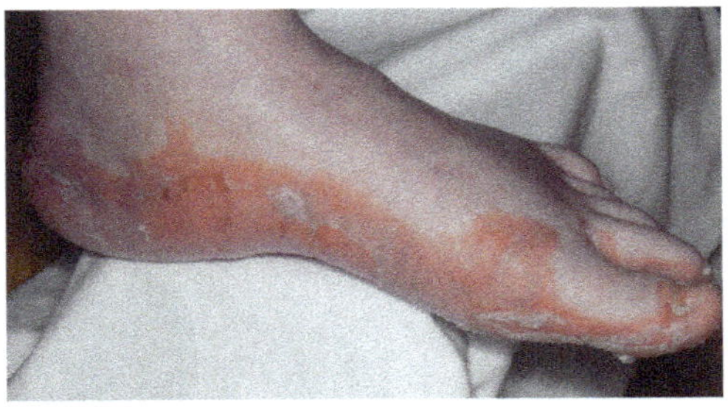

Necrolytic acral erythema
Photograph courtesy of the Mayo Clinic Department of Dermatology, Rochester MN

c. Necrolytic Migratory Erythema

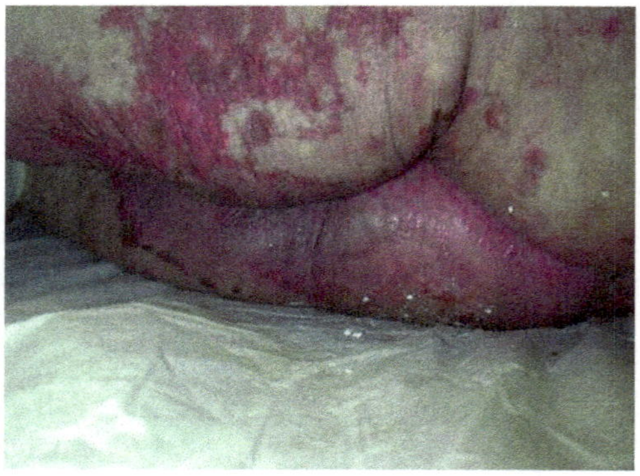

Necrolytic migratory erythema
Photograph courtesy of SpringerImages Database, Springer Publishing Company

Necrolytic migratory erythema

A. Cutaneous manifestation of the glucagonoma syndrome—glucagon-secreting islet cell pancreatic tumor
B. Superficial epidermal necrosis leading to flaccid bullae and crusted erythematous eroded patches and plaques with a circinate, polycyclic, or annular appearance
C. Most commonly occurs on the face (especially perioral), intertriginous areas (perineum, groin, buttocks, thighs), flexural folds, and distal extremities
D. May look like intertrigo or seborrheic dermatitis
E. Remits and recurs over weeks to months
F. Rash precedes tumor in 67 %
G. Angular cheilitis and glossitits (beefy red tongue) may also be seen
H. Most patients are ill at presentation with weight loss, adult-onset diabetes (hyperglycemia), stomatitis, diarrhea, anemia, conjunctivitis

Necrolytic migratory erythema

A. Erythematous, erosive, desquamating plaques

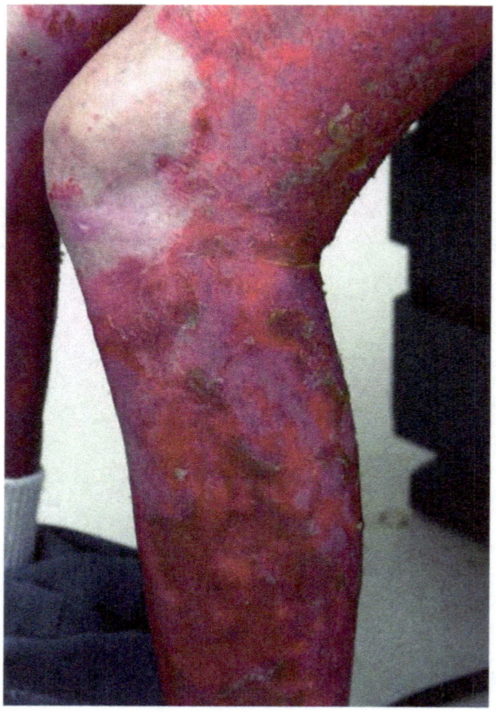

Necrolytic migratory erythema
Photograph courtesy of SpringerImages Database, Springer Publishing Company

Urticarias

102

a. Urticaria

Urticaria

A. Lasts less than 24 hours (transient)
B. May be idiopathic or triggered by infections, foods, medications
C. Wheals: superficial dermal swellings characterized by pruritic edematous pink plaques with central pallor which may be small, large, papular, circinate, polycyclic, or annular

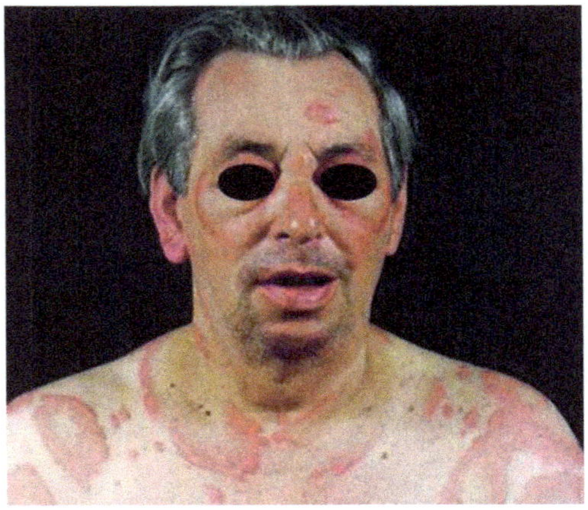

Urticaria
Photograph courtesy of SpringerImages Database, Springer Publishing Company

H.M. Gloster, Jr. et al., *Absolute Dermatology Review: Mastering Clinical Conditions on the Dermatology Recertification Exam*, DOI 10.1007/978-3-319-03218-4_102,

i. Uriticaria – Dermatographism

Dermatographism

A. A type of physical urticaria which is triggered by an external physical stimulus
B. Wheals are usually located on stimulated skin
C. Simple dermatographism—5 % of normal people represents an exaggerated physiological response
D. Symptomatic dermatographism—linear wheals at sites of friction or scratching (figures a and b)

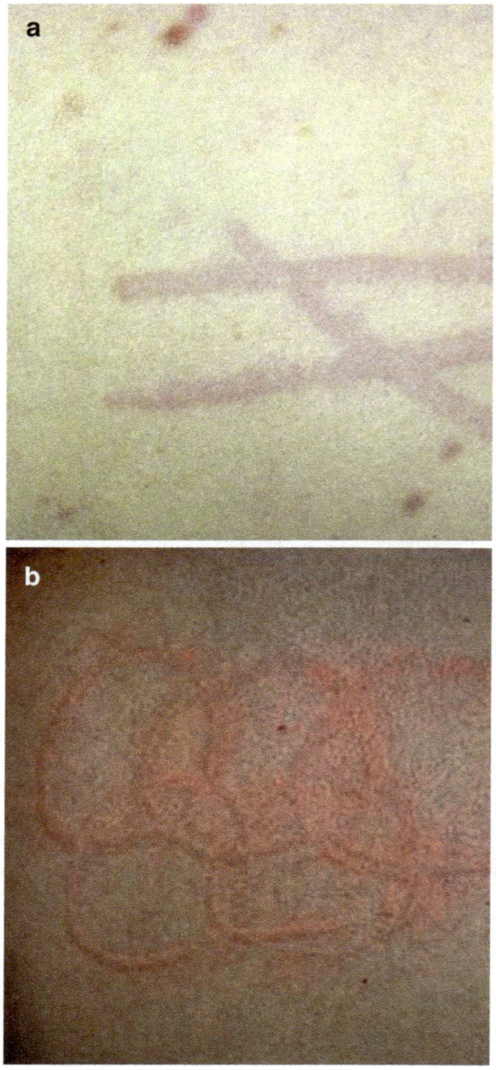

Uriticaria – dermatographism
Photograph courtesy of SpringerImages Database, Springer Publishing Company

ii. Delayed Pressure Urticaria

Delayed pressure urticarial

A. Type of physical urticaria
B. Deep red pruritic painful swellings at sites of sustained pressure after a delay of 30 min to 12 hours and may persist for days
C. Common sites include the waistline below tight clothes, below elastic socks, feet in tight shoes, genitalia after intercourse, palms after manual work, soles after walking

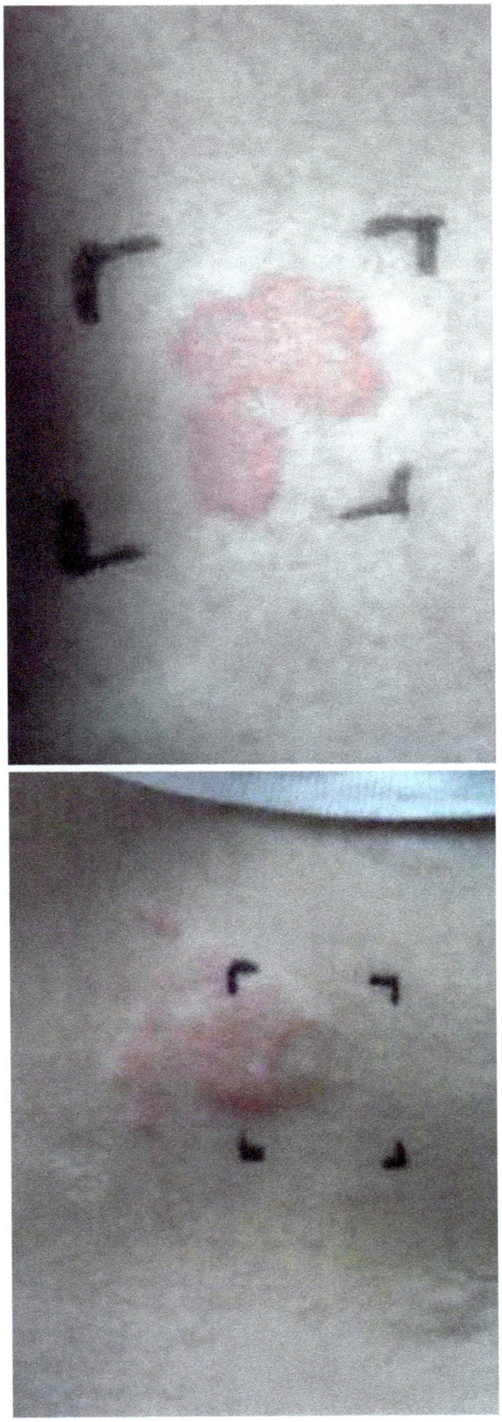

Delayed pressure urticarial
Photograph courtesy of SpringerImages Database, Springer Publishing Company

iii. Cold Induced Urticaria

Cold induced urticaria

A. A type of physical urticaria
B. Whealing within minutes of rewarming after cold exposure such as rainy windy cold weather or after ice cube contact

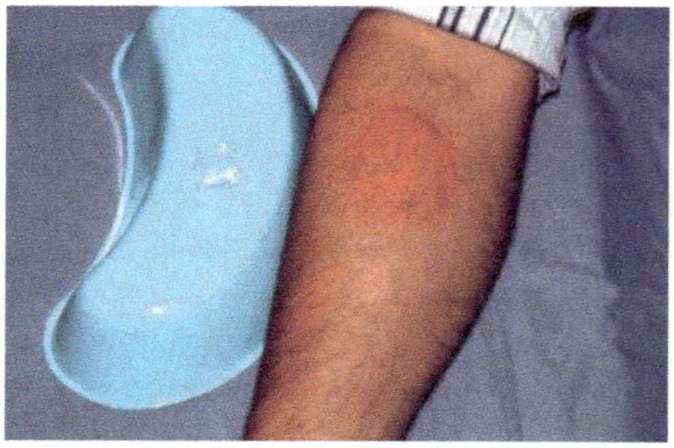

Cold induced urticaria
Photograph courtesy of SpringerImages Database, Springer Publishing Company

iv. Cholinergic Urticaria

Cholinergic (heat induced) urticaria

A. A type of physical urticaria
B. Multiple transient papular monomorphic wheals (2–3 mm in diameter) surrounded by an erythematous flare
C. Occur within 15 min of perspiration-inducing stimuli (e.g., physical exertion, hot baths, sudden emotional distress, alcohol, spicy food)

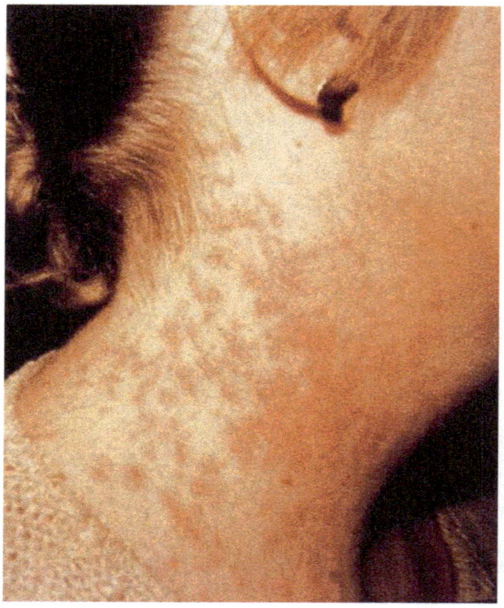

Cholinergic urticaria
Photograph courtesy of SpringerImages Database, Springer Publishing Company

v. Solar Urticaria

Solar urticaria

A. A type of physical urticaria
B. Itching and wheals occur within minutes after exposure to ultraviolet light or visible light on exposed areas

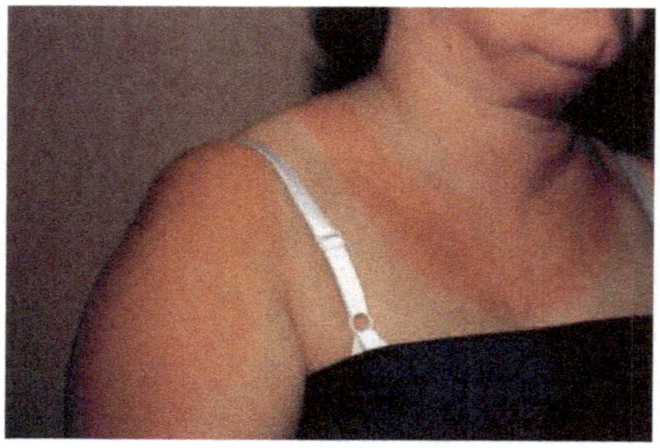

Solar urticaria
Photograph courtesy of SpringerImages Database, Springer Publishing Company

b. Angioedema

Angioedema

1. Acute transient swellings without erythema deep in the dermis and subcutaneous tissue or submucosal tissue
2. Most commonly on the lips and periorbital area

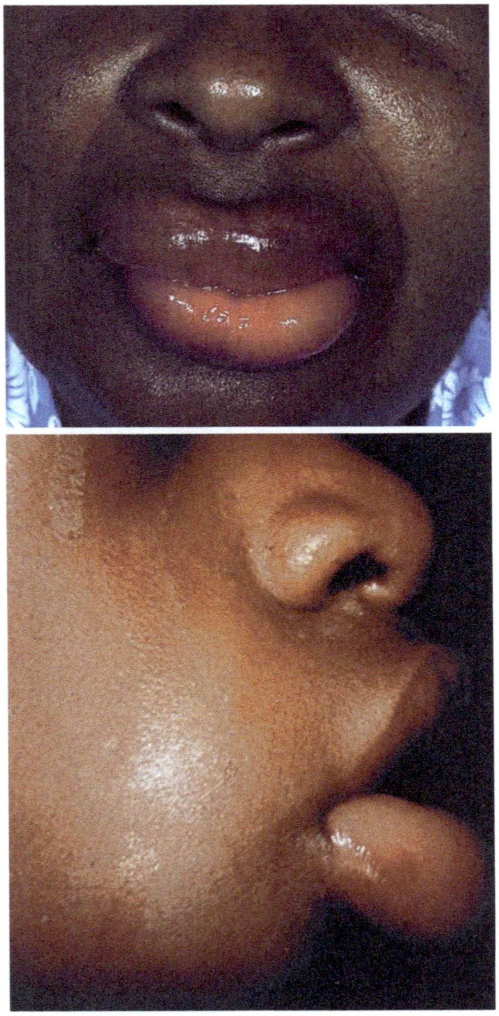

Angioedema
Photograph courtesy of SpringerImages Database, Springer Publishing Company

103 Polymorphic Eruption of Pregnancy

Polymorphic eruption of pregnancy (formerly known as pruritic and urticarial papules and plaques of pregnancy: PUPPP)

A. Pruritic urticarial vesiculopapules and urticarial plaques appear within the abdominal striae with periumbilical sparing (pemphigoid gestationis begins in the umbilical area)
   1. Subsequently spreads to trunk and extremities
   2. Polymorphous features (vesicles, erythema, target lesions, eczematous lesions) appear as disease progresses and spreads
B. Usually begins during the latter portion of the third trimester (85 %) or immediately postpartum (15 %)
C. Usually resolves within 4 weeks and does not recur
D. More common in primigravida women
E. No maternal or fetal risk

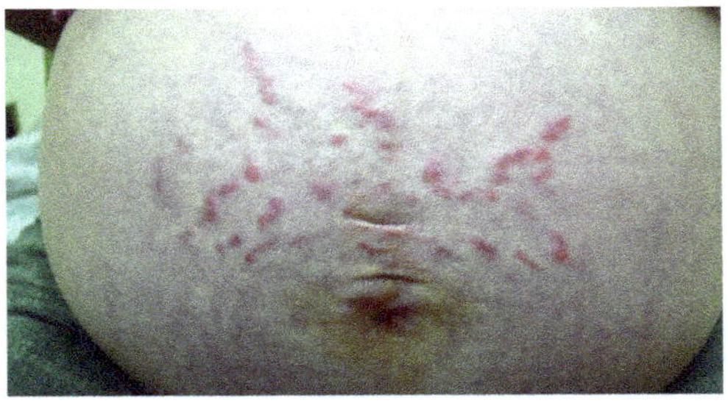

Polymorphic eruption of pregnancy
Photograph courtesy of SpringerImages Database, Springer Publishing Company

Polymorphic eruption of pregnancy (formerly known as pruritic and urticarial papules and plaques of pregnancy: PUPPP)

A. Pruritic urticarial vesiculopapules and urticarial plaques appear within the abdominal striae with periumbilical sparing (figure a)
B. Subsequently spreads to trunk and extremities (figure b)

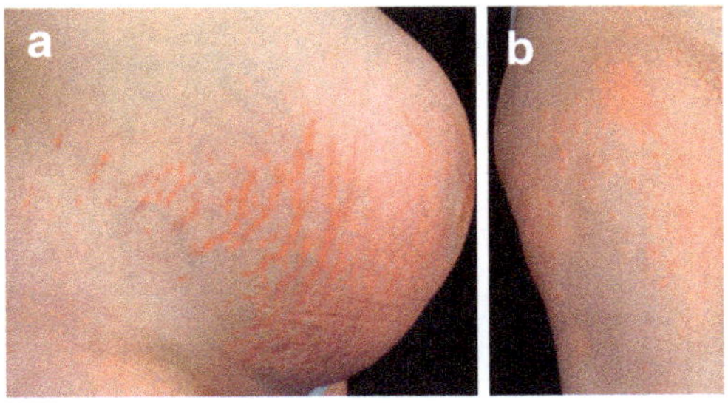

Polymorphic eruption of pregnancy
Photograph courtesy of SpringerImages Database, Springer Publishing Company

H.M. Gloster, Jr. et al., *Absolute Dermatology Review: Mastering Clinical Conditions on the Dermatology Recertification Exam*,
DOI 10.1007/978-3-319-03218-4_103, © Springer International Publishing Switzerland 2016

Chapter XVI

Vascular and Lymphatic Disorders

Telangiectasias

104

a. Spider Angioma

Spider angioma

A. Central, rasied red papule (central feeding arterial vessel) with multiple small radiating dilated vessels
B. Seen in otherwise healthy people, especially women and children
C. Multiple lesions may occur with pregnancy, liver disease, or oral contraceptives

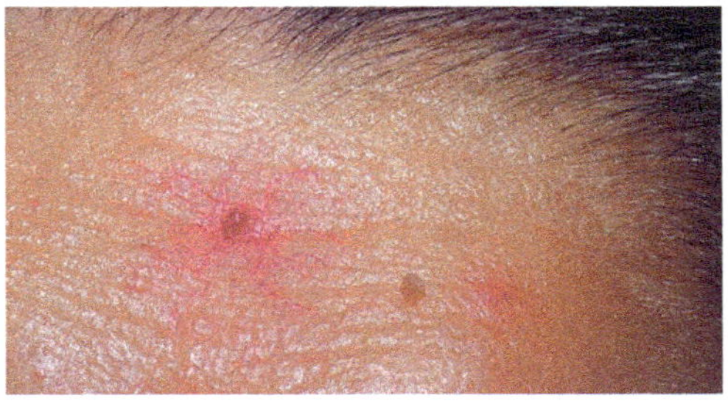

Spider angioma
Photograph courtesy of SpringerImages Database, Springer Publishing Company

b. Generalized Essential Telangiectasia

Generalized essential telangiectasia

A. Adult women usually but occasionally childhood
B. Most commonly occurs on the limbs, especially the distal legs as sheets of telangiectasias (may spread proximally with time as the "upward march")

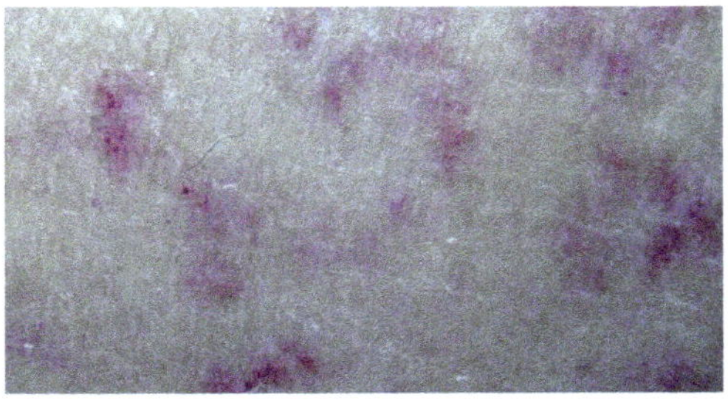

Generalized essential telangiectasia
Photograph courtesy of SpringerImages Database, Springer Publishing Company

c. Unilateral Nevoid Telangiectasia

Unilateral nevoid telangiectasia

A. Segmental unilateral distribution of discrete telangiectasias most commonly located on the area innervated by the trigeminal, cervical, and upper thoracic dermatomes
B. Congenital and acquired forms exist
C. May be related to increased estrogen receptors in blood vessels in the area or increased estrogen levels (pregnancy, liver disease, puberty)

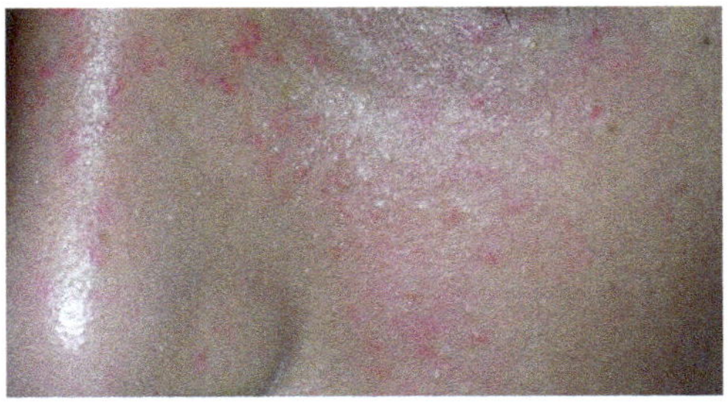

Unilateral nevoid telangiectasia
Photograph courtesy of SpringerImages Database, Springer Publishing Company

H.M. Gloster, Jr. et al., *Absolute Dermatology Review: Mastering Clinical Conditions on the Dermatology Recertification Exam*,
DOI 10.1007/978-3-319-03218-4_104,

d. Livedo Reticularis

Livedo reticularis

A. Common physiological finding consisting of a mottled red to bluish discoloration occurring in a net-like reticulated vascular pattern due to alterations in blood flow through cutaneous microvasculature

B. May be congenital (cutis marmorata telangiectatica congenita), acquired (physiological response to cold), or associated with underlying systemic disease

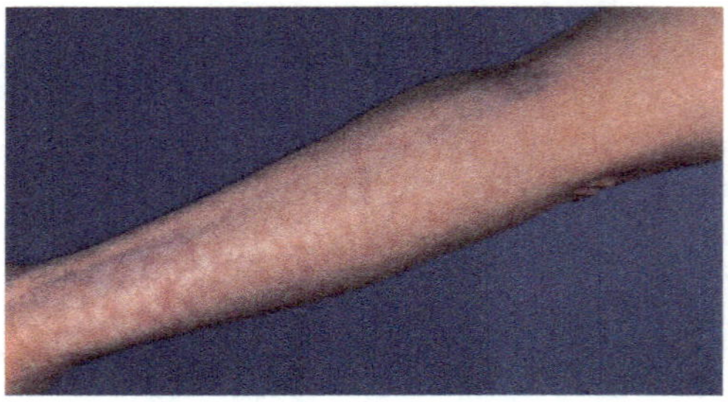

Livedo reticularis
Photograph courtesy of SpringerImages Database, Springer Publishing Company

Livedo reticularis associated with systemic disease

A. Livedo reticularis in a patient with antiphospholipid syndrome

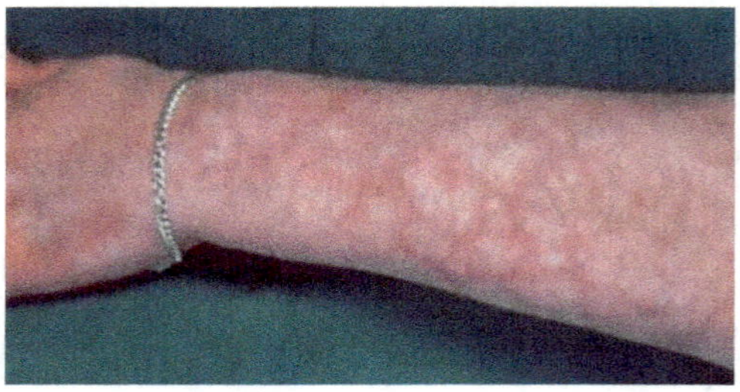

Livedo reticularis
Photograph courtesy of SpringerImages Database, Springer Publishing Company

Livedo reticularis associated with systemic disease

A. Livedo reticularis in a patient with polyarteritis nodosa (figure a)
B. Livedo reticularis in a patient with Sneddon's syndrome (figure b)

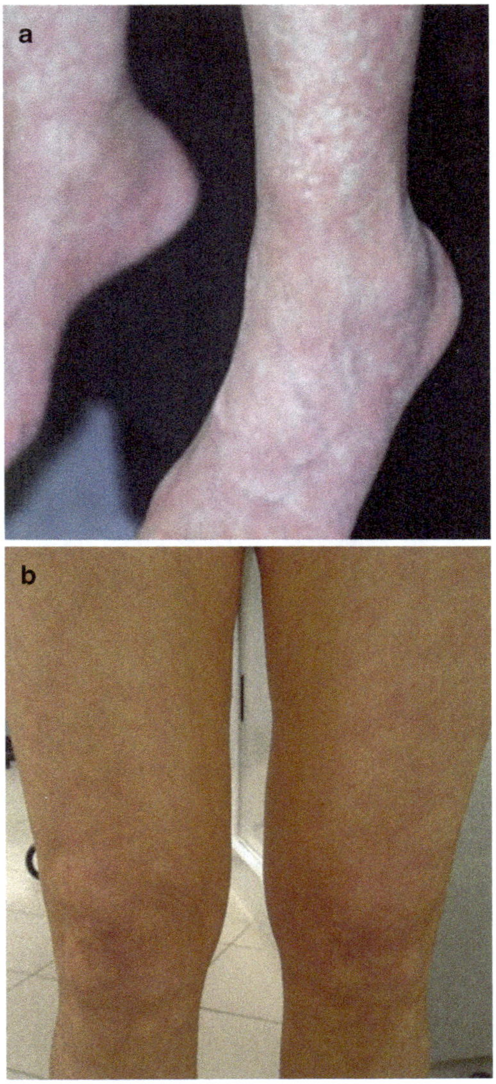

Livedo reticularis
Photograph courtesy of SpringerImages Database, Springer Publishing Company

105 Hemangioma

a. Superficial Hemangioma

Hemangioma

A. Most common soft tissue tumor of infancy
B. Usually appear in the first several weeks of life
C. May occur anywhere but most common on head and neck
D. Red telangiectatic, bluish bruise, or white anemic macule is seen at birth in 50 % of patients
E. Superficial hemangiomas (figures a and b)
   1. Located in superficial dermis
   2. Bright red strawberry-like papules and plaques with a cobblestone, lobulated surface are present during the proliferative phase (strawberry hemangioma)
   3. Most common type

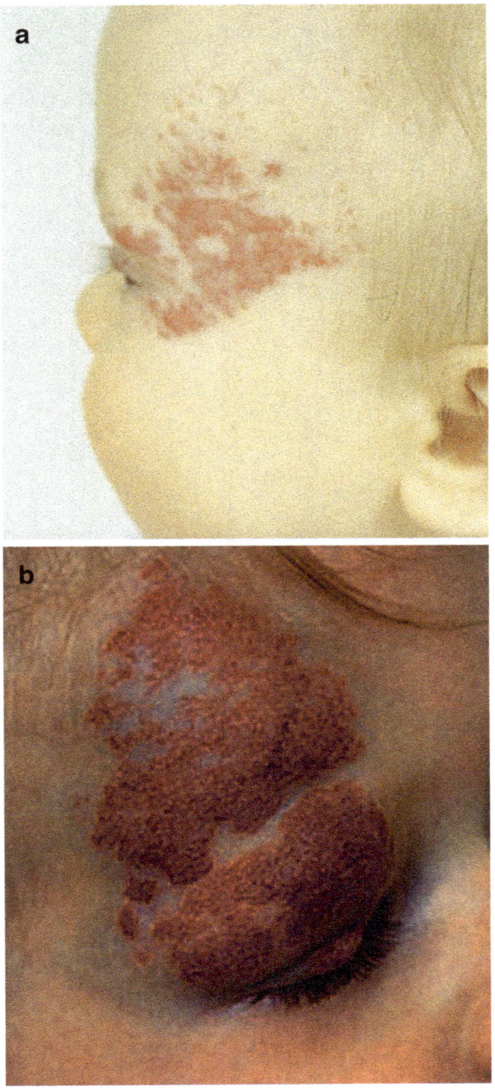

Superficial hemangioma
Photograph courtesy of SpringerImages Database, Springer Publishing Company

H.M. Gloster, Jr. et al., *Absolute Dermatology Review: Mastering Clinical Conditions on the Dermatology Recertification Exam*, DOI 10.1007/978-3-319-03218-4_105, © Springer International Publishing Switzerland 2016

b. Mixed Hemangioma

Hemangioma
- A. Mixed hemangioma
  1. Both superficial and deep components
  2. Second most common type
  3. A well-defined red vascular plaque overlying a larger, poorly circumscribed light blue nodule (figure a)
- B. Typical growth patterns
  1. Proliferation
     - a. Most growth occurs between 3 and 5 months of age
     - b. Early proliferative phase (rapid increase in size)
     - c. Later proliferative phase (continued growth at a slower rate)
  2. Gradual spontaneous involution over several years
     - a. May begin as early as the first year of life and continue for several years
     - b. Regresses by 10 % per year, 50 % regressed by 5 years of age
     - c. Color changes from bright red to gray purple, and 50 % leave fibrofatty tissue, atrophy, and/or telangiectasias (figure b)

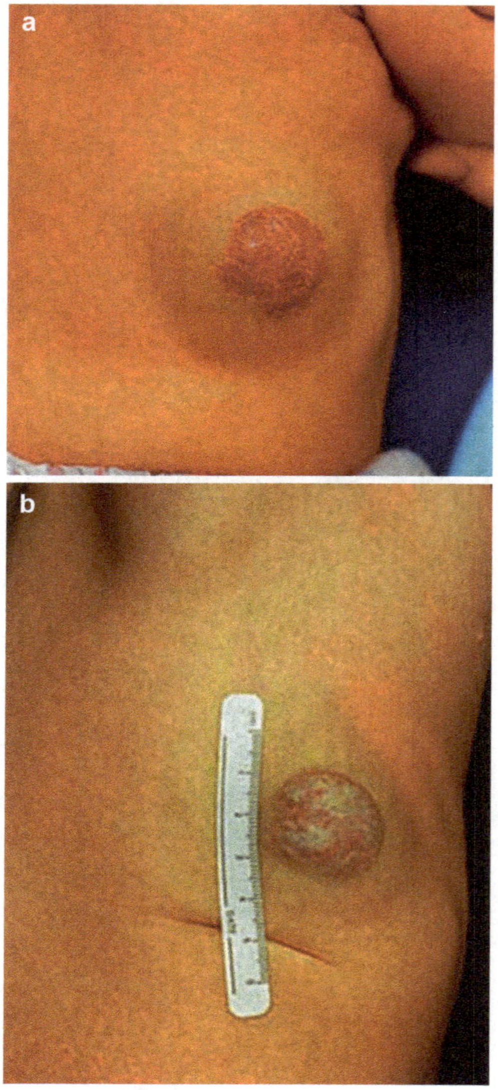

Mixed hemangioma
Photograph courtesy of SpringerImages Database, Springer Publishing Company

c. Deep Hemangioma

Deep hemangioma (cavernous hemangioma)

a. Located in the deep dermis or subcutaneous tissue
b. Not apparent until after a few weeks of age
c. Warm, ill-defined light blue purple rubbery masses with minimal overlying skin changes (figures a and b)

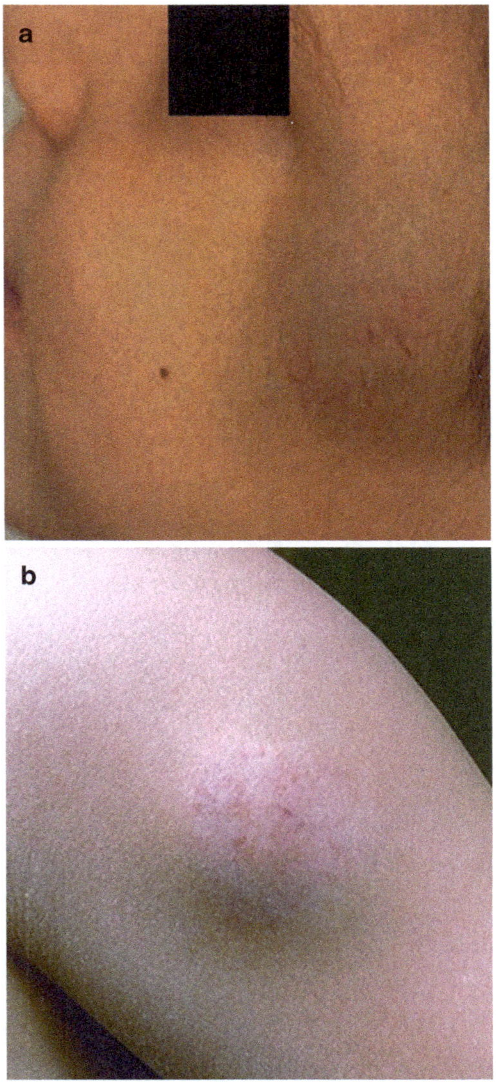

Deep hemangioma
Photograph courtesy of SpringerImages Database, Springer Publishing Company

Vascular Malformations

106

a. Capillary Malformation

i. Port Wine Stain

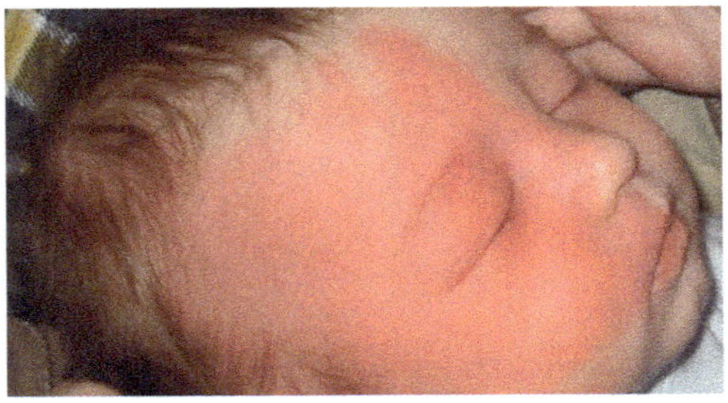

Port wine stain
Photograph courtesy of SpringerImages Database, Springer Publishing Company

Capillary malformation (port wine stain)

A. Red to red purple macular discoloration during infancy (does not have texture in infancy like hemangiomas)
B. Consists of superficial and deep dilated capillaries
C. Port wine stain (PWS)
   a. Type of capillary malformation
   b. Present at birth
   c. Facial PWS may be distributed along the cranial nerve five dermatome
   d. Facial lesions often become purple red during adulthood, and the skin may thicken
   e. Sturge-Weber Syndrome: a facial PWS usually located in the first division of the fifth cranial nerve sensory distribution and may be associated with ipsilateral ocular and leptomeningeal and brain anomalies

ii. Cutis Marmorata Telangiectatica Congenita

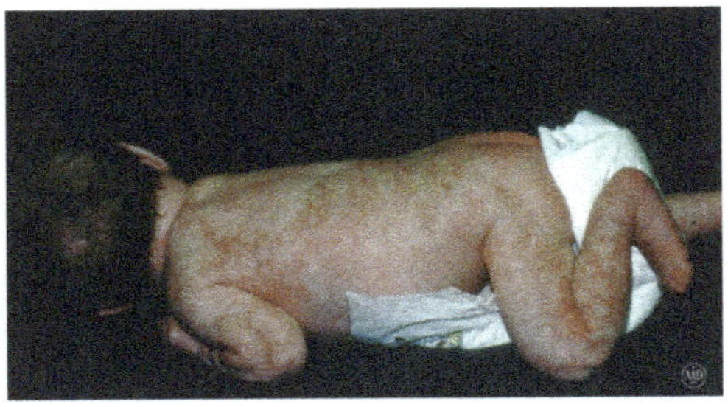

Cutis marmorata telangiectatica congenita
Photograph courtesy of the American Academy of Dermatology

Cutis marmorata telangiectatica congenita

A. Type of capillary malformation
B. Red purple reticulated violaceous patches with telangiectasia and sometimes prominent veins
C. Atrophic depressions and ulcerations may be seen, especially over joints
D. Affects one or more limbs and the corresponding quadrants of the trunk
E. Often present at birth, improves in first few years of life
F. May be associated with other anomalies (vascular malformations, limb asymmetry, neurological or ocular abnormalities)

H.M. Gloster, Jr. et al., *Absolute Dermatology Review: Mastering Clinical Conditions on the Dermatology Recertification Exam*,
DOI 10.1007/978-3-319-03218-4_106, © Springer International Publishing Switzerland 2016

Cutis marmorata telangiectatica congenita

A. Red purple reticulated violaceous patches with telangiectasia on the trunk and limbs

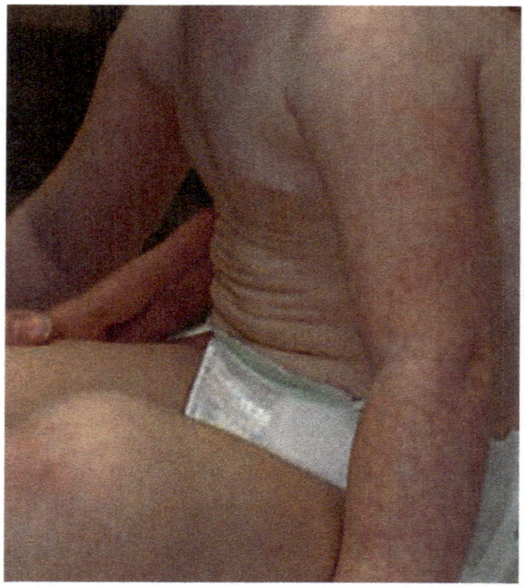

Cutis marmorata telangiectatica congenita
Photograph courtesy of SpringerImages Database, Springer Publishing Company

Cutis marmorata telangiectatica congenita

A. Atrophic depressions and ulcerations may be seen, especially over joints

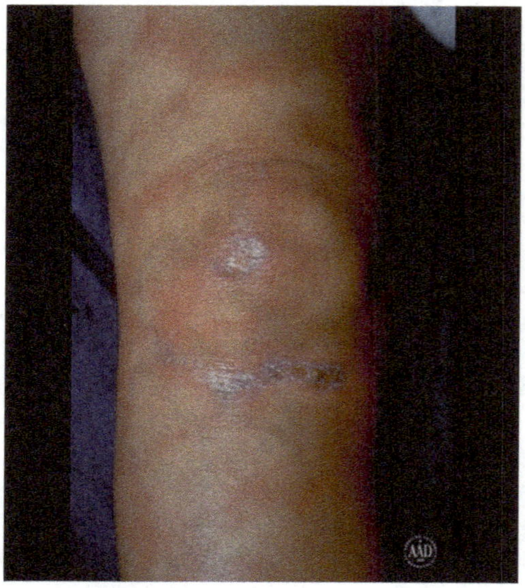

Cutis marmorata telangiectatica congenita
Photograph courtesy of the American Academy of Dermatology

Cutis marmorata telangiectatica congenita

A. Red purple reticulated violaceous patches with telangiectasia on a single limb

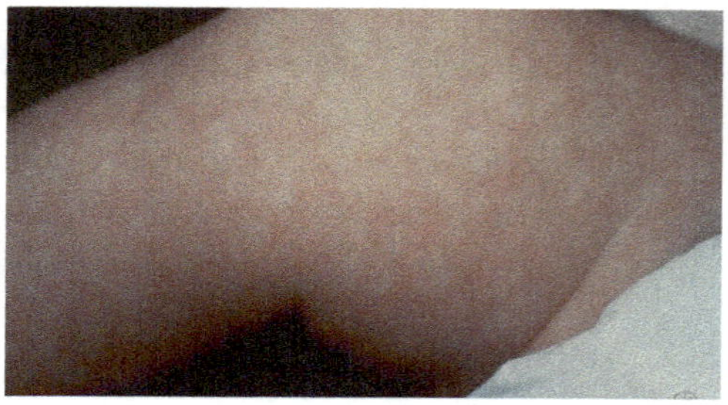

Cutis marmorata telangiectatica congenita
Photograph courtesy of the American Academy of Dermatology

iii. Klippel Trenaunay Syndrome

Kippel-Trenaunay syndrome

A. Limb capillary malformation or capillary lymphatic malformation associated with overgrowth of the affected extremity (soft tissue and bony hypertrophy) and varicocities

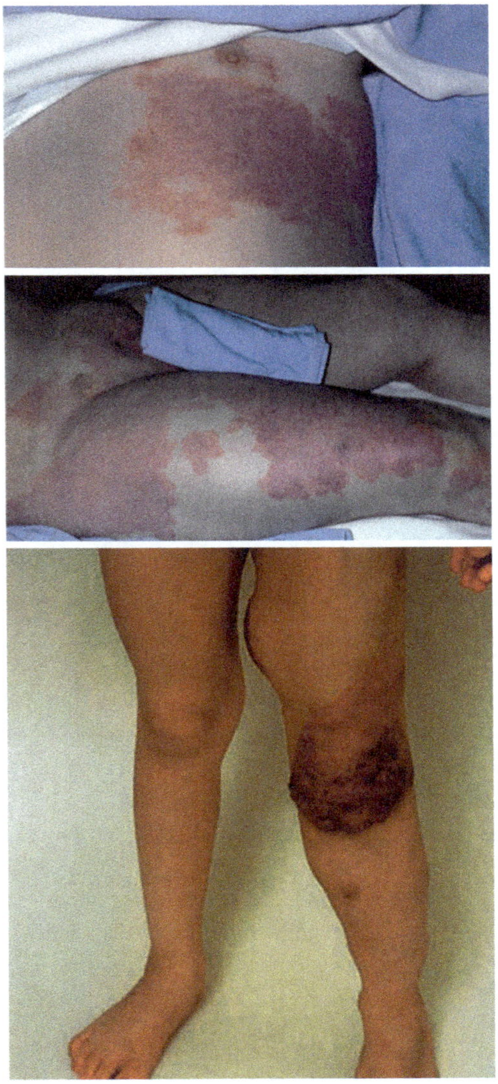

Klippel Trenaunay syndrome
Photograph courtesy of SpringerImages Database, Springer Publishing Company

iv. Hereditary Hemorrhagic Telangiectasia (Osler Weber Rendu)

Hereditary hemorrhagic telangiectasia (Osler Weber Rendu, also see Chap. 16, section 106a (iv))

A. Autosomal dominant
B. Epistaxis in childhood or adolescence
C. Telangiectasias of face, lips, tongue, palms, fingers
D. Visceral arteriovenous malformations of the lungs, brain, gastrointestinal and genitourinary tracts

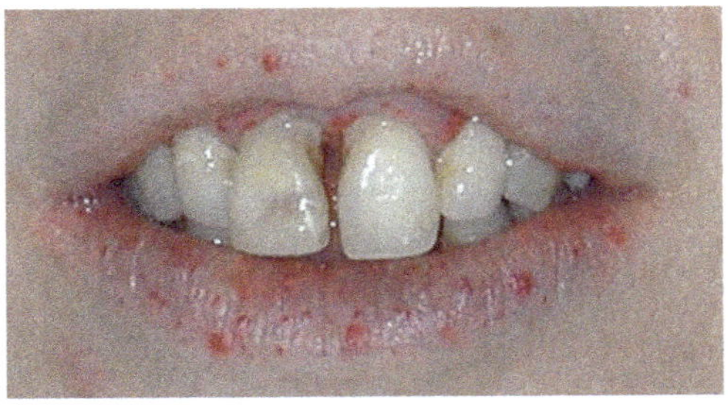

Hereditary hemorrhagic telangiectasia (Osler Weber Rendu)
Photograph courtesy of SpringerImages Database, Springer Publishing Company)

b. Venous Malformations

Venous malformation

A. Blue, soft, compressible and fills with dependency

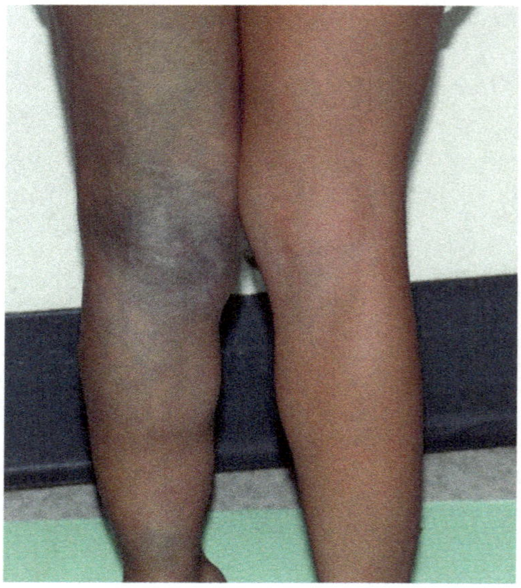

Venous malformation
Photograph courtesy of SpringerImages Database, Springer Publishing Company

i. Blue Rubber Bleb Nevus Syndrome

Blue rubber bleb nevus syndrome

A. Usually occurs sporadically, though autosomal dominant forms have been reported
B. Blue-purple, soft, rubbery, compressible subcutaneous nodules (venous malformations) which refill after being compressed or fill with dependency
C. Gastrointestinal and central-nervous-system vascular malformations may also occur

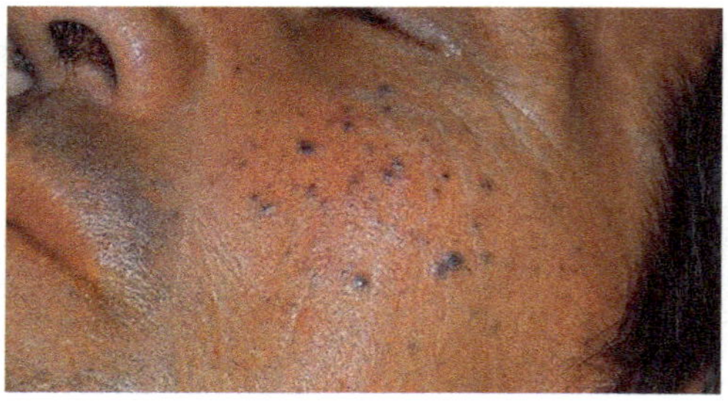

Blue rubber bleb nevus syndrome
Photograph courtesy of SpringerImages Database, Springer Publishing Company

c. Arteriovenous Malformation

Arteriovenous malformation (AVM)

A. Four stages
   1. Dormant: red, warm, macular (mimics capillary malformation) or slightly infiltrated (mimics late involuting infantile hemangioma) (figure b)
   2. Expansion: warm mass with thrill and throbbing, dilated draining veins (figure a)
   3. Destruction: pain, ulceration, occasional bone lysis and fracture
   4. Cardiac decompensation: high-output cardiac failure, also signs of stages 2 and 3

B. 40 % present at birth, 60 % appear later in life

C. Most commonly on the head

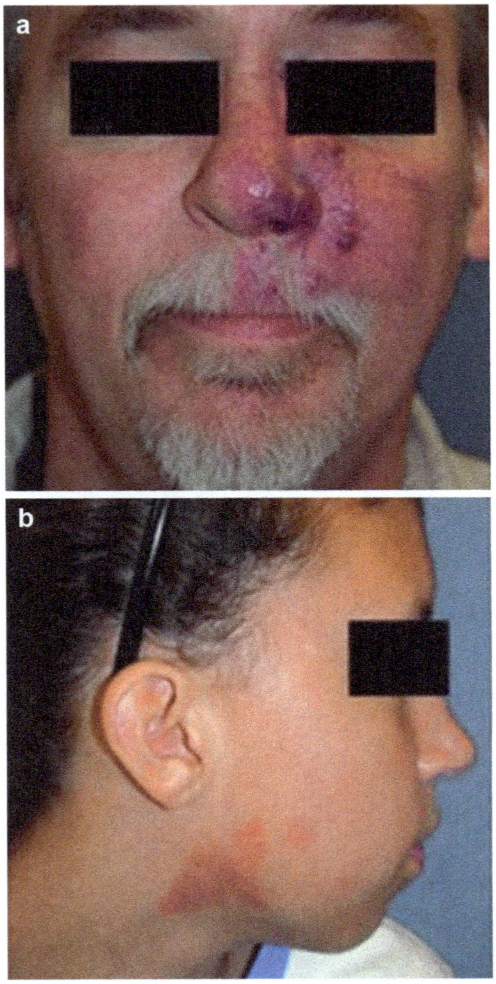

Arteriovenous malformations
Photograph courtesy of SpringerImages Database, Springer Publishing Company

Lymphatic Malformations

a. Lymphangioma Circumscriptum

Lymphangioma circumscriptum

A. Microcystic lymphatic malformation (hyperplasia of lymphatic network forming vesicles)
B. Most common type of lymphatic malformation
C. Plaques whose surface is covered with crops of clear to white ("milky white papules") or hemorrhagic vesicles or red to purple and skin-colored translucent papules resembling frog spawn
D. May occur anywhere on the skin (especially the chest and proximal limbs) and mouth
E. May be much more extensive than they appear

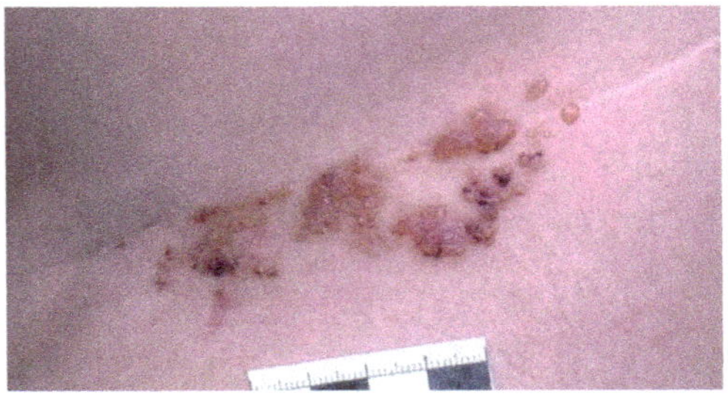

Lymphangioma circumscriptum
Photograph courtesy of SpringerImages Database, Springer Publishing Company

Lymphangioma circumscriptum

A. Clear and hemorrhagic vesicles resembling "frog's spawn" in a linear array

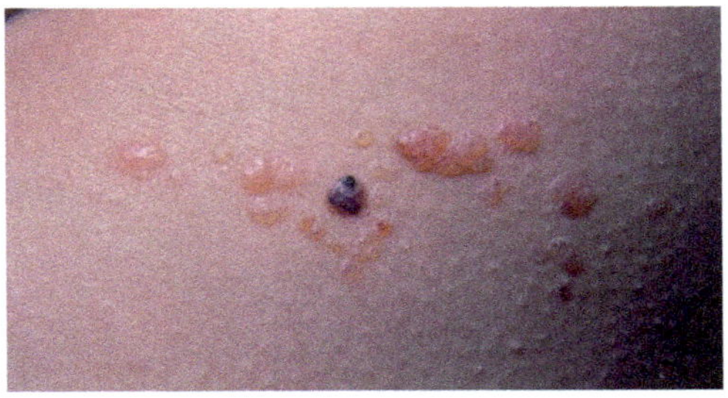

Lymphangioma circumscriptum
Photograph courtesy of SpringerImages Database, Springer Publishing Company

H.M. Gloster, Jr. et al., *Absolute Dermatology Review: Mastering Clinical Conditions on the Dermatology Recertification Exam*,
DOI 10.1007/978-3-319-03218-4_107, © Springer International Publishing Switzerland 2016

b. Cystic Hygroma

Cystic hygroma

A. Macrocystic lymphatic malformation (hyperplasia of lymphatic network forming large cysts)

B. Large, soft translucent mass under normal skin most commonly on the neck, axilla, lateral chest wall

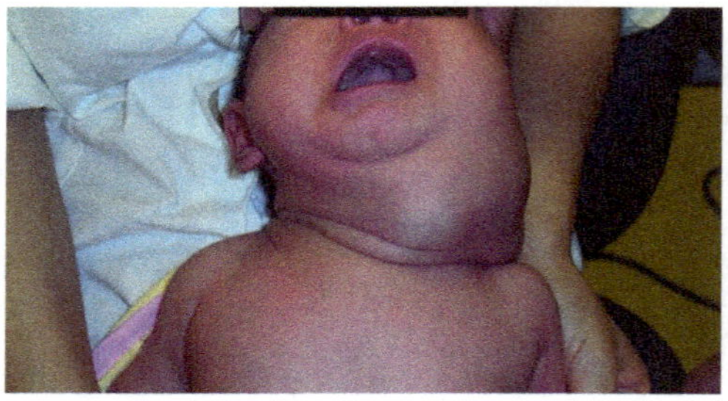

Cystic hygroma
Photograph courtesy of SpringerImages Database, Springer Publishing Company

Chapter XVII

Pigmentary Disorders

108 Vitiligo

Vitiligo

A. Amelanotic depigmented chalk white macules or patches with discrete margins surrounded by normal skin
   1. Ivory white by Wood's light
   2. Enlarge centrifugally over time
   3. May koebnerize (develop at sites of trauma or friction)
   4. Sites of predilection (normally hyperpigmented areas)—face (usually around eyes and mouth, periorificial), neck, extremities (dorsal hands, flexor wrists, digits, elbows, knees, dorsal ankles, shins), nipples, axillae, umbilicus, sacral, anogenital, inguinal
B. Leukotrichia (white hair)
   1. Usually seen along with depigmentation of surrounding epidermis
   2. Vitiligo of the scalp presents as several localized patches of white or gray hair
C. Associated diseases—both are more common in vitiligo patients
   1. Halo nevi
   2. Autoimmune thyroid disease

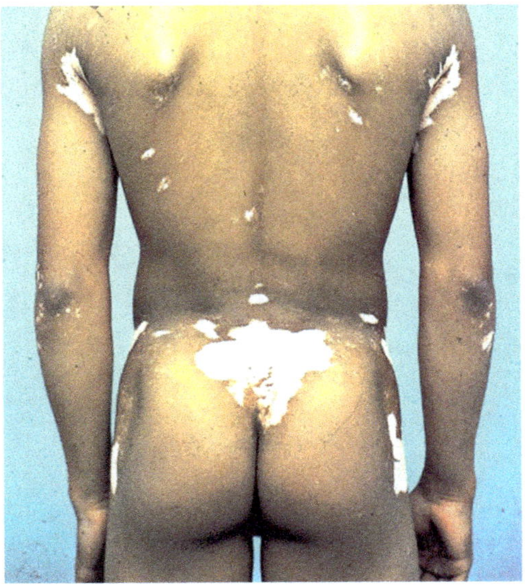

Vitiligo
Photograph courtesy of SpringerImages Database, Springer Publishing Company

H.M. Gloster, Jr. et al., *Absolute Dermatology Review: Mastering Clinical Conditions on the Dermatology Recertification Exam*, DOI 10.1007/978-3-319-03218-4_108, © Springer International Publishing Switzerland 2016

Vitiligo

A. Symmetrical vitiligo of both lower extremities

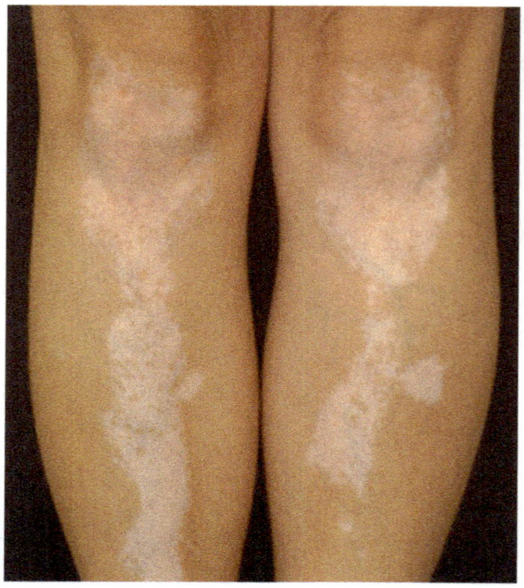

Vitiligo
Photograph courtesy of SpringerImages Database, Springer Publishing Company

a. Vitiligo and Halo Nevi

Halo nevi may be associated with vitilgo

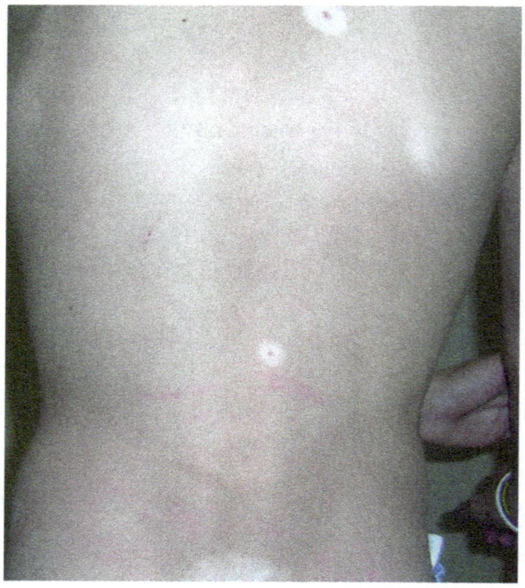

Vitiligo and halo nevi
Photograph courtesy of SpringerImages Database, Springer Publishing Company

b. Unilateral Segmental Vitiligo

Unilateral (segmental) vitilgo

A. More common in children
B. One or more macules involving a unilateral segment of the body
C. Lesions stop abruptly at midline
D. The face is the most common location

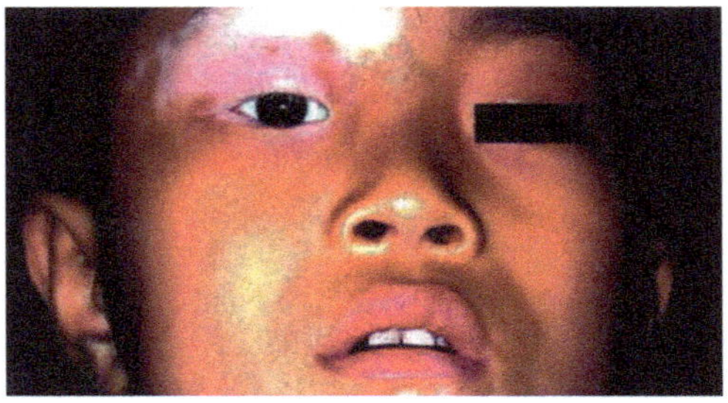

Unilateral segmental vitiligo
Photograph courtesy of SpringerImages Database, Springer Publishing Company

Unilateral (segmental) vitilgo of the chest and abdomen

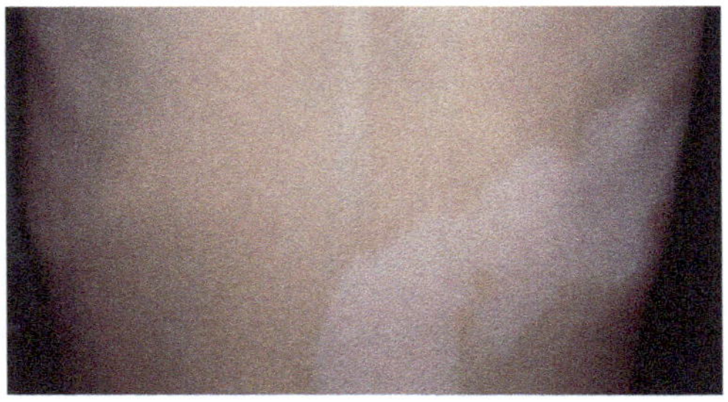

Unilateral Segmental Vitiligo
Photograph courtesy of SpringerImages Database, Springer Publishing Company

109 Postinflammatory Hyperpigmentation

Postinflammatory hyperpigmentation

A. Common in dark skin
B. Inflammation or injury to the skin (preceding inflammation may be transient or subclinical) results in increased melanin in the epidermis or dermis in the form of asymptomatic hyperpigmented macules and patches whose size, shape, and distribution can provide clues to underlying etiology
  1. Epidermal melanin
     a. Usually tan to dark brown
     b. Fades more readily than dermal melanin
     c. Commonly caused by acne atopic dermatitis, psoriasis, pityriasis rosea, pyodermas
     d. More common in skin of color
  2. Dermal
     a. Usually gray brown
     b. Typically caused by disorders characterized by degeneration of basal layer and inflammation at dermal–epidermal junction (lichen planus, lichenoid drug reaction, lupus erythematosus, fixed drug reaction)
     c. Persists longer than epidermal postinflammatory pigmentation and may be permanent

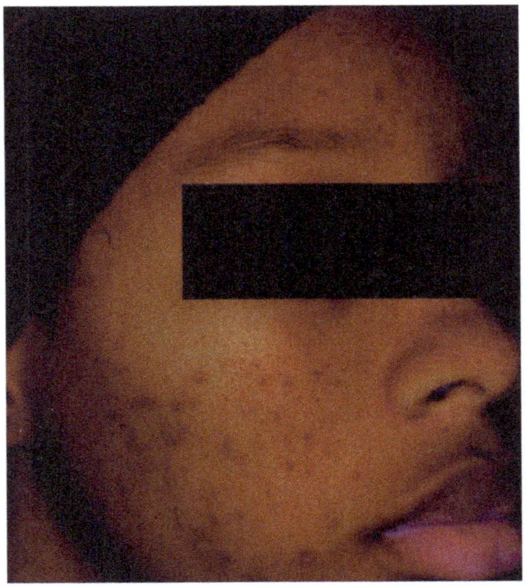

Postinflammatory hyperpigmentation
Photograph courtesy of SpringerImages Database, Springer Publishing Company

Postinflammatory hyperpigmentation

A. Acne vulgaris with postinflammatory hyperpigmentation

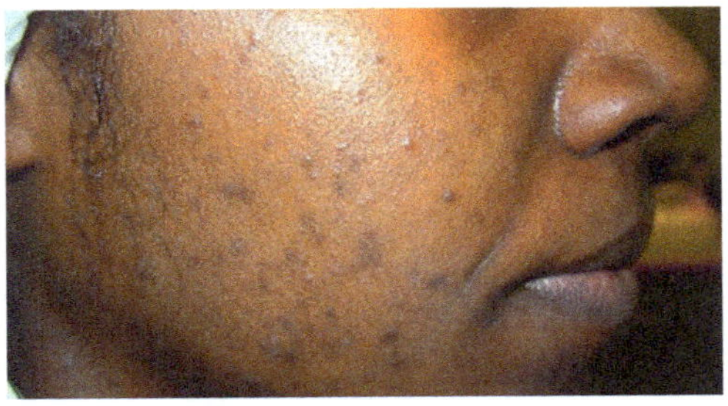

Postinflammatory hyperpigmentation
Photograph courtesy of SpringerImages Database, Springer Publishing Company

H.M. Gloster, Jr. et al., *Absolute Dermatology Review: Mastering Clinical Conditions on the Dermatology Recertification Exam*,
DOI 10.1007/978-3-319-03218-4_109, © Springer International Publishing Switzerland 2016

Chapter XVIII

Neutrophilic Dermatoses

Pyoderma Gangrenosum 110

Pyoderma gangrenosum (also see Chap. 7, section 48 a(iv))

A. The initial lesion is a tender pustule on a red or violaceous base or a red papule or nodule which is often thought to be an insect bite

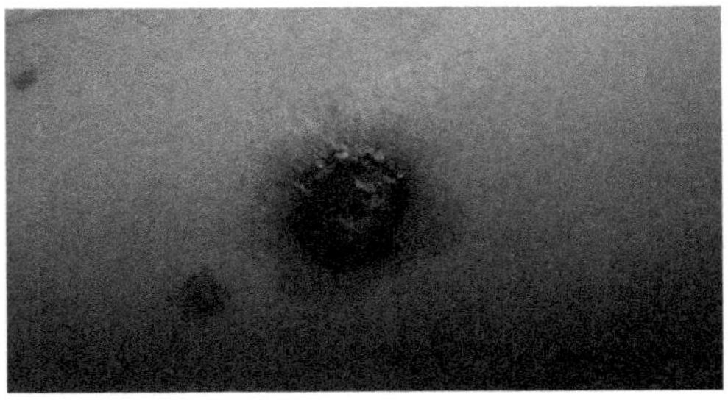

Pyoderma gangrenosum
Photograph courtesy of SpringerImages Database, Springer Publishing Company

H.M. Gloster, Jr. et al., *Absolute Dermatology Review: Mastering Clinical Conditions on the Dermatology Recertification Exam*, DOI 10.1007/978-3-319-03218-4_110, © Springer International Publishing Switzerland 2016

Pyoderma gangrenosum
- A. The initial lesion develops into a painful ulcer with a necrotic undermined and overhanging border, which has a violet-gray gun metal color and inflammatory rim
- B. Base of ulcer may be purulent or vegetative
- C. Ulcer extends centrifugally, may rapidly expand
- D. Satellite violaceous papules which ulcerate may appear distal to the edge of the ulcer
- E. Most commonly occurs on the lower extremities (pretibial area) but may be anywhere
- F. Pathergy is common (trauma initiates and aggravates lesions)
- G. One or multiple lesions may develop
- H. Associated illnesses—seen in 50 % of patients
  1. Inflammatory bowel disease—20–30 %
  2. Arthritis—20 %
  3. Hematologic malignancy—15–25 %
     a. Leukemia
     b. Myelodysplastic syndrome
     c. Monoclonal gammopathies
  4. Drug induced

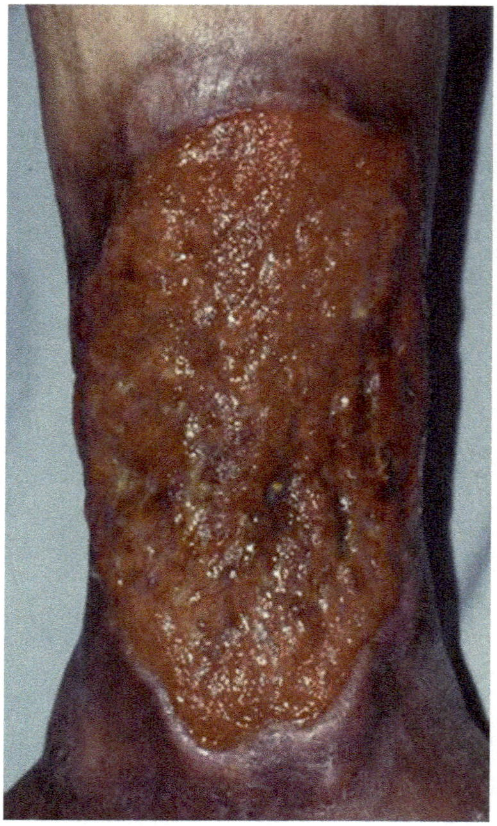

Pyoderma gangrenosum
Photograph courtesy of SpringerImages Database, Springer Publishing Company

Pyoderma gangrenosum
- A. Ulcer on the lower leg with a purulent base and necrotic undermined and overhanging border which has a violet-gray gun metal color and inflammatory rim

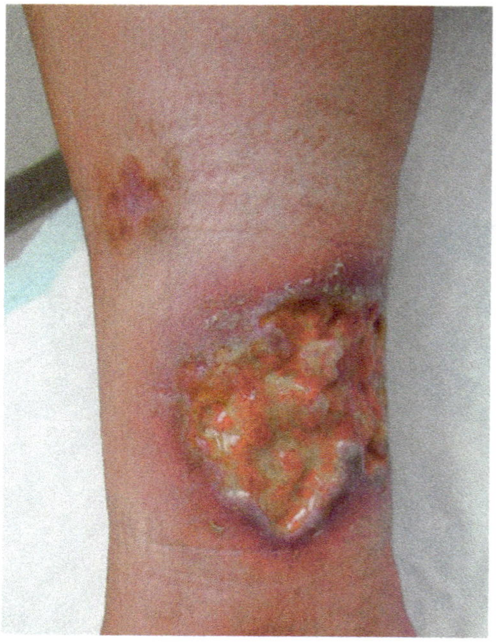

Pyoderma gangrenosum
Photograph courtesy of SpringerImages Database, Springer Publishing Company

Pyoderma gangenosum

A. Ulcer with irregular, necrotic undermined and overhanging borders
B. The edge of ulcer is undermined and often has a violet-gray gun metal color and inflammatory rim with a purulent or vegetative base

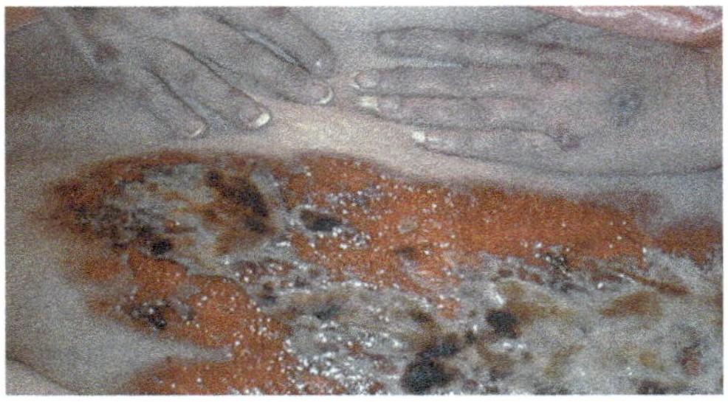

Pyoderma gangrenosum
Photograph courtesy of the American Academy of Dermatology

a. Atypical Pyoderma Gangrenosum

Atypical pyoderma gangrenosum

A. Hemorrhagic bullae and superficial erosions
B. Favors upper extremities (especially the dorsal hands) and face
C. Usually occurs in the setting of leukemia and myelodysplasia
D. Systemic features usually absent

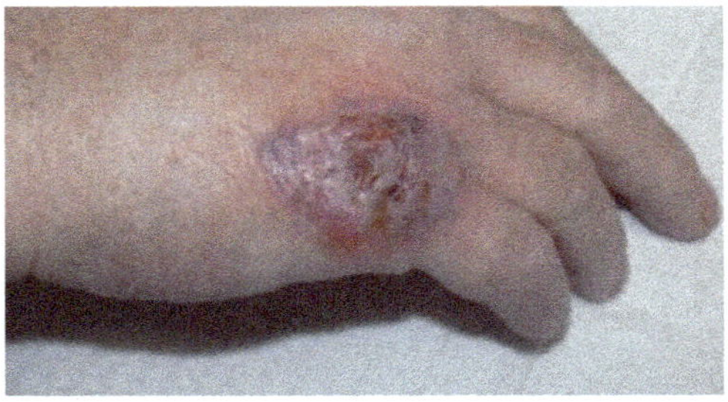

Atypical pyoderma gangrenosum
Photograph courtesy of SpringerImages Database, Springer Publishing Company

b. Superficial Granulomatous (Vegetative) Pyoderma Gangrenosum

Superficial granulomatous (vegetative) pyoderma grangrenosum

A. Localized superficial vegetative, boggy plaque
B. Favors the trunk

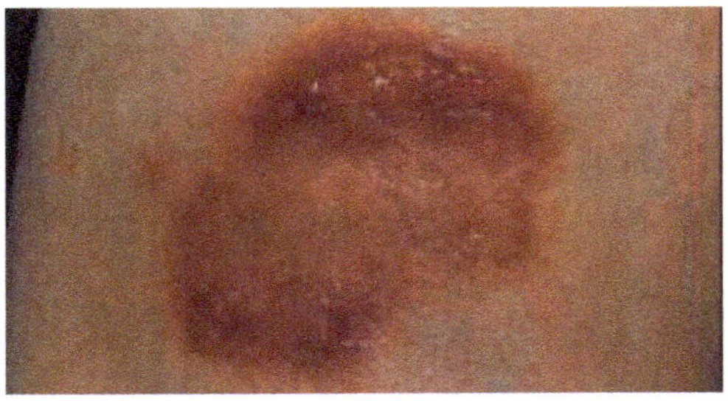

Superficial granulomatous (vegetative) pyoderma grangrenosum
Photograph courtesy of SpringerImages Database, Springer Publishing Company

c. Pyostomatitis Vegetans

Pyostomatis vegetans

A. Chronic, vegetative sterile pyoderma on the labial or buccal mucosa
B. Multiple yellow pustules that often are arranged in linear, serpentine fashion that has been likened to a "snail track"
C. May be associated with vegetative or ulcerative pyoderma gangrenosum
D. Seen in patients with inflammatory bowel disease

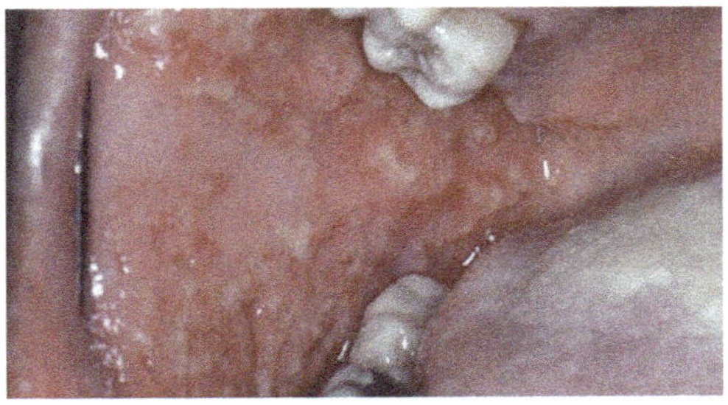

Pyostomatis vegetans
Photograph courtesy of SpringerImages Database, Springer Publishing Company

Acute Febrile Neutrophilic Dermatosis (Sweet's Syndrome)

111

Acute febrile neutrophilic dermatosis (Sweet's Syndrome)

A. Upper respiratory infection or flu-like symptoms frequently precede the syndrome
B. Tender, edematous, erythematous papules and plaques that may develop vesicles, bullae, or pustules within the plaques
C. Vesiculobullous variant most frequently associated with acute myelogenous leukemia and may progress to ulceration resembling pyoderma gangrenosum
D. Favors the head, neck, and extremities (especially dorsal hand)
E. May be widespread in malignancy-associated cases
F. Pathergy is common
G. Resolves spontaneously in 5–12 weeks, recurs in 30 %
H. Associated conditions
    1. Infections—upper respiratory tract infections due to streptococcus, Yersinia
    2. Vaccinations
    3. Malignancies
        a. Hematologic (especially acute myelogenous leukemia), 10–20 %
        b. Solid tumors
    4. Inflammatory bowel disease
    5. Autoimmune disease
    6. Drugs
    7. Pregnancy

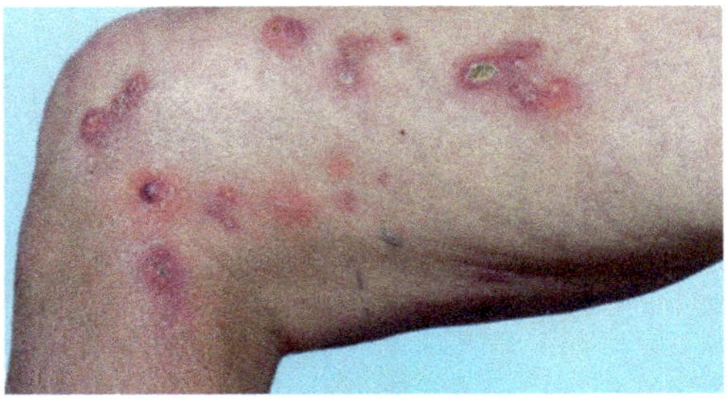

Acute febrile neutrophilic dermatosis (Sweet's Syndrome)
Photograph courtesy of SpringerImages Database, Springer Publishing Company

Acute febrile neutrophilic dermatosis (Sweet's Syndrome)

A. Tender, edematous, erythematous plaques

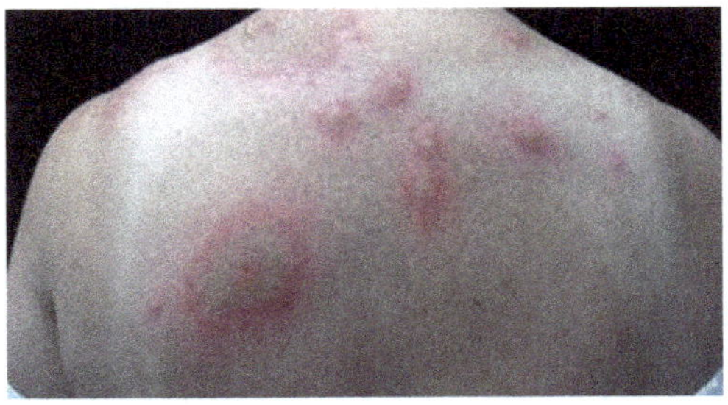

Acute febrile neutrophilic dermatosis (Sweet's Syndrome)
Photograph courtesy of SpringerImages Database, Springer Publishing Company

H.M. Gloster, Jr. et al., *Absolute Dermatology Review: Mastering Clinical Conditions on the Dermatology Recertification Exam*, DOI 10.1007/978-3-319-03218-4_111, © Springer International Publishing Switzerland 2016

Erosive Pustular Dermatosis 112

Erosive pustular dermatosis

A. Sterile pustules, crusts, erosions arising within photodamaged skin of the bald scalp
B. May be related to cutaneous atrophy

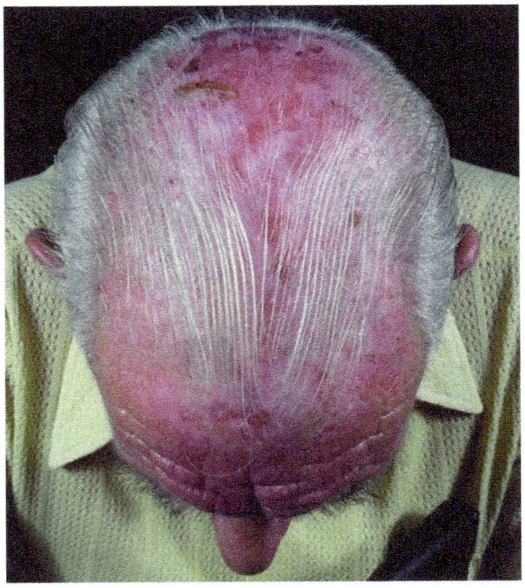

Erosive pustular dermatosis
Photograph courtesy of SpringerImages Database, Springer Publishing Company

H.M. Gloster, Jr. et al., *Absolute Dermatology Review: Mastering Clinical Conditions on the Dermatology Recertification Exam*,
DOI 10.1007/978-3-319-03218-4_112, © Springer International Publishing Switzerland 2016

Chapter XIX

Disoders of Langerhans Cells, Macrophages, and Mast Cells

113 Langerhans Cell Histiocytosis

a. Letterer-Siwe Disease

Letter-Siwe disease

A. Acute diffuse form of Langerhans cell histiocytosis
B. Usually develops before the age of 2
C. Presents with a recalcitrant eruption of 1–2 mm red to yellow-brown petechial papules (petechial and purpuric papules are clues to the diagnosis) topped with scale and crust which may cluster to form an erythematous, weeping, crusted eruption
D. A seborrheic or intertriginous distribution is common (scalp, face, trunk, buttocks), and the eruption is often confused with seborrheic dermatitis, diaper dermatitis, and intertrigo
   1. Scalp lesions may be confused with seborrheic dermatitis, but papules are more discrete with crusting
   2. Pink thin plaques in the inguinal area can also resemble seborrheic dermatitis
   3. Lesions on the perineum may resemble recalcitrant diaper dermatitis, which is a common presenting sign
   4. Visceral and bone lesions may occur (especially osteolytic cranial lesions)

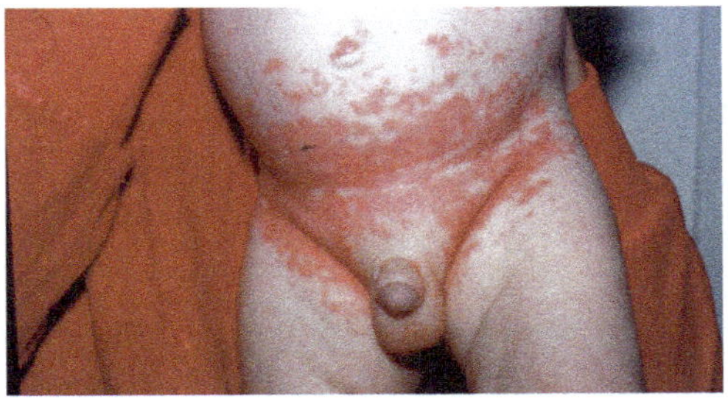

Letter-Siwe disease
Photograph courtesy of the American Academy of Dermatology

Letter-Siwe disease

A. Recalcitrant eruption of 1–2 mm red to yellow-brown petechial papules (petechial and purpuric papules are clues to the diagnosis) topped with scale and crust which may cluster to form an erythematous, weeping, crusted eruption

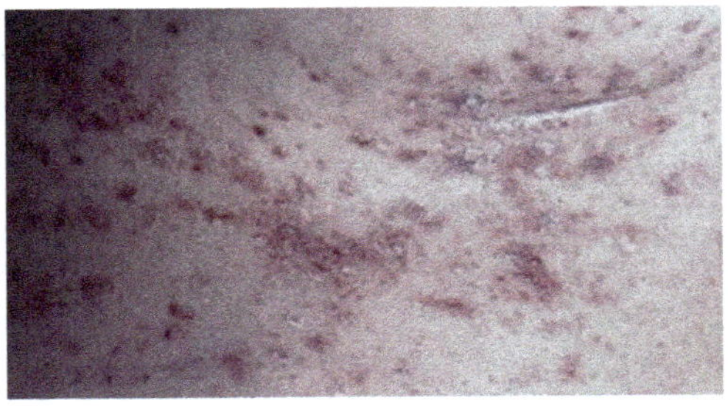

Letter-Siwe disease
Photograph courtesy of SpringerImages Database, Springer Publishing Company

H.M. Gloster, Jr. et al., *Absolute Dermatology Review: Mastering Clinical Conditions on the Dermatology Recertification Exam*, DOI 10.1007/978-3-319-03218-4_113, © Springer International Publishing Switzerland 2016

b. Multicentric Reticulohistiocytosis

Multicentric reticulohistiocytosis

A. Yellow to reddish-brown hard papules on the fingers and hands
   1. Papules may cluster around the nail folds ("coral bead sign")
B. May be associated with polyarthritis and underlying malignancy

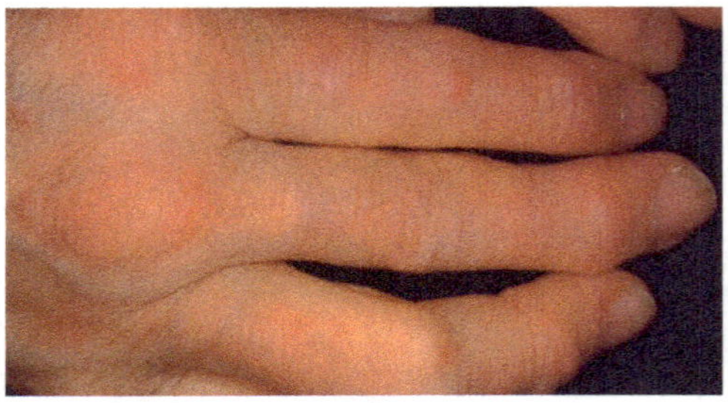

Multicentric reticulohistiocytosis
Photograph courtesy of SpringerImages Database, Springer Publishing Company

114 Xanthogranulomas

a. Juvenile Xanthogranuloma

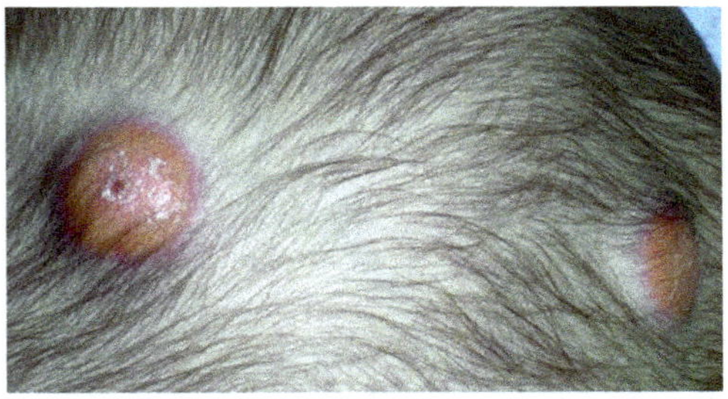

Juvenile xanthogranuloma
Photograph courtesy of SpringerImages Database, Springer Publishing Company

Juvenile xanthogranuloma

A. Most common non-Langerhans cell histiocytosis
B. Touton giant cell is characteristic histological finding
C. Most common in infants and young children
D. Usually occurs on the head and neck
E. Usually regresses after several years
F. Two variants
    1. Small nodular form (micronodular)—numerous 2–5 mm dome-shaped red-brown papules on the upper body which rapidly become yellow
    2. Large nodular form
        a. More common variant
        b. One or a few 1–2 cm nodules
        c. Pink initially, then orange to yellow brown due to accumulation of lipid in histiocytes
G. Extracutaneous lesions
    1. Eye (most common though rare): unilateral, onset under the age of 2, often affects the iris (color change in the iris, anterior chamber hemorrhage, glaucoma)
    2. Lung

H.M. Gloster, Jr. et al., *Absolute Dermatology Review: Mastering Clinical Conditions on the Dermatology Recertification Exam*,
DOI 10.1007/978-3-319-03218-4_114,

Juvenile xanthogranuloma

A. Small nodular form (micronodular)—numerous 2–5 mm dome-shaped red-brown papules on the upper body which rapidly become yellow

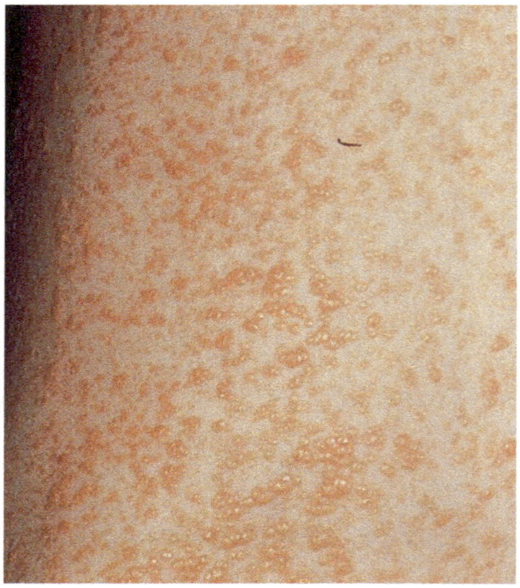

Juvenile xanthogranuloma
Photograph courtesy of SpringerImages Database, Springer Publishing Company

b. Necrobiotic Xanthogranuloma

Necrobiotic xanthgranuloma

A. Most common in the sixth decade
B. Yellow brown indurated papules, nodules, or plaques in a periorbital distribution
C. 80 % have paraproteinemia (IgG monoclonal gammopathy) due to plasma cell dyscrasia or lymphoproliferative disorder
D. Multisystem disease
   1. Plasma cell dyscrasia—multiple myeloma
   2. Ocular disease (50 %)—orbital masses, keratitis, conjunctivitis, iritis, proptosis, ectropion
   3. Hepatosplenomegaly

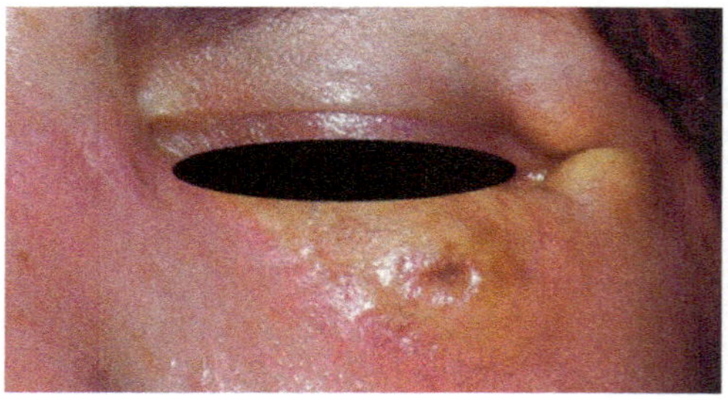

Necrobiotic xanthgranuloma
Photograph courtesy of SpringerImages Database, Springer Publishing Company

Necrobiotic xanthogranuloma

A. Yellow brown indurated plaques in a periorbital distribution

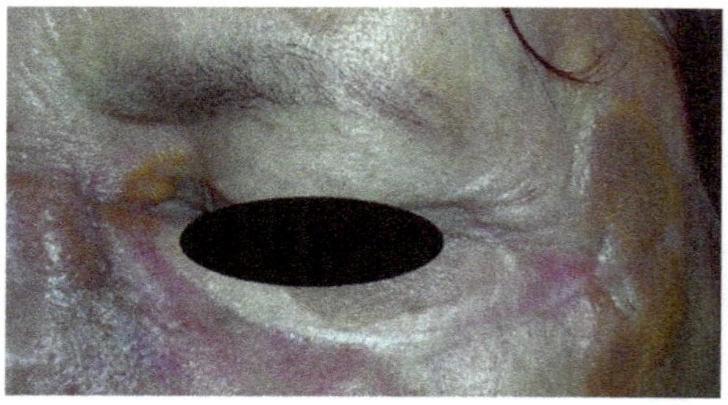

Necrobiotic xanthgranuloma
Photograph courtesy of SpringerImages Database, Springer Publishing Company

Xanthomas

115

a. Xanthelasma

Xanthelasma

A. Plane xanthomas (yellow to orange macules, papules, patches, and plaques) of the eyelids
B. Only 50 % of patients have hyperlipidemia

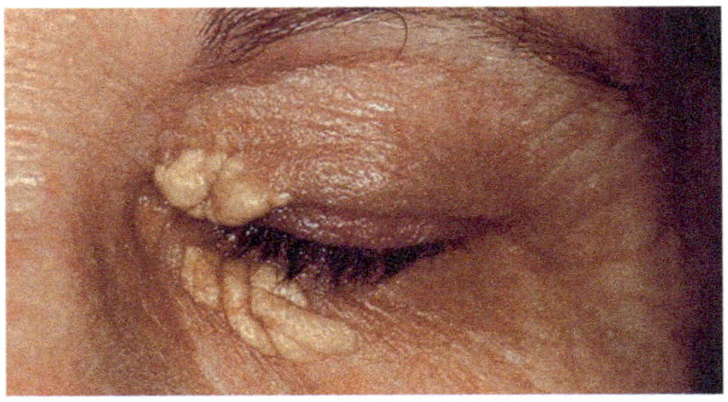

Xanthelasma
Photograph courtesy of SpringerImages Database, Springer Publishing Company

b. Eruptive Xanthoma

Eruptive xanthomas

A. Eruptive yellow-orange to red-brown generalized crops of small (1–5 mm) papules
B. Most commonly occur on the extensor extremities (especially the knees but also elbows), buttocks, and hands
C. May koebnerize
D. May be seen in the setting of primary familial lipid disorders, secondary hyperlipidemia with high triglyceride levels, diabetes, obesity, pancreatitis, chronic renal failure, hypothyroidism, nephrotic syndrome

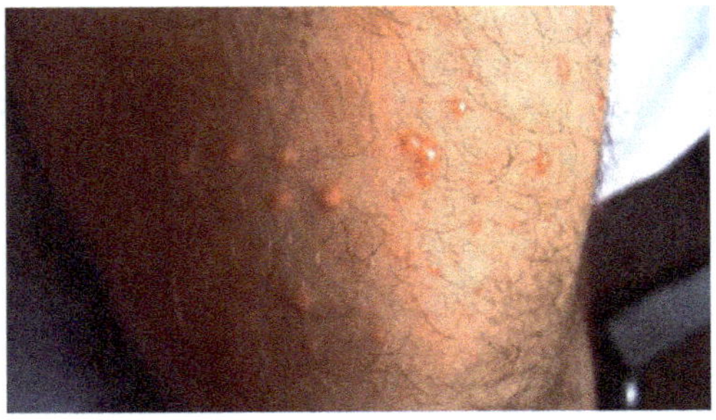

Eruptive xanthoma
Photograph courtesy of SpringerImages Database, Springer Publishing Company

Eruptive xanthomas

A. Eruptive reddish orange generalized small papules on the buttock of a woman with diabetes mellitus and hypertriglyceridemia

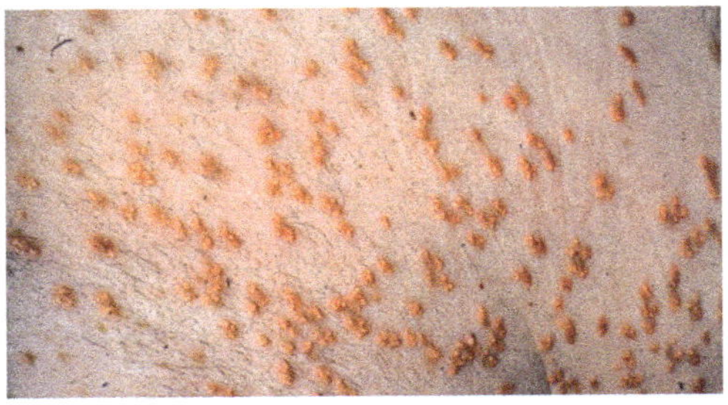

Eruptive xanthoma
Photograph courtesy of SpringerImages Database, Springer Publishing Company

H.M. Gloster, Jr. et al., *Absolute Dermatology Review: Mastering Clinical Conditions on the Dermatology Recertification Exam*, DOI 10.1007/978-3-319-03218-4_115,

c. Tuberous Xanthoma

Tuberous xanthoma

A. Pink yellow papules or nodules usually greater than 3 cm in diameter on the elbows and knees
B. May be seen in hypercholesterolemic states

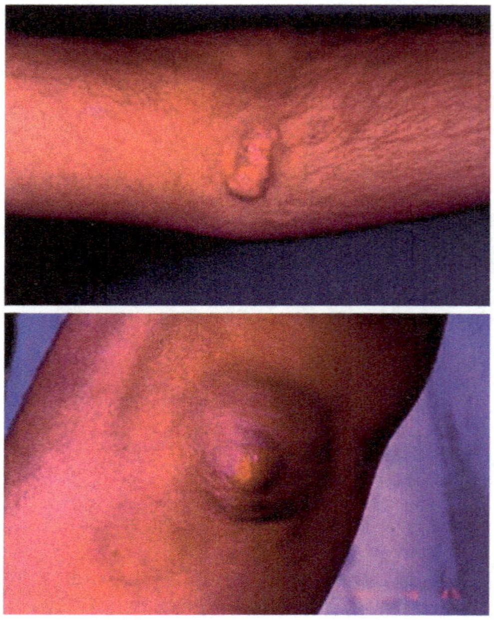

Tuberous xanthoma
Photograph courtesy of SpringerImages Database, Springer Publishing Company

d. Verruciform Xanthoma

Verruciform xanthoma

A. Verrucous, solitary 1–2 cm plaque in the mouth primarily but also anogenital area
B. No associated hyperlipidemia but may be seen with lymphedema, epidermolysis bullosa, pemphigus vulgaris, discoid lupus erythematosus, and graft-versus-host disease

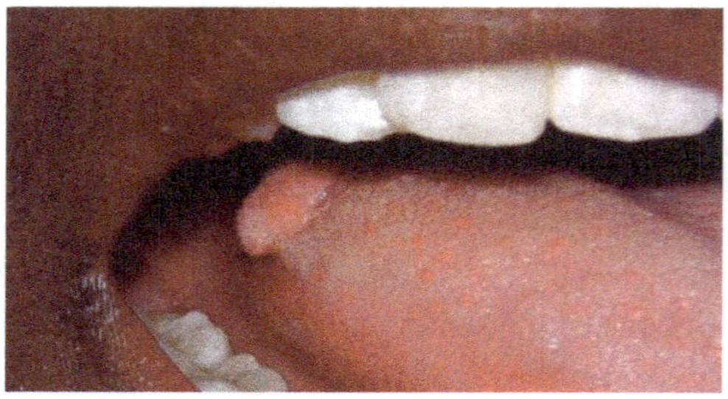

Verruciform xanthoma
Photograph courtesy of SpringerImages Database, Springer Publishing Company

e. Tendinous Xanthoma

Tendinous xanthoma

A. Firm smooth nodular lipid deposits on the Achilles tendon or extensor tendons of the hands, knees, elbows
B. Almost always due to underlying disorder of lipid metabolism, most often seen in familial hypercholesterolemia, an autosomal dominant disorder of lipid metabolism

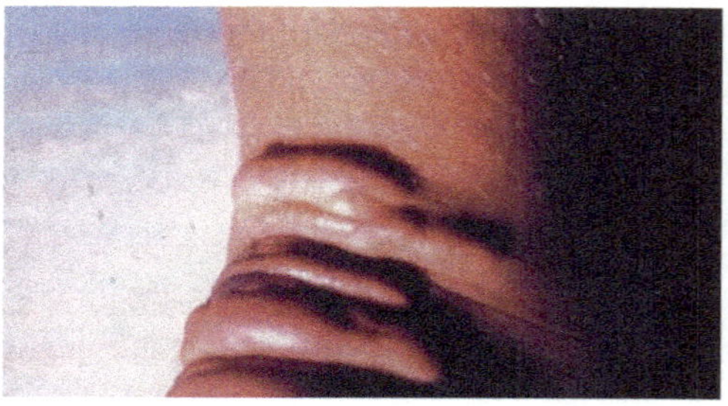

Tendinous xanthoma
Photograph courtesy of SpringerImages Database, Springer Publishing Company

116 Sarcoidosis

Sarcoidosis

A. Systemic granulomatous disorder of unknown origin that most commonly involves the lungs (hilar adenopathy in 90 %)
B. Many other organs may be involved including the liver, spleen, bone, kidney, gastrointestinal tract, lymph nodes, central nervous system, muscle, heart, endocrine, eye
C. Hypercalcemia—10 % of patients
D. Cutaneous manifestations
    1. Seen in 1/3 of patients with systemic sarcoidosis
    2. May be the first or only sign of disease
    3. Red brown to violaceous papules and plaques on face, lips, neck, upper back, extremities
        a. May develop within preexisting scars or sites of prior trauma (e.g., tattoo)
        b. Diascopy (pressure induces blanching) yields a yellow brown "apple jelly" color

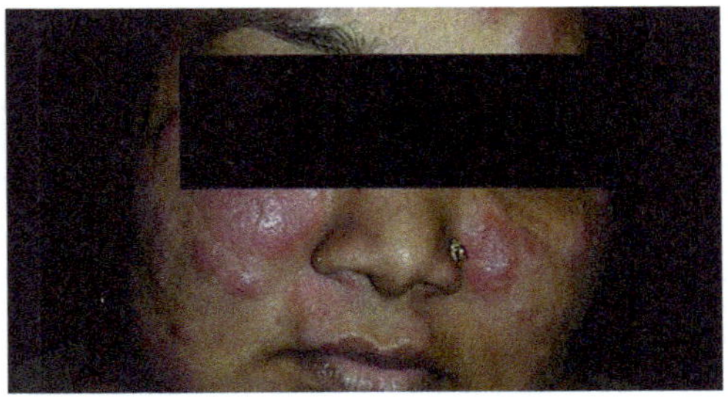

Sarcoidosis
Photograph courtesy of SpringerImages Database, Springer Publishing Company

a. Erythema Nodosum

Erythema nodosum

A. Symmetrical tender red nodules on the pretibial areas
B. May be a nonspecific manifestation of sarcoidosis
C. Lofgren's syndrome
    1. Sarcoidosis manifesting with erythema nodosum, hilar adenopathy, fever, migrating polyarthritis, acute iritis
    2. Good prognosis: associated with subacute transient sarcoidosis which resolves spontaneously within a few years

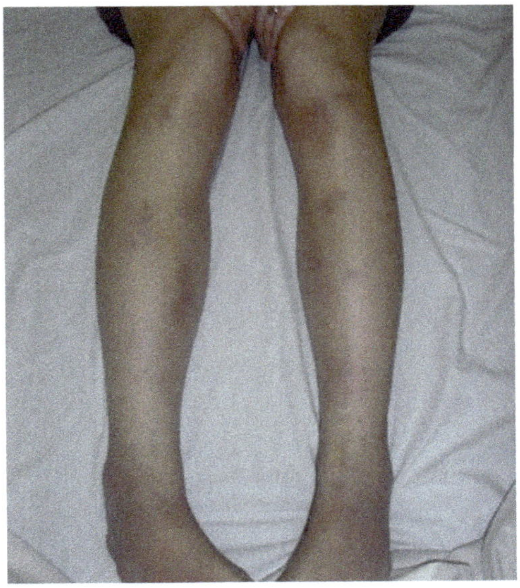

Erythema nodosum
Photograph courtesy of SpringerImages Database, Springer Publishing Company

H.M. Gloster, Jr. et al., *Absolute Dermatology Review: Mastering Clinical Conditions on the Dermatology Recertification Exam*,
DOI 10.1007/978-3-319-03218-4_116, © Springer International Publishing Switzerland 2016

b. Lupus Pernio

Lupus pernio

A. Coalescing red to violaceous smooth shiny papules and plaques on the head and neck, especially the nose (may have a beaded appearance along nasal rim)

B. 75% of patients with nasal rim involvement have chronic sarcoidosis of the lungs, 50 % have sarcoidosis of upper respiratory tract, and cystic bone lesions are more common

C. May also involve other areas more affected by cold (ears, cheeks, lips, forehead)

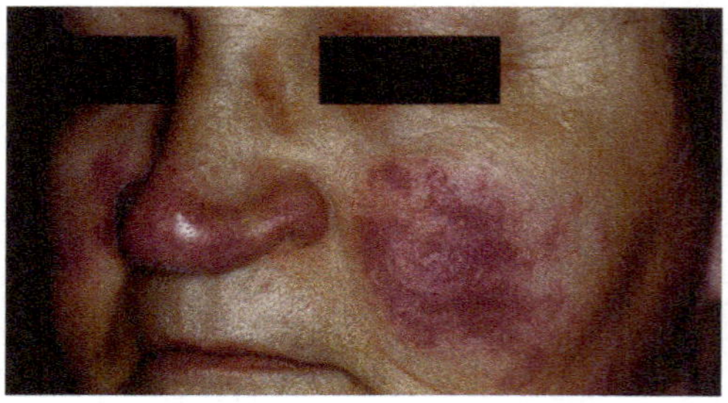

Lupus pernio
Photograph courtesy of SpringerImages Database, Springer Publishing Company

Lupus pernio

A. Coalescing red to violaceous smooth shiny papules and plaques on the nose with a beaded appearance along nasal rim

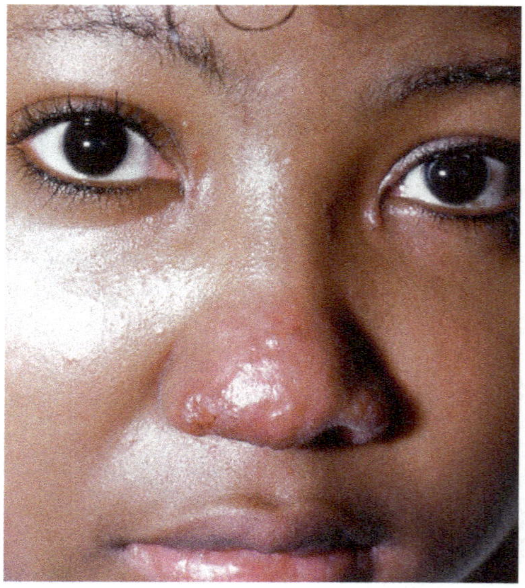

Lupus pernio
Photograph courtesy of the American Academy of Dermatology

117 Granuloma Annulare

a. Localized Granuloma Annulare

Localized granuloma annulare

A. Most common form in children
B. Arciform to annular plaques (plaques are composed of small papules) with central clearing located on the extremities (lateral or dorsal hands most often but also the feet and ankles)—figures a and b
C. 50 % resolve within 2 years, 40 % have recurrences

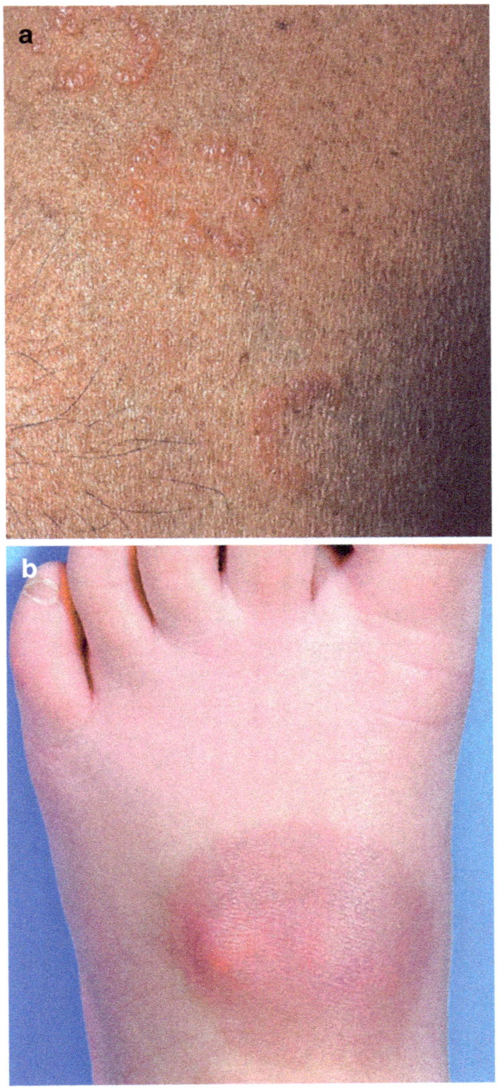

Localized granuloma annulare
Photograph courtesy of SpringerImages Database, Springer Publishing Company

H.M. Gloster, Jr. et al., *Absolute Dermatology Review: Mastering Clinical Conditions on the Dermatology Recertification Exam*,
DOI 10.1007/978-3-319-03218-4_117, © Springer International Publishing Switzerland 2016

b. Papular Granuloma Annulare

Papular granuloma annulare

A. Small papules may have a central dell usually on the extremities

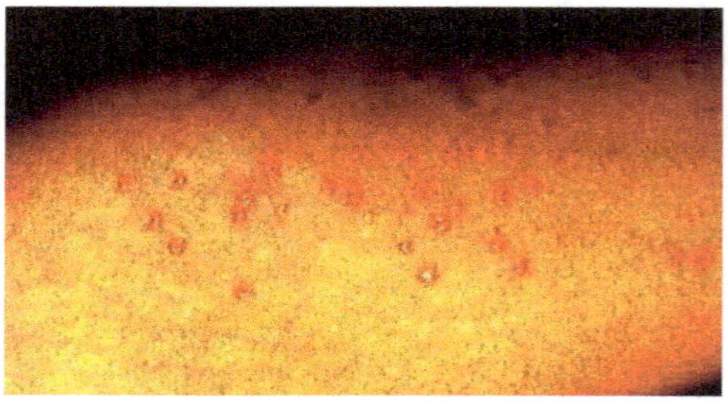

Papular granuloma annulare
Photograph courtesy of SpringerImages Database, Springer Publishing Company

c. Subcutaneous Granuloma Annulare

Subcutaneous granuloma annulare

A. Painless skin-colored nodules usually on the extremities (may resemble rheumatoid nodules)
B. Usually reported in children under 6 years of age

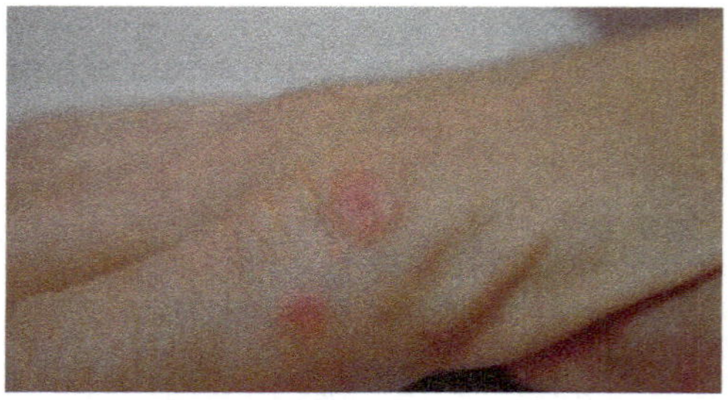

Subcutaneous granuloma annulare
Photograph courtesy of SpringerImages Database, Springer Publishing Company

d. Generalized Granuloma Annulare

Generalized granuloma annulare

A. Numerous small skin-colored pink-violet papules in a symmetric distribution on the trunk and proximal extremities; some papules may coalesce to form annular plaques
B. Later age of onset (usually women in fifth to sixth decade), poorer response to therapy, more chance of lipid abnormalities

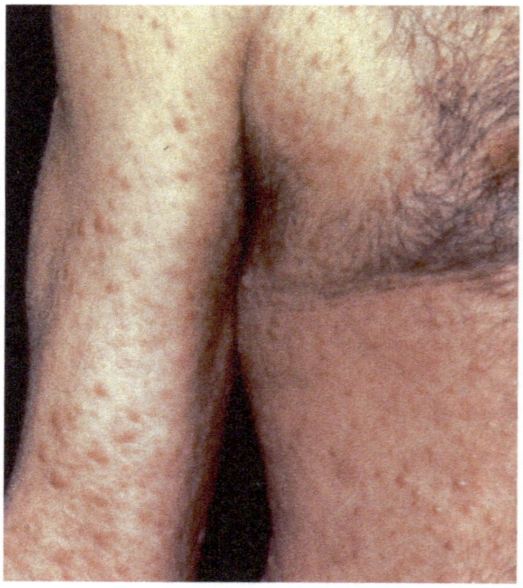

Generalized granuloma annulare
Photograph courtesy of the American Academy of Dermatology

Generalized granuloma annulare

A. Numerous small skin-colored pink-violet papules coalescing to form annular plaques

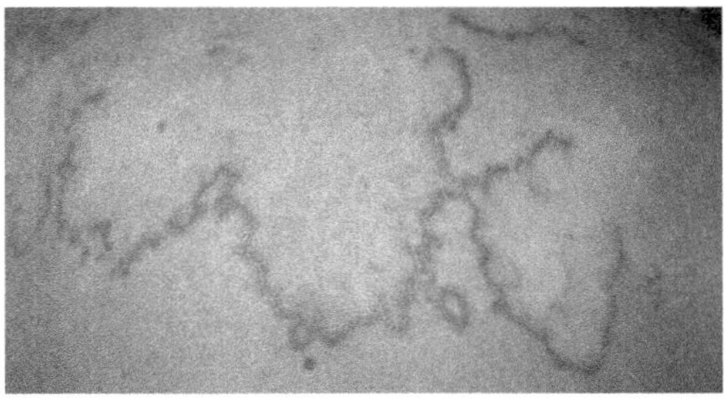

Generalized granuloma annulare
Photograph courtesy of SpringerImages Database, Springer Publishing Company

118 Necrobiosis Lipoidica Diabeticorum

Necrobiosis lipoidica diabeticorum

A. Well-demarcated, typically bilateral plaques with violaceous to red-brown, palpable peripheral borders and waxy, yellow brown atrophic centers with telangiectasias
B. Shins most common site
C. May ulcerate with trauma
D. 15–65 % have diabetes mellitus
E. Most common in young to middle-age adults, women more often than men

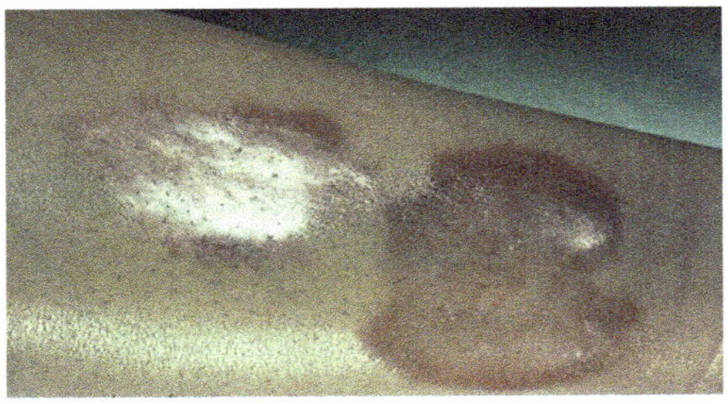

Necrobiosis lipoidica diabeticorum
Photograph courtesy of SpringerImages Database, Springer Publishing Company

Necrobiosis lipoidica diabeticorum

A. Bilateral plaques on the shins with violaceous, palpable borders and waxy, yellow brown atrophic centers with telangiectasias

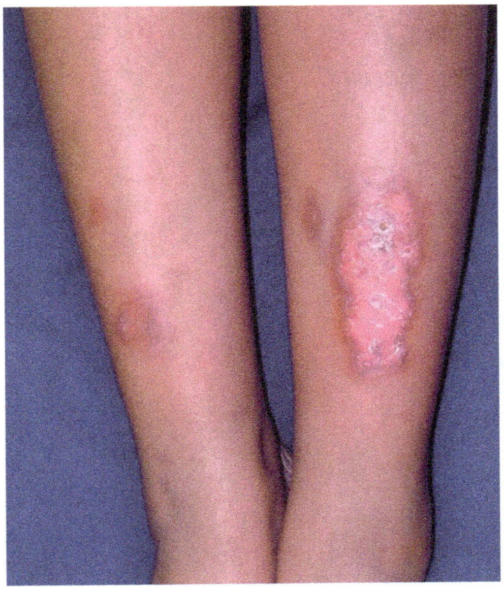

Necrobiosis lipoidica diabeticorum
Photograph courtesy of SpringerImages Database, Springer Publishing Company

H.M. Gloster, Jr. et al., *Absolute Dermatology Review: Mastering Clinical Conditions on the Dermatology Recertification Exam*, DOI 10.1007/978-3-319-03218-4_118,

Foreign Body Granuloma

119

Foreign body granuloma

A. Acute inflammatory response shortly after entry of foreign material, usually resolves, then weeks, months, or years later a chronic inflammatory response occurs with variety of presentations:
   1. Red to red brown papules
   2. Nodules and plaques with or without ulceration
   3. Chronic draining fistula or wound

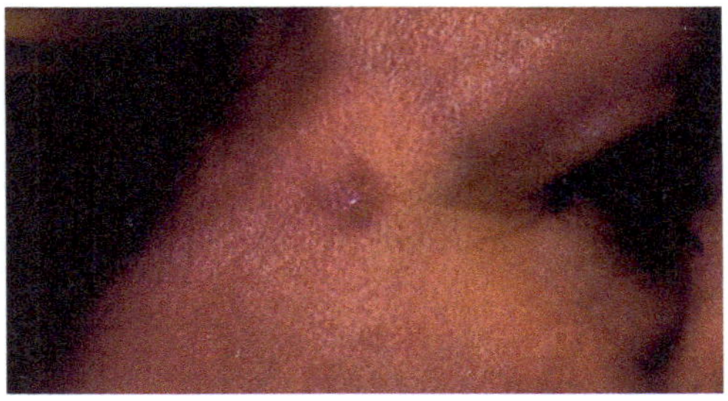

Foreign body granuloma
Photograph courtesy of SpringerImages Database, Springer Publishing Company

H.M. Gloster, Jr. et al., *Absolute Dermatology Review: Mastering Clinical Conditions on the Dermatology Recertification Exam*, DOI 10.1007/978-3-319-03218-4_119,

120 Mastocytosis

a. Urticaria Pigmentosa

Urticaria pigmentosa

A. One or more tan to red brown papules or plaques that appear during early childhood (3–9 months of age) and resolve during late adolescence or early adulthood
B. The papules and plaques form an urticarial wheal upon rubbing (Darier's sign)
C. Usually appear on the trunk, sparing the face, palms, and soles
D. Most common form of childhood mastocytosis

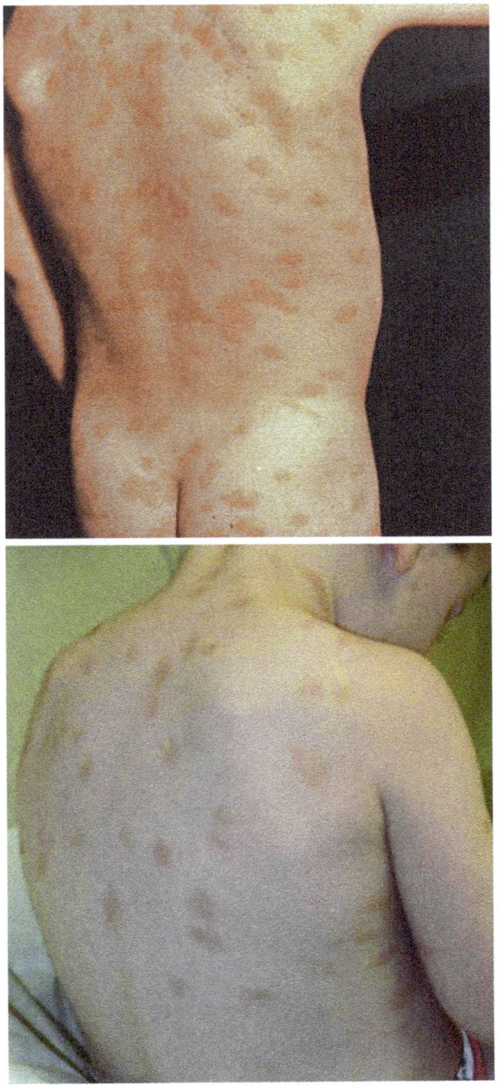

Urticaria pigmentosa
Photograph courtesy of SpringerImages Database, Springer Publishing Company

H.M. Gloster, Jr. et al., *Absolute Dermatology Review: Mastering Clinical Conditions on the Dermatology Recertification Exam*, DOI 10.1007/978-3-319-03218-4_120, © Springer International Publishing Switzerland 2016

b. Solitary Mastocytoma

Solitary mastocytomas

A. Solitary tan, yellow-tan, or brown plaque or nodule that urticates upon rubbing (Darier's sign)
B. Second-most common form of childhood mastocytosis
C. Occurs mainly in children, may be present at birth or appear in early infancy
D. Favors distal extremities

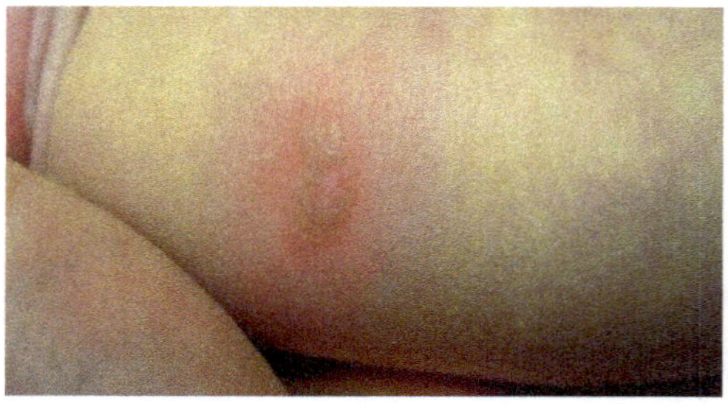

Solitary mastocytoma
Photograph courtesy of SpringerImages Database, Springer Publishing Company

Chapter XX

Dermal Connective Tissue Disorders

121 Keloids

Keloid

A. Firm, irregularly shaped hypertrophic mass resulting from trauma
B. Extends beyond wound margin (site of original injury) into adjacent normal skin, often with claw-like extensions – figures a and b
C. Favors sites of tension (upper back, chest, shoulders) but may occur on sites of minimal tension (earlobe after piercings)

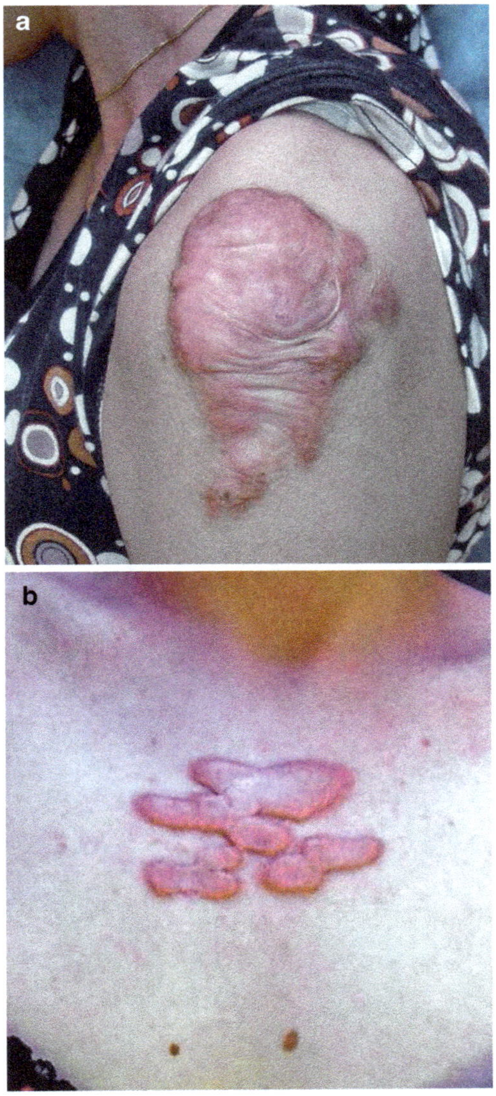

Keloids
Photograph courtesy of SpringerImages Database, Springer Publishing Company

H.M. Gloster, Jr. et al., *Absolute Dermatology Review: Mastering Clinical Conditions on the Dermatology Recertification Exam*, DOI 10.1007/978-3-319-03218-4_121, © Springer International Publishing Switzerland 2016

Keloid

A. Earlobe keloid that arose after a piercing

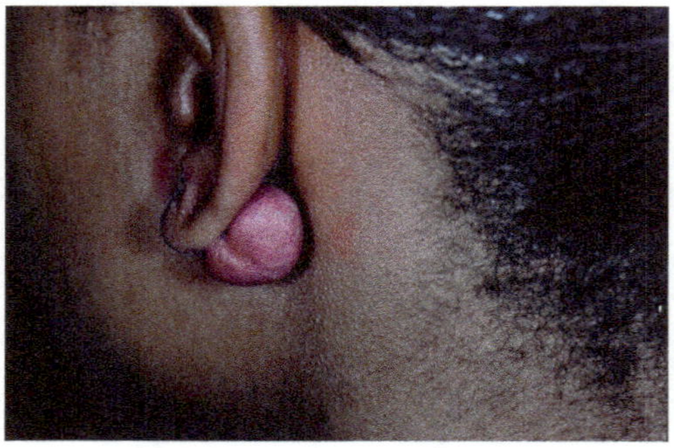

Keloid
Photograph courtesy of Hugh Gloster, MD

Hypertrophic Scar

122

Hypertrophic scar

A. Scar that is raised and confined to the wound margin
B. Favors sites of tension (upper trunk, deltoid)
C. Preceded by injury

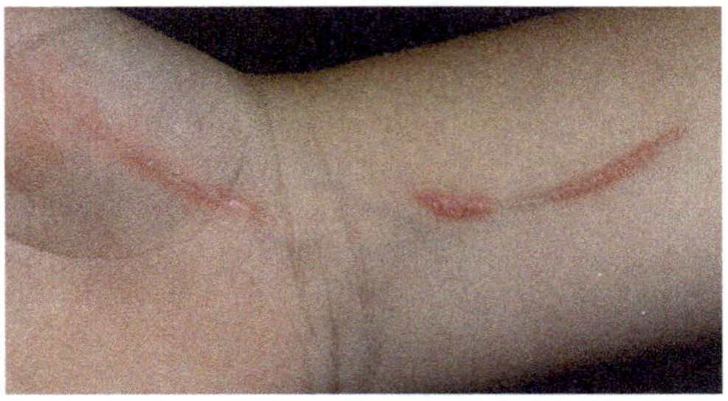

Hypertrophic scar
Photograph courtesy of SpringerImages Database, Springer Publishing Company

H.M. Gloster, Jr. et al., *Absolute Dermatology Review: Mastering Clinical Conditions on the Dermatology Recertification Exam*, DOI 10.1007/978-3-319-03218-4_122, © Springer International Publishing Switzerland 2016

Perforating Dermatoses

123

a. Acquired Perforating Dermatosis (Kyrle's Disease)

Acquired perforating dermatosis (Kyrle's disease)

A. Associated with diabetes (most patients with diabetes have nephropathy) or pruritus of renal failure (most patients have chronic renal failure and are on dialysis)
B. Most commonly on the lower extremities (legs) of adults
C. Pruritic papules and nodules with a central keratotic core
   1. Late lesions are often excoriated papules with central crusted craters or depressed, atrophic, hyperpigmented scars

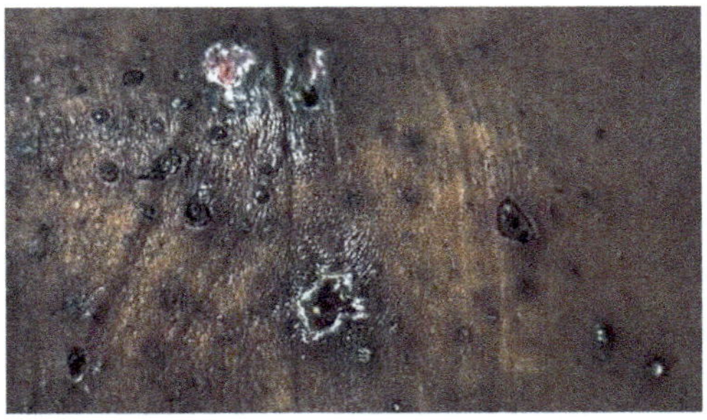

Acquired perforating dermatosis (Kyrle's disease)
Photograph courtesy of SpringerImages Database, Springer Publishing Company

H.M. Gloster, Jr. et al., *Absolute Dermatology Review: Mastering Clinical Conditions on the Dermatology Recertification Exam*, DOI 10.1007/978-3-319-03218-4_123, © Springer International Publishing Switzerland 2016

b. Elastosis Perforans Serpiginosa

Elastosis perforans serpiginosa

A. Begins in childhood or early adulthood, young adult males most common
B. Three forms
    1. Idiopathic
    2. Reactive: 40 % associated with genetic fibrous tissue abnormalities
    3. Drug-induced (penicillamine)
C. Involves elastic tissue (abnormal elastic tissue expelled via transepidermal elimination)
D. Hyperkeratotic 2–5 mm papules arranged in a serpiginous, arciform, or annular pattern that most often occur on the lateral neck (but also face, arms, flexural areas) and may reach several cm in diameter
E. Spontaneous resolution within 6 months – 5 years, often with atrophic scarring

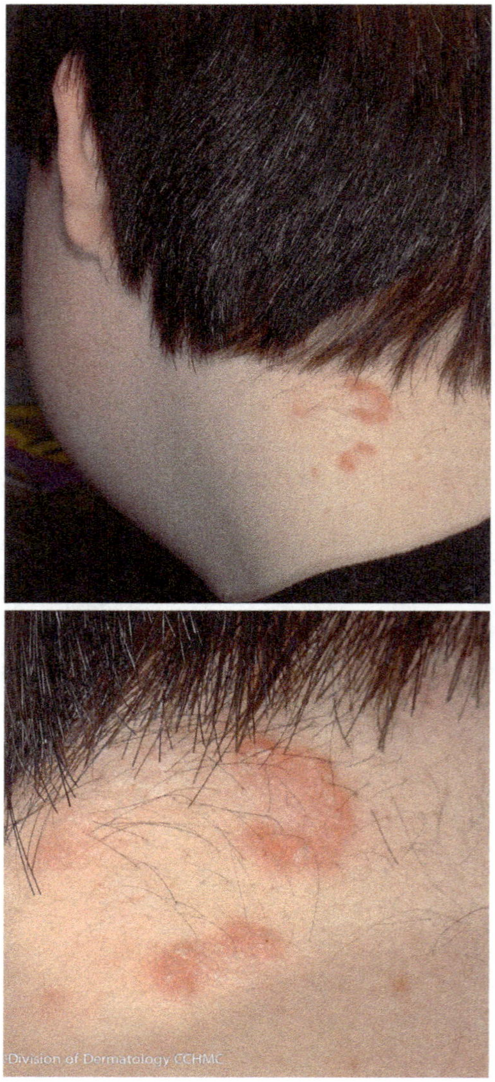

Elastosis perforans serpiginosa
Photograph courtesy of Kara Shaw, MD. Division of Dermatology, CCHMC

Chapter XXI

Panniculitis

Erythema Nodosum

124

Erythema nodosum

A. Bilateral tender red subcutaneous nodules symmetrically on the pretibial areas (figure a)
B. May develop a bruise-like appearance in later stages (figure b)
C. Nodules do not ulcerate and usually resolve within a few days or weeks but may recur
D. May be associated with fever, malaise, and arthralgias
E. Most cases occur in young women
F. May be associated with a wide variety of systemic disorders, but 30 % have no known disease association
   1. Inflammatory bowel disease (especially Crohn's)
   2. Sarcoidosis
      a. Erythema nodosum is associated with a more benign self-limited form of sarcoid – Lofgren's syndrome – a variant of sarcoidosis with bilateral hilar adenopathy and erythema nodosum
   3. Infections
      a. Upper respiratory tract infections – most common infectious cause
      b. Bacterial gastroenteritis (e.g., Yersinia)
      c. Viral upper respiratory infection
      d. Coccidiomycosis
   4. Drugs (e.g., estrogens and oral contraceptives)

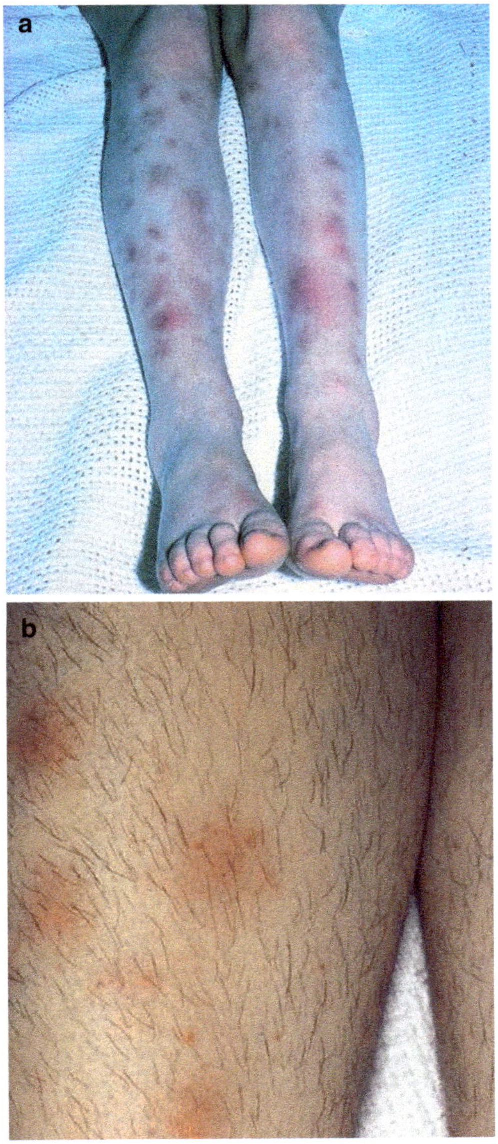

Erythema nodosum
Photograph courtesy of SpringerImages Database, Springer Publishing Company

H.M. Gloster, Jr. et al., *Absolute Dermatology Review: Mastering Clinical Conditions on the Dermatology Recertification Exam*,
DOI 10.1007/978-3-319-03218-4_124, © Springer International Publishing Switzerland 2016

Erythema nodosum

A. Bilateral tender red subcutaneous nodules symmetrically on the pretibial areas

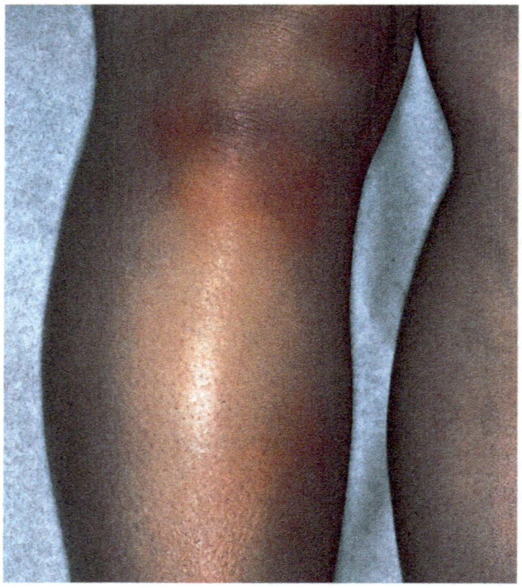

Erythema nodosum
Photograph courtesy of SpringerImages Database, Springer Publishing Company

Lipodermatosclerosis 125

a. Lipodermatosclerosis (Acute Phase)

Lipodermatosclerosis (sclerosis panniculitis or stasis panniculitis), acute phase

A. Favors the medial aspect of lower extremities above the malleolus
B. Develops in the setting of chronic venous insufficiency
C. Acute phase: erythema, warmth, tenderness similar to cellullitis

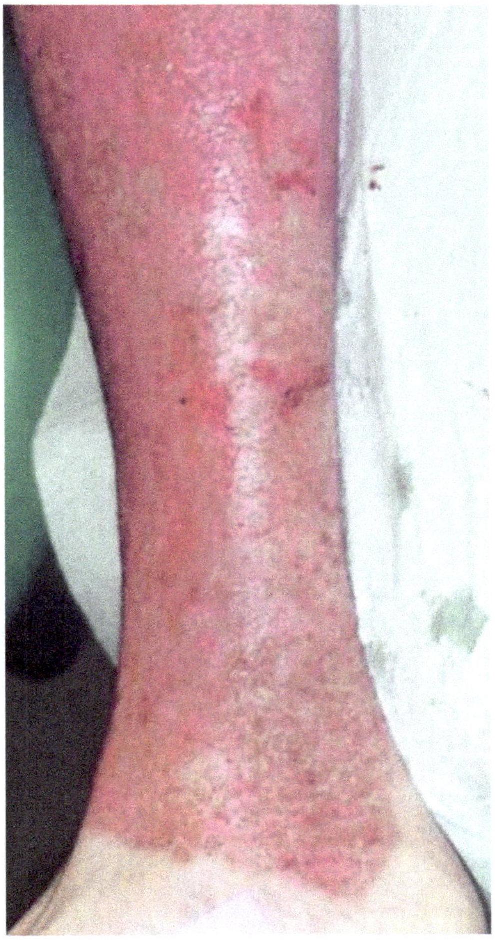

Lipodermatosclerosis (acute phase)
Photograph courtesy of SpringerImages Database, Springer Publishing Company

H.M. Gloster, Jr. et al., *Absolute Dermatology Review: Mastering Clinical Conditions on the Dermatology Recertification Exam*, DOI 10.1007/978-3-319-03218-4_125, © Springer International Publishing Switzerland 2016

b. Lipodermatosclerosis (Chronic Phase)

Lipodermatosclerosis (sclerosis panniculitis or stasis panniculitis), chronic phase

A. Induration with woody bound-down skin due to sclerosis of the dermis and subcutaneous fat that gives the leg the appearance of an "inverted wine bottle"
B. Red, brown, or violet hyperpigmentation is common

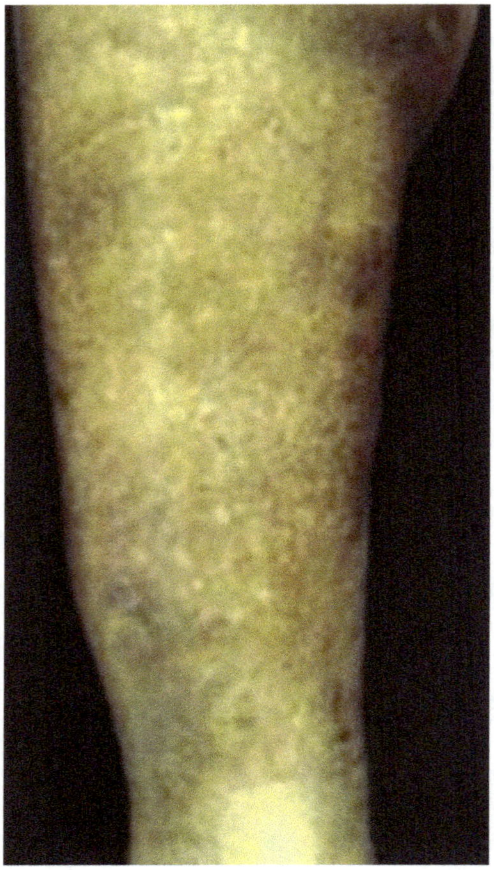

Lipodermatosclerosis (chronic phase)

Index

H.M. Gloster, Jr. et al., *Absolute Dermatology Review: Mastering Clinical Conditions on the Dermatology Recertification Exam*,
DOI 10.1007/978-3-319-03218-4,

CPSIA information can be obtained
at www.ICGtesting.com
Printed in the USA
LVHW060743190119
604298LV00021B/8/P

9 783319 032177